The Interpersonal World
of the Infant

THE

INTERPERSONAL

WORLD

OF THE INFANT

*A View from Psychoanalysis
and Developmental
Psychology*

With a New Introduction by the Author

DANIEL N. STERN

BASIC
BOOKS

A Member of The Perseus Books Group

Lyrics on p. 268 from "Reeling in the Years," words and music by Walter Becker and Donald Fagen. © copyright 1973 by MCA Music, a division of MCA, Inc., New York, NY. Used by permission. All rights reserved.

Excerpt on pp. 140–41 from Daniel N. Stern, "Affect Attunement," in *Frontiers of Infant Psychiatry*, vol. 2, ed. Justin D. Call, Eleanor Galenson, and Robert L. Tyson. Copyright © 1984 by Basic Books, Inc., Publishers. Reprinted by permission of the publisher.

Library of Congress Cataloging in Publication Data

Stern, Daniel N.
 The interpersonal world of the infant.

 Bibliography: p. 278
 Includes index.
 1. Infant psychology. 2. Psychoanalysis.
3. Developmental psychology. I. Title. [DNLM:
1. Child Development. 2. Child Psychology.
3. Infant. 4. Psychoanalysis—in infancy & childhood.
WS 350.5 S839i]
BF719.S75 1985   155.4′22   85-47553
ISBN 0-465-09589-5

CONTENTS

PREFACE   *vii*

INTRODUCTION TO THE PAPERBACK EDITION   *xi*

PART I

THE QUESTIONS AND THEIR BACKGROUND

Chapter 1
*Exploring the Infant's Subjective Experience: A Central Role for
the Sense of Self*   *3*

Chapter 2
Perspectives and Approaches to Infancy   *13*

PART II

THE FOUR SENSES OF SELF

Chapter 3
The Sense of an Emergent Self   *37*

Chapter 4
The Sense of a Core Self: I. Self versus Other   *69*

Chapter 5
The Sense of a Core Self: II. Self with Other   *100*

Chapter 6
The Sense of a Subjective Self: I. Overview   *124*

Chapter 7
The Sense of a Subjective Self: II. Affect Attunement   *138*

v

CONTENTS

Chapter 8
The Sense of a Verbal Self 162

PART III

SOME CLINICAL IMPLICATIONS

Chapter 9
The "Observed Infant" as Seen with a Clinical Eye 185

Chapter 10
*Some Implications for the Theories Behind Therapeutic
Reconstructions* 231

Chapter 11
*Implications for the Therapeutic Process of Reconstructing a
Developmental Past* 256

EPILOGUE 275
BIBLIOGRAPHY 278
INDEX 295

PREFACE

THE PATHS LEADING toward my writing this book have been many and interwoven. When I was a resident in psychiatry and in psychoanalytic training, we were always asked to summarize each case with a psychodynamic formulation, that is, an explanatory historical account of how the patient became the person who walked into your office. The account was to begin as early as possible in the patient's life, to include the preverbal and preoedipal influences operating during infancy. This task was always an agony for me, especially trying to tie the infancy period into a coherent life account. It was agonizing because I was caught in a contradiction. On one side, there was the strong conviction that the past influences the present in some coherent fashion. This fundamental assertion of all dynamic psychologies was one of the things that made psychiatry, for me, the most fascinating and complex of all the branches of medicine. Psychiatry was the only clinical discipline for which development really mattered. But on the other side, my patients knew so little about their earliest life histories and I knew even less about how to ask about them. So I was forced to pick and choose among those few facts about their infancies that best fit the existing theories and from these selected pickings come up with a coherent historical account. The formulations for all of the cases began to sound alike. Yet the people were very different. This exercise was like playing a game with limited moves—or worse, smacked of intellectual dishonesty—in an endeavor that otherwise adhered so closely to what felt to be true. The earliest months and years of life held a firm and prominent place in the theories, but occupied a speculative and obscure role in dealing with a real person. This contradiction has continued to disturb and intrigue me. Addressing this contradiction is one of the major tasks of this book.

A second path began when I discovered the current research in developmental psychology. It promised new approaches and tools for finding out more about that earliest period. And I used those tools for the next fifteen years, together with the clinical approach. This

vii

book attempts to create a dialogue between the infant as revealed by the experimental approach and as clinically reconstructed, in the service of resolving the contradiction between theory and reality.

There was a third path—one that supports the argument that the present is best understood with knowledge of the past. When I was seven or so, I remember watching an adult try to deal with an infant of one or two years. At that moment it seemed to me so obvious what the infant was all about, but the adult seemed not to understand it at all. It occurred to me that I was at a pivotal age. I knew the infant's "language" but also knew the adult's. I was still "bilingual" and wondered if that facility had to be lost as I grew older.

This early incident has a history of its own. As an infant, I spent considerable time in the hospital, and in order to know what was going on, I became a watcher, a reader of the nonverbal. I never did grow out of it. So when halfway through my residency I finally discovered the ethologists, it was with great excitement. They offered a scientific approach to the study of the naturally occurring nonverbal language of infancy. And this struck me as the necessary complement to the analysis of verbal self-report as described by the dynamic psychologies. One has to be "bilingual" to begin to solve the contradiction.

Some may say that research or theory that is determined by highly personal factors should not be trusted. Others will say that no one in their right mind would bother with the arduous business of research without a history of personal reasons. Developmentalists would have to cast their lot with the latter.

The most recent path leading directly to the writing of this book has been influenced by several colleagues and friends to whom I am indebted. They have read all or portions of the manuscript at various stages, offering the kinds of suggestions and criticisms that help both to encourage and to reshape a book. In particular, I am most grateful to Susan W. Baker, Lynn Hofer, Myron Hofer, Arnold Cooper, John Dore, Kristine MacKain, Joe Glick, and Robert Michels.

Three groups have been helpful in shaping specific aspects of this book. For a period of time I was privileged to join in regular meetings with Margaret Mahler and her colleagues Annamarie Weil, John McDevitt, and Anni Bergman. While they will probably not agree with many of the conclusions I have drawn, the discussions we had en route to divergent conclusions were always enriching and deepened my theoretical understandings. The second group, put together by Katherine Nelson to study the crib talk of one child, included Jerome Bruner, John Dore, Carol Feldman, and Rita Watson. Discussions were invaluable in thinking about the interaction between the preverbal and verbal experiences of a child. The third group was brought together by Robert Emde and Arnold Sameroff at the Center for Advanced Study in the Behavioral Sciences to study developmental psychopathology. Discussions with Alan Sroufe, Arnold Sameroff, Robert Emde, Tom Anders, Hawley Parmelee, and Herb Leiderman helped in struggling with the problems of how relational problems get internalized.

I would also like to acknowledge the ubiquitous contributions of the many people who have worked in our Laboratory of Developmental Processes during this period: Michelle Allen, Susan Baer, Cecilia Baetge, Roanne Barnett, Susan Evans, Victor Fornari, Emily Frosch, Wendy Haft, Lynn Hofer, Paulene Hopper, Anne Goldfield, Carol Kaminski, Terrel Kaplan, Kristine MacKain, Susan Lehman, Babette Moeller, Pat Nachman, Carmita Parras, Cathy Raduns, Anne Reach, Michelle Richards, Katherine Shear, Susan Spieker, Paul Trad, Louise Weir, and Yvette Yatchmink.

I also wish to thank those outside of our laboratory with whom I have had the opportunity to collaborate—namely, John Dore at CUNY and Bertrand Cramer in Geneva.

I am especially indebted to Cecilia Baetge for the preparation of this manuscript at all phases and for her administrative skill in making the writing of a book and conducting the rest of my professional life possible.

Jo Ann Miller, my editor at Basic Books, has been wonderful in her encouragement, criticism, ideas, patience, impatience, and deadlines, all mixed together with sensitivity and exquisite timing. Nina Gunzenhauser's clarity of mind and good sense in copy editing were indispensable.

Much of the research related to this book was supported by the Herman and Amelia Ehrmann Foundation, the William T. Grant Foundation, the Fund for Psychoanalytic Research, the National Foundation of the March of Dimes, the National Institute of Mental Health, and Warner Communications, Inc.

Finally, I want to thank all of the parents and infants—my ultimate collaborators—who have let us learn from them.

INTRODUCTION TO THE PAPERBACK EDITION

REVISITING A BOOK WRITTEN fifteen years ago about a rapidly changing field poses a dilemma. Do I rewrite it entirely—or do I let it stand and go ahead with other things? Finding neither alternative satisfactory, I have opted for a third solution, writing an extensive new Introduction. This revision permits me to correct, add to, subtract from, and elaborate on selected issues. It also permits me to step back and evaluate the book's impact and to respond to some of the criticisms that have been directed at it. Finally, it allows me to trace where the book has led my own thinking.

Revisiting Selected Issues

This book has now been in print for fifteen years in ten languages. Four issues seem to have had the greatest impact.

THE LAYERED MODEL OF DEVELOPMENT

In contrast to the conventional stage model(s) whereby each successive phase of development not only replaces the preceding one but also essentially dismantles it, reorganizing the entire perspective, the layered model postulated here assumes a progressive accumulation of senses of the self, socioaffective competencies, and ways-of-being-with-others. No emerging domain disappears; each remains active and interacts dynamically with all the others. In fact, each domain facilitates the emergence of the ones that follow. In this way, all senses of the self, all socioaffective competencies, and all ways-of-being-with-others remain with us throughout the life span, whereas according to the stage model, earlier developmental organization can be accessed only by means of a process-like regression.

The shift to a layered model came about for two reasons. First, the classical Freudian model of psychosexual stages (replete with fixations) had not fulfilled its predictive promise for linkage with later psychopathology even after three-quarters of a century; it was not productive of new ideas and had become less persuasive and less interesting. And second, Piaget's stage model, at the time still the dominant paradigm of development, accounted for the infant's encounter with the inanimate physical world (with space, time, number, volume, weight, etc.), for which task it had been constructed—but it was inadequate to conceptualize the encounter with the richer and more complicated social-emotional human world composed of self and others, which is the world that interests me.

In this book's original 1985 edition, I stated—but without the force of solid conviction (yet)—that the infant's encounter with the human world was, if not primary, certainly not secondary, and that it had to be guided by psychological principles separate and different from those that directed his encounter with the inanimate, physical world. The two encounters proceed in parallel: That was the central point.

It had begun to occur to many working in the field that infants, and adults, had (indeed, had to have) two different, parallel systems of perception, cognition, affectivity, and memory, for encountering and making sense of the physical and human worlds. Of course, the two systems interact dynamically. This new view, a radical departure emphasizing the specificity of local knowledge in the broadest sense of those terms, has been gaining evidence and theoretical strength during the past fifteen years. (See, for example, Braten, 1998; Leslie, 1987; Rochat, 1999; Thelen and Smith,

1994.) Currently, it is proving to be extremely productive for both normal and pathological development (particularly concerning autism).

The layered model is not actually new. (The notion of parallel models is far newer.) It was greatly influenced by other nonsequential models such as the spirals of Werner and Kaplan (1963) and others. Some psychologists continue to criticize it for being essentially a model of growth, not development. There is some truth to this criticism, but a model must fit the data it proposes to embrace, and the layered model outlined here was more appropriate than the stage model to the infant's meeting with the unique features of the human world. In any event, it seems to have helped many to push their thinking further than previous models did—at least when dealing with human interaction.

UNPACKING THE SELF

The book's view that self/other differentiation begins at birth or before has been another source of much discussion, particularly in psychoanalytically influenced circles. If such differentiation is not the work of any special life phase, the "final" disentanglement of self from other cannot be dated in any meaningful sense. So instead of seeing the separation of self from other as a phase-limited developmental task, even the developmental task, this book maintains that self/other differentiation is in place and in process almost from the very beginning. Therefore, the infant's major developmental task is the opposite one, the creation of ties with others—that is, increasing relatedness. It is important to note that the research cited above on parallel (perceptual, cognitive, and affective) systems operating essentially from birth supports the contention of differentiated beginnings for self and other.

This view places more emphasis on strategies and problems in attachment when viewing pathology, and it minimizes, even does away with, the need to conceptualize phases of "normal autism," "primary narcissism," and "symbiosis." This is not to say that vaguely similar phenomena do not exist as pathological entities later in life. They do, but they do not have their points of origin in the first two years; thus they cannot constitute specific sources of the pathogenic mechanism to which regression can occur.

In general, the postulated senses of self were based on the developmental appearance of new world- and self-viewing possibilities that became available with the timed emergence of new infant capacities.

As concerns the first three preverbal senses of self—the sense of an emergent self, the sense of a core self, and the sense of a subjective (intersubjective) self—I am now less convinced that they emerge in a clear temporal sequence, each new one to be added to the others in the layered fashion mentioned above. At this point, I am far more inclined to see all three as emerging together, and largely by virtue of their dynamic interactions with one another. So if I were writing the book today, I would describe them as separate subcategories of a nonverbal sense of self, for reasons that will emerge as we proceed.

DEALING WITH THE NONVERBAL

The focus on nonverbal behavior has also stirred debate and rethinking. Developmentalists working with infants are comfortable dealing with nonverbal communication. Most psychoanalysts, however, are not; they are more at ease with words, narrative interpretation, and meaning. Since this book is in part about bringing together ideas from developmental psychology and psychodynamic psychotherapy, a natural tension—a sort of zone of turbulence—exists where the verbal and the nonverbal meet. Many of the notions and influences of the book flow from this encounter.

First of all, there is the size of the units that make up the data. Observers of babies are forced to work with small behavioral units, on the order of seconds or split seconds; larger units appear thanks to repetition and nestings of the smaller units. The method of such observers is chiefly, but not exclusively, microanalytic. Psychotherapists, on the other hand, deal with larger units composed of coherent, not nested, networks of meaning that take on a unitary sense within the narrative format. One way to (try to) bridge the gap is by finding (or attributing) implicit, narrative-like meaning to the smaller behavioral patterns. This is the path that I and others searching for clinical relevance have chosen. Its advantages and dangers will be taken up further on.

One consequence of the book's application of a narrative perspective to the nonverbal has been the discovery of a language useful to many psychotherapies that rely on the nonverbal. I am thinking particularly of dance, music, body, and movement therapies, as well as existential psychotherapies. This observation came as a pleasant surprise to me since I did not originally have such therapies in mind; my thinking has been enriched by coming to know them better.

Perhaps the most significant result of dealing with the nonverbal world at the appropriate (micro)level of analysis is the light it sheds on framing such questions as What is an internal object? and How does it form?

INTERNALIZATIONS VERSUS WAYS-OF-BEING-WITH

The book took notions that had recently emerged in developmental psychology and applied them to the material of greatest relevance to psychodynamics. This had not been done before.

The central idea that internal objects are constructed from repeated, relatively small interactive patterns derived from the microanalytic perspective. Such internal objects are not people; nor are they parts or aspects of others. Rather, they are constructed from the patterned experience of self in interaction with another: What is inside (i.e., represented internally) comprises interactive experiences.

At various points in the book, these internal objects are referred to as representations of interactions that have been generalized (RIGs). Subsequently, I have preferred to call them ways-of-being-with, deemphasizing the process of formation in favor of describing the lived phenomenon in a more experience-near and clinically useful way.

This view of the internal object world was a departure from most of those prevailing at the time in dynamic psychotherapies. It was criticized as leaving out of the picture the subjective world—in particular, the influence of fantasies (especially "original" or innate fantasies)—and, more generally, as being a behaviorist view that regarded the baby as an accurate reader and con-structor of what was happening to her objectively, as recorded by an observer.

The essence of the actual approach was different. The idea was to survey the data on nonverbal interaction that was then becom-ing accessible, thanks to new methodologies, and to take this data and imagine, on the basis of other available concepts, how an in-fant might mentally construct a subjective world of his experience of self and other. This is not behaviorism but, rather, a technique that involves using new observations of behavior together with informed speculations about how behavior can be mentally con-strued. In encompassing both, it takes a long (and often shaky) step beyond behaviorism.

The intent behind this step was not to replace notions of innate fantasies but to see how clinically relevant a subjective world could be constituted before it became necessary to resort to and explore specific innate features—fantasies, action tendencies, pref-erences, values, and so on. In a sense, the approach could be seen as a defining exercise to better delimit and focus on what as-yet-unknown innate features were requisite. The outcome was the opening up of a wider dialogue on both the nature of the infant's (and adult's) internal world and the process of its formation.

Selected Chapter Discussion

"THE SENSE OF AN EMERGENT SELF" (CHAPTER 3)
The most exciting chapter for some, this has been the most con-fusing for others, due, I suspect, to the often unclear boundary be-tween what is process and what is content. The distinction is probably hardest to make when the focus is on the (subjective) ex-perience of arriving at a mental content.

Chapter 3 describes the several ways that organization can form in the infant's mind. The notion of the process of organiza-tion coming into being is readily graspable; it can even be in-ferred by observing from the outside. It is the next step that is difficult—the experience of the process of organization coming into being. And the emergent sense of self has to do with the experience of this process.

Although there are many examples of kinds of experience (e.g., transmodal), what I now believe is missing from the list is some notion of consciousness. The experience of process must be a discrete, bounded event or moment, a sort of "coming-into-being at the present moment" (Woolf, 1923). If it does not have this feature, there is no way to distinguish the emergent sense of self from all other unattended mental and physical activities that result in the progressive organization of the mind.

The next questions thus become What kind of consciousness are we talking about? And emergence into what kind of moment? I avoided these questions in the original book. To approach them we will need a notion of primary consciousness that is applicable to infants early in life.

Researchers working within the new perspective of an embodied mind, where the traditional sharp separation between body and mind is no longer maintained, have provided insights into the nature of a primary consciousness that is usable in infancy (e.g., Clark, 1997; Damasio, 1999; Varela, Thompson, and Rosch, 1993). Primary consciousness is not self-reflective, it is not verbalized, and it lasts only during a present moment that corresponds to "now."

The basic idea consists of several parts. The first is that all mental acts (perception, feeling, cognition, remembering) are accompanied by input from the body, including, importantly, internal sensations. The internal input includes the momentary states of arousal, activation, tonicity, levels of motivational activation or satiety (in various systems), and well-being. This input is what Damasio (1994, 1999) has called "background feelings," which are similar to the vitality affects introduced in the present book. (See, especially, Damasio 1999, p. 287.) The other input from the body includes all the things the body does or must do to permit, support, amplify (etc.) the ongoing mental activity (perceiving, thinking, etc.), such as postures formed or held, movements (of the eyes, head, or body), displacements in space, and contractions and relaxations of muscular tone. The body is never doing nothing. (Envision Rodin's Thinker. He sits immobile, posing his head on his hand and an elbow on his knee. True, he is not moving, but there is extraordinary tension in his posture, suggesting active, intense proprioceptive feedback from almost every muscle group. This feedback, along with the Thinker's presumably heightened arousal, provides the background feeling against which his specific thoughts are etched. It is the contrast between the foreground and the background that captures the viewer and expresses the message.)

All of these body signals come from the self—an as-yet-unspecified self. Such signals need not be attended to. They need not enter into awareness. Yet they are there in the background. They are the continuous music of being alive. That is why I refer to changes or modulations in this music as vitality affects. It is this music that will permit the emergent self—the "proto-self" in Damasio's (1999) terms—to appear. But first it must be yoked with a mental activity.

The second element, then, is an intentional object, as the notion is used in philosophy. The intentional object is whatever the mind is stretching toward. It is whatever is "in mind." (There need not be an intention in the psychological sense of a motivated goal-directedness.) It could be a red ball, an internal pain, the sensation of the nipple in the mouth, a thought, a memory.

Primary consciousness is the yoking together, in a present moment, of the intentional object and the vital background input from the body. The body input specifies that it is you who is now having the experience of the intentional object. And a sense of the self emerges as the living vital experiencer of the intentional object. This is what I mean by a sense of an emergent self—experiencing being alive while encountering the world (or encountering yourself) at a given moment, an awareness of the process of living an experience. The contents of the experience could be anything.

Each time there is a moment of primary consciousness, the self as experiencer is felt and is situated in the world. At that moment, the sense of an emergent self appears. This must happen many times an hour, or minute. Although these moments of primary consciousness are short and periodic, they offer rehearsings of the continual music of living. The sense of an emergent self is a sort of "pulse," as Damasio (1994) calls it, which continually respecifies the living self in the process of experiencing. Furthermore, the dynamic quality of vitality affects ensures that the experience has a contoured time line.

There is no reason not to believe that dogs and higher animals experience something similar to primary consciousness. And among humans, moments of primary consciousness in early infancy appear to occur most markedly during the states of alert inactivity and alert activity.

Many of the examples given in Chapter 3 concern the yoking together of two different intentional objects. What I want to emphasize is that these yokings must, in themselves, be yoked to the vital bodily feelings and shifting vitality affects of experiencing. With that understood, the chapter can be reread in the light of a more precise definition of what is emerging, and when.

"THE SENSE OF A CORE SELF: I. SELF VERSUS OTHER" (CHAPTER 4)
In Chapter 4, the sense of a core self is described as consisting of four relatively invariant experiences: self-agency, self-coherence, self-history (continuity), and self-affectivity. Today, I would reduce the number to three by eliminating self-affectivity, which is no longer needed because it becomes subsumed by the expanded notion of the emergent self described above and by the sense of continuity described below. (My intent is not, however, to minimize the central and omnipresent role of affect in mental life.)

I would also change the descriptor self-history to self-continuity. History is too rich a term, implying a sense of past and its connectedness to a present. All I really mean is that each time the infant is confronted with herself at moments of primary consciousness, she feels the "same" by virtue of the invariants created from her vital background feelings and her vitality affects and their expression. Continuity as a sense, not as a fact, is actually a consistently refound continuity, since the sensation of going-on-being emerges only when an experience is brought forward into a present moment. Effectively, then, one feels continuous even if most of the time the sense of continuity is nowhere in play. But when it is, one refinds the sense of being the same.

"The Sense of a Core Self with Other" (Chapter 5) and "The Sense of a Subjective Self" (Chapters 6 and 7)

If, as mentioned above, the infant starts life with three partially distinct systems for experiencing self, others, and inanimate objects, certain changes are required in the developmental schema as originally described. A crucial set of findings bears on this issue.

Recent evidence for the presence of mirror neurons and adaptive oscillators along with the deepening literature on early imitation suggest that, probably from the beginning of life, infants have the capacity for what Braten (1998) terms altero-centric participation or what Trevarthen (1979) has long called primary intersubjectivity.

The crucial findings are as follows. In monkeys, mirror neurons have been found in the premotor cortex (Rizzolatti and Arbib, 1998). When one monkey executes a gesture involving the hands and mouth, certain neurons in this area fire. When a second monkey watches the first monkey perform the gesture, mirror neurons in the second monkey's brain fire in the same area as in the performing monkey. Presumably, this phenomenon provides the watching monkey with a neurobiological basis for, in some fashion, feeling in his own body an act that occurred in another's body. The implications for affective resonance, imitation, intersubjectivity, and empathy are evident. These experiments have not yet been repeated in humans. According to Rizzolatti and Arbib (1998), however, when an adult human watches another person make a gesture, the threshold for firing in the same muscles is reduced.

Another set of experiments points in the same direction. Researchers have found adaptive oscillators that permit us to synch our movements to those of others who are moving (McCauley, 1994; Port, Cummins, and McCauley, 1995; Torras, 1985). Apparently, there are "clocks" in different systems within us that fire at a given periodicity but can be reset by an incoming stimulus such as a movement external to us made by another. This resetting permits our system to establish, and remain in, synchrony with the timing of another system. Such findings supply a biological mechanism for the long-observed human (including infant) capacities to feel another's action and to act accordingly, in an age-appropriate way.

Yet another line of research bears on recognition of the self versus the other, the timing of this capacity, and a possible mechanism underlying different perceptual processes for self versus other.

It has been argued that infants have a precocious and exquisite appreciation of contingent relations. Further, they can distinguish perfect contingency from high but imperfect contingency (Watson, 1994). Perfect contingency is the necessary consequence of self-generated behavior, whereas high but imperfect contingent relations are the almost inevitable result of parental mirroring, attuning, and parental responsivity in general.

Other findings suggest that infants orient more to perfect contingencies (i.e., to self-generated events) during the first several months of life, and that after three months of life it is the high but imperfect contingencies (i.e., other-generated events) that become more interesting to the infant. These phenomena occur quite early, indeed (Bahrick and Watson, 1985; Gergely and Watson, 1999; Rochat and Morgan, 1995; Watson, 1994).

The importance of perceiving the different contingency relations as mechanisms for helping to distinguish self from other was noted in the original edition; however, this newer body of research carries such ideas much further, puts them on a more solid footing, and, along with the expanding perspective on early imitation, necessarily alters not only our view of the infant's experiences of self-with-other but also our dating of the onset of intersubjectivity.

I will start with the first of these concerns. Originally, most of the emphasis was placed on the infant's experience of a self-regulating-other. I do not intend to alter the centrality of that experience. What is needed, however, is a more extended repertoire of experiences of self-with-other, which will include the extraordinary yet common situation whereby one's nervous system is captured, so to speak, by the nervous system of another, thanks to mirror neurons and adaptive oscillators, and probably other as-yet-undiscovered mechanisms. At such times, the invariants that specify a core sense of self are not completely co-opted by the other. The core sense of self is not swept away. There is only a partial overlapping. Still, the experience will have its own quality and make up yet another ultimately discernible way of being-with-another. I call this latter phenomenon self-resonating-with-another.

The second modification to the original schema concerns the developmental onset of intersubjectivity. But here I must make a correction. In my references to the sense of a subjective self in Chapters 6 and 7, what I really meant was the sense of an intersubjective self. That is the descriptor I have always used in speaking about it.

The main question is When does intersubjectivity begin? In Chapter 6, I maintain that it begins, properly speaking, around nine months of age with the advent of interattentionality (e.g., pointing), interintentionality (e.g., expecting motives to be read), and interaffectivity (e.g., affect attunement and social referencing). In light of the new evidence on other-centered-participation shown by infants in their many forms of imitation, as well as the new findings on mirror neurons and adaptive oscillators, I am now convinced that early forms of intersubjectivity exist from almost the beginning of life.

This represents a shift in my thinking, especially since I took issue with Trevarthen (in Chapter 6) for positing a "primary intersubjectivity" from birth to around nine months and then a "secondary subjectivity" after nine months (Trevarthen, 1979; Trevarthen and Hubley, 1978). I am now in agreement with these findings on the earlier origins. However, in order to preserve the special features of secondary intersubjectivity (again, as noted in Chapter 6), I will still refer to the secondary intersubjectivity that arises around the ninth month as simply intersubjectivity. (Although there is a fairly clear boundary between primary and secondary intersubjectivity, these terms must be considered provisional until we have a fuller picture of which developmental domains, as they emerge, are encompassed into a coherent intersubjective field, and at what ages.)

In any event, the most important point is that a primary intersubjectivity starts from the beginning, as does the sense of an emergent self, as does the sense of a core self (as reconfigured). Accordingly, the developmental schema in Figure 2.2 (p. 32) needs to be revised.

We now find the following main subcategories of the sense of self-with-other:

- The first is the self-regulating-other, described in Chapter 5, which concerns the regulation of security, attachment, arousal, activation, pleasure, unpleasure, physiological gratification, self-esteem, and so on.

- The second includes the various experiences of primary inter-subjectivity whereby the self is linked to the other by way of other-centric-participation—including self-resonating-with-an-other, as described above.

- The third is the self-in-the-presence-of-the-other. This refers to the being-with that may occur when the infant is perceiving, thinking, or acting, alone but in the physical proximity of a care-giver, whereby the physical presence (without any interactive, psychological presence) serves as a framing environment in which the infant can continue to be psychologically alone, on his own. In a sense, this subcategory is a special variation of the self-regulating-other (Stern, 1995, ch. 6).

- There is yet a fourth subcategory, but the extent to which it ex-pands and elaborates the previous three is still to be clarified. It is the sense of self-with-others, particularly as part of the family triad. Accumulating evidence suggests that the infant (at least by three months) starts to form expectations and representa-tions of self as part of a triadic constellation (Fivaz and Corboz, 1998). This is to be expected when so much time is spent in tri-ads as well as in dyads. But the question remains: To what ex-tent should the sense of self within a triad be seen as parallel to the sense of self in dyads, and how and when do the two influ-ence one another?

Together these senses of self form the main ways-of-being-with-another. As development proceeds, all are in constant dynamic in-teraction, helping to define their separate boundaries.

"The Sense of a Verbal Self (and a Narrative Self)"
(Chapter 8)
In the 1985 edition, the ability to create an autobiographical nar-rative was given a very small role as merely a tag-on to the verbal self. I no longer see it that way. The ability to tell a narrative about your own experience is a separate fundamental capacity, beyond and independent of fashioning words from symbols and thus ver-bally referring to yourself and your world. The narrative capacity

evolves much later (at around three years of age) than language per se (around eighteen months), and it requires different aspects of mind. Granted, an infrastructure of language ability must exist before the telling of a narrative can manifest itself. (A narrative format for perceiving can precede language, however.)

At this writing, I am convinced that the development of the narrative capacity opens the way to completely new domains of the self—namely, the narrative self, or selves, whose importance is evident when the following considerations are taken into account.

1. The narrations told to self and others about your experience become the official history of your life. They constitute your autobiography and, as such, are the primary data of talking therapies that deal with the past—both the past of one minute ago and the far past of childhood.

2. In childhood most autobiographical narratives are co-constructed with others, usually the parents or siblings. Daily history is established by parental questions as ordinary as "What happened at school today?" and "What did you and your brother do this morning?" The narrative that results from these questions is truly a co-construction, whereby the parent and child work together to gather the pieces of the story, order them sequentially, give them a coherence as a story, and then evaluate the story by establishing its emotional highpoints and values. The product becomes the official history shared by the family and a part of family lore.

A new body of research views the process of co-construction between parent and child as a form of regulation having much in common with other forms of regulation (e.g., attachment). Different regulatory styles are now recognized, each having different consequences for the contents of the narration. An important aspect of the co-constructing is that it is highly asymmetric. If the parent weren't there, only the child could know what happened. Still, the parent is more expert in recognizing where pieces of the told story are missing or not likely (etc.) and in creating a coherent whole. The two must negotiate a final product that always has an uncertain relationship with the historical truth (de Roten, 1999; Favez, 1996; Stern, 1990).

Another aspect of creating a narrative of "what happened" is that the process of construction acts as a sort of laboratory in which a narrative self is forged, mistakes are corrected, elaborations added, and adjustments fine-tuned. The resulting narrative self will use implicit and explicit material from all the other senses of self discussed above; it is the one that will be both subject and currency of the clinical process.

In light of the foregoing, I now offer the following revised version of Figure 2.2.

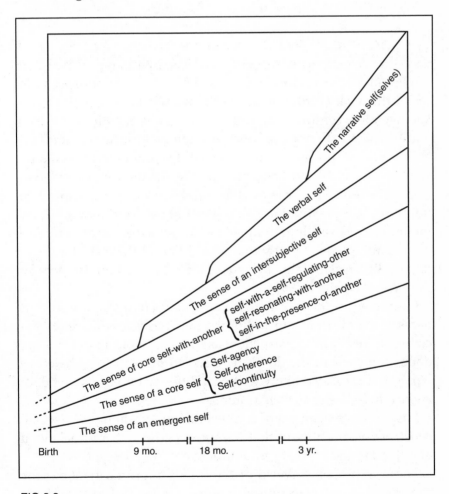

FIG.2.2

"SOME CLINICAL IMPLICATIONS" (CHAPTERS 9, 10, AND 11)
The chapters in Part III concern the clinical implications of Parts I and II. To significantly add to this section requires a second book. In fact, the original plan for The Interpersonal World of the Infant was to break it into two volumes, the second to consist of the clinical implications and applications of the first. This second book is still brewing.

Response to Major Criticisms

THE SOCIAL-CONSTRUCTIONIST CRITIQUE
Social constructionists have criticized The Interpersonal World of the Infant for being decontextualized because I do not specify in detail the local culture in which the work takes place (Western, late twentieth century, middle and upper class, mostly white, etc.) and because I do not examine how the assumptions, methods, and nature of this local culture (which I share) determine the results of the study and hence, ultimately, the theory that emerges from it. Accordingly, I can discover only what I already know. I do not remedy this situation by comparing the local assumptions, methods, and findings with those known from cross-cultural work. And, finally, I imply that what I find in this very local culture is universal and innate because I don't say otherwise (see, for example, Cushman, 1991).

I agree with much of this social-constructionist critique. It is necessary and useful for political as well as scientific reasons. I count on the social constructionists to write about it, but to have done so myself in the depth required to do justice to the effort would have resulted in my writing a different book. So two books are needed—theirs as well as mine.

It is within the context of my general appreciation of the social-constructionist criticism that I want to clarify where I believe it goes too far and becomes unproductive.

The Interpersonal World of the Infant is primarily about the process whereby sociocultural contexts are enacted so as to shape people's behavior, their inner worlds, their relationships. In short, it is about the process of culturally contextualizing the developing infant. The social constructionists, however, seem to ignore what is a very nuanced appreciation on the part of most developmentalists concerning the difference between culture as viewed from the outside, at a distance, and its specific enactment in terms that could influence an infant. For instance, we well know that socioeconomic status in this Western culture is the most potent statistical variable affecting many global outcome measures. But that tells us nothing about how it acts.

In the context of the book's importance, the results of the contextualizing process (which, granted, are locally determined) matter less in the long run than the process itself at this stage of our knowledge. There is not an infinite number of variables through which any culture can be enacted early in life such that they will be perceivable by the infant. The repertoire comprises facial expressions, or the lack thereof; visual regards, or their avoidance; vocalizations, or silences; body orientations; physical distances; gestures; ways of being held; the rhythms, timing, and duration of acts and activities; and so on. No other human alphabet for sociocultural contextualization exists. To continue the analogy: Different cultures can make different sentences with this same alphabet, but first we must examine how such an alphabet can (not must) work. I'd have thought that the social constructionists would have been delighted to find an alphabet—and a way of using it—so systematically described.

Suppose that at the very beginning of the book I had written a clear disclaimer, something like "The role played by the study's population, methods, hypotheses, and basic assumptions in determining the study's findings will not be examined. I assume that the readers are deeply familiar with white, middle- and upper-class, late-twentieth-century Western society. This book is about how, given our basic assumptions, our infants develop into people like us. Obviously, then, no conclusions drawn here need pertain to any other culture." (All of which I, too, believe—and take for granted—and probably should have said to avoid any confusion.) Would that disclaimer have satisfied the social-constructionist critics? Would the book, even with the disclaimer, still have been criticizable on political grounds as a description that inevitably obscures a proscription—and is thus a concealed political act? To avoid this outcome, how often must the disclaimer be recalled to the reader? Or must all the cultural variations be put into play and examined? And if they were, would it not then be another book, possibly a lesser one? To what extent is the social-constructionist critique primarily "politically correct," overly confining, and only secondarily helpful?

Cushman (1991) states that because I do not specify and examine my context, my findings and resulting theory are implied to be universally applicable, when in fact they apply only to the local context I work in. This implication, he claims, gives a misleading and unjustifiable weight to predesign, to the innate.

In this book I have tried to indicate whenever there appears to be an innate preference, or tendency, or capacity, or timing of appearance. These factors are viewed as guidelines within which different specific uses can be created under different (cultural or other) conditions. But Cushman misunderstands my broad use of the term predesign when he states, for example, that I have no evidence that the process of attunement is predesigned. His argument would be that attunement is not seen in the same form, or perhaps not at all, in another culture. But what I mean by predesigned is that there is an innate human capacity to feel the effortful, temporal form of another's action. For example, the aforementioned findings regarding mirror neurons and adaptive oscillators supply a biologically based mechanism for the human capacity to feel another's action. The fact that this capacity can take different cultural forms does not make the capacity less innate; it only suggests how different cultures might use it. This was very clearly the sense in which I was using the term predesign. Misunderstanding that could only be in the service of another agenda.

There is yet another aspect of context that developmentalists must be sensitive to. Although the culture may be present in all human behaviors, to the infant the cultural manifestations of some behaviors are more opaque and those of others more transparent. The infant also has less access to the entire culture than adults do. Most cultural elements of a society have to be filtered and varied through subgroups, then through individual family or kin groupings, and finally through the immediate caregiver(s) and peers. Only then does the cultural enactment reach the young infant's effective immediate surround.

As the infant develops, her exposure and access to cultural features undergo changes. Accordingly, the very nature of the cultural element is, in itself, a developmental variable. Language is a good example. In the beginning the paralinguistics carry the cultural enactments. Later, the arbitrary sound symbols do so as well. (This is why I insist that a sharp distinction be made between language as music and language as lyrics—not because one is cultural and the other isn't, as Cushman suggests, but because the cultural penetration, or surroundedness, is different in depth, breadth, and nature.)

THE RELEVANCE OF INFANT OBSERVATION FOR PSYCHOANALYSIS

Green (1997), whose field is psychoanalysis, and Wolff (1996), in infant research, both conclude that infant research and observation have no relevance for psychoanalysis. Aspects of their position are similar inasmuch as Green has relied heavily on Wolff's criticisms.

The first question ought to be Relevant for which psychoanalysis? Psychoanalysis is many things to many people. Wolff chooses to define its domain in the limited terms of the early, traditional, Freudian psychoanalysis of roughly seventy-five years ago—one that embodies the unconscious, particularly unconscious fantasies, and whose goal is making the unconscious conscious. But that definition leaves out many issues of major concern to more modern psychoanalysis, especially the world of object relations, inasmuch as they concern internal representations, transference, intersubjectivity, and the creation of narratives—even though it is in exactly these areas that infant research has been most pertinent and helpful to psychoanalysts. In effect, Wolff's definition precludes the possibility of relevance.

Green has imposed different but equally strict boundaries on what psychoanalysis is and, accordingly, what can possibly matter to it. He chooses to accept as psychoanalytic only data that have been gathered within, and ideas that have directly emerged from, the tightly defined psychoanalytic situation and its technique.

Given these constraints, infant observation could have only indirect relevance at best, and even then no more than anthropology, say, or literature. So minimalist a position jeopardizes the relationship of psychoanalysis to all other knowledge of human beings. The result is a severely isolated field of dwindling interest and pertinence to other sciences and humanities.

Green disqualifies the relevance of infant observation on another basis as well, insisting that the data of psychoanalysis consist of words, symbols, narratives, and meanings, all outside the infant's capacity. The infant's raw experience cannot be reorganized après coup—that is, by deferred action—because that would require the mediation of language. Yet deferred action is the central point of interest in psychoanalysis.

This position does not take into account the fact that the infant starts to accumulate nonverbal, nonsymbolic, implicit knowledge about his object relations, and that such knowledge is now recognized as containing far more elaborate representations than previously thought possible. These early representations form the basis for later conscious and unconscious object relationships, including what surfaces in the transference.

Green, along with and following Wolff, also claims that the approach taken in The Interpersonal World of the Infant is in many respects pseudoscientific, circular, or heavily saturated with theory that directs observation—even that it is anthropomorphic and pathomorphic. (See also Barratt, 1996; Wilson, 1996). Both argue that I had a preexisting theory of infant experience based on my view of adult psychopathology and that I selectively identified a few developmental research findings to prove what I already assumed. Such reasoning would indeed have been circular, but it is not what I did.

Rather, I did the following. I explored all the scientific observations in the developmental literature as of 1984. My aim was to describe which capacities the scientific community thought were available to infants at different ages. (Recall that this was time when the explosion of research about infants had been in full swing for almost two decades, although most psychoanalysts and other psychotherapists were unfamiliar with the domain.) Toward this end I established an objective set of limiting (and starting) conditions that could inform inferences about what infants could conceivably do or not do in constructing their subjective experience. This phase was the outgrowth of more than twenty years of reading and contributing to the literature on infant development—hardly a matter of picking and choosing a few findings that supported some preconceptions. It is pertinent to point out that there are over 400 references in the book, mostly to the work of others, on the basis of which I attempted to determine the consensus of the field so as to set parameters for making inferences and perhaps offer new possibilities. These sources were largely independent of psychoanalytic theory and considerations of psychopathology in general.

Such an approach constitutes a necessary and valid way to use the findings in one domain of knowledge to inform another. It is not circular up to this point. Yet Green and Wolff ignore or dismiss this essential first step of defining the context in which inferences, speculations, and hypotheses can be generated.

The second step in my work is the more problematic one: drawing inferences or hypotheses from the objective constraints. There is no way that inferences about another's subjective experience can escape at least some contamination from the experiences and beliefs of the person doing the inferring. But Wolff is incorrect in diagnosing the origins of that inevitable contamination in my work. It arose not from my clinical experience with patients but, rather, from the totality of my empathic, acculturated understanding of normal human behavior, of which my knowledge gained from patients is only a very small part.

We are stuck with circular contamination in our inferences about others' subjective experience. This is an old dilemma endemic to all theorizing, psychoanalytic or otherwise. The problem cannot be avoided, only confined and recognized. However, when we have been broadly inclusive rather than highly selective in identifying consensual objective constraints, and when we have used the totality of our human experience as opposed to the tenets of any preexisting theory in the process of inference making, then we have skirted circularity scientifically insofar as this is possible. There are not many such partial escapes in our common endeavor to understand human subjective experience.

Both critics also failed to make the crucial distinction between the criteria acceptable for hypothesis generating and those acceptable for hypothesis testing. The Interpersonal World of the Infant is an attempt to define the former. The real question now is whether the hypotheses generated in the book have anything of interest to say for the ongoing psychoanalytic and psychotherapeutic discourse and vice versa. In the minds of most, it does.

The Book as a Map to Future Work

A book such as this foreshadows the direction of one's own future work. Below are some of the threads, some clearly visible and others less so, that I have picked up and developed further during the fifteen years since its writing.

STUDIES ON CHILDREN'S NARRATIVES

As it became more and more evident that the narrative sense of self/selves was key to later clinical issues, and as the co-constructing process increasingly showed itself to be crucial, several colleagues and I initiated a study of children's narratives (Favez et al., 1994). (A move in this direction had already been stimulated by the group put together by Katherine Nelson [1989] to analyze the bedtime monologues of a two-year-old.) Children from four to six were engaged in a highly novel and emotionally charged standard play situation, each session of which was televised. Half the mothers watched the session through a one-way mirror; the other half did not see what happened. Immediately after the session, each child and mother reconstructed a narrative of the events just experienced by the child, who simply reported "what happened and what he felt." We could thus compare the narration with the objective record. Indeed, it is important that we could know objectively what happened and how the child reacted, because in much of the research on narrative reconstruction there is no objective referent.

The most striking results were those that showed how different were the styles of negotiating the reconstruction. Some mothers went mainly after the facts and the sequence of events, with less emphasis on the coherence of the story and the emotional evaluation of what happened. Others were more interested in the coherence and emotional evaluation. Still others were altogether passive, in the sense of being nondirective. As might be expected, the style of co-narration was a powerful determinant of the form and content of the final narrative, regardless of whether it was inconsistent with what actually happened. Distorted or not, the co-narratives remained relatively stable over several months (Favez et al., 1994; Favez, 1996).

Each type of co-narration was found to be associated with specific dyadic interactive patterns during the process of co-construction (Favez et al., 1994; de Roten, 1999). The style of co-construction emerged as a regulatory strategy that demanded an integration of cognitive, affective, and nonverbal action. The co-construction of autobiographical history can thus be added to the list of crucial dyadic activities—such as attachment, free-play, and feeding—that demand coordinated strategy to accomplish. Different such strategies exist, and each has potentially different clinical consequences.

Turning to the Mother's Experience

Although its emphasis is on the infant, The Interpersonal World of the Infant is all about dyadic interaction at the interpersonal and intrapsychic levels. The conceptualization of the dyad is symmetrical, providing the basic model for exploring mothers' overt interactive behaviors and the mental representations in constant silent dialogue with them. Over the years, I had treated many mothers both with and without their babies, and had observed many others while doing research with the infants. Ultimately, for reasons that are not entirely clear to me, the mothers in the background of The Interpersonal World of the Infant came to the foreground as the subject of a focused reflection.

The most surprising consequence of this reflection was the realization that mothers create a new mental/psychic organization upon becoming mothers—a phenomenon I call the motherhood constellation. This constellation was a unique, independent, fundamental organization of mind, and not, as many people have assumed, a derivative or new version of old complexes, or a coloration added to a previously operating organization in the mothers' life. The resulting book (Stern, 1995) concluded with an examination of that constellation.

THE TRIAD

Since infants appear to live in triads, quartets, and so on, as well as in dyads, I deemed it necessary to expand the dyadic work to include the triad at least. This might seem a simple task, but first it was necessary to grapple with a fundamental question: Is the triad, for an infant, a set of three interrelated dyads, or is it an entity in itself that can be represented? Through the work of Fivaz and Corboz (1998) I was convinced that the triad is a unit in itself. This conclusion led to a series of collaborations exploring the infant's ability to deal with different triadic configurations and their transitions. Our observations suggested that, between three and six months of age, infants start to form schemas of the triadic configurations of which they are a part (Fivaz et al., 1995; Stern and Fivaz-Depeursinge, 1997).

THE WORLD OF SUBJECTIVE EXPERIENCE

The problem of how we can know the nature of the infant's subjective experience is always lurking in The Interpersonal World of the Infant. Of course we can't know it. And even with the onset of speech, any close mapping of narration to experience is uncertain and fraught with difficulties. The solution opted for in the book was to hypothesize, conservatively and not too specifically, about the infant's subjective life based on the aggregate of available objective findings and on the scientific zeitgeist on such questions.

Despite the need for great caution in such an endeavor, I decided to go even further in The Diary of a Baby (Stern, 1990). This was a "fun" book, written during the relocation of my laboratory—a sort of "pony" of The Interpersonal World of the Infant, intended mostly for parents. However, for that project, I could no longer be conservative and nonspecific. There could be no story if there were no specific happenings and specific experiences. So I made up these happenings and experiences. I was guided by accepted objective data, but I made them up nonetheless. This exercise in imagination proved fascinating and useful. It pushed my own thinking further in terms of exploring the question of how narrated accounts are in fact mapped onto lived experience. And what is lived experience, anyway? These ponderings led to the next line of inquiry, the microanalytic interview.

The Microanalytic Interview

Since there is no direct route to subjective lived experience other than later narrative, I decided to apply a variant of the microanalytic techniques from which we have learned so much about second-by-second interactive behavior. With this variant as a model, I developed the microanalytic interview, which attempts to describe the nature of instant-by-instant lived experience, but as told after the fact.

This type of interview has already been briefly discussed (Stern, 1995). In essence, the subject is asked to describe what was experienced during an event (e.g., a child at play) that had occurred only minutes or hours before. A short segment, usually a minute or less in duration and with a clear beginning and end, is autoselected. Then, a one- to two-hour interview is conducted in an effort to reconstruct the constituent experiences and the timing of their unfolding.

The subject is asked to describe what she thought, felt, and did. She is asked about the position her body was in and about her shifts in position and in bodily orientation. She is asked to make a "movie" with me of the event: I am the cameraman and she must direct me as to when a new "take" (i.e., a scene-shift) is necessary and what kind of shot (e.g., close-up, wide-angle) best captures each segment. Most important, the subject is asked to assign a duration to each element, and to draw a time curve of the event.

During the interview, we make many passes over the same material, each time adding new elements or correcting or adjusting others. The process is over when the subject feels that the event as reconstructed has reached a point of verisimilitude with the lived experience that cannot be improved upon.

Great attention is paid to the distinction between elements that were actually experienced and those that the subject knows must have happened. By the same token, all associations and memories that emerged during the telling but not as part of the experience are excluded. Finally, no suggestions of what may have happened come from the interviewer.

Among the most important findings were those showing the richness of daily experience, with multiple events occurring simultaneously. The polyphonic and polyrhythmic aspects of such experience are in perfect accord, subjectively validating the mind's parallel processing. Fascinatingly, the narrative form given to the lived moments-as-recounted corresponded to life concerns of the subject that reached well beyond the short experience—much like the world revealed in a grain of sand.

But a crucial question remains: How good is the correspondence between the lived experience and the reconstructed narrative? Given the availability of sophisticated brain imaging techniques, this question can be partially answered. At least the identification and timing of certain categories of mental events, such as movements, visual attention, perhaps even memories, can be ascertained. My colleagues and I are currently planning such research.

EXPLORING THE PRESENT MOMENT

The progressive interest in subjective experience, in both infants and adults, has led me to explore the nature of the present moment as lived. After all, life is lived in the present moment, which, in turn, is the temporal stage on which memories and future anticipations play. Even verbal reconstructions after the fact are occurring "now" in a present moment of their own.

Despite this obvious fact, psychology in general has paid insufficient attention to describing and conceptualizing the present moment. (That has been left largely to the philosophers, whose domain it traditionally has been.) An exploration of the present moment and its implications for psychology, psychoanalysis, and the neurosciences is the subject of a book I have begun to write. And a working group in Boston of which I am a member has begun to examine the nature of various kinds of subjective present moments in psychotherapy (present moments, now moments, moments of meeting), particularly in terms of what role they play in bringing about change (Stern et al., 1998).

I am continuing the line of research referred to as the microanalytic interview to help define the fact that, phenomenologically, we live only in the present. Our descriptions and theories of psychological processes must come to reflect that reality.

෧ᠻᢀ   ෧ᠻᢀ   ෧ᠻᢀ

One final personal word about *The Interpersonal World of the Infant*. Probably the most gratifying and validating comments about the book have identified it as a catalyst for bringing together people from different disciplines to discuss the issues it has raised. Psychotherapists and developmental psychologists from the same institution have come together for the first time as a working group; anthropologists, psychoanalysts, and developmentalists have formed interdisciplinary discussion groups; and psychotherapists of different schools have joined forces. It is a particular source of pride that the book has been instrumental in bridging gulfs between isolated fields and facilitating reciprocally enriching exchanges.

References

Bahrick, L. R., and Watson, J. S. (1985). Detection of intermodal proprioceptive-visual contingency as a potential basis of self-perception in infancy. Developmental Psychology, 21, 963–973.

Barratt, B. R. (1996). The relevance of infant observation for psychoanalysis. Journal of the American Psychoanalytic Association, 44, 2.

Braten, S. (1998). Infant learning by altero-centric participation: The reverse of egocentric observation in autism. In S. Braten (Ed.), Intersubjective communication and emotion in early ontogeny. Cambridge: Cambridge University Press.

Clark, A. (1997). Being there: Putting brain, body, and world together again. Cambridge, Mass.: MIT Press.

Cushman, P. (1991). Ideology obscured: Political uses of the self in Daniel Stern's Infant. American Psychologist, 46; 201–219.

Damasio, A. (1994). Decartes' error: Emotion, reason and the human brain. New York: Putnam.

_____. (1999). The feeling of what happens. New York: Basic Books.

de Roten, Y. (1999). L'interaction mère-enfant dans la narration d'un événement d'ordre émotionnel. Doctoral thesis, Faculté de Psychologie et Sciences d'Education, Université de Genève (Thèse No. 282).

Favez, N. (1996). Modes maternels de régulation émotionnelle du point-culminant des narrations autobiographiques d'enfants en âge préscolaire. Doctoral thesis, Faculté de Psychologie et Sciences d'Education, Université de Genève (Thèse No. 233).

Favez, N., Gertsch-Bettens, C., Heinze, X., Koch-Spinelli, M., Muhlebach, M.-C., Valles, A., and Stern, D. N. (1994). Réalité historique et réalité narrative chez le jeune enfant: Présentation d'une stratégie de recherche. Revue Suisse de Psychologie, 53(2), 98–103.

Fivaz, E., and Corboz, A. (1998). The primary triangle. New York: Basic Books.

Fivaz-Depeursinge, E., Maury, M., Bydlowski, M., and Stern, D. N. (1995). Une consultation mère-nourrisson: Entrerien clinique, micro-analyses et méthod interprétatives. In O Bourguignon and M. Bydlowski (Eds.), La recherche clinique en psychopathologie: Perspectives critiques. Paris: Presses Universitaires de France (Le Fils Rouge).

Gergely, G., and Watson, J. S. (1999). Early social-emotional development: Contingency perception and the social biofeedback model. In P. Rochat (Ed.), Early social cognition (pp. 101–136). Hillsdale, N.J.: Erlbaum.

Green, A. (1997). How far is empirical research relevant to psychoanalytic theory and practice? The example of research in infancy. A discussion with Daniel Stern at the Psychoanalysis Unit. London: University College London.

McCauley, J. (1994). Finding metrical structure in time. In E. Moser et al. (Eds.), Proceedings of the 1993 Connectionist Models Summer School. Hillsdale, N.J.: Erlbaum.

Nelson, K. (Ed.). (1989). Narratives from the crib. Cambridge, Mass.: Harvard University Press.

Port, R., Cummins, F., and McCauley, J. (1995). Naive time, temporal patterns and human audition. In R. Port and T. van Gelder (Eds.), Mind as motion. Cambridge, Mass.: MIT Press.

Rizzolatti, G., and Arbib, M. A. (1998). Language within our grasp. Trends in Neuroscience, 21, 188–194.

Rochat, P. (Ed.). (1999). Early social cognition. Hillsdale, N.J.: Erlbaum.

Rochat, P., and Morgan, R. (1995). The function and determinants of early self-exploration. In P. Rochat (Ed.), The self in infancy: Theory and research. Advances in psychology, Vol. 112 (pp. 395–415). Amsterdam: North Holland/Elsevier Science Publishers.

Stern, D. N. (1990). The diary of a baby. New York: Basic Books.

_____. (1995). The motherhood constellation. New York: Basic Books.

Stern, D. N., and Fivaz-Depeursinge, E. (1997). Construction du réel et affect: Points de vue développmentaux et systemiques. In M. Elkaim (Ed.), Construction du réel et éthique en psychothérapie familiale. Paris/Bruxelles: De Boeck & Larcier.

Stern, D. N., Sander, L. W., Nahum, J. P., Harrison, A. M., Lyons-Ruth, K., Morgan, A. C., Bruschweiler-Stern, N., and Tronick, E. Z. (1998). Non-interpretive mechanisms in psychoanalytic therapy: The "something more" than interpretation. International Journal of Psycho-Analysis, 79, 903–921.

Thelen, E., and Smith, L. (1994). A dynamic systems approach to the development of cognition and action. Cambridge, Mass.: MIT Press.

Torras, C. (1985). Temporal-pattern learning in neural models. Amsterdam: Springer-Verlag.

Trevarthen, C. (1979). Communication and cooperation in early infancy: A description of primary intersubjectivity. In M. M. Bullowa (Ed.), Before speech: The beginning of interpersonal communication. New York: Cambridge University Press.

Trevarthen, C., and Hubley, P. (1978). Secondary intersubjectivity: Confidence, confiders and acts of meaning in the first year. In A. Lock (Ed.), Action, gesture and symbol. New York: Academic Press.

Varela, F. J., Thompson, E., and Rosch, E. (1993). The embodied mind. Cambridge, Mass.: MIT Press.

Watson, J. S. (1994). Detection of self: The perfect algorithm. In S. Parker, R. Mitchell, and M. Boccia (Eds.), Self-awareness in animals and humans: Developmental perspectives (pp. 131–149). Cambridge, Mass.: Cambridge University Press.

Werner, H., and Kaplan, B. (1963). Symbol formation: An organismic-developmental approach to language and expression of thought. New York: Wiley.

Wilson, A. (1996). The relevance of infant observation for psychoanalysis. Journal of the American Psychoanalytic Association, 44(2).

Wolff, P. H. (1996). The irrelevance of infant research for psychoanalysis. Journal of the American Psychoanalytic Association, 44(2), 369–392.

Woolf, V. (1923). Diary. August 30, 1923.

PART I

THE QUESTIONS
AND THEIR
BACKGROUND

Chapter 1

Exploring the Infant's Subjective Experience: A Central Role for the Sense of Self

ANYONE CONCERNED with human nature is drawn by curiosity to wonder about the subjective life of young infants. How do infants experience themselves and others? Is there a self to begin with, or an other, or some amalgam of both? How do they bring together separate sounds, movements, touches, sights, and feelings to form a whole person? Or is the whole grasped immediately? How do infants experience the social events of "being with" an other? How is "being with" someone remembered, or forgotten, or represented mentally? What might the experience of relatedness be like as development proceeds? In sum, what kind of interpersonal world or worlds does the infant create?

Posing these questions is something like wondering what the universe might have been like the first few hours after the big bang. The universe was created only once, way out there, while interpersonal worlds are created, in here, every day in each new infant's mind. Yet both events, at almost opposite frontiers, remain remote and inaccessible to our direct experience.

Since we can never crawl inside an infant's mind, it may seem pointless to imagine what an infant might experience. Yet that is at the heart of what we really want and need to know. What we imagine infant experience to be like shapes our notions of who the infant is. These notions make up our working hypotheses about infancy. As such, they serve as the models guiding our clinical concepts about psychopathology: how, why, and when it begins. They are the wellspring of ideas for experiments about infants: what do they think and feel? These working theories also determine how we, as parents, respond to our own infants, and ultimately they shape our views of human nature.

Because we cannot know the subjective world that infants inhabit, we must invent it, so as to have a starting place for hypothesis-making. This book is such an invention. It is a working hypothesis about infants' subjective experience of their own social life.

The proposed working theory arises now, because the enormous research advances of the recent past have put in our hands whole new bodies of information about infants, as well as new experimental methods to inquire about their mental life. The result is a new view of the infant as observed.

One aim of this book is to draw some inferences about the infant's subjective life from this new observational data. This has not been done before, for two reasons. On the one hand, developmentalists, who are creating this new information, generally work within the tradition of observational and experimental research. In keeping with that approach, they choose not to make inferential leaps about the nature of subjective experience. Their emphasis on objective phenomena, even in clinical matters, is in line with the phenomenological trend now prevalent in American psychiatry, but it places severe limits on what can be embraced as clinical reality—objective happenings only, not subjective happenings. And just as importantly, this approach remains unresponsive to the basic questions about the nature of the infant's experience.

Psychoanalysts, on the other hand, in building their developmental theories continually make inferences about the nature of the infant's subjective experiences. This has been both a liability and a great strength. It has permitted their theories to embrace a larger clinical reality that includes life as subjectively experienced (and that is why it works clinically). But they have made their inferential leaps on the basis of reconstructed clinical material alone, and in the light of older and outdated views of the infant as observed. The new observational data has not yet been fully addressed by psychoanalysis, although important attempts in that direction have begun (see, for example, Brazelton 1980; Sander 1980; Call, Galenson, and Tyson 1983; Lebovici 1983; Lichtenberg 1981, 1983).

I have worked for some years as both a psychoanalyst and a developmentalist, and I feel the tension and excitement between these two points of view. The discoveries of developmental psychology are dazzling, but they seem doomed to remain clinically sterile unless one is willing to make inferential leaps about what they might mean for the subjective life of the infant. And the psychoanalytic developmental theories about the nature of infant experience, which are essential for guiding clinical practice, seem to be less and less tenable and less interesting in light of the new information about infants. It is against this background, which I know to be shared by many others, that I will attempt to draw inferences about the infant's subjective social experience from this new data base. The aims of this book, then, are to use these inferences to describe a working hypothesis of the infant's experience and to evaluate their possible clinical and theoretical implications.

Where can we start inventing infants' subjective experience of their own social life? I plan to start by placing the sense of self at the very center of the inquiry.

The self and its boundaries are at the heart of philosophical speculation on human nature, and the sense of self and its counterpart, the sense of other, are universal phenomena that profoundly influence all our social experiences.

While no one can agree on exactly what the self is, as adults we still have a very real sense of self that permeates daily social experience. It arises in many forms. There is the sense of a self that is a single, distinct, integrated body; there is the agent of actions, the experiencer of feelings, the maker of intentions, the architect of plans, the transposer of experience into language, the communicator and sharer of personal knowledge. Most often these senses of self reside out of awareness, like breathing, but they can be brought to and held in consciousness. We instinctively process our experiences in such a way that they appear to belong to some kind of unique subjective organization that we commonly call the sense of self.

Even though the nature of self may forever elude the behavioral sciences, the sense of self stands as an important subjective reality, a reliable, evident phenomenon that the sciences cannot dismiss. How we experience ourselves in relation to others provides a basic organizing perspective for all interpersonal events.

The reasons for giving the sense of self a central position, even—or especially—in a study of the preverbal infant, are many. First, several senses of the self may exist in preverbal forms, yet these have been relatively neglected. We comfortably assume that at some point later in development, after language and self-reflexive awareness are present, the subjective experience of a sense of self arises and is common to everyone, providing a cardinal perspective for viewing the interpersonal world. And certainly a sense of self is readily observable after self-reflexive awareness and language are present. A crucial question for this book is, does some kind of preverbal sense of self exist before that time? There are three possibilities. Language and self-reflection could act simply by *revealing* senses of the self that had already existed in the preverbal infant, that is, by making them evident as soon as the child can give an introspective account of inner experiences. Alternatively, language and self-reflection could *transform* or even *create* senses of the self that would only come into existence at the very moment they became the subject matter of self-reflection.

It is a basic assumption of this book that some senses of the self do exist long prior to self-awareness and language. These include the senses of agency, of physical cohesion, of continuity in time, of having intentions in mind, and other such experiences we will soon discuss. Self-reflection and language come to work upon these preverbal existential senses of the self and, in so doing, not only reveal their ongoing existence but transform them into new experiences. If we assume that some preverbal senses of the self start to form at birth (if not before), while others require the maturation of later-appearing capacities before they can emerge, then we are freed from the partially semantic task of choosing criteria to decide, a priori, when a sense of self *really* begins. The task becomes the more familiar one of describing the developmental continuities and changes in something that exists in some form from birth to death.

Some traditional psychoanalytic thinkers dismiss the whole issue of a preverbal subjective life as outside the pale of legitimate inquiry on both the methodological and the theoretical grounds just mentioned. They are joined in this position by many developmental experimentalists. Legitimate inquiry about human experience would, in that view, preclude the study of its very origins.

And that is exactly what we wish to study. Accordingly, it must be asked, what kind of a sense of self might exist in a preverbal infant? By "sense" I mean simple (non-self-reflexive) awareness. We are speaking at the level of direct experience, not concept. By "of self" I mean an invariant pattern of awarenesses that arise only on the occasion of the infant's actions or mental processes. An invariant pattern of awareness is a form of organization. It is the organizing subjective experience of whatever it is that will later be verbally referenced as the "self." This organizing subjective experience is the preverbal, existential counterpart of the objectifiable, self-reflective, verbalizable self.

A second reason for placing the sense of self, as it may exist preverbally, at the center of this inquiry is the clinical one of understanding normal interpersonal development. I am mostly concerned with those senses of the self that are essential to daily social interactions, not to encounters with the inanimate world. I will therefore focus on those senses of the self that if severely impaired would disrupt normal social functioning and likely lead to madness or great social deficit. Such senses of the self include the sense of agency (without which there can be paralysis, the sense of non-ownership of self-action, the experience of loss of control to external agents); the sense of physical cohesion (without which there can be fragmentation of bodily experience, depersonalization, out-of-body experiences, derealization); the sense of continuity (without which there can be temporal disassociation, fugue states, amnesias, not "going on being," in Winnicott's term); the sense of affectivity (without which there can be anhedonia, dissociated states); the sense of a subjective self that can achieve intersubjectivity with another (without which there is cosmic loneliness or, at the other extreme, psychic transparency); the sense of creating organization (without which there can be psychic chaos); the sense of transmitting meaning (without which there can be exclusion from the culture, little socialization, and no validation of personal knowledge). In short, these senses of the self make up the foundation for the subjective experience of social development, normal and abnormal.

A third reason for placing the sense of self at the center of a developmental inquiry is that recently there have been renewed attempts to think clinically in terms of various pathologies of the self (Kohut 1971, 1977). As Cooper (1980) points out, however, it is not that the self has been newly discovered. The essential problem of the self has been crucial to all clinical psychologies since Freud and for a variety of historical reasons has culminated in a psychology of the self. It has also been central to many of the dominant strains in academic psychology (for example, Baldwin 1902; Cooley 1912; Mead 1934).

The final reason to focus upon the sense of self in infancy is that it fits with a strong clinical impression about the developmental process. Development occurs in leaps and bounds; qualitative shifts may be one of its most obvious features. Parents, pediatricians, psychologists, psychiatrists, and neuroscientists all agree that new integrations arrive in quantum leaps. Observers also concur that the periods between two and three months (and to a lesser degree between five and six months), between nine and twelve months, and around fifteen to eighteen months are epochs of great change. During these periods of change, there are quantum leaps in whatever level of organization one wishes to examine, from electroencephalographic recordings to overt behavior to subjective experience (Emde, Gaensbauer, and Harmon 1976; McCall, Eichhorn, and Hogarty 1977; Kagan, Kearsley, and Zelazo 1978; Kagan 1984). Between these periods of rapid change are periods of relative quiessence, when the new integrations appear to consolidate.

At each of these major shifts, infants create a forceful impression that major changes have occurred in their subjective experience of self and other. One is suddenly dealing with an altered person. And what is different about the infant is not simply a new batch of behaviors and abilities; the infant suddenly has an additional "presence" and a different social "feel" that is more than the sum of the many newly acquired behaviors and capacities. For instance, there is no question that when, sometime between two and three months, an infant can smile responsively, gaze into the parent's eyes, and coo, a different social feel has been created. But it is not these behaviors alone, or even in combination, that achieve the transformation. It is the altered sense of the infant's subjective experience lying behind these behavioral changes that makes us act differently and think about the infant differently. One could ask, which comes first, an organizational change within the infant or a new attribution on the part of the parent? Does the advent of new infant behaviors such as focal eye contact and smiling make the parent attribute a new persona to the infant whose subjective experience has not as yet changed at all? In fact, any change in the infant may come about partly by virtue of the adult interpreting the infant differently and acting accordingly. (The adult would be working within the infant's proximal zone of development, that is, in an area appropriate to infant capacities not yet present but very soon to emerge.) Most probably, it works both ways. Organizational change from within the infant and its interpretation by the parents are mutually facilitative. The net result is that the infant appears to have a new sense of who he or she is and who you are, as well as a different sense of the kinds of interactions that can now go on.

Another change in sense of self is seen at about age nine months, when suddenly infants seem to sense that they have an interior subjective life of their own and that others do too. They become relatively less interested in external acts and more interested in the mental states that go on "behind" and give rise to the acts. The sharing of subjective experience becomes possible, and the subject matter for interpersonal exchanges is altered. For example, without using any words, the infant can now communicate something like "Mommy, I want you to look over here (alter your focus of attention to match my focus of attention), so that you too will see how exciting and delightful this toy is (so that you can share my subjective experience of excitement and pleasure)." This infant is operating with a different sense of self and of other, participating in the social world with a different organizing subjective perspective about it.

Given the sense of self as the starting point for this inquiry into the infant's subjective experience of social life, we will examine the different senses of self that appear to emerge as the maturation of capacities makes possible new organizing subjective perspectives about self and other. And we will examine the implications of such a developmental process for clinical theory and practice. The following is a summary of the major points of our examination.

Infants begin to experience a sense of an emergent self from birth. They are predesigned to be aware of self-organizing processes. They never experience a period of total self/other undifferentiation. There is no confusion between self and other in the beginning or at any point during infancy. They are also predesigned to be selectively responsive to external social events and never experience an autistic-like phase.

During the period from two to six months, infants consolidate the sense of a core self as a separate, cohesive, bounded, physical unit, with a sense of their own agency, affectivity, and continuity in time. There is no symbiotic-like phase. In fact, the subjective experiences of union with another can occur only after a sense of a core self and a core other exists. Union experiences are thus viewed as the successful result of actively organizing the experience of self-being-with-another, rather than as the product of a passive failure of the ability to differentiate self from other.

The period of life from roughly nine to eighteen months is not primarily devoted to the developmental tasks of independence or autonomy or individuation—that is, of getting away and free from the primary caregiver. It is equally devoted to the seeking and creating of intersubjective union with another, which becomes possible at this age. This process involves learning that one's subjective life—the contents of one's mind and the qualities of one's feelings—can be shared with another. So while separation may proceed in some domains of self-experience, new forms of being with another are proceeding at the same time in other domains of self-experience. (Different domains of self-experience refer to experiences that occur within the perspective of different senses of the self.)

This last point highlights a more general conclusion. I question the entire notion of phases of development devoted to specific clinical issues such as orality, attachment, autonomy, independence, and trust. Clinical issues that have been viewed as the developmental tasks for specific epochs of infancy are seen here as issues for the lifespan rather than as developmental phases of life, operating at essentially the same levels at all points in development.

The quantum shifts in the social "presence" and "feel" of the infant can therefore no longer be attributed to the departure from one specific developmental task-phase and the entrance into the next.

Instead, the major developmental changes in social experience are attributed to the infant's acquisition of new senses of the self. It is for this reason that the sense of self looms so large in this working theory. The sense of self serves as the primary subjective perspective that organizes social experience and therefore now moves to center stage as the phenomenon that dominates early social development.

Four different senses of the self will be described, each one defining a different domain of self-experience and social relatedness. They are the sense of an *emergent self*, which forms from birth to age two months, the sense of a *core self*, which forms between the ages of two and six months, the sense of a *subjective self*, which forms between seven to fifteen months, and a sense of a *verbal self*, which forms after that. These senses of self are not viewed as successive phases that replace one another. Once formed, each sense of self remains fully functioning and active throughout life. All continue to grow and coexist.

Infants are seen as having a very active memorial and fantasy life, but they are concerned with events that actually happen. ("Seductions," as Freud first encountered them in clinical material, are real events at this stage of life. There are no wish fulfilling fantasies.) The infant is thus seen as an excellent reality-tester; reality at this stage is never distorted for defensive reasons. Further, many of the phenomena thought by psychoanalytic theory to play a crucial role in very early development, such as delusions of merger or fusion, splitting, and defensive or paranoid fantasies, are not applicable to the infancy period—that is, before the age of roughly eighteen to twenty-four months—but are conceivable only after the capacity for symbolization as evidenced by language is emerging, when infancy ends.

More generally, many of the tenets of psychoanalysis appear to describe development far better after infancy is over and childhood has begun, that is, when speech is available. This observation is not meant as a disconfirmation of psychoanalytic theory; it is a suggestion that psychoanalytic theory has been misapplied to this earlier period of life, which it does not describe well. On the other hand, academic working theories that describe the infancy period do not give adequate importance to subjective social experience. The emphasis in this account on the development of the sense of self is a step in the direction of gradually finding theories that better fit the observable data and that will ultimately prove of practical import in dealing with subjective experience.

Finally, one of the major clinical implications of the proposed working hypothesis is that clinical reconstructions of a patient's past can best use developmental theory to help locate the origin of pathology in one of the domains of self-experience. Since the traditional clinical-developmental issues such as orality, autonomy, and trust are no longer seen as occupying age-specific sensitive periods but as being issues for the life span, we can no longer predict the actual developmental point of origin of later-emerging clinical problems involving these issues, as psychoanalysis has always promised. We can, however, begin to make predictions about the origins of pathology in the various domains of self-experience. The result is a greater freedom in therapeutic exploration.

These, then, are the general outlines of the working theory that will result from making clinically informed inferences from the newly available infancy data. Because the different senses of the self are so central to this account, separate chapters of part 2 of this book are devoted to describing how each new sense of self comes about, what maturing capacities and abilities make it possible, what new perspective it adds to the infant's social world view, and how this new perspective enhances the infant's capacity for relatedness. Part 3 then looks at some clinical implications of this working theory, from differing viewpoints. Chapter 9 looks at the "observed infant" with a clinical eye. Chapter 10 reverses that perspective and looks at the reconstructed infant of clinical practice with the eye of an observer of infants. And the last chapter looks at the implications of this developmental viewpoint for the therapeutic process of reconstructing a patient's past.

First, however, it seems essential to explain in greater detail the nature of my approach and its problems. Chapter 2 will address those issues, in particular the advantages and limitations of combining data from experimental and clinical sources; the rationale for placing the sense of self at the center of a developmental account of social experience; and the conceptualization of the developmental progression of senses of the self.

Chapter 2

Perspectives and Approaches to Infancy

THE PICTURE of infant experience suggested in this book has both differences from and similarities to the pictures currently drawn by psychoanalysis and developmental psychology. Since the approach I have adopted borrows methods and findings from developmental psychology and insights from clinical practice, it is important to discuss in greater detail the assumptions of each discipline and the problems of using both approaches together.

The Observed Infant and the Clinical Infant

Developmental psychology can inquire about the infant only as the infant is observed. To relate observed behavior to subjective experience, one must make inferential leaps. Clearly, the inferences will be more accurate if the data base from which one is leaping is extensive and well established. The study of intrapsychic experience must be informed by the findings of direct observation, as the source of most new information about infants continues to be naturalistic and experimental observations. But at best, the observations of an infant's available capacities can only help to define the limits of subjective experience. To render a full account of that experience, we require insights from clinical life, and a second approach is needed for this task.

In contrast to the infant as observed by developmental psychology, a different "infant" has been reconstructed by psychoanalytic theories in the course of clinical practice (primarily with adults). This infant is the joint creation of two people, the adult who grew up to become a psychiatric patient and the therapist, who has a theory about infant experience. This recreated infant is made up of memories, present reenactments in the transference, and theoretically guided interpretations. I call this creation the *clinical infant,* to be distinguished from the *observed infant,* whose behavior is examined at the very time of its occurrence.

Both of these approaches are indispensable for the present task of thinking about the development of the infant's sense of self. The clinical infant breathes subjective life into the observed infant, while the observed infant points toward the general theories upon which one can build the inferred subjective life of the clinical infant.

Such a collaboration was not conceivable before the last decade or so. Up to that point, the observed infant concerned mostly nonsocial encounters: physical landmarks like sitting and grasping or the emergence of capacities for perceiving and thinking about objects. The clinical infant, on the other hand, has always concerned the social world as subjectively experienced. So long as these two infants involved different issues, they could go their own ways. Their coexistence was nonproblematic, and their collaborative potential was small.

But this is no longer the case. Observers of infants have recently begun to inquire about how and when infants might see, hear, interact with, feel about, and understand other persons as well as themselves. These efforts are bringing the observed infant in line with the clinical infant to the extent that both concern versions of the infant's lived social experience, including the infant's sense of self. Their coexistence now invites comparisons and cooperation.

The problem raised by drawing upon these two differently derived infants is, to what extent are they really about the same thing? To what extent do they share common ground, so that they can be joined for one purpose? At first glance, both viewpoints appear to be about the real infant's social experience. If this is so, then each should be able to validate or invalidate the claims of the other. However, many believe that the two versions are not at all about the same reality and that the conceptualizations of one are impervious to the findings of the other. In that case, there would exist no common meeting ground for comparison, and possibly not even for cooperation (Kreisler and Cramer 1981; Lebovici 1983; Lichtenberg 1983; Cramer 1984; Gautier 1984).

The dialogue between these two views of infancy and how they may influence one another is a secondary theme of this book. The way in which they together can illuminate the development of the infant's sense of self is the primary theme. For both purposes, it is important to examine each view more fully.

A clinical infancy is a very special construct. It is created to make sense of the whole early period of a patient's life story, a story that emerges in the course of its telling to someone else. This is what many therapists mean when they say that psychoanalytic therapeutics is a special form of story-making, a narrative (Spence 1976; Ricoeur 1977; Schafer 1981). The story is discovered, as well as altered, by both teller and listener in the course of the telling. Historical truth is established by what gets told, not by what actually happened. This view opens the door for the possibility that any narrative about one's life (especially one's early life) may be just as valid as the next. Indeed, there are competing theories, or potential narratives, about what early life was actually like. The early life narratives as created by Freud, Erikson, Klein, Mahler, and Kohut would all be somewhat different even for the same case material. Each theorist selected different features of experience as the most central, so each would produce a different felt-life-history for the patient.

Viewed in this way, can any narrative account ever be validated by what was thought to have happened in infancy? Schafer (1981) argues that it cannot. He suggests that therapeutic narratives do not simply explicate or reflect what may actually have happened back then; they also create the real experience of living by specifying what is to be attended to and what is most salient. In other words, real-life-as-experienced becomes a product of the narrative, rather than the other way around. The past is, in one sense, a fiction. In this view, the notion of mutual validation between the clinical (narrated) infant and the observed infant is out of the question. No meeting ground exists.[1]

Ricoeur (1977) takes a less extreme position. He does not believe, as does Schafer, that no meeting ground for external validation exists. If that were so, he argues, it would "turn psychoanalytic statements into the rhetoric of persuasion under the pretext that it is the account's acceptability to the patient that is therapeutically effective" (p. 862).

Ricoeur suggests that there are some general hypotheses about how the mind works and how it develops that exist independently of the many narratives that could be constructed—for example, the developing sequence of psychosexual stages or the developing nature of object- or person-relatedness. These general hypotheses can be potentially tested or strongly supported by direct observation or by evidence existing outside of any one particular narrative and outside of psychoanalysis. One advantage of Ricoeur's position is that it provides the clinical infant with greatly needed independent sources of information to help examine the implicit general hypotheses that go into the construction of the life narrative. The observed infant might be such a source.

I am in full agreement with Ricoeur's position, which provides much of the rationale for proceeding as I do in this book, but with the understanding that this position applies to metapsychology, or the constraints of developmental theory, not to any one patient's reconstructed felt-history.

There is a third consideration that bears on this issue of contrasting, partially incompatible viewpoints. The current scientific Zeitgeist has a certain persuasive and legitimizing force in determining what is a reasonable view of things. And at this moment the Zeitgeist favors observational methods. The prevailing view of the infant has shifted dramatically in the past few years and will continue to shift. It will ultimately be a cause for uneasiness and questioning if the psychoanalytic view of infancy becomes too divergent and contradictory relative to the observational approach. As related fields, presum-

---

1. The two infants live at different levels of epistemological discourse. For Schafer, therefore, the issue of the validity of a narrative is strictly an internal matter. The issue is never a question of whether the life narrative was observably true back when, but of whether the life story "appear(s) [to the narrator] after careful consideration to have the virtues of coherence, consistency, comprehensiveness, and common sense" (p. 46).

ably about the same subject matter even though from different perspectives, they will not tolerate too much dissonance, and it currently appears that it is psychoanalysis that will have to give way. (This position may seem overly relativistic, but science advances by shifting paradigms about how things are to be seen. These paradigms are ultimately belief systems.) Thus, the mutual influence between the observed and the clinical infants will result both from a direct confrontation about those specific issues that the two views can contest, as implied by Ricoeur, and from the evolving sense of the nature of infancy, to which both views contribute. This process will gradually determine what feels acceptable, tenable, and in accord with common sense.

The observed infant is also a special construct, a description of capacities that can be observed directly: the ability to move, to smile, to seek novelty, to discriminate the mother's face, to encode memories, and so on. These observations themselves reveal little about what the "felt quality" of lived social experience is like. Moreover, they tell us little about higher organizational structures that would make the observed infant more than a growing list of capacities that is organized and reorganized. As soon as we try to make inferences about the actual experiences of the real infant—that is, to build in qualities of subjective experience such as a sense of self—we are thrown back to our own subjective experience as the main source of inspiration. But that is exactly the domain of the clinical infant. The only storehouse of such information is our own life narratives, what it has felt like to live our own social lives. Here, then, is the problem: the subjective life of the adult, as self-narrated, is the main source of inference about the infant's felt quality of social experience. A degree of circularity is unavoidable.

Each view of the infant has features that the other lacks. The observed infant contributes the capacities that can be readily witnessed; the clinical infant contributes certain subjective experiences that are fundamental and common features of social life.[2]

The partial joining of these two infants is essential for three

2. The potential dangers of adultomorphizing are real. Therefore, it is important that the subjective experiences chosen are not those seen exclusively or particularly in adult psychopathological states, nor those that come to be acceptable and reasonable only after much psychodynamic self-exploration. They should be apparent to anyone and a normal part of common experience.

reasons. First, there must be some way that actual happenings—that is, observable events ("mother did this, and that . . .")—become transformed into the subjective experiences that clinicians call intrapsychic ("I experienced mother as being . . ."). It is this crossover point that involves the participation of both the observed infant and the clinical infant. While the two perspectives do not overlap, they do touch one another at certain points to create an interface. One can never understand the genesis of psychopathology without this interface. Second, the therapist who is better acquainted with the observed infant may be in a position to help patients create more appropriate life narratives. Third, the observer of infants who is better acquainted with the clinical infant may be prompted to conceive of new directions for observation.[3]

Perspectives on the Subject Matter of Development

THE PSYCHOANALYTIC PERSPECTIVE

Developmental psychology views the maturation of new capacities (such as hand-eye coordination, recall memory, and self-awareness) and their reorganization as the appropriate subject matter of developmental shifts. For the sake of clinical utility and a subjective account, psychoanalysis has had to take a further step and define the progressive reorganizations in terms of larger organizing principles of development, or mental life. Freud's developmental progression from oral to anal to genital stages was seen as the sequential reorganization of drive, or the nature of the id. Erikson's developmental progression from trust to autonomy to industry was seen as the sequential reorganization of ego and character structures. Similarly, Spitz's progression of organizing principles concerned a sequential restructuring of ego precursors. Mahler's developmental progression

---

3. Even those who are decidedly committed to the approach of psychopharmacology will ultimately (when further advances in neurochemical understanding have been made and assimilated) have to re-confront or confront for the first time the level of subjective experience in the light of their new understandings. At the moment, the level of subjective experience may seem like a thing of the past from the chemical viewpoint, but soon enough it will be the wave of the future, if and when (and only if and when) chemical psychiatry fulfills its promise.

from normal autism to normal symbiosis to separation-individuation concerned the restructuring of ego and id, but in terms of the infant's experience of self and other. Klein's developmental progression (depressive, paranoid, and schizoid positions) also concerns the restructuring of the experience of self and other, but in a very different manner.

The developmental account described in this book, in which new senses of the self serve as organizing principles of development, is closest to the accounts of Mahler and Klein in that its central concern, like theirs, is for the infant's experience of self and other. The differences lie in what the nature of that experience is thought to be, in the order of the developmental sequence, and in my focus on the development of the sense of self, not encumbered with or confused with issues of the development of the ego or id.

Psychoanalytic developmental theories share another premise. They all assume that development progresses from one stage to the next, and that each stage is not only a specific phase for ego or id development but also specific for certain proto-clinical issues. In effect, developmental phases concern the infant's initial dealing with a specific type of clinical issue that can be seen in pathological form in later life. This is what Peterfreund (1978) and Klein (1980) mean by a developmental system that is both pathomorphic and retrospective. More specifically, Peterfreund speaks of "two fundamental conceptual fallacies, especially characteristic of psychoanalytic thought: the adultomorphization of infancy and the tendency to characterize early states of normal development in terms of hypotheses about later states of psychopathology" (p. 427).

It is in this way that Freud's phases of orality, anality, and so on refer not only to stages of drive development but to potential periods of fixation—that is, to specific points of origin of pathology—that will later result in specific psychopathological entities. Similarly, Erikson sought in his developmental phases the specific roots of later ego and character pathology. And in Mahler's theory, the need to understand later clinical phenomena such as childhood autism, symbiotic psychosis of childhood, and overdependency initially led to postulating the occurrence of these entities in some preliminary form earlier in development.

These psychoanalysts are developmental theorists working backward in time. Their primary aim was to aid in understanding the development of psychopathology. This in fact was a task of therapeutic urgency, a task that no other developmental psychology was dealing with. But it forced them to position pathomorphically chosen clinical issues seen in adults in a central developmental role.

In contrast, the approach taken here is normative rather than pathomorphic and prospective rather than retrospective. While disruptions in the development of any sense of self may prove to be predictive of later pathology, the different senses of self are designed to describe normal development and not to explain the ontogeny of pathogenic forms (which does not mean that ultimately they may not be helpful in that task).

Psychoanalytic theories make yet another assumption, that the pathomorphically designated phase in which a clinical issue is being worked on developmentally is a sensitive period in ethological terms. Each separate clinical issue, such as orality, autonomy, or trust, is given a limited time slot, a specific phase in which the designated phase-specific clinical issue "comes to its ascendancy, meets its crisis, and finds its lasting solution through a decisive encounter with the environment" (Sander 1962, p. 5). In this way each age or phase becomes a sensitive, almost critical, period for the development of a single phase-specific clinical issue or personality feature. Freud's, Erikson's, and Mahler's sequences are examples par excellence. In such systems, each issue (for example, symbiosis, trust, or orality) ends up with its own distinct epoch. The result is a parade of specific epochs, in which each of the most basic clinical issues of life passes by the grandstand in its own separate turn.

Do these clinical issues really define age-specific phases? Does the succession of different predominant clinical issues explain the quantum leaps in social relatedness that observers and parents readily note? From the point of view of the developmental psychologist, there are serious problems with using clinical issues to describe developmental phases meaningfully. The basic clinical issues of autonomy and independence provide a good example.

How does one identify the crucial events that might define a phase that is specific to the issues of autonomy and independence? Both Erikson (1950) and Freud (1905) placed the decisive encounter for this clinical issue around the independent control of bowel functioning at about twenty-four months. Spitz (1957) placed the decisive encounter in the ability to say "no" at fifteen months or so. Mahler

(1968, 1975) considered the decisive event for autonomy and independence to be infants' capacity to walk, to wander away from mother on their own initiative, beginning at about twelve months. The timing of these three different decisive encounters disagrees by a whole year, half the two-year-old child's life. That is a big disagreement. Which author is right? They are all right, and that is both the problem and the point.

In fact, there are other behaviors that can equally well be identified as criteria for autonomy and independence. The interaction between mother and infant as carried on with gaze behavior during the three- to six-month period, for instance, is strikingly like the interaction between mother and infant as carried out with locomotor behaviors during the twelve- to eighteen-month period. During the three- to five-month period, mothers give the infant control—or rather the infant takes control—over the initiations and terminations of direct visual engagement in social activities (Stern 1971, 1974, 1977; Beebe and Stern 1977; Messer and Vietze, in press). It must be recalled that during this period of life the infant cannot walk and has poor control over limb movements and eye-hand coordination. The visual-motor system, however, is virtually mature, so that in gazing behavior the infant is a remarkably able interactive partner. And gazing is a potent form of social communication. When watching the gazing patterns of mother and infant during this life period, one is watching two people with almost equal facility and control over the same social behavior.[4]

In this light, it becomes obvious that infants exert major control over the initiation, maintenance, termination, and avoidance of social contact with mother; in other words, they help to regulate engagement. Furthermore, by controlling their own direction of gaze, they self-regulate the level and amount of social stimulation to which they are subject. They can avert their gaze, shut their eyes, stare past, become glassy-eyed. And through the decisive use of such gaze behaviors, they can be seen to reject, distance themselves from, or defend themselves against mother (Beebe and Stern 1977; Stern

4. The same can of course be said of any dyad of infant and caregiver. Throughout this book, "mother," "parent," and "caregiver" are generally used interchangeably to mean the primary caregiver. Similarly, "the dyad" denotes infant and primary caregiver. The exceptions should be fairly obvious: references to breast-feeding, to specific cases, and to research focusing on maternal behavior.

1977; Beebe and Sloate 1982). They can also reinitiate engagement and contact when they desire, through gazing, smiling, and vocalizing.

The manner in which infants regulate their own stimulation and social contact through gaze behavior is quite similar, for the generic issue of autonomy and independence, to the manner in which they accomplish the same thing nine months later by walking away from and returning to mother's side.[5] Why, then, should we not consider the period from three to six months also as phase-specific for the issue of autonomy and independence, both as displayed in overt behavior and as experienced subjectively?[6]

Mothers know quite well that infants can assert their independence and say a decisive "NO!" with gaze aversions at four months, gestures and vocal intonation at seven months, running away at fourteen months, and language at two years. The basic clinical issue of autonomy or independence is inherently operating in all social behaviors that regulate the quantity or quality of engagement. The decision, then, as to what constitutes a decisive event that makes autonomy or independence *the* phase-specific issue appears to have more to do with maturational leaps in cognitive level or motor capacities that are outside the considerations of autonomy and independence *per se.* It is these abilities and capacities that are the real desiderata in each theoretician's definition of a phase. And each theoretician uses a different criterion.

Those who are persuaded that there do exist basic clinical issues, time-locked specific phases, would argue that all clinical issues are of course being negotiated all of the time, but that there is still the feature of predominance, that one life-issue is relatively more prominent at one life period. Certainly, at a given point in development the new behaviors that are used to conduct ongoing issues can be more dramatic (for example, the forms that autonomy and independence take in the "terrible twos"), and these new forms can also require more socializing pressure that attracts much more attention

5. Messer and Vietze (in press) point out that the dyadic gazing patterns become far less regulatory of the interaction at one year, when infants have acquired other ways (such as locomotion) of regulating the interaction and their own level of tension.

6. One could argue that not until twelve months do infants have sufficient intentionality, object permanence, and other cognitive capacities to make the notion of autonomy or independence meaningful. But one could also argue that not until eighteen to twenty-four months do infants have enough symbolic functions or self-awareness to make these notions meaningful. Both arguments have been made.

to them. But the need for more socializing pressure is largely culturally determined.[7] The "terrible twos" are not terrible in all societies.

It therefore seems likely that a relative predominance of protoclinical issues in a particular age period is illusory and emerges from theoretical, methodological, or clinical needs and biases in conjunction with cultural pressures. It is in the eyes of the beholder, not in the infant's experience. Further, if one picks out one basic life-issue and devotes a developmental epoch to its decisive resolution, the picture of the developmental process will necessarily be distorted. It will portray potential clinical narratives, not observable infants. There are no convincing grounds, from the observational point of view, for considering basic clinical issues as adequate overall definers of phases or stages of development.[8]

Clinical issues are issues for the life span, not phases of life. Consequently, clinical issues fail to account for the developmental changes in the social "feel" of the infant or in the infant's subjective perspective about social life.

There is an additional problem with making these traditional clinical-developmental issues the subject matter of sequential sensitive phases of life. In spite of the fact that these views have been prevalent for many decades, there have as yet been no prospective longitudinal studies that support the very clear predictions of these theories. Psychological insults and trauma at a specific age or phase should result in predictably specific types of clinical problems later on. No such evidence exists.[9]

7. Sameroff (1983) provides a systems-theory model for explaining the interaction between society and the parent-infant dyad in determining "predominance" of an issue, that is, how events at the societal level can make an issue more salient for the dyad.

8. Pine (1981) has offered a compromise accounting for the fact commonly observed by mothers that infants are "in" many clinical issue-specific phases at the same time (for example, attaching, while becoming autonomous, while developing mastery). He suggests that the infant has many significant "moments" in any day or hour when different clinical issues are dominant. The problem with this solution is twofold. Significant "moments" appear to be chosen partly on the basis of preconception about the predominant phase (that is, circularly), and such moments are organized around high-intensity experiences. The privileged organizing capacity of high-intensity compared to medium- or low-intensity moments is an open empirical issue. Nonetheless, the impressions that led Pine to this particular solution attest to the widespread recognition of the problem.

9. One of the problems with the implicit or explicit predictions that psychoanalytic theory has made about the ontogeny of pathology is that they were perhaps too specific. Recent thinking about developmental psychopathology (Cicchetti and Schnieder-Rosen, in press; Sroufe and Rutter 1984) stresses that the manifestations of pathology may be very different at

THE PERSPECTIVE OF CLINICALLY ORIENTED DEVELOPMENTALISTS

For those who observe infants directly, there certainly do appear to be phases of development. These phases, however, are not seen in terms of later clinical issues, but rather in terms of current adaptive tasks that arise because of maturation in the infant's physical and mental capacities. The result is a progression of developmental issues that the dyad must negotiate together for adaptation to proceed. It is from this perspective that Sander (1964) has described the following phases: physiological regulation (zero to three months); regulation of reciprocal exchange, especially social-affective modulation (three to six months); the joint regulation of infant initiation in social exchanges and in manipulating the environment (six to nine months); the focalization of activities (ten to fourteen months); and self-assertion (fifteen to twenty months). Greenspan (1981) has evolved a somewhat similar sequence of stages, except that his stray further from readily observable behavior and incorporate some of the abstract organizing principles of psychoanalysis and attachment theory. The stages he proposes are thus more heterogeneous: homeostasis (zero to three months); attachment (two to seven months); somatopsychological differentiation (three to ten months); behavioral organization, initiative, and internalization (nine to twenty-four months); and representational capacity, differentiation and consolidation (nine to twenty-four months).

Most observers of parent-infant interactions would agree that such descriptive systems more or less capture many of the important developmental changes. While several specifics of these descriptive systems are arguable, the systems are helpful clinically in evaluating and treating parent-infant dyads in distress. The central point here is not the validity of these descriptions but the nature of the perspective they take. They view the dyad as the unit of focus and they view it in terms of adaptive tasks. This is at a great remove from any consideration of the infant's likely subjective experience. Infants go about their business of growing and developing, and abstract entities such as homeostasis, reciprocal regulation, and the like are not a

---

different ages. Even most normal developmental issues are now thought to undergo considerable transformation in manifestation across age. This has been an accumulating impression about the paradox of developmental discontinuity within continuity (Waddington 1940; Sameroff and Chandler 1975; Kagan, Kearsley, and Zelazo 1978; McCall 1979; Garmenzy and Rutter 1983; Hinde and Bateson 1984).

24

conceivably meaningful part of their subjective social experience. Yet it is exactly with the infant's subjective experience that we are most concerned in this inquiry.

Attachment theory as it has grown from its origins in psychoanalysis and ethology (Bowlby 1969, 1973, 1980) to include the methods and perspectives of developmental psychology (Ainsworth and Wittig 1969; Ainsworth et al. 1978) has come to embrace many levels of phenomena. At various levels, attachment is a set of infant behaviors, a motivational system, a relationship between mother and infant, a theoretical construct, and a subjective experience for the infant in the form of "working models."

Some levels of attachment, such as the behavior patterns that change to maintain attachment at different ages, can be seen readily as sequential phases of development, while others, such as the quality of the mother-infant relationship, are life-span issues (Sroufe and Waters 1977; Sroufe 1979; Hinde 1982; Bretherton and Waters, in press).

Most attachment theorists, perhaps because of their grounding in academic psychology, have been slow to pick up on Bowlby's notion that while attachment is a perspective on evolution, on the species and on the individual dyad, it is also a perspective on the subjective experience of the infant in the form of the infant's working model of mother. Only recently have researchers readdressed Bowlby's notion of the working model of the mother in the infant's mind. Currently several researchers (Bretherton, in press; Main and Kaplan, in press; Osofsky 1985; Sroufe 1985; Sroufe and Fleeson 1985) are reaching further to make the construct of attachment meaningful at the level of the infant's subjective experience.[10]

THE PERSPECTIVE OF THE DEVELOPING SENSES OF THE SELF

The present account, even in the form of a working hypothesis, shares many features with both traditional psychoanalytic theory and attachment theory. Higher order constructs are needed to serve as the organizing principles of development. In this respect, the account is completely in line with both theories. It differs from them in that the organizing principle concerns the subjective sense of self. While

---

10. Attachment theory is both normative and prospective. Yet interestingly it is proving to be specifically predictive—and strongly so—of later behaviors, some of which are pathological. (The research findings will be discussed in detail in chapters 5 and 9.)

Self Psychology is emerging as a coherent therapeutic theory that places the self as a structure and process at the center, there have as yet been no systematic attempts to consider the sense of self as a developmental organizing principle, although some speculations in that direction have been made (for example, Tolpin 1971, 1980; Kohut 1977; Shane and Shane 1980; Stechler and Kaplan 1980; Lee and Noam 1983; Stolerow et al. 1983). And it is not yet clear how compatible the present developmental view will be with the tenets of Self Psychology as a clinical theory for adults.

Certainly, Mahler and Klein and the object relations school have focused upon the experience of self-and-other, but mainly as the fall out of, or secondary to, libidinal or ego development. Those theorists never considered the sense of self as the primary organizing principle.

This account, centering on the sense of self-and-other, has as its starting place the infant's inferred subjective experience. It is unique in that respect. Subjective experiences themselves are its main working parts, in contrast to the main working parts of psychoanalytic theories, which are the ego and id from which subjective experiences are derived.

The Developmental Progression of the Sense of Self

As new behaviors and capacities emerge, they are reorganized to form organizing subjective perspectives on self and other. The result is the emergence, in quantum leaps, of different senses of the self. These will be outlined briefly here. In part 2 separate chapters are devoted to each.

There is, for one, the physical self that is experienced as a coherent, willful, physical entity with a unique affective life and history that belong to it. This self generally operates outside of awareness. It is taken for granted, and even verbalizing about it is difficult. It is an experiential sense of self that I call the *sense of a core self*.[11] The sense of a core self is a perspective that rests upon the working of many

---

11. The sense of a core self includes the phenomena that are encompassed in the term "body ego" as used in the psychoanalytic literature. However, it includes more than that, and it is conceptualized differently without recourse to the entity ego. The two are not strictly comparable. It is also more than a sensorimotor schema, since it includes affective features.

interpersonal capacities. And when this perspective forms, the subjective social world is altered and interpersonal experience operates in a different domain, a *domain of core-relatedness*. This developmental transformation or creation occurs somewhere between the second and sixth months of life, when infants sense that they and mother are quite separate physically, are different agents, have distinct affective experiences, and have separate histories.

That is only one possible organizing subjective perspective about the self-and-other. Sometime between the seventh and ninth months of life, infants start to develop a second organizing subjective perspective. This happens when they "discover" that there are other minds out there as well as their own. Self and other are no longer only core entities of physical presence, action, affect, and continuity. They now include subjective mental states—feelings, motives, intentions—that lie behind the physical happenings in the domain of core-relatedness. The new organizing subjective perspective defines a qualitatively different self and other who can "hold in mind" unseen but inferable mental states, such as intentions or affects, that guide overt behavior. These mental states now become the subject matter of relating. This new *sense of a subjective self* opens up the possibility for intersubjectivity between infant and parent and operates in a new domain of relatedness—the *domain of intersubjective relatedness*—which is a quantum leap beyond the domain of core-relatedness. Mental states between people can now be "read," matched, aligned with, or attuned to (or misread, mismatched, misaligned, or misattuned). The nature of relatedness has been dramatically expanded. It is important to note that the domain of intersubjective relatedness, like that of core-relatedness, goes on outside of awareness and without being rendered verbally. In fact, the experience of intersubjective relatedness, like that of core-relatedness, can only be alluded to; it cannot really be described (although poets can evoke it).

The sense of a subjective self and other rests upon different capacities from those necessary for a sense of a core self. These include the capacities for sharing a focus of attention, for attributing intentions and motives to others and apprehending them correctly, and for attributing the existence of states of feeling in others and sensing whether or not they are congruent with one's own state of feeling.

At around fifteen to eighteen months, the infant develops yet a

27

third organizing subjective perspective about self and other, namely the sense that self (and other) has a storehouse of personal world knowledge and experience ("I know there is juice in the refrigerator, and I know that I am thirsty"). Furthermore, this knowledge can be objectified and rendered as symbols that convey meanings to be communicated, shared, and even created by the mutual negotiations permitted by language.

Once the infant is able to create shareable meanings about the self and the world, a *sense of a verbal self* that operates in the *domain of verbal relatedness* has been formed. This is a qualitatively new domain with expanding, almost limitless possibilities for interpersonal happenings. Again, this new sense of self rests on a new set of capacities: to objectify the self, to be self-reflective, to comprehend and produce language.

So far we have discussed three different senses of the self and other, and three different domains of relatedness that develop between the age of two months and the second year of the infant's life. Nothing has yet been said about the period from birth to two months. It can now be filled in.

During this earliest period, a sense of the world, including a sense of self, is emergent. Infants busily embark on the task of relating diverse experiences. Their social capacities are operating with vigorous goal-directedness to assure social interactions. These interactions produce affects, perceptions, sensorimotor events, memories, and other cognitions. Some integration between diverse happenings is made innately. For instance, if infants can feel a shape by touching an object, they will know what the object should look like without ever having seen it before. Other integrations are not so automatic but are quickly learned. Connectedness forms rapidly, and infants experience the emergence of organization. A *sense of an emergent self* is in the process of coming into being. The experience is that of the emergence of networks becoming integrated, and we can refer to its domain as the *domain of emergent relatedness*. Still, the integrative networks that are forming are not yet embraced by a single organizing subjective perspective. That will be the task of the developmental leap into the domain of core-relatedness.

The four main senses of self and the domains of relatedness that have been described will occupy much of this book. The four senses of the self conform in their time of emergence to the major developmental shifts that have been noted. The change in the social feel of an infant with the emergence of each sense of self is also in accord with the nature of these shifts. So is the predominant "action" between parent and child, which shifts from the physical and actional to the mental events that underlie the overt behavior and then to the meanings of events. Before examining these senses and domains further, however, we must address the issue of sensitive periods and make clear that we are dealing not only with successive phases but also with simultaneous domains of self-experience.

As the four domains of relatedness develop successively, one after the other, what happens to each domain when the next comes along? Does each sense of self remain intact in the presence of the new ones, so that they coexist? Or does the emergence of each new sense of self eclipse the existing ones, so that sequential phases wax and wane?

The traditional picture of both the clinical infant and the observed infant leans toward a view of sequential phases. In both developmental systems, the infant's world view shifts dramatically as each new stage is ushered in, and the world is seen dominantly, if not exclusively, in terms of the organization of the new stage. What happens, then, to the previous phases, to the earlier world views? Either they are eclipsed and drop out or, as Werner (1948) suggests, they remain dormant but become integrated into the emergent organization and thereby lose much of their previous character. As Cassirer (1955) puts it, the advent of a higher stage "does not destroy the earlier phase, rather it embraces it in its own perspective" (p. 477). This also happens in Piaget's system.

In these developmental progressions of phases, it is possible to return to something like an earlier phase. But special processes and conditions are needed to pull the person back, in developmental time, to experience the world in a manner similar to the way it was experienced earlier. In clinical theories, regression serves that purpose. In Werner and Kaplan's system (1963), one can move up and down the ontogenic spiral. These returns to previous and more global modes of experience are thought to occur mainly under conditions of challenge, stress, conflict, failure of adaptation, or fatigue, and in dream states, psychopathological conditions, or drug states. With the exception of these regressions, developing world views are mainly successive and sequential, not simultaneous. Current organizations of

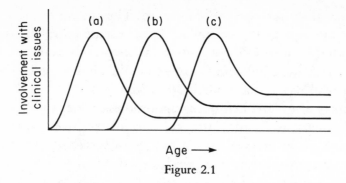

Figure 2.1

experience subsume earlier ones. They do not coexist with them. This developmental progression is schematized in figure 2.1, in which (a) could represent orality, trust, normal autism; (b) anality, autonomy; (c) genitality, and so on.

This view of development may be the most reasonable when one is considering the developmental progression of certain mental abilities or cognitive capacities, but that is not the present task. We are trying to consider the sense of self as it occurs in interpersonal encounters, and in that subjective sphere simultaneity of senses of the self appears to be closer to common experience. And no extraordinary conditions or processes need be present to permit the movement back and forth between experiences in different domains, that is, between different senses of the self.

An illustration from adult experience will help us to understand this simultaneity of senses of self. Making love, a fully involving interpersonal event, involves first the sense of the self and the other as discrete physical entities, as forms in motion—an experience in the domain of core-relatedness, as is the sense of self-agency, will, and activation encompassed in the physical acts. At the same time it involves the experience of sensing the other's subjective state: shared desire, aligned intentions, and mutual states of simultaneously shifting arousal, which occur in the domain of intersubjective relatedness. And if one of the lovers says for the first time "I love you," the words summarize what is occurring in the other domains (embraced in the verbal perspective) and perhaps introduce an entirely new note about the couple's relationship that may change the meaning of the history that has led up to and will follow the moment of saying it. This is an experience in the domain of verbal relatedness.

What about the domain of emergent relatedness? That is less

readily apparent, but it is present nonetheless. One may, for example "get lost in" the color of the other's eye, as if the eye were momentarily not part of the core other, unrelated to anyone's mental state, newly found, and outside of any larger organizing network. At the instant the "colored eye" comes again to belong to the known other, an emergent experience has occurred, an experience in the domain of emergent relatedness.[12]

We see that the subjective experience of social interactions seems to occur in all domains of relatedness simultaneously. One can certainly attend to one domain for a while to the partial exclusion of the others, but the others go on as distinct experiences, out of but available to awareness. In fact, much of what is meant by "socializing" is directed at focusing awareness on a single domain, usually the verbal, and declaring it to be the official version of what is being experienced, while denying the experience in the other domains ("unofficial" versions of what is happening). Nonetheless, attention can and does shift with some fluidity from experience in one domain to that in another. For instance, language in interpersonal service is largely the explication (in the verbal domain) of concomitant experiences in other domains, plus something else. If you ask someone to do something, and that person answers "I'd rather not. I'm surprised you asked!" he may at the same time raise his head and throw it back slightly, raise his eyebrows, and look down his nose a bit. The meaning of this nonverbal behavior (which is in the domain of core-relatedness and intersubjective relatedness) has been well rendered in language. Still these physical acts retain distinctive experiential characteristics. Performing or being the target of them involves experiences that reside outside of language itself.

All domains of relatedness remain active during development. The infant does not grow out of any of them; none of them atrophy, none become developmentally obsolete or get left behind. And once all domains are available, there is no assurance that any one domain will necessarily claim preponderance during any particular age period. None has a privileged status all of the time. Since there is an orderly temporal succession of emergence of each domain during develop-

12. These emergent experiences are descriptively disassociated from organizing perspectives. However, they are not the product of "disassociation" as a psychic process defined by psychoanalysis any more than is the initial impression of an isolated feature of a work of art viewed in the contemplative mode.

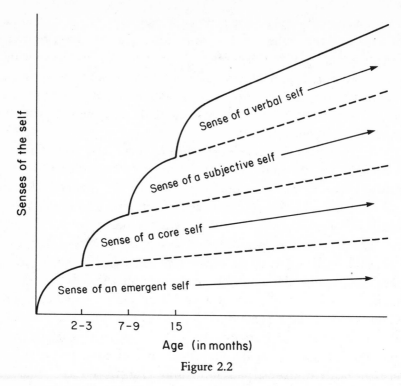

Figure 2.2

ment—first emergent, then core, then subjective, then verbal—there will inevitably be periods when one or two domains hold predominance by default. In fact, each successive organizing subjective perspective requires the preceding one as a precursor. Once formed, the domains remain forever as distinct forms of experiencing social life and self. None are lost to adult experience. Each simply gets more elaborated. It is for this reason that the term *domains* of relatedness has been chosen, rather than *phases* or *stages*.[13] The developmental situation as described is depicted in figure 2.2.

We can now return to the issue of sensitive periods. It seems that the initial period of formation for many developing psychological (and neurological) processes is a relatively sensitive one in the sense that an event occurring early will have a greater impact and its influence will be more difficult to reverse than an event occurring later. This general principle presumably applies to the formative

13. "Domains" seems preferable over "levels," because "levels" implies a hierarchical status that is accurate ontogenetically but need not pertain in the sphere of social life as subjectively experienced.

32

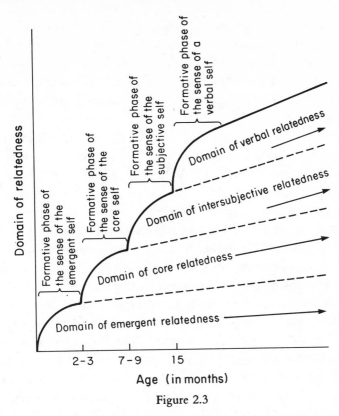

Figure 2.3

phase of each sense of the self. The timing of the formative phases is schematized in figure 2.3.

This view permits us to consider the formative phase for each sense of self as a sensitive period. The clinical implications of doing so will be considered in chapters 9 and 11.

What happens to the important clinical issues of autonomy, orality, symbiosis, individuation, trust, attachment, mastery, curiosity, and so on—the issues that occupy center stage in the therapeutic creation of the clinical infant? These clinical issues do not drop out of the picture at all. They simply hand over their role as primary organizers of subjective experience to the changing senses of self. Life-course clinical issues such as autonomy and attachment are worked on equally in all the domains of relatedness that are available at any given time. During each formative phase of relatedness, the arena of interpersonal action in which the issues get played out will change as the self and other are sensed as different. Accordingly, different forms of the same life-course issue develop in succession: for example,

33

physical intimacy during core-relatedness, subjective (empathic-like) intimacy during intersubjective relatedness, and the intimacy of shared meanings during verbal relatedness. Thus, each life-course clinical issue has its own developmental line, and a slightly different contribution to that developmental line is made in each domain of relatedness.[14]

In summary, the subjective social life of the infant will be viewed as having the following characteristics. The infant is endowed with observable capacities that mature. When these become available, they are organized and transformed, in quantum mental leaps, into organizing subjective perspectives about the sense of self and other. Each new sense of self defines the formation of a new domain of relatedness. While these domains of relatedness result in qualitative shifts in social experience, they are not phases; rather, they are forms of social experience that remain intact throughout life. Nonetheless, their initial phase of formation constitutes a sensitive period of development. Subjective social experience results from the sum and integration of experience in all domains. The basic clinical issues are seen as issues for the life span and not as issues of developmental phases. A different contribution is made to the ontogeny of the developmental lines of all clinical issues as each domain of self-experience emerges.

With this much of the point of view and approach in hand, we can turn in the next section of this book to a closer look at the four senses of self and their four domains of relatedness. We will bring together the observational and clinical evidence that argues for this view of the development of the infant's subjective social experience.

14. This treatment of lines of development is an extreme version of the same idea put forward by A. Freud (1965). However, she did not fully abandon the notion of libidinal phase specificity. The present suggestion is a rejection of that notion. Here, all clinical issues become developmental lines, and no hidden or ultimately clinical issues remain anchored to any given developmental epochs.

PART II

THE FOUR SENSES
OF SELF

Chapter 3

The Sense of an Emergent Self

THE AGE of two months is almost as clear a boundary as birth itself. At about eight weeks, infants undergo a qualitative change: they begin to make direct eye-to-eye contact. Shortly thereafter they begin to smile more frequently, but also responsively and infectiously. They begin to coo. In fact, much more goes on during this developmental shift than what is reflected by increased overt social behaviors. Most learning is faster and more inclusive. Strategies for paying attention to the world shift in terms of altered visual scanning patterns. Motor patterns mature. Sensorimotor intelligence reaches a higher level, as Piaget has described. Electroencephalograms reveal major changes. Diurnal hormonal milieu stabilizes, along with sleep and activity cycles. Almost everything changes. And all observers of infants, including parents, agree on this (Piaget 1952; Sander 1962; Spitz 1965; Emde et al. 1976; Brazelton et al. 1979; Haith 1980; Greenspan and Lourie 1981; Bronson 1982).

Until this developmental shift occurs, the infant is generally thought to occupy some kind of presocial, precognitive, preorganized life phase that stretches from birth to two months. The central questions of this chapter are, how might the infant experience the social world during this initial period? And what might be the

37

infant's sense of self during this time? I conclude that during the first two months the infant is actively forming a sense of an emergent self. It is a sense of organization in the process of formation, and it is a sense of self that will remain active for the rest of life. An overarching sense of self is not yet achieved in this period, but it is coming into being. To understand how this conclusion was reached, it is necessary to understand the likely nature of infant experience at this age.

In the last fifteen years a revolution has occurred in observing and thereby evaluating infants. One result of this revolution is that the infant's subjective social life during the first two months has had to be reconsidered.

Observing the Young Infant: A Revolution in Infancy Research

The following description of the revolution in infancy research is intended to serve several purposes: to show some of the infant capacities that bear on forming a sense of self, capacities that no one imagined to be present so early one or two decades ago; to provide a common vocabulary and set of concepts for what is to follow; and, perhaps most important, to expand the frame of reference about infants that is commonly prevalent among clinicians and others who have not been able to keep up with the rapidly growing literature on infancy. Knowledge of the newly discovered infant capabilities will in itself do the expanding.

People have always had questions they would like to have asked of infants. What do infants see, smell, feel, think, want? Good questions abounded, but answers were scarce. How could an infant answer? The revolution in research consisted of turning the situation on its head, by asking not, what is a good question to pose to an infant? but, what might an infant be able to do (like sucking) that would serve as an answer? With this simple turn-around, the search for infant abilities that could be made into answers (response measures) began, and the revolution was set in motion.

One other change in view was required. This was the realization that newborns are not always in a state of sleep, hunger, eating, fussing, crying, or full activity. If that were the case, all potential behavioral "answers" would always be either already in action or precluded by another activity or state. But it is not the case. Starting from birth, infants regularly occupy a state called alert inactivity, when they are physically quiet and alert and apparently are taking in external events (Wolff 1966). Furthermore, alert inactivity can last several minutes, sometimes longer, and recurs regularly and frequently during wakefulness. Alert inactivity provides the needed time "window" in which questions can be put to newborns and answers can be discerned from their ongoing activity.

The issue at stake is, how can we know what infant's "know"? Good infant "answers" have to be readily observable behaviors that are frequently performed, that are under voluntary muscular control, and that can be solicited during alert inactivity. Three such behavioral answers immediately qualify, beginning at birth: head-turning, sucking, and looking.

The newborn does not have good control of his or her head and cannot hold it aloft in the upright position. But when lying on their backs so that their heads are supported, newborns do have adequate control to turn the head to the left or right. Head-turning became the answer to the following question: can infants tell the smell of their own mothers' milk? MacFarlane (1975) placed three-day-old infants on their backs and then placed breast pads taken from their nursing mothers on one side of their heads. On the other side, he placed breast pads taken from other nursing women. The newborns reliably turned their heads toward their own mothers' pads, regardless of which side the pads were placed on. The head-turning answered MacFarland's question in the affirmative: infants are able to discriminate the smell of their own mothers' milk.

Newborns are good suckers. Life depends on sucking, a behavior that is controlled by voluntary muscles. When not nursing (nutritive sucking), infants engage in a great deal of non-nutritive sucking on anything they can get hold of, including their own tongues. Non-nutritive sucking occurs during the newborn's periods of alert inactivity, making it a potentially good "answer." Infants can rapidly be trained to suck to get something to happen. It is done by placing a pacifier with an electronically bugged nipple—that is, one with a pressure transducer inside it—in the infant's mouth. The transducer is hooked up to the starter mechanism of a tape recorder or slide carousel, so that when the infant sucks at certain specified rates the recorder goes on or the carousel turns over a new slide. In that way infants control what they hear or see by maintaining some rate of sucking (Siqueland and DeLucia 1969). Sucking was used to determine whether infants are especially interested in the human voice, in preference to other sounds of the same pitch and loudness. The infants' sucking rates answered the question affirmatively (Friedlander 1970).

Newborns arrive with a visual motor system that is mature in many respects. They see reasonably well at the right focal distance, and the reflexes controlling the eye movements responsible for object fixation and visual pursuit are intact at birth. Infant looking patterns are thus a third potential "answer." Fantz (1963), in a series of pioneering studies, used infant visual preferences to answer the question, do infants prefer looking at faces rather than at various other visual patterns? They do indeed, though the reasons are complicated. (Note that all three questions asked in these studies concern interpersonal or social issues and attest to the early responsiveness of infants to their social world.)

To yoke these "answers"[1] to more interesting questions, several paradigms have been developed and elaborated. To learn whether an infant prefers one thing over another, one need only put the two stimuli in competition in a "paired comparison preference paradigm" and see which stimulus wins out for attention. For instance, if an infant is shown a symmetrical pattern in which the left side is the mirror image of the right side, and next to it is shown the same pattern lying on its side, so the top half is the mirror image of the bottom half, the infant will look longer at the left-right mirror images than at the top-bottom mirror images (see Sherrod 1981). Conclusion: infants prefer symmetry in the vertical plane, characteristic of human faces, to symmetry in the horizontal plane. (Note that parents automatically tend to align their faces to the infant's in the vertical plane.)

But suppose there is no preference for one thing over another. Can we still find out if the infant can tell them apart? To determine if infants can discriminate one thing from another, some form of the "habituation/dishabituation" paradigm is used. This method is based

---

1. Heart rate change and evoked potentials as psychological responses to external events also can be used as answers, either alone or to validate the behavioral answers.

on the notion that if the same thing is presented to infants repeatedly, they will respond to it progressively less. Presumably, this reaction of habituation is due to the fact that the original stimulus becomes less and less effective as it loses its novelty. In effect, the infant gets bored with it (Sokolov 1960; Berlyne 1966). If one wishes to know, for example, if infants can discriminate a smiling face from a surprise face, one presents the smiling face six or so times as the infants look at it progressively less. The surprise face of the same person is then substituted for the next expected presentation of the smiling face. If the infants notice the substitution they will dishabituate, that is, look at it a lot, as they did the smiling face at its first presentation. If they cannot tell the surprise face from the smiling one, then they will continue to habituate, that is, look at it as little as they had come to look at the smiling face after seeing it repeatedly.

These procedures tell only if infants can make a discrimination or not. They do not tell whether they have formed any concept or representation of the properties that generally make up a smile. To know that, one must take an additional step. It must be shown, for example, that an infant will discriminate a smile regardless of whose face it is on. One then can say that the infant has an abstract representation of the invariant (unchanging) properties that constitute smiles regardless of variant (changing) properties such as whose face is wearing the smile.

Using these kinds of experimental paradigms and these methods of eliciting "answers" from infants, an impressive body of information has been gathered. The examples given not only explain how one inquires about infants and hint at the capacities that infants are being found to have; they also help in laying out the information from which we can draw some general principles about infant perception, cognition, and affect that will be needed for the arguments in this chapter and elsewhere (see Kessen et al. 1970; Cohen and Salapatek 1975; Kagan et al. 1978; Lamb and Sherrod 1981; Lipsitt 1983; Field and Fox, in press). These, in brief, are:

1. Infants seek sensory stimulation. Furthermore, they do it with the preemptory quality that is prerequisite to hypothesizing drives and motivational systems.
2. They have distinct biases or preferences with regard to the sensations they seek and the perceptions they form. These are innate.

3. From birth on, there appears to be a central tendency to form and test hypotheses about what is occurring in the world (Bruner 1977). Infants are also constantly "evaluating," in the sense of asking, is this different from or the same as that? How discrepant is what I have just encountered from what I have previously encountered (Kagan et al. 1978)? It is clear that this central tendency of mind, with constant application, will rapidly categorize the social world into conforming and contrasting patterns, events, sets, and experiences. The infant will readily discover which features of an experience are invariant and which are variant—that is, which features "belong" to the experience (J. Gibson 1950, 1979; E. Gibson 1969). The infant will apply these same processes to whatever sensations and perceptions are available, from the simplest to the ultimately most complex— that is, thoughts about thoughts.

4. Affective and cognitive processes cannot be readily separated. In a simple learning task, activation builds up and falls off. Learning itself is motivated and affect-laden. Similarly, in an intense affective moment, perception and cognition go on. And, finally, affective experiences (for example, the many different occasions of surprise) have their own invariant and variant features. Sorting these is a cognitive task concerning affective experience.

This view of the young infant, made possible by the revolution in research, is mainly cognitive and determined in large part by the nature of experimental observations. But what about the young infant as viewed by clinicians or parents, and what about the more affective infant with motivations and appetites that force the infant out of the state of alert inactivity? It is here that the divergence between the observed and clinical infant may begin.

The Clinical and Parental View of the Young Infant

The vast majority of the mother's time during the infant's first two months is spent in regulating and stabilizing sleep-wake, day-night, and hunger-satiation cycles. Sander (1962, 1964) has called the primary task of this early period that of physiological regulation, and Greenspan (1981) that of homeostasis.

When the baby first comes home from the hospital, the new parents live from minute to minute, attempting to regulate the newborn. After a few days they may be able to see twenty minutes into the future. By the end of a few weeks, they have the luxury of a future that is predictable for stretches of time as long as an hour or two. And after four to six weeks, regular time clumps of three to four hours are possible. The tasks of eating, getting to sleep, and general homeostasis are generally accompanied by social behaviors by the parents: rocking, touching, soothing, talking, singing, and making noises and faces. These occur in response to infant behaviors that are also mainly social, such as crying, fretting, smiling, and gazing. A great deal of social interaction goes on in the service of physiological regulation. Sometimes parents fail to appreciate that social interactions are happening when they so realistically have their eye on the goal of the activity, such as soothing the baby; the ends seem all important, and the means to those ends go unnoticed as moments of interpersonal relatedness. At other times, parents do focus on the social interaction and act, from the beginning, as though the infant had a sense of self. Parents immediately attribute their infants with intentions ("Oh, you want to see that"), motives ("You're doing that so Mommy will hurry up with the bottle"), and authorship of action ("You threw that one away on purpose, huh?"). It is almost impossible to conduct social interaction with infants without attributing these human qualities to them. These qualities make human behavior understandable, and parents invariably treat their infants as understandable beings, that is, as the people they are about to become, by working in the infant's zone of proximal development.[2]

Parents thus view young infants on the one hand as physiological systems in need of regulation and, on the other hand, as fairly developed people with subjective experiences, social sensibilities, and a sense of self that is growing, if not already in place.

Classical psychoanalysis has focused almost exclusively on physiological regulation during this early period, while seeing right past the fact that much of this regulation was actually conducted via the mutual exchange of social behaviors. This approach has resulted in

2. While parents are consummate experts at this alignment with the future states of being of their infants, there is a related phenomenon in therapy. Friedman (1982) points out that "it is not necessary for the analyst to know the exact nature of the development he is encouraging. It is sufficient that he treats the patient as though he were roughly the person he is about to become. The patient will explore being treated that way, and fill in the personal details" (p. 12).

the picture of a fairly asocial infant, but it has also provided a rich description of the infant's inner life as it is affected by changes in physiological state. For instance, Freud (1920) saw infants shielded from relatedness by the "stimulus barrier" that protected them from having to register and deal with external stimulation, including other people. Mahler, Pine, and Bergman (1975) have viewed infants as occupying a state of "normal autism," essentially unrelated to others. In both of these views infants are related to others only indirectly, to the extent that the others influence their internal states of hunger, fatigue, and so on. In these views, infants remain in a prolonged state of undifferentiation, in which no social world exists, subjectively, to help them discover a sense of self or of other. On the other hand, the fluctuating affects and physiological tensions that befall infants are seen as the wellspring of experiences that will ultimately define a sense of self. These experiences occupy center stage for the first two months.

The British object relations "school" and H. S. Sullivan, an American parallel, were unique among clinical theorists in believing that human social relatedness is present from birth, that it exists for its own sake, is of a definable nature, and does not lean upon physiological need states (Balint 1937; Klein 1952; Sullivan 1953; Fairbairn 1954; Guntrip 1971). Currently, the attachment theorists have further elaborated this view with objective data (Bowlby 1969; Ainsworth 1979). These views consider the infant's *direct* social experience, which parents have always intuited to be part of the infant's subjective life, to be the central focus of concern.

All these clinical theories have a common assertion: that infants have a very active subjective life, filled with changing passions and confusions, and that they experience a state of undifferentiation by struggling with blurred social events that presumably are seen as unconnected and unintegrated. These clinical views have identified some of the salient experiences of internal state fluctuations and social relatedness that could contribute to a sense of self, but they have not been in a position to discover the mental capacities that might lead the infant to use these experiences to differentiate a sense of self or of other. That is where the experimental work of developmentalists makes its contribution. It permits us to look at how the infant might experience the worlds of affect and changes in

44

tension state as well as the perceptions of the external world that accompany affect and tension changes. After all, it is the integration of all of these that will constitute the infant's social experience.

The Nature of the Emergent Sense of Self: the Experience of Process and Product

We can now return to the central question: what kind of sense of self is possible during this initial period? The notion that it exists at all at these very early ages is generally dismissed or not even broached, because the idea of a sense of self is usually reserved for some overarching and integrating schema, concept, or perspective about the self. And clearly, during this early period infants are not capable of such an overview. They have separate, unrelated experiences that have yet to be integrated into one embracing perspective.

The ways in which the relations between disparate experiences can come into being have been the basic subject matter of much of the works of Piaget, the Gibsons, and associational learning theorists. Clinical theorists have lumped all these processes together and described them metaphorically as the forming of "islands of consistency" (Escalona 1953). They describe the leaps that make up this development of organization in terms of the cognitions at each progressive step or level. They thus tend to interpret the *product* of those integrating leaps as the sense of self. But what about the *process* itself—the very experience of making the leaps and creating relations between previously unrelated events or forming partial organizations or consolidating sensorimotor schemas. Can the infant experience not only the sense of an organization already formed and grasped, but the coming-into-being of organization? I am suggesting that the infant can experience the *process* of emerging organization as well as the result, and it is this experience of emerging organization that I call the *emergent sense of self*. It is the experience of a process as well as a product.

The emergence of organization is no more than a form of learning. And learning experiences are powerful events in an infant's life. As we have already noted, infants are predesigned to seek out and engage in learning opportunities. All observers of learning, in any form, have been impressed with how strongly motivated (that is, positively reinforcing) is the creation of new mental organizations. It has been proposed that the early learning described by Piaget that results in the consolidation of sensorimotor schemes such as thumb-to-mouth is intrinsically motivated (Sameroff 1984). The experience of forming organization involves both the motivated process and the reinforcing product; I will focus here more on the process.[3]

But first, can infants also experience non-organization? No! The "state" of undifferentiation is an excellent example of non-organization. Only an observer who has enough perspective to know the future course of things can even imagine an undifferentiated state. Infants cannot know *what* they do not know, nor *that* they do not know. The traditional notions of clinical theorists have taken the observer's knowledge of infants—that is, relative undifferentiation compared with the differentiated view of older children—reified it, and given it back, or attributed it, to infants as their own dominant subjective sense of things. If, on the other hand, one does not reify undifferentiation as an attribute of the infant's subjective experience, the picture looks quite different. Many separate experiences exist, with what for the infant may be exquisite clarity and vividness. The lack of relatedness between these experiences is not noticed.

When the diverse experiences are in some way yoked (associated, assimilated, or connected in some other way), the infant experiences the emergence of organization. In order for the infant to have any formed sense of self, there must ultimately be some organization that is sensed as a reference point. The first such organization concerns the body: its coherence, its actions, its inner feeling states, and the memory of all these. That is the experiential organization with which the sense of a core self is concerned. Immediately prior to that, however, the reference organization for a sense of self is still forming; in other words, it is emergent. The sense of an emergent self thus concerns the process and product of forming organization. It concerns the learning about the relations between the infant's sensory experiences. But that is essentially what all learning is about.

3. The self-organizing tendencies of many systems have been noted, and Stechler and Kaplan (1980) have applied these notions to the self in development. The concern here is, however, with the subjective experience of forming organization.

Learning is certainly not designed for the exclusive purpose of forming a sense of self, but a sense of self will be one of the many vital byproducts of the general learning capacity.

The sense of an emergent self thus includes two components, the products of forming relations between isolated experiences and the process. The products will be discussed in greater detail in the next chapter, on the sense of a core self, which describes which products come together to form the first encompassing perspective of the self. In this chapter I will focus more sharply on the process, or the experience of organization-coming-into-being. To do so, I will examine the various processes available to the young infant for creating relational organization and the kinds of subjective experiences that might evolve from engaging in these processes.

Processes Involved in Forming the Sense of an Emergent Self and Other

AMODAL PERCEPTION

In the late 1970s, the findings of several experiments raised profound doubts about how infants learn about the world, that is, how they connect experiences. What was at stake was the long-standing philosophical and psychological problem of perceptual unity—how we come to know that something seen, heard, and touched may in fact be the same thing. How do we coordinate information that comes from several different perceptual modalities but emanates from a single external source? These experiments drew widespread attention to the infant's capacity to transfer perceptual experience from one sensory modality to another and did so in an experimental format open to replication.

Meltzoff and Borton's experiment (1979) lays out the problem and issue clearly. They blindfolded three-week-old infants and gave them one of two different pacifiers to suck on. One pacifier had a spherical-shaped nipple and the other was a nipple with nubs protruding from various points around its surface. After the baby had had some experience feeling (touching) the nipple with only the mouth, the nipple was removed and placed side by side with the other kind of nipple. The blindfold was taken off. After a quick visual comparison, infants looked more at the nipple they had just sucked.

These findings seemed to run counter to current accounts of infant learning and world knowledge. On theoretical grounds, infants should not have been able to do this task. A Piagetian account would have required that they first form a schema of what the nipple felt like (a haptic schema) and a schema of what the nipple looked like (a visual schema); then these two schemas would have to have some traffic or interaction (reciprocal assimilation), so that a coordinated visual-haptic schema would result (Piaget 1952). Only then could the infants accomplish the task. Clearly, the infants did not in fact have to go through these steps of construction. They immediately "knew" that the one they now saw was the one they had just felt. Similarly, a strict learning theory or associationist account of these findings would be at a total loss to explain them, since the infants had had no prior experience to form the required associations between what was felt and what was seen. (For fuller accounts of the problem in its theoretical context, see Bower 1972, 1974, 1976; Moore and Meltzoff 1978; Moes 1980; Spelke 1980; Meltzoff and Moore 1983.) While this haptic-visual transfer of information appears to improve and get faster as infants get older (Rose et al. 1972), it is clear that the capacity is present in the first weeks of life. Infants are predesigned to be able to perform a cross-modal transfer of information that permits them to recognize a correspondence across touch and vision. In this case the yoking of the tactile and visual experiences is brought about by way of the innate design of the perceptual system not by way of repeated world experience. No learning is needed initially, and subsequent learning about relations across modalities can be built upon this innate base.

The correspondence just described occurred between touch and vision, and it concerned shape. What about other modalities, and what about other qualities of perception, such as intensity and time? Are infants equally gifted in recognizing these cross-modal equivalences? Using heart rate as an outcome measure in a habituation paradigm, Lewcowicz and Turkewitz (1980) "asked" three-week-old infants which levels of light intensity (luminescence of white light) corresponded best with certain levels of sound intensity

THE SENSE OF AN EMERGENT SELF

(decibels of white noise). The infant was habituated to one level of sound, and attempts at dishabituation were then made with various levels of light, and vice versa. In essence, the results revealed that these young infants did find that certain absolute levels of sound intensity corresponded with specific absolute levels of light intensity. Furthermore, the matches of intensity level across modes that the three-week-olds found to be most correspondent were the same matches that adults chose. Thus, the ability to perform audio-visual cross-modal matching of the absolute level of intensity appears to be well within infants' capacity by three weeks of age.

How about time? At present, few experiments bear directly on the question of whether an infant can translate temporal information across perceptual modalities (see Allen et al. 1977; Demany et al. 1977; Humphrey et al. 1979; Wagner and Sakowitz 1983; Lewcowicz, in press; and Morrongiello 1984). Using heart rate and behavior as the respondent measures, these investigators show that infants recognize that an auditory temporal pattern is correspondent with a similar visually presented temporal pattern. It is almost certain that in the near future there will be many more such experiments demonstrating infants' capacities to transfer, intermodally, the properties of duration, beat, and rhythm, as specifically defined. These temporal properties are readily perceived in all modalities and are excellent candidates as properties of experience that can be transferred cross-modally, because it is becoming clearer that the infant from early in life is exquisitely sensible of and sensitive to the temporal features of the environment (Stern and Gibbon 1978; DeCasper 1980; Miller and Byrne 1984).

Of all these transfers of properties between modes, the hardest to imagine is how an infant might be able to transfer information about shape between the visual and auditory modes. Shape is not usually conceived of as an acoustic event; the shape transfer is easier to imagine across the tactile and visual modes. But speech itself, in a natural situation, is a visual as well as an acoustic configuration, because the lips move. Intelligibility goes up considerably when the lips are in view. By six weeks, babies tend to look more closely at faces that speak (Haith 1980). Moreover, when the actual sound produced is in conflict with the lip movements seen, the visual information unexpectedly predominates over the auditory. In other words, we hear what we *see*, not what is *said* (McGurk and MacDonald 1976).[4]

The question then seems irresistible: can infants recognize the correspondence between auditorily and visually presented speech sounds? That is, can they detect the correspondence between the configuration of a sound as heard and the configuration of the articulatory movements of the mouth that produce the sound as seen? Two separate laboratories working simultaneously on this problem came up with a positive answer (MacKain et al. 1981, 1983; Kuhl and Meltzoff 1982). The two experiments used a similar paradigm but different stimuli. They both presented the infant with two faces seen simultaneously. One face articulated one sound and the second face articulated a different sound, but only one of the two sounds was actually produced for the infant to hear. The question was whether the infant looked longer at the "right" face. MacKain et al. used a variety of disyllables as stimuli (mama, lulu, baby, zuzu), while Kuhl and Meltzoff used single vowels "ah" and "ee." Both experiments found that the infants did recognize the audio-visual correspondences.[5] The concordant results of the two experiments greatly strengthen the finding.

How about the sensation of one's own movement or position, that is, the modality of proprioception? In 1977, it was shown that three-week-old infants would imitate an adult model in sticking out their tongues and opening their mouths (Meltzoff and Moore 1977). While the ability to perform these early imitations had been observed previously and commented upon (Maratos 1973; Uzgiris 1974; Trevarthan 1977), the strongest possible inferences had not been made—namely, that there was an innate correspondence between what infants saw and what they did. Subsequent experiments showed that even the protrusion of a pencil or the like could also produce infant tongue protrusion.

Later, the issue was removed to the sphere of affect expression. Field et al. (1982) reported that newborn infants, age two days, would reliably imitate an adult model who either smiled, frowned,

4. For instance, if one views a mouth articulating (silently) the sound "da" and hears a voice-over with the sound "ba," one will experience "da" or sometimes an intermediate sound "ga."

5. MacKain et al. found that this particular audio-visual matching task was facilitated by left hemispheric activation, but discussion of that finding is beyond the scope of this book.

or showed a surprise face. The problems presented by these findings are manifold. How do babies "know" that they have a face or facial features? How do they "know" that the face they see is anything like the face they have? How do they "know" that specific configurations of that other face, as only seen, correspond to the same specific configurations in their own face as only felt, proprioceptively, and never seen? The amount of cross-modal fluency in terms of predesign is extraordinary. This is a special case, however, because one does not know whether the infant's response is imitative or reflex-like. Does the sight of a specific visual configuration of the other's face correspond to a proprioceptive configuration in the infant's own face? In this case one can talk about cross-modal correspondence (vision-proprioception). Or does the specific configuration on the other's face trigger a specific motor program to perform the same act? In that case one is talking about a specific innate social releasing stimulus. At present, it is not possible to make a definitive choice (see Burd and Milewski 1981).

Infants thus appear to have an innate general capacity, which can be called *amodal perception,* to take information received in one sensory modality and somehow translate it into another sensory modality. We do not know how they accomplish this task. The information is probably not experienced as belonging to any one particular sensory mode. More likely it transcends mode or channel and exists in some unknown supra-modal form. It is not, then, a simple issue of a direct translation across modalities. Rather, it involves an encoding into a still mysterious amodal *representation,* which can then be recognized in any of the sensory modes.

Infants appear to experience a world of perceptual unity, in which they can perceive amodal qualities in any modality from any form of human expressive behavior, represent these qualities abstractly, and then transpose them to other modalities. This position has been strongly put forth by developmentalists such as Bower (1974), Moore and Meltzoff (1978), and Meltzoff (1981), who posit that the infant, from the earliest days of life, forms and acts upon abstract representations of qualities of perception. These abstract representations that the infant experiences are not sights and sounds and touches and nameable objects, but rather shapes, intensities, and temporal patterns—the more "global" qualities of experience. And the need and ability to form abstract representations of primary qualities of perception and act upon them starts at the beginning of mental life; it is not the culmination or a developmental landmark reached in the second year of life.

How might amodal perception contribute to a sense of an emergent self or a sense of an emergent other? Take the infant's experience of the mother's breast as an example. Does the baby initially experience two unrelated "breasts," the "sucked breast" and the "seen breast"? A Piagetian account would have said yes, as would most psychoanalytic accounts, since they have adopted Piagetian or associationist assumptions. The present account would say no. The breast would emerge as an already integrated experience of (a part of) the other, from the unlearned yoking of visual and tactile sensations. The same is true for the infant's finger or fist, as seen and sucked, as well as for many other common experiences of self and other. Infants do not need repeated experience to begin to form some of the pieces of an emergent self and other. They are predesigned to forge certain integrations.

While amodal perceptions will help the infant integrate potentially diverse experiences of self and other, a sense of an emergent self is concerned not only with the product but with the process of integration, as we saw earlier. Ultimately, the breast as seen and the breast as sucked will become related, whether by amodal perception, by assimilation of schemas, or by repeated association. What might the particular experience of amodally derived integration be like as an emergent experience, compared with an integration brought about by assimilation or association? Each process of relating diverse events may constitute a different and characteristic emergent experience.

For instance, the actual experience of looking for the first time at something that, on the basis of how it felt to the touch, should look a certain way and having it, indeed, look that way is something like a déjà vu experience. The infant presumably does not anticipate how an object should look and therefore has no experience of cognitive confirmation. Many would suggest that such an experience would go totally unnoticed, or that at most it would be registered nonspecifically as "all-rightness" with smooth functioning. They would further suggest that the experience would take on specific qualities only if sight happened to disconfirm the tactile information—again a cognitive perspective on the matter. I suggest that at a preverbal level (outside of awareness) the experience of finding a cross-modal match (especially the first time) would feel like a correspondence or imbuing of present experience with something prior or familiar. Present experience would feel related in some way to experience from elsewhere. This primitive form of a déjà vu event is quite different from the process of making associational linkages, which may have more the quality of a discovery—that two things already apprehended belong together. It is likely that in this domain of emergent experience there is also the experience of premonition of a hidden future in the process of revealing a structure that can only be sensed opaquely. A typology of such events at the experiential level rather than at a conceptual level is greatly needed.

"PHYSIOGNOMIC" PERCEPTION

Heinz Werner (1948) proposed a different kind of amodal perception in the young infant, which he called "physiognomic" perception. In Werner's view, the amodal qualities that are directly experienced by the infant are categorical affects rather than perceptual qualities such as shape, intensity, and number. For instance, a simple two-dimensional line or a color or a sound is perceived to be happy ($\sim$), sad ($\diagdown$), or angry ($\wedge\wedge$). Affect acts as the supra-modal currency into which stimulation in any modality can be translated. This is a kind of amodal perception too, since an affect experience is not bound to any one modality of perception. All of us engage in "feeling perception"—but is it frequent, continuous, or otherwise? It is likely to be a component (though usually unconscious) of every act of perception. Its mechanism, however, remains a mystery, as does the mechanism of amodal perception in general. Werner suggested that it arose from experience with the human face in all its emotional displays, hence the name "physiognomic" perception. To date there is no empirical evidence, only speculation, about its existence or nature in young infants.

"VITALITY AFFECTS"

We have so far considered two ways in which the infant experiences the world about him. The experiments on cross-modal capacities suggest that some properties of people and things, such as shape, intensity level, motion, number, and rhythm, are experienced directly as global, amodal perceptual qualities. And Werner suggests that some aspects of people and things will be experienced directly as categorical affects (angry, sad, happy, and so on).

There is a third quality of experience that can arise directly from encounters with people, a quality that involves vitality affects. What do we mean by this, and why is it necessary to add a new term for certain forms of human experience? It is necessary because many qualities of feeling that occur do not fit into our existing lexicon or taxonomy of affects. These elusive qualities are better captured by dynamic, kinetic terms, such as "surging," "fading away," "fleeting," "explosive," "crescendo," "decrescendo," "bursting," "drawn out," and so on. These qualities of experience are most certainly sensible to infants and of great daily, even momentary, importance. It is these feelings that will be elicited by changes in motivational states, appetites, and tensions. The philosopher Suzanne Langer (1967) insisted that in any experience-near psychology, close attention must be paid to the many "forms of feeling" inextricably involved with all the vital processes of life, such as breathing, getting hungry, eliminating, falling asleep and emerging out of sleep, or feeling the coming and going of emotions and thoughts. The different forms of feeling elicited by these vital processes impinge on the organism most of the time. We are never without their presence, whether or not we are conscious of them, while "regular" affects come and go.

The infant experiences these qualities from within, as well as in the behavior of other persons. Different feelings of vitality can be expressed in a multitude of parental acts that do not qualify as "regular" affective acts: how the mother picks up baby, folds the diapers, grooms her hair or the baby's hair, reaches for a bottle, unbuttons her blouse. The infant is immersed in these "feelings of vitality." Examining them further will let us enrich the concepts and vocabulary, too impoverished for present purposes, that we apply to nonverbal experiences.

A first question is, why do these important experiences not fit into the terms and concepts of already existing affect theories? Usually one thinks of affective experience in terms of discrete categories of affect—happiness, sadness, fear, anger, disgust, surprise, interest, and perhaps shame, and their combinations. It was Darwin's great contribution (1892) to postulate that each of these had an innate discrete facial display and a distinct quality of feeling and that these

54

innate patterns evolved as social signals "understood" by all members to enhance species survival.[6] Each discrete category of affect is also generally thought to be experienced along at least two commonly agreed upon dimensions: *activation* and *hedonic tone*. Activation refers to the amount of intensity or urgency of the feeling quality, while hedonic tone refers to the degree to which the feeling quality is pleasurable or unpleasurable.[7]

Vitality affects do not comfortably fit into these current theories of affect, and for that reason they require a separate name. Yet they are definitely feelings and belong within the domain of affective experience. They will be tentatively called *vitality affects*, to distinguish them from the traditional or Darwinian *categorical affects* of anger, joy, sadness, and so on.

Vitality affects occur both in the presence of and in the absence of categorical affects. For example, a "rush" of anger or of joy, a perceived flooding of light, an accelerating sequence of thoughts, an unmeasurable wave of feeling evoked by music, and a shot of narcotics can all feel like "rushes." They all share similar envelopes of neural firings, although in different parts of the nervous system.

6. These seven or eight discrete expressions, taken alone or in combinatory blends, account for the entire emotional repertoire of facial expressiveness in man. This has come to be known as the "discrete affect hypothesis." And this hypothesis has proven very robust for over one hundred years. Well-known cross-cultural studies indicate fairly convincingly that photographs of the basic facial expressions will be similarly recognized and identified in all cultures tested (Ekman 1971; Izard 1971). Universality in the face of wide socio-cultural differences argues for innateness. Similarly, it is now well known that a child born blind shows the normally expected repertoire of facial expressions until about three to four months (Freedman 1964; Fraiberg 1971), strongly suggesting that these discrete display patterns are innate, emerging without the need of learning provided by the feedback of vision. However, when we inquire about the subjective quality of feeling associated with any facial expression, the cross-cultural fit appears to be present but less tight. The *central* sensation of sadness can have its own distinctive qualities as verbally expressed by one people compared with another people (Lutz 1982). We share the same finite set of affect expressions, but not necessarily the same set of feeling qualities.

7. Some affect categories such as happiness or sadness are always pleasurable or unpleasurable, but to varying degrees others, like surprise, are not. Generally, activation and hedonic tone are seen as dimensions along which categories of affects are experienced. For example, exuberant joy is the happiness category of affect experienced at the high end of the activation dimension, in contrast to, say, contemplative bliss, which is also in the happiness category but experienced at the low end of activation. Both feelings, however, could be judged to be equally pleasurable in hedonic tone. Conversely, pleasant surprise and unpleasant surprise fall at different ends of the hedonic tone dimension but could be at the same level on the activation dimension. There are other dimensions along which affect categories are thought to fall (see Arnold 1970; Dahl and Stengel 1978; Plutchik 1980).

The felt quality of any of these similar changes is what I call the vitality affect of a "rush."

Expressiveness of this kind is not limited to categorical affect signals. It is inherent in all behavior. Various activation contours or vitality affects can be experienced not only during the performance of a categorical signal, such as an "explosive" smile, but also in a behavior that has no inherent categorical affect signal value; for example, one can see someone get out of a chair "explosively." One does not know whether the explosiveness in arising was due to anger, surprise, joy, or fright. The explosiveness could be linked to any of those Darwinian feeling qualities, or to none. The person could have gotten out of the chair with no specific category of affect but with a burst of determination. There are a thousand smiles, a thousand getting-out-of-chairs, a thousand variations of performance of any and all behaviors, and each one presents a different vitality affect.

The expressiveness of vitality affects can be likened to that of a puppet show. The puppets have little or no capacity to express categories of affect by way of facial signals, and their repertoire of conventionalized gestural or postural affect signals is usually impoverished. It is from the way they move in general that we infer the different vitality affects from the activation contours they trace. Most often, the characters of different puppets are largely defined in terms of particular vitality affects; one may be lethargic, with drooping limbs and hanging head, another forceful, and still another jaunty.

Abstract dance and music are examples par excellence of the expressiveness of vitality affects. Dance reveals to the viewer-listener multiple vitality affects and their variations, without resorting to plot or categorical affect signals from which the vitality affects can be derived. The choreographer is most often trying to express a way of feeling, not a specific content of feeling. This example is particularly instructive because the infant, when viewing parental behavior that has no intrinsic expressiveness (that is, no Darwinian affect signal), may be in the same position as the viewer of an abstract dance or the listener to music. The manner of performance of a parent's act expresses a vitality affect, whether or not the act is (or is partially colored with) some categorical affect.

One can readily imagine, in fact, that the infant does not initially perceive overt acts as such, as do adults. (This act is a reach for the bottle. That act is the unfolding of a diaper.) Rather, the infant is far more likely to perceive directly and begin to categorize acts in terms of the vitality affects they express. Like dance for the adult, the social world experienced by the infant is primarily one of vitality affects before it is a world of formal acts. It is also analogous to the physical world of amodal perception, which is primarily one of abstractable qualities of shape, number, intensity level, and so on, not a world of things seen, heard, or touched.

Another reason for separating vitality affects from categorical affects is that they cannot be adequately explained by the concept of level of activation. In most accounts of affects and their dimensions, what are here called vitality affects might be subsumed under the all-purpose, unswerving dimension of level of activation or arousal. Activation and arousal certainly occur, but they are not experienced simply as feelings somewhere along, or at some point on, this dimension. They are experienced as dynamic shifts or patterned changes within ourselves. We can use the dimension of arousal-activation only as a general index of level of arousal-activation. We need to add an entirely new categorization of this aspect of experience, namely, vitality affects that correspond to characteristic patterned changes. These patterned changes over time, or activation contours, underlie the separate vitality affects.[8]

Because activation contours (such as "rushes" of thought, feeling, or action) can apply to any kind of behavior or sentience, an activation contour can be abstracted from one kind of behavior and can exist in some amodal form so that it can apply to another kind

8. All the different activation contours can be described in terms of intensity of sensation as a function of time. Changes in intensity over time are adequate to explain "explodings," "fadings," "rushes," and so on, no matter what actual behavior or neural system is the source of these changes. That is why vitality affects have been hidden within the dimension of activation-arousal. However, the activation-arousal dimension needs to be broken apart and viewed not only as a single dimension but also as more momentary patterned changes of activation in time—that is, activation contours that exist in some amodal form. These contours of activation give rise to vitality affects at the level of feeling.

This account of vitality affects is greatly indebted to the work of Schneirla (1959, 1965) and particularly of Tompkins (1962, 1963, 1981). However, Tompkins concluded that discrete patterns of neural firing (density × time)—what are here called activation contours—result in discrete Darwinian affects, while I conclude that they result in a distinct form of affective experience, or vitality affects. Nonetheless, Tompkins's work is the basis for the present account.

of overt behavior or mental process.[9] These abstract representations may then permit intermodal correspondences to be made between similar activation contours expressed in diverse behavioral manifestations. Extremely diverse events may thus be yoked, so long as they share the quality of feeling that is being called a vitality affect. An example of such a correspondence may be the basis for a metaphor as seen in Defoe's novel *Moll Flanders*. When the heroine is finally caught and imprisoned after a life of crime, she says, "I had . . . no thought of heaven or hell, at least that went any farther than a bare flying touch. . . ." ([New York: Signet Classics, 1964], p. 247). The activation contour of her ideation reminds her of the activation contour of a particular physical sensation, a fleeting touch. And they evoke the same vitality affect.

If young infants experience vitality affects, as is being suggested, they will often be in a situation analogous to that of Moll Flanders, in which a variety of diverse sensory experiences with similar activation contours can be yoked—that is, they can be experienced as correspondent and thereby as creating organization. For instance, in trying to soothe the infant, the parent could say, "There, there, there . . . ," giving more stress and amplitude on the first part of the word and trailing off towards the end of the word. Alternatively, the parent could silently stroke the baby's back or head with a stroke analogous to the "There, there" sequence, applying more pressure at the onset of the stroke and lightening or trailing it off toward the end. If the duration of the contoured stroke and the pauses between strokes were of the same absolute and relative durations as the vocalization-pause pattern, the infant would experience similar activation contours no matter which soothing technique was performed. The two soothings would feel the same (beyond their sensory specificity) and would result in the same vitality affect experience.

If this were so, the infant would be a step up in the process of experiencing an emergent other. Instead of one distinct stroking-mother and a second and separate "There, there"-mother, the infant would experience only a single vitality affect in soothing activities—

9. All of this assumes that infants are early endowed with pattern- or sweep-detectors that can identify such contours. Suggestive evidence exists that they are. Fernald (1984), for example, showed that infants can readily discriminate a rising pitch contour from a falling one, even though the two are the same voice making the same vowel sound with the same pitch range and amplitude and differing only in temporal pattern. New research in this area is crucial.

a "soothing vitality affective mother." In this fashion the amodal experience of vitality affects as well as the capacities for cross-modal matching of perceived forms would greatly enhance the infant's progress toward the experience of an emergent other.[10]

The notion of activation contours (as the underlying feature of vitality affects) suggests a possible answer to the mysterious question of what form the amodal representation resides in when it is held abstracted from any particular way of perceiving it. The amodal representation could consist of a temporal pattern of changes in density of neural firing. No matter whether an object was encountered with the eye or the touch, and perhaps even the ear, it would produce the same overall pattern or activation contour.

The notion of vitality affects may prove helpful in imagining some of the infant's experiences of forming organization in yet another way. The consolidation of a sensorimotor schema provides an illustration. The thumb-to-mouth schema is a good one, since it occurs quite early. Following the suggestion of Sameroff (1984), we can describe the initial consolidation of the thumb-to-mouth schema as something like this. The infant initially moves his hand toward the mouth in a poorly coordinated, loosely directed, jerky manner. The entire pattern—thumb-to-mouth—is an intrinsically motivated, species-specific behavioral pattern that tends to completion and smooth functioning as the goals. During the initial part of a successful trial, while the thumb is getting closer but is not yet in the mouth, the pattern is incomplete and there is increased arousal. When the thumb finally finds its way into the mouth, there is a falloff in arousal, because the pattern is consummated and "smooth functioning" of sucking (an already consolidated schema) takes over. Along with the decrease in arousal there is a relative shift toward positive hedonic tone upon the resumption of smooth functioning. This thumb-finding-the-mouth and mouth-finding-the-thumb occurs over and over until it is smoothly functioning, that is, until adaptation of the pattern is accomplished through assimilation/accommodation of the sensorimotor schema. When this happens and the scheme is fully

10. There are infinite possible activation contours. One can only assume that they organize into recognizable groupings, so that we can recognize families of contours for which relatively discrete vitality affects are the felt component and can even designate words—"surgings," "fadings," "resolutions," and so on to some of these families. The differentiation into a greater number of more discrete families is an empirical developmental issue.

consolidated, the thumb-to-mouth behavior is no longer accompanied by arousal and hedonic shifts. It then goes unnoticed as "smooth functioning." But during the initial trials, when the schema is still being consolidated, the infant experiences, for each precariously successful attempt, a specific contour of arousal buildup as the hand is uncertainly finding its way to the mouth and then a falloff in arousal and a shift in hedonic tone when the mouth is found and secured. In other words, each consolidating trial is accompanied by a characteristic vitality affect associated with sensations from the arm, hand, thumb, and mouth—all leading to consummation.

The product of this development—a smoothly functioning thumb-to-mouth schema—may go unnoticed once formed. But the process of formation, itself, will be quite salient and the focus of heightened attention. This is an experience of organization in formation. This example is not different in principle from the more familiar case of the buildup of hunger (tension, arousal), consummation in the act of feeding (arousal reduction and hedonic shift), and sensations and perceptions about self and others. However, the thumb-in-mouth case is different in that it concerns a sensorimotor schema, not a physiological need state, that its motivation is conceptualized somewhat differently, and most important for our purposes, that it gives rise to a different vitality affect associated with different body parts and different contexts.

There are many different sensorimotor schemas that need to be adapted, and the consolidation process for each of them involves a subjective experience of somewhat different vitality affects associated with different body parts and sensations in different contexts. It is these subjective experiences of various organizations in formation that I am calling the sense of an emergent self. The particular experiences of the consolidation of a sensorimotor schema may have more of a quality of tension resolution than of déjà vu or of discovery as already described for some of the other senses of an emergent self.

We have now examined three processes involved in forming a sense of an emergent self and other: amodal perception, physiognomic perception, and the perception of corresponding vitality affects. All three are forms of direct, "global" perception, in which the yoking of diverse experiences is accompanied by distinctive subjective experiences. However, that is not the only way the world of related experiences comes into being. There are also constructionist processes that provide the infant with different ways to experience an emergent self and other. These processes are associated with a different approach to infant experience, but one that is complementary to the approach just discussed.

CONSTRUCTIONIST APPROACHES TO RELATING SOCIAL EXPERIENCES

The constructionist view assumes that the infant perceives the human form initially as one of many arrays of physical stimuli, not essentially different from various other arrays, such as windows, cribs, and mobiles. It further assumes that the infant first detects separate featural elements of persons: size, motion, or vertical lines. These featural elements, which could by themselves belong to any stimulus array, are then progressively integrated until a configuration, a whole form, is synthesized into a larger constructed entity—first, a face, and gradually a human form.

The processes that form the constructionist view are assimilation, accommodation, identifying invariants, and associational learning. The emergence of the sense of self is therefore described more in terms of discoveries about the relations between peviously known disparate experiences than in terms of the process itself. While learning in one form or another, is the underlying process of a constructionist approach, what can and will be learned is channeled by innate predilections common to the species. Humans are born with preferences or tendencies to be attentive to specific features within a stimulus array. This is true for stimulation in any sensory modality. There is a developmental sequence in which the infant detects or finds most salient different features at different ages. This progression is best studied in vision. From birth to two months, infants have a tendency to seek out the stimulus features of movement (Haith 1966), size, and contour density, the number of contour elements per unit area (Kessen et al. 1970; Karmel, Hoffman, and Fegy 1974; Salapatek 1975). After two months of age, curvature, symmetry, complexity, novelty, aperiodicity, and ultimately config- urations (form) become more salient stimulus features (See Hainline 1978; Haith 1980; Sherrod 1981; Bronson 1982).

Infants also come into the world with attentional (potential information-gathering) strategies that have their own maturational unfolding. Again, these have been best studied in vision. Up to two months of age, infants predominantly scan the periphery or edges of objects. After that age, they begin to shift their gaze to look at the internal features (Salapatek 1975; Haith et al. 1977; Hainline 1978). When the object is a face, there are two important exceptions to this general progression of attentional strategy. When some auditory stimulation such as speaking is added, even infants younger than two months tend to shift their gaze from the periphery to the internal features of the face (Haith et al. 1977). The same tendency has been observed when there is movement of the facial features (Donee 1973).

Using this information to predict how the human face will be experienced in constructionist terms, we could predict roughly the following progression. During the first two months, infants should find the face no different from other objects that move, that are roughly the same size, and that have similar contour density. Infants would acquire much familiarity with the features that make up the border areas, such as the hairline, but little familiarity with the internal features of the face: the eyes, nose, mouth—in short, all the features that taken together make up its configuration or "faceness." After the age of about two months, when attentional strategy shifts to internal scanning, infants would first pay attention to those features with more of the stimulus properties they preferred: curvature, contrast, vertical symmetry, angles, complexity, and so on. These preferences would lead them to be attentive first to the eyes, then to the mouth, and last to the nose. After considerable experience with these features and their invariant spatial relationships, they would have constructed a schema or identified the invariants of the configuration that designates "faceness."

Indeed, it is readily demonstrable that by the age of five to seven months infants can remember for over a week the picture of a particular face that has been seen only once and for less than a minute (Fagan 1973, 1976). This feat of long-term recognition memory requires a representation of the unique form of a particular face. It is unlikely that it is done on the basis of feature recognition. The fact that faces make sounds and that their internal parts move in talking and expressing should push the constructionist timetable somewhat earlier, but it does not change the sequence in which the construction of form perception progresses.

This constructionist approach could be applied equally well to audition, touch, and the other modalities of human stimulation. If one accepts the constructionist picture and timetable for the earliest perceptual encounter with human stimuli, one must conclude that the infant is not related in any distinctive or unique way to other persons. Interpersonal relatedness does not yet exist as distinct from relatedness to things. The infant is asocial, but by virtue of being indiscriminate, not by virtue of being unresponsive, as suggested by psychoanalytic formulations of a stimulus barrier that protects the infant for the first few months of life. One can entertain a notion of relatedness to isolated stimulus features or properties, but that is a weak notion indeed. The idea of relatedness to circles or spheres (or to "part objects," in psychoanalytic terms) does not seem to carry one far into the domain of the interpersonal.

The problem is, then, how and when do these constructions become related to human subjectivity, so that selves and others emerge? Before dealing with that problem, we should note that some evidence suggests that infants never experience any salient human form (face, voice, breast) as nothing more than a particular physical stimulus array among others, but rather that they experience persons as unique forms from the start. The evidence is of several kinds: (1) By the age of one month, infants do show appreciation of more global (nonfeatural) aspects of the human face such as animation, complexity, and even configuration (Sherrod 1981). (2) Infants gaze differently when scanning live faces than when viewing geometric forms. They are less captured by single featural elements and scan more fluidly during these first months (Donee 1973). (3) When scanning live faces, newborns act differently than when scanning inanimate patterns. They move their arms and legs and open and close their hands and feet in smoother, more regulated, less jerky cycles of movement. They also emit more vocalizations (Brazelton et al. 1974, 1980). (4) The recent finding of Field et al. (1982), that two- to three-day-old infants can discriminate and imitate smiles, frowns, and surprise expressions seen on the face of a live interactant, clearly indicates that the infant not only is perceiving internal facial features but appears to be discriminating some of their different configurations.[11] (5) The recognition of a specific individual's face or voice is supportive evidence for some kind of specialness attached to

11. It can, however, be argued that the discrimination of expressive configurations is based on the detection of a single feature necessary and sufficient for each configuration.

that person's stimuli. The evidence is convincing that the neonate can discriminate the mother's voice from another woman's voice reading the exact same material (DeCasper and Fifer, 1980).[12] The evidence for recognition of individual faces prior to two months is less secure. Many researchers continue to find it, but a larger number do not (see Sherrod 1981). Despite these qualifications of the constructionist view, there is little question that infants do construct relationships as well as perceive them directly.

Approaches to an Understanding of the Infant's Subjective Experience

Amodal perception (based on abstract qualities of experience, including discrete affects and vitality affects) and constructionistic efforts (based on assimilation, accommodation, association, and the identification of invariants) are thus the processes by which the infant experiences organization. While these processes have been most studied in perception, they apply equally well to the formation of organization in all domains of experience: motor activity, affectivity, and states of consciousness. They also apply to the yoking of experiences across different domains (sensory with motor, or perceptual with affective, and so on).

One of the most pervasive problems in understanding infants continues to be the difficulty in finding unifying concepts and language that will include the formation of organization as it occurs in the various domains of experience. For instance, when speaking about the yoking of diverse perceptions to form higher-order perceptions, we can talk in cognitive terms. When speaking about the yoking of sensory experience and motor experience, we can adopt Piaget's conceptual system and talk in terms of sensorimotor schemas. When speaking about the yoking of perceptual and affective experience, we are thrown back on more experiential concepts that are less systematized, such as those employed in psychoanalysis. All of these

12. The pitch range and general stress patterns do not appear to be the distinctive features that permit the infant to make this discrimination. Voice quality may be the best bet (Fifer, personal communication, 1984).

yokings must draw upon the same basic processes that we have discussed, yet we tend to act as if the formation of organization follows its own unique laws in each domain of experience. And to some extent it may. But the commonalities are likely to be far greater than the differences.

There is no reason to give any one domain of experience primacy and make it the point of departure to approach the infant's organization of experience. Several approaches can be described, all of them valid, all of them necessary, and all of them equally "primary."[13]

The infant's actions. This is the route implied in Piaget's work. Self-generated action and sensations are the primary experiences. The emergent property of things, in the beginning, is an action-sensation amalgam in which the object is first constructed in the mind by way of the actions performed on it; for example, there are things that can be grasped and things that can be sucked. While learning about the world, the infant necessarily identifies many invariants of subjective experience of self-generated actions and self-sensations—in other words, of emergent self experiences.

Pleasure and unpleasure (hedonic tone). This is the route that Freud initially explored. He stated that the most salient and unique aspect of human experience is the subjective experience of pleasure (tension reduction) and unpleasure (tension or excitation buildup). This is the basic assumption of the pleasure principle. He assumed that visual perceptions of the environment such as the breast or face or tactile sensations or smells associated with pleasures (such as feeding) or unpleasure (such as hunger) become affect-imbued. It is in this way that affective and perceptual experiences are yoked. On the surface it is an associationist's view, but Freud's version of this view was slightly different. Affects not only make perceptions relevant by way of association; they also provide the ticket of admission for perceptions even to get into the mind. Without the experience of hedonic tone, no perceptions would be registered at all. Hedonic tone did for Freud what self-generated action did for Piaget. They both "created" perceptions as mental phenomena and yoked these perceptions to primary experiences.

Do infants experience hedonic tone in the first months of life? When watching an infant in distress or contentment, one finds it very hard not to believe so. Emde (1980a, 1980b) has postulated that hedonic tone is the first experience of affect. Biologists have generally assumed that from an evolutionary standpoint, pain and pleasure or approach and withdrawal should be the primary affective experiences, for their value to survival.

---

13. One could argue that some experiences are more crucial for survival then others, but that is outside of considerations of subjective experience.

Further, evolution built the experience of categories of affect upon the foundation of hedonic tone (Schneirla 1965; Mandler 1975; Zajonc 1980). Emde et al. (1978) suggests that ontogeny may recapitulate phylogeny in the progression of affective experience. In this light it is interesting that Emde et al. report that in interpreting the facial expressions of the youngest infants, mothers feel most confident about their attribution of hedonic tone, somewhat less confident about level of activation, and least confident about the discrete category of affect seen on the infant's face.

Discrete categories of affect. Even if hedonic tone emerges earlier or faster as an affective experience, the study of infants' faces also makes clear that they express (whether or not they feel) discrete categories of affect. Using detailed film analysis, Izard (1978) observed that newborns show interest, joy, distress, disgust, and surprise. Facial displays of fear appear at about six months (Cicchetti and Sroufe 1978), and shame appears much later. Affect is expressed not only in the face, in the beginning. Lipsitt (1976) has described how newborns express anger by moving the face, arms, and whole body in concert when they experience lack of air from nasal occlusion at the breast. In a similar vein, Bennett (1971) has described how the infant's entire body expresses pleasure; there are quiverings of pleasure as well as smiles.

We simply do not know if infants are actually feeling what their faces, voices, and bodies so powerfully express to us, but it is very hard to witness such expressions and not to make that inference. It is equally hard theoretically to imagine that infants would be provided initially with an empty but convincing signal, when they need the feelings they express to regulate themselves, to define their very selves, and to learn with.[14]

Infant states of consciousness. In the first months of life, the infant cycles dramatically through the sequence of states first described by Wolff (1966): drowsiness, alert inactivity, alert activity, fuss-cry, regular sleep, and paradoxical sleep. It has been suggested that the different waking states of consciousness may also serve the role of an organizing focus for all other experiences, and accordingly they provide a primary approach for describing early infant subjective experience (Stechler and Carpenter 1967; Sander 1983a, 1983b).

Perceptions and cognitions. This is the route most often taken by experimentalists. It results in a view of the infant's social experience as a

---

14. During the last decade, developmental psychologists have tended to stress the cognitive capacities required for an infant to have an affective experience (Lewis and Rosenblum 1978). The result has been an overemphasis on the linkage between the development of cognitive structure and affect. The realization is now occurring that not all affective life is the handmaiden to cognition, either for infants or for adults, and that infants' *feelings*, especially in the beginning, can and must be considered irrespective of what they *know*. (See Demos [1982a, 1982b]; Fogel et al. [1981]; and Thoman and Acebo [1983] for a discussion of this issue in relation to infants, and Zajonc [1980] and Tompkins [1981] in relation to adults.)

subset of perception and cognition in general. Social perception and social cognition follow the same rules applicable to all other objects.

The problem with each of these approaches is that infants do not see the world in these terms (that is, in terms of our academic subdisciplines). Infant experience is more unified and global. Infants do not attend to what domain their experience is occurring in. They take sensations, perceptions, actions, cognitions, internal states of motivation, and states of consciousness and experience them directly in terms of intensities, shapes, temporal patterns, vitality affects, categorical affects, and hedonic tones. These are the basic elements of early subjective experience. Cognitions, actions, and perceptions, as such, do not exist. All experiences become recast as patterned constellations of all the infant's basic subjective elements combined.

This is what Spitz (1959), Werner (1948), and others had in mind when they spoke of global and coenesthetic experience. What was not recognized at the time of their formulations was the extent of the infant's formidable capacities to distill and organize the abstract, global qualities of experience. Infants are not lost at sea in a wash of abstractable qualities of experience. They are gradually and systematically ordering these elements of experience to identify self-invariant and other-invariant constellations. And whenever any constellation is formed, the infant experiences the emergence of organization. The elements that make up these emergent organizations are simply different subjective units from those of adults who, most of the time, believe that they subjectively experience units such as thoughts, perceptions, actions, and so on, because they must translate experience into these terms in order to encode it verbally.

This global subjective world of emerging organization is and remains the fundamental domain of human subjectivity. It operates out of awareness as the experiential matrix from which thoughts and perceived forms and identifiable acts and verbalized feelings will later arise. It also acts as the source for ongoing affective appraisals of events. Finally, it is the ultimate reservoir that can be dipped into for all creative experience.

All learning and all creative acts begin in the domain of emergent relatedness. That domain alone is concerned with the coming-into-being of organization that is at the heart of creating and learning. This domain of experience remains active during the formative period of each of the subsequent domains of sense of self. The later senses of self to emerge are products of the organizing process. They are true, encompassing perspectives about the self—about the physical, actional self, about the subjective self, about the verbal self. The process of forming each of these perspectives, the creative act concerning the nature of self and others, is the process that gives rise to the sense of an emergent self, which will be experienced in the process of forming each of the other senses of the self, to which we can now turn.

Chapter 4

The Sense of a Core Self:
I. Self versus Other

AT THE AGE of two to three months, infants begin to give the impression of being quite different persons. When engaged in social interaction, they appear to be more wholly integrated. It is as if their actions, plans, affects, perceptions, and cognitions can now all be brought into play and focused, for a while, on an interpersonal situation. They are not simply more social, or more regulated, or more attentive, or smarter. They seem to approach interpersonal relatedness with an organizing perspective that makes it feel as if there is now an integrated sense of themselves as distinct and coherent bodies, with control over their own actions, ownership of their own affectivity, a sense of continuity, and a sense of other people as distinct and separate interactants. And the world now begins to treat them as if they are complete persons and do possess an integrated sense of themselves.

In spite of this very distinctive impression, the prevailing views of clinical developmental theory do not reflect the image of an infant with an integrated sense of self. Instead, it is widely held that infants go through an extended period of self/other undifferentiation and that only very slowly, sometime towards the end of the first year of life, do they differentiate a sense of self and other. Some psychoanalytic developmental theories, of which Mahler provides the most influential example, propose that during the undifferentiated phase infants experience a state of fusion or "dual-unity" with mother. This is the phase of "normal symbiosis," lasting roughly from the second to the seventh or ninth month. This state of dual-unity is proposed as the background from which the infant gradually separates and individuates to arrive at a sense of self and of other. Academic theories have not differed basically from the psychoanalytic theories in the sense that both propose a slow emergence of self after a long period of undifferentiation.

Recent findings about infants challenge these generally accepted timetables and sequences and are more in accord with the impression of a changed infant, capable of having—in fact, likely to have—an integrated sense of self and of others. These new findings support the view that the infant's first order of business, in creating an interpersonal world, is to form the sense of a core self and core others. The evidence also supports the notion that this task is largely accomplished during the period between two and seven months. Further, it suggests that the capacity to have merger- or fusion-like experiences as described in psychoanalysis is secondary to and dependent upon an already existing sense of self and other. The newly suggested timetable pushes the emergence of the self earlier in time dramatically and reverses the sequencing of developmental tasks. First comes the formation of self and other, and only then is the sense of merger-like experiences possible.

Before examining the new evidence, we must ask, what kind of a sense of self is the infant likely to discover or create, beyond the sense of an emergent self that appeared in the first two months?

The Nature of an Organized Sense of Self

The first organizing subjective perspective about the self must be at a fairly basic level.[1] A tentative list of the experiences available to the infant, and needed to form an organized sense of a core self

---

1. This discussion will generally concern sense of self. The sense of other is most often the opposite side of the same coin and is implied.

includes (1) *self-agency,* in the sense of authorship of one's own actions and nonauthorship of the actions of others: having volition, having control over self-generated action (your arm moves when you want it to), and expecting consequences of one's actions (when you shut your eyes it gets dark); (2) *self-coherence,* having a sense of being a nonfragmented, physical whole with boundaries and a locus of integrated action, both while moving (behaving) and when still; (3) *self-affectivity,* experiencing patterned inner qualities of feeling (affects) that belong with other experiences of self; and (4) *self-history,* having the sense of enduring, of a continuity with one's own past so that one "goes on being" and can even change while remaining the same. The infant notes regularities in the flow of events.

These four self-experiences, taken together, constitute a sense of a core self. This sense of a core self is thus an experiential sense of events. It is normally taken completely for granted and operates outside of awareness. A crucial term here is "sense of," as distinct from "concept of" or "knowledge of" or "awareness of" a self or other. The emphasis is on the palpable experiential realities of substance, action, sensation, affect, and time. Sense of self is not a cognitive construct. It is an experiential integration. This sense of a core self will be the foundation for all the more elaborate senses of the self to be added later.[2]

These four basic self-experiences seem to be reasonable choices from a clinical point of view as well as from a developmental point of view, in that they are necessary for adult psychological health. It is only in major psychosis that we see a significant absence of any of these four self-experiences. Absence of agency can be manifest in catatonia, hysterical paralysis, derealization, and some paranoid states in which authorship of action is taken over. Absence of coherence can be manifest in depersonalization, fragmentation, and psychotic experiences of merger or fusion. Absence of affectivity can be seen in the anhedonia of some schizophrenias, and absence of continuity can be seen in fugue and other disassociative states.

A sense of a core self results from the integration of these four basic self-experiences into a social subjective perspective. Each of these self-experiences can be seen as self-invariant. An invariant is that which does not change in the face of all the things that do

---

2. It is reasonable to believe that many higher nonhuman animals form such a sense of a core self. That in no way diminishes this achievement.

change. To be persuaded that a sense of a core self is likely to form during the first half year of life as a primary social task, one would want to be assured that the infant has the appropriate opportunities to find the necessary self-invariants (agency, coherence, and so on) in daily social life, the capacities to identify these self-invariants, and the ability to integrate all of these self-invariants into a single subjective perspective. Let us begin with the opportunities.

The Natural Opportunities for Identifying Self-Invariants

The period roughly from two to six months is perhaps the most exclusively social period of life. By two or three months the social smile is in place, vocalizations directed at others have come in, mutual gaze is sought more avidly, predesigned preferences for the human face and voice are operating fully, and the infant undergoes that biobehavioral transformation resulting in a highly social partner (Spitz 1965; Emde et al. 1976). Before these changes at two months, the infant is relatively more engaged with social behaviors directly bearing on the regulation of physiological needs—sleep and hunger. And after six months the infant changes again and becomes fascinated by, and proficient in, manipulating external objects; coordination of limbs and hand-to-eye have improved rapidly, and an interest in inanimate objects sweeps the field. When in physiological and affective equilibrium, the infant becomes relatively more engaged with things than with people. So it is in between these two shifts at two and six months of age that the infant is relatively more socially oriented. This short period of intense and almost exclusive sociability results both from default and design.

Given this honeymoon period of intense sociability, how are the interpersonal interactions mutually constructed so that the infant is in a position to identify the invariants ("islands of consistency") that will come to specify a core self and a core other? This has been discussed in greater detail elsewhere (Stern 1977), but the highlights for our purposes are as follows:

First, the caregivers' social behaviors elicited by the infant are generally exaggerated and moderately stereotypic. "Baby talk," the example par excellence, is marked by raised pitch, simplified syntax, reduced rate, and exaggerated pitch contours (Ferguson 1964; Snow 1972; Fernald 1982; Stern, Spieker, and MacKain 1983). "Baby faces" (the often odd but effective faces made automatically by adults towards infants) are marked by exaggeration in fullness of display, longer duration, and slower composition and decomposition of the display (Stern 1977). Similarly, gaze behaviors are exaggerated, and adults tend to "work in closer" to proximate positions best suited for the infant to focus on and attend exclusively to the adult's behavior. The social presence of an infant elicits variations in adult behavior that are best suited to the infant's innate perceptual biases; for example, infants prefer sounds of a higher pitch, such as are achieved in "baby talk." The result is that the adult's behavior is maximally attended by the infant.

Ultimately, it is these same caregiver behaviors that are the stimuli from which the infant must pick out the many invariants that specify an other. The matching of caregiver behavioral variations and infant predelictions gives the infant the optimal opportunity to perceive those behavioral invariants that identify self or other.

Caregivers typically perform these exaggerated behaviors in a theme and variation format. An example of this format in verbal behavior might go something like this:

Hey, *honey* . . . Yeah, *honey* . . . Hi, *honey* . . . Watcha doing, *honey?* . . . Yeah, what*cha doing?* . . . what are *ya doing?* . . . what are *ya doing* there? . . . *ya doing* nothing?

There are two themes, "honey" and "ya doing." Each theme is restated several times, with minor variations in language or paralanguage.

The same kind of theme and variations format is also the rule for repetitious facial displays or body-touching games. For example, the general game "I'm going to get you," when played in the tickle form of "walking fingers," consists of repeated finger marches up the infant's legs and torso, ending up with a neck or chin tickle as the punch line. It is played over and over, but each finger march is distinctly different from the previous one in speed, in suspense, in vocal accompaniment, or in some other way. The longer the caregiver can introduce an optimal amount of novelty into the performance of each successive round, the longer the infant will stay entranced.

There are two reasons why caregivers engage in this kind of varied repetitiveness (though they generally are not conscious of their reasons). First, if the caregiver did the exact same thing at each repeat, the infant would habituate and loose interest. Infants rapidly determine if a stimulus is the same as those seen or heard immediately before; if it is, they soon stop responding to it. So the caregiver who wishes to maintain a steady high level of interest must constantly change the stimulus presentation a little bit to prevent the baby from habituating. The caregiver's behavior must keep changing, to keep the baby in the same place; it cannot be exact repeats. But then why not do something completely different each time? Why use variations on a theme? This leads to the second reason, the importance of order and repetitiveness.

One of the central tendencies of mind that infants readily display is the tendency to order the world by seeking invariants. A format in which each successive variation is both familiar (the part that is repeated) and novel (the part that is new) is ideally suited to teach infants to identify interpersonal invariants. They get to see a complex behavior and observe which parts of it, so to speak, can be deleted and which parts must remain for it to be the same. They are getting lessons in identifying the invariant features of interpersonal behavior.

The use of exaggerated infant-elicited behaviors and their organization into a theme-and-variation format are not done by caregivers to teach the infant about interpersonal invariants. That is a by-product. They are done to help regulate the infant's level of arousal and excitation within a tolerable range (and to keep the parents from getting bored).

Each infant has an optimal level of excitation that is pleasurable. Beyond that level of excitation the experience becomes unpleasurable, and below a certain level the experience becomes uninteresting and stops being pleasurable. The optimal level is actually a range. Both partners adjust to keep the infant within it. On the one side, the caregiver regulates the level of activity in facial and vocal expressions, gestures, and body movements—the stimulus events that determine the infant's level of excitation. Corresponding to each infant's optimal range of excitation is an optimal range of stimulation. By sensitively gearing the level of such behaviors as the extent of exaggeration and the amount of variation to the infant's current level of excitation and the direction of its predictable drift, the caregiver achieves the optimal range of stimulation.

On the other side, the infant also regulates the level of excitation, using gaze aversion to cut out stimulation that has risen above the optimal range and gaze and facial behaviors to seek out and invite new or higher levels of stimulation when the level of excitation has fallen too low (Brazelton et al. 1974; Stern 1974a, 1975; Fogel 1982). When one watches infants play their role in these mutual regulations, it is difficult not to conclude that they sense the presence of a separate other and sense their capacity to alter the behavior of the other as well as their own experience.

With this kind of mutual regulation, infants in effect get extensive experience with self-regulation of their own level of excitation and with regulation, through signals, of a responsive caregiver's level of stimulation. This amounts to an early coping function. Infants also get extensive experience with the caregiver as a regulator of their levels of excitation, that is, of being with an other who helps them self-regulate. All this can be best observed in the fairly stereotypic parent-infant games of this life period (Call and Marschak 1976; Fogel 1977; Schaffer 1977; Stern et al. 1977; Tronick et al. 1977; Field 1978; Kaye 1982).

It is important to note that during this period of life, these social interactions are in no way purely cognitive events. They mainly involve the regulation of affect and excitation. Perceptual, cognitive, and memorial events play a considerable role in these regulatory events, but they are all about affect and excitement. It must also be recalled that during this period, when face-to-face social interactions are one of the main forms of interpersonal engagement, the major emotional peaks and valleys of social life now occur during these encounters and not during activities such as feeding, when physiological regulation is uppermost. These social matters concern both the infant's cognitive and affective experience.

But how about the extreme affective states related to physiological and bodily needs—distress and crying because of hunger or discomfort, and contentment due to satiation? Do these present an entirely different social situation for the infant insofar as discovery of self and other are concerned? No. Parental behavior in these situations follows the same general rules that it does during social play. Behaviors are exaggerated, repeated with appropriate variation, and stereotypic. Imagine an attempt to soothe a distressed baby. The facial, vocal, and tactile behaviors are greatly exaggerated and repeated with constant variations until success is achieved. Soothing, comforting, putting to sleep, and so on are rituals that follow a narrowly prescribed repertoire of themes and variations. (Unsuccessful soothing consists of a series of uncompleted, broken up, ineffective rituals, but it is ritual nonetheless.) And during these events the infant is of course experiencing affective changes that vary along with the parents' behavioral themes and variations.

These, then, are the daily life events that offer up the opportunities from which the infant must identify the invariants that specify a core self and, complementarily, those that specify a core other. We can now turn to the capacities the infant would need in order to be able to discover the basic invariants that will specify a core self and other.

The Identification of Self-Invariants

First of all, the intrinsic motivation to order one's universe is an imperative of mental life. And the infant has the overall capacity to do so, in large part by identifying the invariants (the islands of consistency) that gradually provide organization to experience. In addition to this general motivation and capacity, the infant needs specific capacities to identify the invariants that seem most crucial in specifying a sense of a core self. Let us look closely at the four crucial invariants.

AGENCY

Agency, or authorship of action, can be broken down into three possible invariants of experience: (1) the sense of volition that precedes a motor act, (2) the proprioceptive feedback that does or does not occur during the act, and (3) the predictability of consequences that follow the act. What capacities does the infant have for identifying these features of agency?

The invariant of volition may be the most fundamental invariant of core self-experience. All movements of voluntary (striated) muscles that are organized at a level higher than the reflex are preceded by the elaboration of a motor plan, which is then executed by the muscle groups (Lashley 1951). Exactly how these motor plans are registered in sentience is not clear, but it is commonly accepted that there is some mental registration (usually out of awareness) of the existence of a motor plan prior to action. The existence of the plan can reach awareness quite readily when its execution is inhibited or when for some reason the motor execution misfires and fails to match the original plan (the thumb hits the cheek instead of going into the mouth, for example). We expect our eyes and hands and legs to do what we have planned for them. The presence of the motor plan as it exists in mind allows for the sense of volition or will. Even when we are unaware of the motor plan, the sense of volition makes our actions seem to belong to us and to be self-acts. Without it, an infant would feel what a puppet would "feel" like, as the nonauthor of its own immediate behavior.

One expects to find motor plans from the very beginning of life, at least as soon as voluntary motor skills become evident. And this, of course, occurs in the first month of life, with hand-to-mouth skills, gazing skills, and sucking skills. Later, a four-month-old reaching for an object of a certain size will begin to shape finger position and degree of hand opening to fit the size of the object to be grasped (Bower et al. 1970). These hand adjustments are made en route to the object; they are accommodations to the size of the object as seen and not yet felt. What must be occurring is that the motor plan for the hand-shaping-during-reach is being formed on the basis of visual information.

One could argue that the achievement of a motor plan such as handshaping is simply a match/mismatch operation with goal-correcting feedback. But such arguments still do not address the initiating mental event that forms the motor plan. That is where volition resides. The execution of match/mismatch operations determines only the liklihood of the original plan being successful or not, or brought to awareness or not.

The reality and importance of motor plans as mental phenomena, particularly as these apply to skilled actions such as talking or playing the piano, were beautifully argued by Lashley. Recently, another illustration of this phenomenon was pointed out to me (Hadiks, personal communication, 1983). If subjects are asked to write their signatures twice, first very small on a piece of paper and then in very large script on a blackboard, the two signatures will be remarkably alike when adjusted for size. What is interesting about this example is that entirely different muscle groups are used to render the two signatures. In the first signing, on paper, the elbow and shoulder are fixed and all action occurs in the fingers and wrist. In the second signing, on the blackboard, the fingers and wrist are fixed and all action occurs in the movements at the elbow and shoulder. The motor program for the signature thus in no way resides in the muscles required for the signing. It resides in the mind and is transferable from one set of muscles to a completely different set of muscles for its execution. Volition in the form of motor plans exists as a mental phenomenon that can be combined with a variety of different muscle groups for execution. This is what Piaget had in mind when he spoke of sensorimotor schemas and the ability of the infant to marshal different means to accomplish the same ends. These considerations lead to a clinical vignette.

Several years ago a pair of "Siamese twins" (Xiphophagus conjoint twins) were born at a hospital near the university where I teach. These were only the sixth set of twins of their kind reported in the world literature. They were connected on the ventral surface between the umbilicus and the bottom of the sternum, so that they always faced one another. They shared no organs, had separate nervous systems, and shared essentially no blood supply (Harper et al. 1980). It was noticed that very frequently one would end up sucking on the other's fingers and vice versa, and neither seemed to mind. About one week before they were to be surgically separated at four months of age (corrected for prematurity), Rita Harper, Director of the Neonatal Nursery, called me because of the potential psychological interest of this pair. Susan Baker, Roanne Barnett, and I had an opportunity to do a number of experiments before surgical separation. One experiment bears on volitional motor plans and the self. When twin A (Alice) was sucking on her *own* fingers, one of us placed one hand on her head and the other hand on the arm that she was sucking. We gently pulled the sucking arm away from her mouth and registered (in our own hands) whether her arm put up resistance to being moved from her mouth and/or whether her head strained forward to go after the retreating hand. In this situation, Alice's arm resisted the interruption of sucking, but she did not give evidence of straining forward with her head. The same procedure was followed when Alice was sucking on her sister Betty's fingers rather than her own. When Betty's hand was gently pulled from Alice's mouth, Alice's arms showed no resistance or movement, and Betty's arm showed no resistance, but Alice's head did strain forward. Thus when her own hand was removed, the plan to maintain sucking was put into execution by the attempt to bring her arm back to the mouth, while when another person's hand was removed the plan to maintain sucking was put into execution with the movement of her head forward. Alice seemed, in this case, to have no confusion as to whose fingers belonged to whom and which motor plan would best reestablish sucking.

We were fortunate to come upon several occasions when Alice was sucking on Betty's fingers while Betty was sucking on Alice's fingers. The same interruption of sucking manipulation was performed, except doubly and simultaneously. The results indicated that each twin "knew" that one's own mouth sucking a finger and one's own finger being sucked do not make a coherent self. Two invariants are missing, volition (of the arm) as we have been talking about it, although this cannot be proved, and predictable consequences, which we shall address below.[3]

This aspect of agency, the sense of volition, must occur very early during the newborn period, since the infant's repertoire of action is not all reflexive even at birth. To the extent that the newborn's behaviors are to a considerable extent reflexive, the sense of volition will not be an invariant of movement. Sometimes it will be there, seen in such voluntary movements as some head-turns, some sucking, most gazing behaviors, and some kickings. Sometimes it will not be there, when a behavior is fired off reflexively; such behaviors include many arm movements (tonic neck reflexes), head movements (rooting), and so on. Until the proportion of all self-action that is reflexive becomes quite small, the sense of volition will be an "almost invariant" of self-action. By the second month of life, when core-relatedness begins, this is certainly the case.

The second invariant property specifying agency is proprioceptive feedback. This is a pervasive reality of self-action whether the action

3. This example is in part an unusual case of "single touch" versus "double touch." Double touch is when you touch yourself and the touched part in turn touches the touching part.

is initiated by self or passively manipulated by another. It is clear that infant motor acts are guided by proprioceptive feedback from the earliest days, and we have very reason to assume that proprioception is developmentally a constant invariant of self-agency, even when the infant is not acting but is holding any antigravity posture. The Papoušeks (1979) have commented on this point, which was also central for Spitz (1957).

Given just these two invariants, volition and proprioception, it becomes clearer how the infant could sense three different combinations of these two invariants: self-willed action of self, (bringing thumb up towards own mouth), in which both volition and proprioception are experienced; other-willed action of other (mother bringing pacifier up towards infant's mouth), in which neither volition nor proprioception are experienced; or other-willed action on self (mother holds baby's wrists and plays "clap hands" or "pat-a-cake," at a point when the child does not yet know the game), in which proprioception but not volition will be experienced. It is in this way that the infant is in a position to identify those invariants that specify a core self, core other, and the various amalgams of these invariants that specify self-with-other. As we add more invariant interpersonal properties, the possibilities expand greatly.

The third invariant that potentially can specify agency is consequence of action. Self events generally have contingent relations very different from events with another. When you suck your finger, your finger gets sucked—and not just generally sucked, but with a sensory synchrony between the tongue and palate sensations and the complementary sensations of the sucked finger. When your eyes close, the world goes dark. When your head turns and eyes move, the visual sights change. And so on.

For virtually all self-initiated actions upon the self, there is a felt consequence. A constant schedule of reinforcement results. Conversely, acts of the self upon the other generally provide less certain consequences and result in a quite variable schedule of reinforcement. The infant's ability to sense contingent relations alone will be of no help in self/other differentiation. What will help, however, will be the infant's ability to tell one schedule of reinforcement from another, since only self-generated acts are constantly reinforced.

Recent experiments show that infants have considerable ability to discriminate different schedules of reinforcement (Watson 1979, 1980). Using a paradigm in which infants must turn their heads against a pressurized pillow to get a mobile to turn, Watson has demonstrated that infants by the age of three months can distinguish between schedules of constant reinforcement (each head-turn is rewarded), a fixed ratio of reinforcement (every third head-turn, say, is reinforced) and a variable schedule (where head-turns are less predictably rewarded). The implications for self/other differentiation are clear. This discrimination provides the needed leverage for the problem at hand. Most classes of action by the self upon the self necessarily have a constant reinforcement schedule. (Arm motions always result in proprioceptive sensations. Vocalization always results in unique resonance phenomena from neck and chest and skull. And so on.)

By contrast, actions of the self upon others are usually variably rewarded. The variable and unpredictable nature of maternal responses to infant actions has been documented often (see Watson 1979). For instance, a three-month-old infant who vocalizes has a 100 percent likelihood of feeling the chest resonance of the sound but the likelihood of mother vocalizing back is only probabilistic (Stern et al. 1974; Strain and Vietze 1975; Schaffer et al. 1977). Similarly, if the three-and-one-half-month-old infant gazes toward mother, it is certain she will come into view, but the odds are only high, not certain, that she will look back (Stern 1974b; Messer and Vietze 1982).

In examining the basis of causal inference in infancy, Watson (1980) suggests that there are three features of causal structure available to the infants by three to four months of age: an appreciation of temporal relations between events; an appreciation of sensory relations, that is, the ability to correlate intensity or duration of a behavior and its effect; and an appreciation of spatial relations, the ability to take into account the spatial laws of a behavior and the laws of its effects. These three dimensions of information about causal structure, which we will examine in more detail in the next section, presumably act additively or interactively in providing the infant with rudimentary knowledge of different occasions or conditions of causality. This knowledge in turn should help to separate the world into self-caused and other-caused effects.

The sense of agency is certainly a major specifier of self versus other. But there is a parallel question of equal magnitude. Must the infant not have a sense of a coherent, dynamic physical entity to which the sense of agency can belong?

SELF-COHERENCE

What are the invariant properties of interpersonal experience that might specify that the self versus the other is a single, coherent, bounded physical entity? And what are the infant's capacities to identify them? Without a sense of self and other as coherent entities unto themselves, a sense of a core self or core other would not be possible, and agency would have no place of residence.

There are several features of experience that could help in establishing self-coherence:

Unity of locus. A coherent entity ought to be in one place at one time, and its various actions should emanate from one locus. It has long been known that infants visually orient to the source of a sound at birth (Worthheimer 1961; Butterworth and Castillo 1976; Mendelson and Haith 1976). Part of the problem of discovering unity of locus is thus already solved by predesign of the nervous system. By the age of three months, infants expect that the sound of a voice should come from the same direction as the visual location of the face.

Because infants' relexes and expectations assure that they will be watching what they are listening to and vice versa (under most natural conditions), infants are in a good position to notice that the behaviors specific to an other occupy a separate locus of origin from the locus occupied by the behaviors specific to themselves. Real life interactions, however, confound this picture, and common locus of origin as an identifiable property of self versus other is often violated. For instance, at the close range of face-to-face interactions, the mother's mouth, face, and voice obey the invariant of common locus of origin, but her hands may be holding or tickling the baby. In that case the mother's hands are as far from her face as is the infant's body. Her hands violate the unity of locus of her facial behaviors just as much as any part of the baby's body might be seen to. Unity of locus certainly plays a role as an interpersonal invariant, but by itself it can take the infant only so far in specifying core self and other. It is very helpful when mother is across the room, but of limited help at close range.

Coherence of motion. Things that move coherently in time belong together. Mother as an object seen moving across the room or against any stationary backdrop will be experienced as having coherence because all of her parts are moving relative to some background (Gibson 1969). Ruff (1980) argues that the continuous optical transformations of a moving object (mother) provide the infant with unique kinds of information to detect structural invariants. Because the mind can extract invariants from dynamic events, Ruff deals with the fact that both the infant and the object may be in motion and puts this fact to use. But the problems with motion as an invariant identifying mother as a core other entity are similar to those encountered for unity of locus. First, when she is quite close, the infant observes that parts of her are moving relatively faster than others. This generally means that parts of her become the background, relatively speaking, for other parts of her. When this occurs, and it occurs often, one arm might appear to be a different entity from the other arm, or from the body. The second problem is that infants experience greater coherence if all parts are moving as if associated by rigid connections (Spelke 1983). This is not often the case with a socially interacting mother. Her hand, head, mouth, and body movements may be far too fluidly related ever to give the impression that they all belong to the same whole.

Coherence of motion alone, then, as an invariant would be of limited value in detecting core entities. Happily, human actions have other properties that can serve as more reliable invariants.

Coherence of temporal structure. Time provides an organizing structure that helps identify different entities. The many behaviors that are invariably performed simultaneously by one person share a common temporal structure. Condon and Ogston (1966) have labeled this self-synchrony, not to be confused with interactional synchrony, which will be discussed later in this section. Self-synchrony refers to the fact that separate parts of the body such as limbs, torso, and face tend to move—in fact, must move—together synchronously to a split second, in the sense that starts, stops, and changes in direction or speed in one muscle group will occur synchronously with starts, stops, and changes in other muscle groups. This does not mean that the two arms must be doing the same thing at the same time, nor that the face and leg, for example, start and stop moving together. It permits each body part to trace its own pattern and to start and stop independently, so long as they all adhere to a basic temporal structure such that changes in one body part occur, if they are going to, only in synchrony with changes in other parts. In addition, these changes in movement occur synchronously with natural speech boundaries at the phonemic level, such that the temporal structure of self-synchronous behavior is like an orchestra, in which the body is the conductor and the voice the music. (Try to pat your head, rub your belly, and count all at the same time. Violating temporal coherence in this activity can be done, but only with great concentration.) In short, all of the stimuli (auditory, visual, tactile, proprioceptive) emanating from the self share a common temporal structure, while all of those emanating from an other share a different temporal structure. Furthermore, Stern (1977) has found that all features of maternal self-synchronous behavior are highlighted or exaggerated, and Beebe and Gerstman (1980) have observed that the "packaging" of maternal behaviors into synchronous bursts or units is especially tight. Both of these observations suggest that mothers act to make the temporal structure of their behavior especially obvious.

There is a potential problem with all of this. Condon and Sander (1974) have suggested that in addition to self-synchrony, there also exists between mother and baby "interactional synchrony," in which the infant's movements are in perfect synchrony with the mother's voice. If this were true, then each partner's behavior would not in fact have a separate and distinct temporal structure, because the timing of the behavior would be largely determined by that of the partner. Since the original publication, however, there have been several unsuccessful attempts to replicate the original demonstration of interactional synchrony. There have also been unsuccessful attempts to demonstrate the same phenomenon using other and more precise methods. In spite of the rapid and wide initial acceptance of the phenomenon of interactional synchrony—its appeal is obvious—it has not stood the test of time, and we do not need to consider it. Self-synchrony does seem to have stood up, and we are left with two persons who, most of the time, have different and distinct temporal patterns common to their individual behavior.

If the infant were equipped with the ability to perceive a common temporal structure in that which is seen and heard, the task of differentiating self from other, and the task of differentiating this other from that other, would be greatly facilitated. Recent evidence strongly suggests that infants do indeed have such a capacity and that it is observable by four months of age, if not earlier.

Spelke (1976, 1979) has reported that infants are responsive to temporal congruity between auditory and visual stimuli, with a tendency to match events that are synchronous in time across sensory modality. She presented four-month-old infants with two animated cartoon films projected side by side, with the sound track appropriate (that is, synchronous) to only one of the films emanating from a speaker placed midway between the two images. The infants could tell which film was synchronous with the sound track and preferred to look at the sound-synchronous film. Through a variety of similar experiments, researchers have found that infants can recognize common temporal structure. It does not matter whether the two synchronous events are in the same modality (both visual) or in mixed modes (one auditory and one visual); infants will spot the two that share the same temporal structure (Spelke 1976; Lyons-Ruth 1977; Lawson 1980). Moreover, infants will notice a discrepancy of 400 milliseconds between a sight and sound that are expected to be paired, such as in lip reading (Dodd 1979).

This work suggests that temporal structure is a valuable invariant in identifying core entities. Infants act as though two events sharing the same temporal structure belong together. Taking the step from experimental stimuli to the stimuli provided by natural human behavior, it seems more than likely that infants should readily perceive that the sounds and sights (voice, movements, and expressions) that share a common temporal structure belong to an entity (self or other) that is distinct by virtue of its unique temporal organization (Spelke and Cortelyou 1981; Sullivan and Horowitz 1983). While there have as yet been no experiments that have extended these findings to the proprioceptive or tactile senses, the weight of evidence is increasing that infants inhabit a sensory world in which they integrate cross-modal experience, recognizing the patterns of sounds, sights, and touches that come from self and those that come from an other as separate phenomena, each with its own singular temporal structure.

If we assume that the infant can identify coherent entities (such as mother's behavior) that have a common temporal structure, will the temporal structure that identifies her be destroyed or interfered with by the infant's own behavior? Will the performance by the infant of an arm movement or a vocalization get mixed up in the mother's temporal structure, or set up a competing temporal structure that obscures it? Can the infant exert selective auditory and visual attention to the temporal structure of the stimuli emanating from one member of the pair, without being distracted or having that structure disorganized by the behavior of the other member?

A recent experiment bears on this question. Walker et al. (1980) demonstrated the ability of four-month-old infants to be selectively inattentive to competing visual events with different time structures. The infants were placed in front of a rear projection screen. Two films of different events were projected on the same area of the screen, one superimposed upon the other. The sound track that was played was synchronous with only one of the films. The images of the two films were then gradually separated, so that they were seen side by side on the screen. After a moment's hesitation, the infants looked at the film that was not synchronous with the sound. They acted as though the film not accompanied by the sound track were a novel event, not noticed before; even though they had been watching it all along during the superimposition. The authors concluded that "perceptual selection is not accomplished through special mechanisms constructed in the course of cognitive development, but is a feature of the art of perceiving early on" (p. 9). The problem of one partner's disrupting the temporal structure of another partner's behavior and thus confusing the discrimination of a core self from a core other may be a theoretical problem for us, but it is not a practical problem for infants in real life.

Coherence of intensity structure. Another invariant identifying the behavior of a separate and distinct person is a common intensity structure. In the separate behaviors that emanate from one person, the modulations in the intensity gradient of one behavior or modality generally match the gradations in the intensity in another behavior. In an angry outburst, for example, the loudness of a vocalization is generally matched by the speed or forcefulness of an accompanying movement, not only absolutely but as the intensity of the behaviors is contoured during their performance. This match of intensity structure is true for the infant's own behavior and the infant's perception of that behavior. For example, as an infant's distress builds and the cry builds in intensity (as an acoustic event), so do the proprioceptive sensations in the chest and vocal cords and the sight and proprioception of a forcefully flailing arm. In short, all the stimuli (auditory, visual, tactile, proprioceptive) emanating from the self (versus other) may share a common intensity structure.

Is it possible that the infant utilizes the perception of levels of intensity to discriminate self and others? Recent experimental work, already mentioned in chapter 3, provides a clue that infants may be able to perceive common intensity level across modalities, just as they can perceive common shape or temporal structure across modalities, and that they can use this information to determine the source (self versus other) of interpersonal events. Lewcowicz and Turkewitz (1980) showed that infants in a laboratory setting can match the intensity of a stimulus experienced in one modality (light) with the intensity of a stimulus experienced in another modality (sound). Intensity-matching across modalities (the seeking of cross-modal equivalence of intensity) is thus another way in which infants are aided in distinguishing self from other.[4]

Coherence of form. The form (or configuration) of the other is an obvious property that "belongs" to someone and can serve to identify that person as an enduring and coherent entity. Infants of two to three months of age have no trouble recognizing the particular facial configuration that belongs to still photographs of their own mothers. Two questions arise. What happens when a face changes expression? And what happens when a face or head changes its angle or position of presentation? First, how does the infant handle internal changes in form? Whenever a face changes its emotional expression, its configuration changes. Does the infant identify different expressional configurations as many different faces, resulting in a "happy mother," a "sad mother," a "surprised mother," and so on, each a separate and unrelated entity? Spieker has results suggesting that infants "know" that the same face showing happiness, surprise, or fear is

4. Several authors have recently stressed that gradient or dimensional information, as opposed to categorical information (brightness vs. pattern, or loudness vs. phonemic structure), has greater importance for the infant than for the adult (Emde 1980a; Stern et al. 1983). Given that young infants may be particularly attentive to the quantitative variations in stimulation, especially variations in intensity, in preference to qualitative variation, the ability to match intensities across modalities will be most helpful in dscriminating whether a particular stimulus (such as the loudness of a vocalization or the speed of forcefulness of a movement) belongs to one or the other member of the dyad in which the infant is participating.

still the same face (1982). They conserve the identity of a particular face across the various transformations of that face in different facial expressions.[5]

The second question is, how do infants handle external changes in form? The boundary form of the face changes as the head is turned, so that the face is seen full on, in a three-quarter presentation, and in profile. Similarly, as a person comes forward or goes away, the size of the face changes, even though the configuration is not transformed. Is a "new" entity revealed to the infant with each of these changes? Are there small mothers, large mothers, full-faced mothers, profile mothers?

The infant's perceptual system (given some experience with the world) seems able to keep track of the identity of an object in spite of changes in its size or distance, its orientation or position of presentation, its degree of shading, and so on. While different theories abound as to how the infant can maintain the identity of inanimate objects across these kinds of changes (see, for example, Gibson 1969; Cohen and Salapatek 1975; Ruff 1980; and Bronson 1982). All agree that the infant can do it. These abilities certainly apply to human stimuli as well as inanimate ones. For example, Fagan finds that five- to seven-month-old infants can recognize the never-before-seen profile of a face after a short familiarization with the full face, or even better with the three-quarter view of the face (Fagan 1976, 1977).[6]

Sometimes these abilities may be enhanced by cues provided by the infant's abilities at cross-modal matching. Walker-Andrews and Lennon (1984) showed that when five-month-old infants were shown two movies side by side, one of a Volkswagen approaching and one of the same car receding, they would look at the approaching car if at the same time they heard the sound of a car getting

5. Spieker also found that when looking at strange faces an infant also conserves the identity of a given expression across different faces displaying that expression. While the infants could conserve both identity and expression, when dealing with strangers they acted as though the facial expression rather than the facial identity was more salient: "If you don't know them, you'd better know what their affect is, rather than who they are." When dealing with a very familiar face, we assume the reverse is the case: "It is still that person, but wearing a different expression."

6. Fagan found that infants extracted the most information about the invariants of configuration from a three-quarter face presentation, compared with a full or profile presentation. So do adults, according to police department experts in criminal identification.

progressively louder, and they would look at the receding car if the sound got progressively softer. The comings and goings of parents must provide innumerable similar examples.

The evidence thus suggests that distance and positional and expressional (internal) changes, which normally accompany the interactive behavior of an other, need not be seen as problematic for the infant. The infant recognizes that form survives these changes, and early in the infant's life, the invariant of form provides yet another means of discriminating one other from all others.

So far, we have discussed five different potential invariant properties that specify a coherent self entity. Many of these invariants are not truly invariant—that is, always nonvarying—but it is likely that their effect is cumulative in the task of discovering the separate organizations that constitute a core self and a core other. A remaining problem concerns whose organization belongs to whom. How, for instance, does the infant sense that a particular coherent organization of behaviors actually is his or her own, and not an other's? The most ready answer is to assume that only the infant's own organization is accompanied by the invariants of agency, especially volition and proprioception.

SELF-AFFECTIVITY

By the age of two months or so, the infant has had innumerable experiences with many of the affects—joy, interest, and distress and perhaps surprise and anger. For each separate emotion, the infant comes to recognize and expect a characteristic constellation of things happening (invariant self-events): (1) the proprioceptive feedback from particular motor outflow patterns, to the face, respiration, and vocal apparatus; (2) internally patterned sensations of arousal or activation; and (3) emotion-specific qualities of feeling. These three self-invariants, taken together, become a higher-order invariant, a constellation of invariants belonging to the self and specifying one category of emotion.

Affects are excellent higher-order self-invariants because of their relative fixity: the organization and manifestation of each emotion is well fixed by innate design and changes little over development (Izard 1977). The facial display (and therefore the proprioceptive feedback from the facial muscles) is invariant in configuration for each discrete affect. If the preliminary evidence of Ekman et al. (1983) is confirmed, each discrete affect also has a specific profile of autonomic firing with its concomitant discrete constellation of internal feelings, at least in adults. And finally, the quality of subjective feeling is specific to each emotion. Therefore, with each separate emotion there occurs the invariant coordination of three discrete self-invariant events.

The self-invariant constellation belonging to each discrete emotion occurs, for any infant, in a number of contexts and usually with different persons. Mother's making faces, grandmother's tickling, father's throwing the infant in the air, the babysitter's making sounds, and uncle's making the puppet talk may all be experiences of joy. What is common to all five "joys" is the constellation of three kinds of feedback: from the infant's face, from the activation profile, and from the quality of subjective feeling. It is that constellation that remains invariant across the various contexts and interacting others. Affects belong to the self, not to the person who may elicit them.

While we have been concerned so far in this discussion only with the categorical affects, a similar case can be made for the vitality affects. The infant experiences a multitude of crescendos, for example, in diverse actions, perceptions, and affects. All of them trace a similar family of activation contours that create a familiar internal state despite the variety of eliciting events. The subjective quality of feeling remains as the self-invariant experience.

SELF-HISTORY (MEMORY)

A sense of a core self would be ephemeral if there were no continuity of experience. Continuity or historicity is the crucial ingredient that distinguishes an interaction from a relationship, with self as well as with an other (Hinde 1979). It is the ingredient that accounts for Winnicott's sense of "going on being" (1958). The infant capacity necessary for this form of continuity is memory. Is the infant's memory up to the task of maintaining a core self-history—a self continuous in time? Is the infant capable of remembering the three different kinds of experience that make up the other main core self-invariants—agency, coherence, and affect? Does an infant of the age of two to seven months have a "motor memory" for experiences of agency, a "perceptual memory" for the experiences of coherence, and an "affect memory" for the affective experiences?[7]

The issues of agency mainly involve motor plans and acts and their consequences. It has long been assumed that infants must have excellent motor memories. Bruner (1969) has called such memory "memory without words." It refers to memories that reside in voluntary muscular patterns and their coordinations: how to ride a bicycle, throw a ball, suck your thumb. Motor memory is one of the more obvious features of infant maturation. Learning to sit, to perform hand-eye coordinations, and so on require some component of motor memory. Piaget implied exactly this (and more) in his concept of a sensorimotor schema.

It is now clear that there are recall memory "systems" that are not language-based and that operate very early (see Olson and Strauss 1984). Motor memory is one of them. Rovee-Collier and Fagen, and their colleagues have demonstrated long-term cued recall for motor memories in three-month-olds (Rovee-Collier et al. 1980; Rovee-Collier and Fagen 1981; Rovee-Collier and Lipsitt 1981). The infants were placed in a crib with an attractive overhead mobile. A string was tied connecting the infant's foot to the mobile, so that each time the infant kicked, the mobile would move. The infants quickly learned to kick to make the mobile move. Several days after the training session, the infants were placed in the same crib with an overhead mobile but without the attaching string. The context of room, personnel, crib, mobile, and so on recalled the motor act, and the infants began to kick at a high rate, even though there was no string and therefore no movement of the mobile. If a different mobile was used during the memory test session, the infant kicked less than with the original mobile; that is, it was a poorer cue for retrieving or recalling the motor act. Similarly, a change in the design of the crib guard, a peripheral visual attribute of the whole episode, altered

7. For the moment, the distinction between recognition memory (in the presence of the object to be remembered) and recall or evocative memory (in the absence of the object) will be overlooked. The dichotomy between recall and recognition memory has been overdrawn. There is probably no such thing as a memory that is spontaneously evoked (pure recall). Some association or cue, regardless of how farflung, must have triggered it. There is a continuum of recall cues, from farflung and slight, as occurs in some free association, to something fairly close to but not identical with the original, to the reappearance of the original itself, which brings us back to recognition memory (see also Nelson and Greundel 1981). The sharp distinction was partially due to the older assumption that recall memory systems had to be language- or symbol-based (Fraiberg 1969).

the infant's cued recall (Rovee-Collier, personal communication, 1984).

One can argue that cued recall is neither truly evocative memory nor recognition memory. The cue is not the same as the original, nor is the memory spontaneously recalled in vacuo. But that is immaterial. The point is that cued recall for motor experiences can be experimentally demonstrated, as well as inferred from natural behavior, and that these motor memories assure self-continuity in time. They thus constitute another set of self-invariants, part of the "motor self."

The issue of coherence mainly involves the infant's perceptions and sensations. What evidence exists for the infant's capacity for remembering perceptions? It is well established that infants by five to seven months have extraordinary long-term recognition memory for visual perceptions. Fagan (1973) has shown that an infant who is shown the picture of a strange person's face for less than one minute will be able to recognize the same face more than one week later. How early does this perceptual memory begin? Perhaps in the womb. DeCasper and Fifer (1980) asked mothers to talk to their fetuses, that is, to direct speech to their pregnant bellies during the last trimester of pregnancy. He gave each a particular script to speak many times each day. The scripts used (for example, passages from stories by Dr. Seuss) had distinctive rhythmic and stress patterns. Shortly after birth the infants were "asked" (using sucking as the response) whether the passage they had heard in utero was more familiar than a control passage. The infants treated the passage they had been exposed to as familiar. In a similar vein, Lipsitt (personal communication, 1984) presented pure tones to fetuses just prior to a caesarian delivery. The tones were treated as familiar by the newly born infants. Thus, for some events, recognition memory appears to operate across the birth gap.

The recognition memory for the smell of the mother's milk and for the mother's face and voice has already been mentioned. It is clear that the infant has an enormous capacity for registering perceptual events in memory. Furthermore, whenever recognition memory of external events occurs, it is not only continuity of the external world that is affirmed, but also continuity of the mental percepts or schemas that permit recognition to begin with. The likelihood that recognition memory is experienced as self-affirming, as well as world-affirming, is suggested by the well-known "smile of recognition," which may be more than pleasure at successful effortful assimilation. ("My mental representation works—that is, it applies to the real world—and that is pleasurable!") In this light, the act of memory itself can be seen as a self-invariant.

Finally, what evidence exists for the infant's capacity to recognize or recall affective experiences? Emde has recently spoken of an affective core to the prerepresentational self (1983). This is exactly what we mean by the continuity of affective experience, in the form of constellations of self-invariants, that contributes to the sense of continuity of self. Affects, as we have seen, are well suited to this task because after two months emotions as displayed and presumably felt change very little from day to day or from year to year. Of all human behavior, affects perhaps change the least over the life span. The muscles that the two-month-old uses to smile or cry are the exact same ones that the adult uses. Accordingly, the proprioceptive feedback from smiling or crying remains the same from birth to death. For this reason, "our affective core guarantees our continuity of experience across development in spite of the many ways we change" (Emde 1983, p. 1). But this does not answer the question of whether the specific conditions that elicit particular affective experiences can be remembered at these ages.

To answer this question experimentally, Nachman (1982) and Nachman and Stern (1983) made six- to seven-month-old infants laugh with a hand puppet that moved, "spoke," and played peek-a-boo, disappearing and reappearing. When the infants were shown the puppet a week later, the sight of it made them smile.[8] This response is considered cued recall because the sight alone of the unmoving, silent puppet made them smile; in other words, it activated an affective experience. Moreover, they smiled at the puppet only after they had had the game experience. Cued recall memory for affective experience as well as motor experience thus seems not to have to await the development of linguistic encoding vehicles. A different form of encoding is involved. This should hardly be surprising to most psychoanalytic theorists, who have always assumed

---

8. This was not a smile of recognition, because another group of infants were shown unmoving puppets that did not make them smile. When this group returned one week later they recognized the test puppet in a paired comparison procedure, but they never smiled at it in spite of their recognition.

that affect memories were laid down from the first moments, or at least weeks, of life and have in fact described the first year of this process (McDevitt 1979).

Gunther describes an example of cued recall memory for an affective experience in the first days of life (1967). A newborn whose breathing is accidentally occluded by the breast during a feeding will be "breast shy" for the next several feedings. Clearly, the infant has the memorial capacities to register, recognize, and recall affective experiences so that continuity of the affective self is assured.

In short, the infant has the abilities to maintain an updated history for his "motor," "perceptual," and "affective" selves—that is, for his agency, coherence and affectivity.

Integrating the Self-Invariants

How do agency, coherence, affectivity, and continuity all become integrated into one organizing subjective perspective? Memory may provide the answer to the extent that it is a system or process for integrating the diverse features of a lived experience. An experience as lived in real time does not have a completed structure until it is over. Its structure is then immediately reconstituted in memory. It is in this sense that the structure of experience as it is lived and as it is remembered may not be so different, and a closer look at what is called *episodic memory* is now crucial for understanding how the different self-invariants embedded in lived experience are integrated.

Episodic memory, as described by Tulving (1972), refers to the memory for real-life experiences occurring in real time. These episodes of lived experience range from the trivial—what happened at breakfast this morning, what I ate, in what order, where I was sitting—to the more psychologically meaningful—what I experienced when they told me my father had had a stroke. Episodic memory has the great advantage, for our purposes, of being able to include actions, perceptions, and affects as the main ingredients or attributes of a remembered episode. It is therefore the view on memory that is most relevant to our inquiry about infant experience. It attempts to render the daily personal events of a life in memorial and representational terms (Nelson 1973, 1978; Shank and Abelson 1975, 1977; Nelson and Greundel 1979, 1981; Nelson and Ross 1980; Shank 1982).

The basic memorial unit is the episode, a small but coherent chunk of lived experiences. The exact dimensions of an episode cannot be specified here; they represent an ongoing problem in the field. There is agreement, however, that an episode is made of smaller elements or attributes. These attributes are sensations, perceptions, actions, thoughts, affects, and goals, which occur in some temporal, physical, and causal relationship so that they constitute a coherent episode of experience. Depending on how one defines episodes, there are no lived experiences that do not clump to form episodes, because there are rarely, if ever, perceptions or sensations without accompanying affects and cognitions and/or actions. There are never emotions without a perceptual context. There are never cognitions without some affect fluctuations, even if only of interest. An episode occurs within one single physical, motivational setting; events are processed in time and causality is inferred, or at least expectations are set up.

An episode appears to enter into memory as an indivisable unit. The different pieces, the attributes of experience that make up an episode, such as perceptions, affects, and actions, can be isolated from the entire episode of which they are attributes. But in general the episode stands as a whole.

Let us say that an infant has experienced a specific episode once, an episode with the following attributes: being hungry, being positioned at the breast (with accompanying tactile, olfactory, and visual sensations and perceptions), rooting, opening mouth, beginning to suck, getting milk. Let us call that a "breast-milk" episode. The next time a similar "breast-milk" episode occurs, if the infant can recognize that most of the important attributes of the current "breast-milk" episode are similar to the past "breast-milk" episode, two *specific* "breast-milk" episodes will have occurred. Two may be enough, but surely if several more occur with detectable similarities and only minor differences, the infant will soon begin to form a *generalized* "breast-milk" episode. This generalized memory is an individualized, personal expectation of how things are likely to proceed on a moment-to-moment basis. The generalized breast-milk episode is not in itself a specific memory any more; it is an abstraction of many specific memories, all inevitably slightly different, that produces one generalized memory structure. It is, so to speak, averaged experience made prototypic. (In this sense it is now potentially part of semantic memory.)

Now, suppose that the next time a specific breast-episode begins, a deviation from the generalized episode happens. For example, at the moment the infant takes the nipple, the infant's nose gets occluded by the breast. The infant cannot breathe, feels distress, flails, averts head from breast, and regains breath. This new specific episode ("breast-occlusion" episode) is similar to, yet importantly and recognizably different from, the anticipated generalized "breast-milk" episode. It becomes a remembered specific episode. Shank (1982) calls the memory of this specific "breast-occlusion" episode the result of a failed expectation. Memory is failure-driven in that the specific episode is only relevant and memorable as a piece of lived experience to the extent that it violates the expectations of the generalized episode.[9] An episode need not be so deviant as this to be memorable as a specific instance of the generalized episode, so long as it is distinctive enough to be discriminated from the prototype.

At this point, one of three things can happen. The "breast-occlusion" experience may never recur, in which case it will persist enshrined as a specific episodic memory. Gunther (1961) has reported that one episode of breast-occlusion appears to influence newborn behavior for several feedings afterwards. The episode then probably becomes part of long-term, cued recall memory. Or the breast-occlusion experience may recur again and again. In that case the specific episodes become generalized to form a new generalized episode, which we can call the generalized "breast-occlusion" episode. Once this has formed, specific instances of these episodes will be memorable as actual episodes only if they are detectably distinctive from the averaged generalized breast-occlusion episode.

Finally, after the first "breast-occlusion" experience, the infant may never again experience an actual specific instance of the generalized "breast-milk" episode. That is to say, there may continue to be feeding trouble, so that the mother has to switch to a bottle. In this case, the original "breast-milk" generalized episode will after a time no longer be a normal, expected part of daily living and may

9. The occlusion episode would be memorable for other reasons, too. But the concern here is mainly with the relations between relative events.

cease to be an active (even retrievable) memory structure.

There are several points to be made about generalized episodes. The generalized episode is not a specific memory. It does not describe an event that actually ever happened exactly that way. It contains multiple specific memories, but as a structure it is closer to an abstract representation, as that term is used clinically. It is a structure about the likely course of events, based on average experiences. Accordingly, it creates expectations of actions, of feelings, of sensations, and so on that can either be met or be violated.

Exactly what events make up these generalized episodes? Nelson and Greundel (1981), in their study of preschoolers, have focused on what might best be called external events (verbally reported as a rule) such as what happens at a birthday party. The actions that make up the episode are: decorate cake, greet guests, open presents, sing "Happy Birthday," blow candles, cut cake, eat cake. These actions occur predictably and in predictable temporal and causal sequence. Children as young as two years construct generalized episodes about these happenings. Nelson and Greundel have called these general schemes (with variable elements but structured wholes) Generalized Event Structures (GERs) and consider them to be basic building blocks of cognitive development as well as of autobiographical memory.

Our concern, in contrast, is with preverbal infants and with different happenings such as what happens when you are hungry and at the breast, or what happens when you and mom play an exciting game. Moreover, our interest concerns not only the actions but also the sensations and affects. What we are concerned with, then, are episodes that involve interpersonal interactions of different types. Further, we are concerned with the interactive experience, not just the interactive events. I am suggesting that these episodes are also averaged and represented preverbally. They are Representations of Interactions that have been Generalized (RIGs).

We do know that infants have some abilities to abstract, average, and represent information preverbally. A recent experiment on the formation of prototypes is instructive in describing the infant's capacities for the kind of process involved. Strauss (1979) showed ten-month-old infants a series of schematic face drawings. Each face was different in length of the nose or placement of the eyes or ears. After the whole series was shown, the infants were asked (in terms of the detection of novelty) which single drawing best "represented" the entire series. They chose a drawing that they had, in fact, never seen. It was a picture that averaged all of the facial feature sizes and placements previously seen, but this "averaged face" was not part of the series and had not been shown before. The conclusion is that infants have a capacity to aggregate experiences and distill (abstract out) an averaged prototype. I suggest that when it comes to more familiar and important matters, such as interactive experiences, the infant's ability to abstract and represent such experiences as RIGs, begins much earlier.

RIGs can thus constitute a basic unit for the representation of the core self. RIGs result from the direct impress of multiple realities as experienced, and they integrate into a whole the various actional, perceptual, and affective attributes of the core self.[10] RIGs can get organized in terms of particular attributes, just as attributes can get organized in terms of RIGs. Any one attribute, such as hedonic feeling tone, will set limits on what kinds of RIGs are likely to occur when that attribute is present.

Somehow, the different invariants of self-experience are integrated: the self who acts, the self who feels, and the self who has unique perceptions about the self's own body and actions all get assembled. Similarly, the mother who plays, the one who soothes, and the ones that are perceived when the infant is happy and distressed all get disentangled and sorted. "Islands of consistency" somehow form and coalesce. And it is the dynamic nature of episodic memory using RIGs as a basic memory unit that makes it happen.

The advantage of an episodic memory system similar to the one that has been briefly described here is that it permits the indexing and reindexing and the organizing and reorganizing of memorial events about self-invariants (or other invariants) in a fluid and dynamic fashion. It allows one to imagine attributes of many different kinds, interrelating in different ways and resulting in a growing and

10. Nelson and Greundel (1981) have argued that the task of forming generalized episodes is of obvious primary importance in infancy and young childhood and that a specific (episodic) memory only forms if it is an unusual example, that is, a partial violation of the generalized episode (Shank's failure-driven memory). She suggests that much of "infantile amnesia" can be explained by the fact that generalized episodes are insufficiently formed or still in formation, so that specific deviations (specific episodic memories) will not get encoded until the generalizing process is further advanced. In other words, there is nothing to remember against. Some of the real problems of reconstruction in treatment may have to do with the fact that specific memories are deviant examplars of a class of events.

integrating network of organized self-experience. (This is what Shank [1982] means by a dynamic memory.)

It is presumably in this way that the different major self-invariants of agency, coherence, and affectivity become sufficiently integrated (with continuity in the form of memory acting as part of the integrating process) that all together they provide the infant with a unified sense of a core self, suggest that during this life period, age two to seven months, the infant gains enough experience with the separate major self-invariants, and the integrating processes reflected in episodic memory advance far enough, that the infant will make a quantum leap and create an organizing subjective perspective that can be called a sense of a core self. (One would assume that a sense of a core other emerges in parallel via complementary processes.) During this period the infant has the capacities to recognize those events that will identify a self and an other. The social interactive situation offers multiple opportunities to capture those events. And the integrative processes are present to organize these subjective events. The combination of capacities, opportunities, and integrative ability, along with the clinical impression of a changed infant as a more complete person, makes it reasonable to conclude that a firm sense of a core self and a core other emerge during this period.

Chapter 5

The Sense of a Core Self: II. Self with Other

SOMETHING of importance is missing from the last chapter. We have discussed the infant's sense of self versus other, but not the sense of self *with* other. There are many ways that being with an other can be experienced, including some of the most widely used clinical concepts, such as merging, fusion, a haven of safety, a security base, the holding environment, symbiotic states, self-objects, transitional phenomena, and cathected objects.

The sense of being with an other with whom we are interacting can be one of the most forceful experiences of social life. Moreover, the sense of being with someone who is not actually present can be equally forceful. Absent persons can be felt as potent and almost palpable presences or as silent abstractions, known only by trace evidence. In the mourning process, as Freud (1917) pointed out, the one who has died almost rematerializes as a presence in many different felt forms. Falling in love provides a different normal example. Lovers are not simply preoccupied with one another. The loved other is often experienced as an almost continual presence, even an aura, that can change almost everything one does—heighten one's perceptions of the world or reshape and refine one's very movements. How can experiences such as these be accounted for in the present framework? How can the ultimately social nature of the infant's and the adult's experience be captured?

In Winnicott's, Mahler's, and many other theoretical renditions, the various important experiences of being with mother are founded on the assumption that the infant cannot adequately differentiate self from other. Self/other fusion is the background state to which the infant constantly returns. This undifferentiated state is the equilibrium condition from which a separate self and other gradually emerge. In one sense, the infant is seen as totally social in this view. Subjectively, the "I" is a "we." The infant achieves total sociability by not differentiating self from other.

In contrast to these views, the present account has stressed the very early formation of a sense of a core self and core other during the life period that other theories allot to prolonged self/other undifferentiation. Further, in the present view, experiences of being with an other are seen as active acts of integration, rather than as passive failures of differentiation. If we conceive of being-with experiences as the result of an active integration of a distinct self with a distinct other, how can we conceive of the subjective social sense of being with an other? It is now no longer a given, as it was in Mahler's undifferentiated "dual-unity."

Clearly, the infant is deeply embedded in a social matrix, in which much experience is the consequence of others' actions. Why, then, is it not reasonable to think, from the infant's subjective viewpoint, in terms of a merged "self/other" or of a "we self" in addition to the solitary self and other? Is not the infant's initial experience thoroughly social, as the British object relations school has taught us? From the objective viewpoint there do appear to be amalgam-like events between self and other. How will these be experienced? Let us approach this problem of the social self by first considering the nature of the self with the social other as an objective event.

Self with Other as an Objective Event

The infant can be with an other such that the two join their activities to make something happen that could not happen without the commingling of behaviors from each. For example, during a "peek-a-boo" or "I'm going to getcha" game, the mutual interaction generates in the infant a self-experience of very high excitation, full of joy and suspense and perhaps tinged with a touch of fear. This feeling state, which cycles and crescendos several times over, could never be achieved by the infant alone at this age, neither in its cyclicity, in its intensity, nor in its unique qualities. Objectively, it is a mutual creation, a "we" or a self/other phenomenon.

The infant is with an other who regulates the infant's own self-experience. In this sense, the other is a *self-regulating other* for the infant.[1] In games like peek-a-boo, it is the regulation of the infant's arousal that is mainly involved. We can speak of a self-arousal-regulating other. Arousal, however, is only one of many possible self-experiences that others can regulate.

Affect intensity is another infant self-experience of arousal that is almost continually regulated by caregivers. For instance, in smiling interactions the dyad can increase by increments the level of intensity of the affect display. One partner increases a smile's intensity, eliciting an even bigger smile from the other partner, which ups the level yet again, and so on, producing a positive feedback spiral. (See Beebe [1973], Tronick et al. [1977], and Beebe and Kroner [1985] for fuller descriptions of these leadings and followings.)

Security or attachment is another such self-experience. All the events that regulate the feelings of attachment, physical proximity, and security are mutually created experiences. Cuddling or molding to a warm, contoured body and being cuddled; looking into another's eyes and being looked at; holding on to another and being held—these kinds of self-experiences with an other are among the most totally social of our experiences, in the straightforward sense that they can never occur unless elicited or maintained by the action or presence of an other. They cannot exist as a part of known self-experience without an other. This is true even if the self-regulating other is fantasied rather than actual. (The experience of hugging demands a partner even in fantasy, or else it can only be performed but not fully experienced. This applies to hugging pillows as well as people. The issue is not whether the pillow hugs back, only that the pillow be physically present or the sensation of it be imagined. In this sense there is no such thing as half a hug or half a kiss.)

1. "Self" is used here not reflexively but, as elsewhere in the book, to denote the infant's self. A self-regulatory other is thus one who regulates the infant, not the other.

Attachment theorists have stressed the indispensable role played by others in the regulation of security. While attachment is of enormous importance as an index of the quality of the parent/child relationship, it is not however, synonymous with the entire relationship. There are many other self-experiences regulated by others that fall outside the proper boundaries of attachment. Excitation has already been described, and others will be described later.

Parents can also regulate what affect category the infant will experience. Such regulation may involve interpreting the infant's behavior, asking questions like, "Is that face to be taken as funny or surprising?" "Is that cup-banging to be taken as amusing or hostile or bad?" In fact, from two to seven months an enormous sector of the entire affective spectrum an infant can feel is possible only in the presence of and through the interactive mediation of an other, that is, by being with another person.

Both infant and caregiver also regulate the infant's attention, curiosity, and cognitive engagement with the world. The caregiver's mediation greatly influences the infant's sense of wonder and avidity for exploration.

Historically most notable, others regulate the infant's experiences of somatic state. These experiences are the ones that have traditionally preoccupied psychoanalysis, namely, the gratification of hunger and the shift from wakeful fatigue to sleep. In all such regulations, a dramatic shift in neurophysiological state is involved. One of the reasons why these events have received such attention in psychoanalysis, which eclipsed for a long while the ability to discern the importance of the other ways of being with a self-regulating other, is undoubtedly that they were more readily explicable in terms of libido shifts and the energetic model, which the other forms of being-with are not. And this way of being-with is clearly of great importance. It is these experiences and their representation, more than any others, that have been thought to approximate most closely the feeling of total merging, of obliterating self/object boundaries and fusing into a "dual-unity." There is no reason, however, why satiation of hunger or falling into sleep should be construed as passing into a state of dual-unity unless one assumes that "symbiosis" is the lived experience of having excitation fall to zero, when subjective experience of any import effectively stops, as is described and implied in the pleasure principle. Most traditional theories do in fact assume just that, and we will examine this assumption in detail in chapter 9. It is just as likely, however, that experiences of hunger reduction and other somatic state regulations are mainly experienced as dramatic transformations in self-state that require the physical mediation of an other (Stern 1980). In that case, the predominant experience would be being with a somatic-state-regulating other rather than merging.

There have now been enough observations of well-fed institutionalized infants and kibbutz babies, as well as of primate behavior, to make it clear that strong feelings and important representations are forged not necessarily by the very acts of being fed or put to sleep (that is, by somatic-state-regulating others) but rather by the manner in which these acts are performed. And the manner is often best explained by the previously listed forms of self-regulation by others. The great advantage of the feeding experience is that it puts into play and brings together, at one time, so many different forms of self-regulation. Finally, Sander (1964, 1980, 1983a, 1983b) has continued to point out that the infant's states of consciousness and activity are ultimately socially negotiated states, taking their form, in part, through the mediation of self-regulating others.

It is clear that the social action of self-regulating others is a pervasive objective fact bearing on the infant's experience, but how may this be experienced subjectively?

Self with Other as a Subjective Experience

Somehow the infant registers the objective experience with self-regulating others as a subjective experience. These experiences are the same ones that have been called mergings, fusings, security gratifications, and so on.

Psychoanalysis has made a distinction between primary mergers and secondary mergers, and the experience we are considering presumably falls into one or the other type. Primary fusions are those experiences of boundary absence, and therefore sensing oneself to be part of an other, because of a maturational inability—that is, the failure to differentiate self from other. Secondary mergers are those experiences of losing one's perceptual and subjective boundaries after they have been formed and, so to speak, being engulfed by or dissolving into an other's semipermeable personhood. These secondary merger experiences are thought to be re-editions of primary mergers, brought about by regression secondary to some wish-related defensive operation.[2]

In the position taken here, these important social experiences are neither primary nor secondary mergers. They are simply the actual experience of being with someone (a self-regulatory other) such that self-feelings are importantly changed. During the actual event, the core sense of self is not breached: the other is still perceived as a separate core other. The change in self-experience belongs to the core self alone. The changed core self also becomes related (but not fused) with the core other. The self-experience is indeed dependent upon the presence and action of the other, but it still belongs entirely to the self. There is no distortion. The infant has accurately represented reality. Let us examine these assumptions in the form of several questions.

First, why does the experience with a self-regulating other not breach or confuse the sense of a core self and a core other? To address this question, let us return to the earlier example of the infant's experience of excitation as regulated by an other in a peek-a-boo game. Why does the infant continue to experience the cycles of anticipation and joy as belonging to the core self? Similarly, why do the wonderful disappearing-reappearing antics belong to mother, as a core other? Why are neither selfhood nor otherness breached or dissolved?

The core senses of self and other do not get disrupted for several reasons. Under normal conditions, the infant has experienced similar joyful cycles of suspense buildup and punch line in other, slightly

---

2. The idea of subjective states of fusion was born of two quite separate concepts. The first concept embraced pathological states seen in older children (*symbiotic psychosis*), in which the child experiences the dissolution of self/other boundaries and resultant feelings of fusion. It also embraces the wish for merger and the fear of engulfment, which are not uncommon clinical features in adult patients. The second concept is the now-familiar assumption that the infant experiences a protracted period of self/other undifferentiation. It was not a long retrospective leap backward in time to assume that if infants could not discriminate self from other, they too would experience states of self/other unity of merger like those reported by older patients. In this way, the notion of primary fusion experiences was historically inspired by the observation of secondary fusion experiences. Primary fusion was a pathomorphic, retrospective, secondary conceptualization.

different situations: "I'm gonna get you" games, "walking fingers," "tickle the tummy," and a host of other suspense games that are standard fare at this age. The infant is also likely to have experienced a dozen or more variations of the peek-a-boo game to begin with: diaper over baby's face, diaper over mother's face, mother's face gets covered by baby's feet as they are brought together, her face rises above and sets below the horizon of the bed, and so on. No matter how mother does it, the infant experiences her antics as belonging to her as a core other; this is only one of the many ways of experiencing her organization, cohesion, and agency.

Moreover, the same general feeling state is engendered in the infant, regardless of which way the mother plays the game. And it is likely that this family of games has been played with the infant by others—father, babysitter, and so on. The particular affect, then, remains, despite variations in the interaction and changes in the interactants. It is only the feeling state that belongs to the self, that is a self-invariant.

Variety is what permits the infant to triangulate and identify what invariants belong to whom. And normal parent/infant interactions are, of course, necessarily extremely variable. To highlight the crucial role of variety of experience in distinguishing self-invariants from other-invariants, imagine the following:

Suppose that an infant experienced joyful cycles of anticipation and resolution only with mother, and that mother always regulated these cycles in the *exact* same way (virtually impossible). That infant would be in a tricky spot. In this particular, unchanging activity, mother would be sensed as a core other because her behavior would obey most of the laws (agency, coherence, continuity) that specify others as against selves. However, the infant could not be sure to what extent his or her feeling state was an invariant property of self or of mother's behavior since both would invariably accompany this feeling. (This is close to the picture of self/other undifferentiation assumed by many, except that we have derived it from the mother's limitations rather than from the infant's.)

Under the normal conditions of inevitable variety, then, the infant should have no trouble in sensing who is who and what belongs to whom in these kinds of encounters. There are, however, many games and routines in which a great degree of similarity of behavior between parent and infant is the rule. May not these present a more difficult task for the infant in distinguishing self from other and from "us"? These include early forms of pat-a-cake, where mother makes her hands and the infant's hands do the same thing, various imitation routines, affect leading and following as in the mutual escalation of smiles, and many more. One could imagine that at such times the cues that specify self-invariants and other-invariants could partially break down, because in imitative interactions, the behavior of the other may be isomorphic (similarly contoured as far as intensity and vitality affects are concerned) and often simultaneous or even synchronous with the behavior of the infant. One might expect that these experiences are the ones that come closest to the notions of merging or of dissolution of self/other boundaries, at least on perceptual grounds (Stern 1980).

Even under these conditions, however, it is quite unlikely that enough of the differentiating cues can be obliterated. Infants' timing capacities are superb. They can detect split-second deviations from simultaneity. For instance, if a mother's face is shown to an infant of three months on a television screen but her voice is delayed by several hundred milliseconds, the infant picks up the discrepancy in synchrony and is disturbed by it, as by a badly dubbed movie (Trevarthan 1977; Dodd 1979). Similarly, it is the ability to estimate time in the split-second range that permits the infant to distinguish the sounds /ba/ and /pa/, which differ only in timing of voice onset (Eimas et al. 1971, 1978). Even if the parent could act like a perfect mirror, the memorial continuity of a core sense of self could not be obliterated.[3]

What happens to the sense of self in those mutual interactions

3. Moments of self/other similarity tend to occur at times of high arousal and retain throughout life their ability to establish a strong feeling of connectedness, similarity, or intimacy, for good or ill. Lovers assume similar postures and tend to move toward and away from one another roughly simultaneously, as in a courting dance. In a political discussion that divides a group into two camps, those of the same opinion will be found to share postural positions (Scheflin 1964). Mothers and infants, when feeling both happy and excited, will tend to vocalize together. This has been given several different names: coacting, chorusing, matching, and mimicking (Stern et al. 1975; Schaffer 1977).

On the negative side, staring, facial or postural mimicking, and "shadow-talking" are all used by children to infuriate peers or adults. There is something intolerably invasive in the sense of negative intimacy in these particular experiences of self/other similarity (not self/other unity). However, this sense of negative intimacy could not arise in infants in the domain of core-relatedness. It requires the assumption of the existence of separate other minds with intentions, and that is not available until the domain of intersubjective relatedness opens up later.

involving the regulation of the infant's security or state transformations? While these interactions are no more devoted to affective
alterations than the interactions already discussed, they are historically
considered more conducive to experiences of mergers. During these
experiences, the parent's behaviors are complementary to the infant's
(holding the infant, who is being held). In this sense, each partner
is generally doing something quite different from the other. The
intactness of self and other is therefore readily maintained, since the
perceptual cues reveal the other to be following a different temporal,
spatial, intensity, and/or movement organization from the self. In
other words, all the cues that specify self-invariants or other-
invariants (discussed in chapter 4) are undisturbed, so that no
confusion in the sense of self versus sense of other need occur at the
level of core-relatedness. It is thus reasonable that the sense of a core
self and a core other need not be breached by the presence of self-
regulating others, even when the experience concerns the infant's
affect state.

A second question now arises. What is the relationship between
the altered self-experience and the regulating role of the other who
helped alter the infant's self-experience? Or, more to the point, how
is that relationship experienced by the infant? We can answer for an
adult or older child. Sometimes it screams out and seems to fill the
entire attentional field, as in the powerful feelings of being with
someone when you are insecure or scared, being enfolded in that
person's arms and engulfed in something like security, of almost
falling into the other's personhood (what a normal "merger" experience is purportedly like).

At other times, the relationship between the altered self-experience
and the regulatory role of the other is silent and goes unnoticed.
This situation is analogous to the silent or invisible presence of the
"self-other" as well expressed in the terminology of Self Psychology
by Wolf (1980) and Stechler and Kaplan (1980).

> Setting aside, for the moment, any particular age-appropriate form of
> the selfobject need, one may compare the need for the continuous
> presence of a psychologically nourishing selfobject milieu with the
> continuing physiological need for an environment containing oxygen. It
> is a relatively silent need of which one becomes aware sharply only when
> it is not being met, when a harsh world compels one to draw the breath
> in pain. And so it goes also with the selfobject needs. As long as a person

is securely embedded in a social matrix that provides him with a field in which he can find, but does not have to be actually utilizing the needed mirroring responses and the needed availability of idealizable values, he will feel comfortably affirmed in his total self and, paradoxically, relatively self-reliant, self-sufficient, and autonomous. But, if by some adversity of events this person would find himself transported into a strange environment, it will be experienced as alien and even hostile, no matter how friendly it might be disposed toward him. Even strong selves tend to fragment under such circumstances. One can feel loneliest in a crowd. Solitude, psychological solitude, is the mother of anxiety. (Wolf 1980, p. 128)

Whether the relationship between altered self-experience and the regulating role of the other is obvious or unobtrusive, the alteration in self-experience always belongs entirely to the self. Even in the obvious situation of a security need being met, the other may appear to provide—may actually even seem to possess—the "security" before enfolding you. But the feeling of becoming secure belongs only to the self. In those situations when the regulatory role of the other goes unnoticed, the experience of self-alteration belongs only to the self by default.

The previous discussion addressed the question of who subjectively owns, so to speak, the alteration in self-experience—the self, the other, or some "we" or fused amalgam. The answer seems to be that it falls completely within the domain of the sense of self. This issue of subjective ownership, however, leaves unanswered the question of how the relationship is sensed.

Some relationship must come to exist between the change in self-experience and the regulating role, obvious or unobtrusive, of the other, simply because they tend to occur together. They become related as do any attributes of a repeated lived experience. They are not elements that are fused or confused; they are simply related. They are two of the more salient elements (that is, attributes) of any particular lived experience with a self-regulating other. Merger experiences at this age are simply a way of being with someone, but someone who acts as a self-regulating other. Any such lived experience includes: (1) significant alterations in the infant's feeling state that seem to belong to the self even though they were mutually created by self with an other, (2) the other person, as seen, heard, and felt at the moment of the alteration, (3) an intact sense of a core self and core other against which all this occurs, and (4) a variety of contextual and situational events. How can all of these be yoked to form a subjective unit that is neither a fusion nor a we-self nor a cool cognitive association between distinct selves and others? This yoking occurs in the form of an actual episode of life as lived. The lived episode—just as in memory—is the unit that locks the different attributes of the experience into relationships one with the other. The relationships are those that prevailed at the actual happening.

Viewed this way, the altering self-experiences and the regulatory role of the other are not simply associated in a learned way. Rather, they are embraced by a larger common unit of subjective experience, the episode, that includes them both along with other attributes and preserves their natural relations. Similarly, the altering self-experience and the perceptions of the other do not have to collapse into one another and become fused or confused. Rather, they can remain as distinct and separate components of the larger subjective unit, the episode.

Lived episodes immediately become the specific episodes for memory, and with repetition they become generalized episodes as described in chapter 4. They are generalized episodes of interactive experience that are mentally represented—that is, representations of interactions that have been generalized, or RIGs. For example, after the first game of peek-a-boo the infant lays down the memory of the specific episode. After the second, third, or twelfth experience of slightly different episodes, the infant will have formed a RIG of peek-a-boo. It is important to remember that RIGs are flexible structures that average several actual instances and form a prototype to represent them all. A RIG is something that has never happened before exactly that way, yet it takes into account nothing that did not actually happen once.

The experience of being with a self-regulating other gradually forms RIGs. And these memories are retrievable whenever one of the attributes of the RIG is present. When an infant has a certain feeling, that feeling will call to mind the RIG of which the feeling is an attribute. Attributes are thus recall cues to reactivate the lived experience. And whenever a RIG is activated, it packs some of the wallop of the originally lived experience in the form of an active memory.

I am suggesting that each of the many different self-regulating other relationships with the same person will have its own distinctive RIG. And when different RIGs are activated, the infant re-experiences different forms or ways of being with a self-regulating other. The activation of different RIGs can influence different regulatory functions, ranging from the biological and physiological to the psychic.[4]

Another question concerns the issue of being with self-regulating others who are present as compared with those who are absent, which in turn brings up the issue of "internalized" relationships. If the lines of argument presented here are followed, the distinction between present and absent self-regulating other does not loom so large, because in both cases infants must deal with their history with others. And this involves the subjective experience of being with an historical self-regulating other that may best be captured by the notion of being with an *evoked companion*.

Evoked Companions

Whenever a RIG of being with someone (who has changed self-experience) is activated, the infant encounters an evoked companion. This can be conceptualized as shown schematically in figure 5.1.

Suppose that the infant has already experienced six roughly similar specific episodes of a type of interaction with a self-regulating other. These specific episodes will be generalized and encoded as a Repre-

---

4. In discussing the psychobiology of bereavement in light of animal experimentation, Hofer remarks,

> Could the elements of the inner life that we experience with people who are close to us come to serve as biological regulators, much the way the actual sensorimotor interactions with the mother act for the infant animal in our experiments? And could this link internal object relations to biological systems? I think this may be possible. Certainly associative or Pavlovian conditioning is a well-known mechanism by which symbolic cues, and even internal time sense, can come to control physiological responses. Thus, it seems possible that the regulating action of important human relationships upon biological systems may be transduced, not only by sensorimotor and temporal patterning of the actual interactions, but also by the internal experiences of the relationship as it is carried out in the minds of the people involved. A permanent loss is sustained at both levels of organization, so that both representational and actual interactions are affected by the reality of the event. (Hofer 1983, p. 15)

Field (in press), in her work on the response of infants to extended maternal separation, reaches toward a similar conclusion as Reite et al. (1981) in their work on infant monkeys.

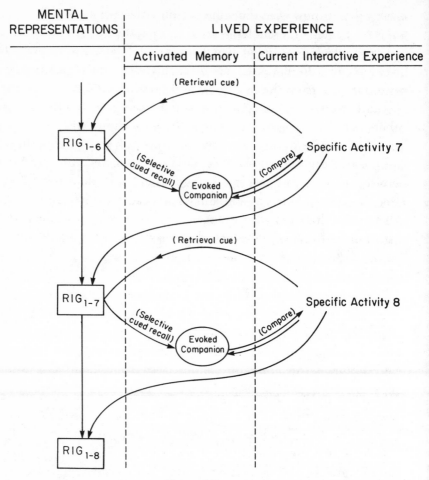

Figure 5.1

sentation of Interaction that has been Generalized (RIG_{1-6}). When a similar but not identical specific episode is next encountered (specific episode #7), some of its attributes act as a retrieval cue to the RIG_{1-6}. The RIG_{1-6} is a representation and not an activated memory. The retrieval cue evokes from the RIG an activated memory which I will call an *evoked companion*. The evoked companion is an experience of being with, or in the presence of, a self-regulating other, which may occur in or out of awareness. The companion is evoked from the RIG not as the recall of an actual past happening, but as an active exemplar of such happenings. This conceptualization seems necessary to explain the form in which such events are encountered in clinical and everyday life—to put some experiential flesh on an abstract representation. Abstract representations such as RIGs are not experienced in the form of life as lived. They must be instantiated in the form of an activated memory that can be part of lived experience.[5] (The evoked companion is not a companion in the sense of a comrade but in the sense of a particular instance of one who accompanies another.)

The evoked companion functions to evaluate the specific ongoing interactive episode. The current interactive experience (specific episode #7) is compared with the simultaneously occurring experience with the evoked companion. This comparison serves to determine what new contributions the current specific episode (#7) can make in revising the RIG_{1-6}. To the extent that specific episode #7 is unique, it will result in some alteration in the RIG, from RIG_{1-6} to RIG_{1-7}. The RIG will thus be slightly different when it is later encountered by the next specific episode (#8), and so on. In this fashion RIGs are slowly updated by current experience. However, the more past experience there is, the less relative impact for change any single specific episode will have. History builds up inertia. (This is essentially what Bowlby means in stating that working models of mother, a different unit of representation from RIGs, are conservative.)

Evoked companions can also be called into active memory during episodes when the infant is alone but when historically similar episodes involved the presence of a self-regulating other. For instance, if a six-month-old, when alone, encounters a rattle and manages to grasp it and shake it enough so that it makes a sound, the initial pleasure may quickly become extreme delight and exuberance, expressed in smiling, vocalizing, and general body wriggling. The extreme delight and exuberance is not only the result of successful mastery, which may account for the initial pleasure, but also the historical result of similar past moments in the presence of a delight- and exuberance-enhancing (regulating) other. It is partly a social response, but in this instance it occurs in a nonsocial situation. At such moments, the initial pleasure born of successful mastery acts as a retrieval cue to activate the RIG, resulting in an imagined interaction with an evoked companion that includes the shared and mutually induced delight about the successful mastery. It is in this way that

5. Psychoanalysis also struggles with the same problems in considering representations. Are they to be treated as images in memory, concepts, abstractions, or a report on overall mental functioning about a focus of interest (see Friedman 1980)?

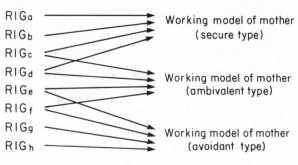

Figure 5.2

an evoked companion serves to add another dimension to the experience, in this case, extra delight and exuberance. So that even if actually alone, the infant is "being with" a self-regulating other in the form of an activated memory of prototypic lived events. The current experience now includes the presence (in or out of awareness) of an evoked companion.

The notion of RIGs and evoked companions bears important similarities to and differences from other postulated phenomena, such as the "working models of mother" in attachment theory, the selfobjects in Self Psychology, merger experiences in Mahlerian theory, early proto-forms of internalization in classical psychoanalytic theory, and "we" experiences (Stechler and Kaplan 1980). All these notions have arisen to fill a clinical need and a theoretical void.

The concept of the RIG and the evoked companion and the working model of attachment are different in several respects. First, they are of a different size and order. An individual RIG concerns the representation of a specific type of interaction. A working model concerns an assembly of many such interactions into a larger representation of a person's repertoire under certain conditions. The RIG can be conceptualized as the basic building block from which working models are constructed. This is shown schematically in figure 5.2.

Working models, as a larger construct, change as new RIGs are included and others are deleted and as the hierarchical structure of RIGs that constitute the working model are reorganized. Nonetheless, there has recently been a remarkable confluence of concern with the nature of the earliest representations or internal working models of mother. The current work of Sroufe (1985), Sroufe and Fleeson (1985), Bretherton (in press), and Main and Kaplan (in press) is all consistent with the general outlines of this approach. They have also found it necessary to turn to episodic memory as a fundamental process in the formation of these personal representations.

Second, RIGs are different from the working model of attachment theory in that working models, at least historically, concern expectations about the regulation primarily of security-attachment states. RIGs embody expectations about any and all interactions that can result in mutually created alterations in self-experience, such as arousal, affect, mastery, physiological state, state of consciousness, and curiosity, and not just those related to attachment.

Finally, the working model is conceived in highly cognitive terms and operates much like a schema that detects deviations from average expectation. The evoked companion as an activated RIG is conceived in terms of episodic memory and lends itself better to the affective nature of being with others, since the affective attributes of the lived and retrieved experience do not get transformed into cognitive terms that simply appraise and guide. In this sense, also, the evoked companion comes closer to the vividness of subjective experience, rather than taking the more experientially remote position of a guiding model. Nonetheless, evoked companions function like working models in two respects. First, they are prototypic memories that are not restricted to one past occurrence. Rather they represent the accumulated past history of a type of interaction with an other. Second, they serve a guiding function in the sense of the past creating expectations of the present and future.

The concept of the RIG and evoked companion differs importantly from selfobjects and mergers, in that the integrity of core sense of self and other is never breached in the presence of an evoked companion. It is also distinct from a "we" experience in that it is felt as an I-experience *with* an other. Finally, it differs from internalizations in that these in their final form are experienced as internal signals (symbolic cues), rather than as lived or reactivated experiences.

At some point in development there is no longer the necessity to retrieve the evoked companion and get a dose of the lived experience. The attribute alone serves as a cue that alters behavior, without a reliving of the generalized event. (This is no different from Pavlov's concepts of secondary signals in classical conditioning.) It remains an empirical question when this happens developmentally and whether, or under what circumstances, the secondary signal (the attribute) is really acting all alone or whether it usually activates the evoked companion to some extent. In either case, evoked companions never disappear. They lie dormant throughout life, and while they are always retrievable, their degree of activation is variable. In states of great disequilibrium such as loss, activation is very manifest.

Evoked companions operate during actual interactions with another person, as well as in the absence of others. They operate by becoming activated, so that a self-regulating other becomes "present" in the form of an active memory. Even during such interactions, in the presence of an other, evoked companions function to tell the infant what is now happening. They are a record of the past informing the present. For instance, if a mother plays a game of peek-a-boo in a very different manner from usual (let's say she is depressed and just going through the motions), the infant will use the companion evoked from the peek-a-boo RIG as a standard against which to check whether the current episode is something significantly changed, to be marked as a special variation, or an entirely new type of self-regulating-other experience. In this way evoked companions help to evaluate expectations and perform a stabilizing and regulating function for self-experience. This sounds like a working model in operation. But the detection of deviation may come about subjectively, in differences in the "presence" and "feel" of the evoked companion compared with the "actual" partner.

So far, we have discussed the use of RIGs mainly in the presence of the other, in fact, during an actual episode with the other. When that is the case, the infant needs only recognition memory to call to mind the evoked companion that is stored in memory, since the actual episode is happening now before the infant. But what about the retrieval of evoked companions in the absence of the other? This, after all, is when the concept of internalization is most generally needed for clinical purposes. The lived episode of being with an other must be recalled when the other is no longer present, requiring recall or evocative memory. It has traditionally been assumed that the infant's recall memory is not adequate to evoke the presence of someone absent until the age of nine to twelve months or so, as evidenced by separation reactions. Some theorists place the timing for evoking absent partners even later, in the second year, when symbolic functioning is available to be enlisted in the task of evocation. That would put these matters beyond the age period we are now considering. From what has already been said (see chapter 3), however, the evidence supports the view that the infant is capable of acts of cued recall memory beginning in the third month of life and perhaps before.[6]

In light of the infant's cued recall memory and memory for interpersonal happenings in terms of RIGs, it seems likely that the

6. It is generally assumed that the infant's elaboration of a "separation response" at nine months or so is the first major evidence of recall memory for interpersonal events. In addition to the other evidence of prior recall memory, there are several problems with this assumption. Schaffer et al. (1972), Kagan et al. (1978), and McCall (1979), among others, have criticized the more traditional view that separation distress comes about solely because the maturation of memory processes permits an internal representation of mother, so that at her departure the infant can evoke her memory and compare it against the condition of her absence, which reveals the infant's aloneness. Kagan et al. (1978), most notably, have raised such questions as, Why does the infant cry as the mother is moving away but still in sight? Why does the baby not cry when she leaves to go into the kitchen for the hundredth time that morning?

An alternate interpretation, basically similar to that proposed by Schaffer et al. (1972), suggests that two processes must come to maturation in order to produce separation distress. The first is the necessary, but not sufficient, condition that the infant has an enhanced ability to retrieve and hold a schema of past experience, that is, to evoke with recall memory an internal representation of the other. The traditional explanation stops here. The second necessary maturational ability to emerge at this age is the ability to generate anticipations of the future-representations of possible events. Kagan et al. (1978) describe this new capacity as the "disposition to attempt to predict future events and to generate response to deal with discrepant situations" (p. 110). If the child cannot generate a prediction or an instrumental response to deal with the prediction, uncertainty and distress result.

It may prove more helpful to break these two processes necessary for the separation reactions into three distinct processes: an improved recall (evocative) memory; the ability to generate future-representations of possible events; and the ability to generate communicative or instrumental responses to deal with the uncertainty and distress that are caused by incongruencies between present events and future representations of events. It is generally agreed that recall or evocative memory improves greatly toward the end of the first year of life. However, it is also clear that some recall memory is functioning long before the advent of separation distress at nine months. The notion, then, of "out of sight, out of mind" until nine months or so and "out of sight, but potentially in mind," thanks to recall memory (for people) after nine months, is not as clearcut as it seems.

In holding this view, we are closer both to Freud's original notion (1900) of the "hallucinated breast," in which he essentially invokes the newborn's use of cued recall memory (without calling it that), and to the recent findings on cued recall we have already alluded to. What Freud called the "hallucinated breast" could be called an attribute of a generalized episode of feeding. We would say that hunger acted as the cue to recall the other attribute, the breast. Freud would say that hunger created the tension that pushed for discharge, and in the face of a blocked motor discharge pathway, the impulse backed up and sought discharge through a sensory pathway, resulting in the hallucination. The sensory discharge was adaptive in that it would momentarily relieve the hunger, by the same amount as the sensory discharge reduced the tension.

Instead of emphasizing the discharge value of using a prototypic episode, we stress its organizing and regulating value. And instead of emphasizing the use of prototypic episodes under the presence of an acute need, we emphasize its continuous use in regulating and stabilizing all ongoing experience by providing continuity, that is, by contextualizing every experience in a history that is always being upgraded.

infant has almost constant rememberings (out of awareness) of previous interactions, both in the actual presence and in the absence of the other person involved in the interactions. I suggest that Freud's original model of the "hallucinated breast" was descriptively right, although it relied on the wrong mechanism. Whenever an infant encounters one part or attribute of a lived episode, the other attributes of that generalized episode (RIG) will be called to mind. Various evoked companions will be almost constant companions in everyday life. Is it not so for adults when they are not occupied with tasks? How much time each day do we spend in imagined interactions that are either memories, or the fantasied practice of upcoming events, or daydreams?

Another way to put all of this is that the infant's life is so thoroughly social that most of the things the infant does, feels, and perceives occur in different kinds of relationships. An evoked companion or internal representation or working model or fantasied union with mother is no more or less than the history of specific kinds of relationships (in Bowlby's terms, 1980) or the prototypic memory of many specific ways of being with mother, in our terms. Once cued recall memory has begun to function, subjective experiences are largely social, regardless of whether we are alone or not. In fact, because of memory we are rarely alone, even (perhaps especially) during the first half-year of life. The infant engages with real external partners some of the time and with evoked companions almost all the time. Development requires a constant, usually silent, dialogue between the two.

This view of being almost continuously with real and evoked companions encompasses what is generally meant when one says that the infant has learned to be trustful or secure in exploring the surrounding world. What could create trust or security in exploring, initially, if not the memory of past experiences with self and other in exploratory contexts? The infant is, in subjective fact, not alone but accompanied by evoked companions, drawn from several RIGs, who operate at various levels of activation and awareness. The infant is therefore trustful. This is a more subjective and more experience-near version of a working model.

The notion of self-with-other as a subjective reality is thus almost pervasive. This subjective sense of being-with (intrapsychically and extrapsychically) is always an active mental act of construction, however, not a passive failure of differentiation. It is not an error of maturation, nor a regression to earlier periods of undifferentiation. Seen in this way, the experiences of being-with are not something like the "delusion of dual-unity" or mergers that one needs to grow out of, dissolve, and leave behind. They are permanent, healthy parts of the mental landscape that undergo continual growth and elaboration. They are the active constitutions of a memory that encodes, integrates, and recalls experience, and thereby guides behavior.

BRIDGING THE INFANT'S SUBJECTIVE WORLD AND THE MOTHER'S SUBJECTIVE WORLD

We have discussed only the infant's subjective world and its relation to those interactive events that are observable to all. This was schematized in figure 5.1. But that is only half of the story. The mother also participates in the same observable interactive episodes, and she too brings her own history to influence her subjective experience of the ongoing observable interaction. In effect, the observable interaction in which both partners participate is the bridge between two potentially quite separate subjective worlds. In principle the dyadic system is symmetrical. The observable interaction acts at the interface. It is not symmetrical in practice, however, because the mother brings so much more personal history to each encounter. She has not only a working model of her infant, but a working model of her own mother (see Main 1985), a working model of her husband (who the baby may frequently remind her of), and various other working models, all of which will come into play.

Accordingly, we can expand figure 5.1 to include the mother's half as shown in figure 5.3. For the purpose of this expansion, what was called the "evoked companion" of the infant in figure 5.1 will be called more generically the "subjective experience of the observable event." To illustrate how this schematization might work, imagine a specific interactive episode: a baby boy, Joey, makes repeated attempts for attention, while mother ignores or refuses to acknowledge his appeals. This specific episode will evoke from the memories of both infant and mother a subjective experience in light of which the currently occurring interactive episode is apprehended. On the mother's side assume that the specific episode has evoked a particular RIG_k that is part of the mother's working model of her own mother (as indicated in figure 5.3). RIG_k, for example, is the

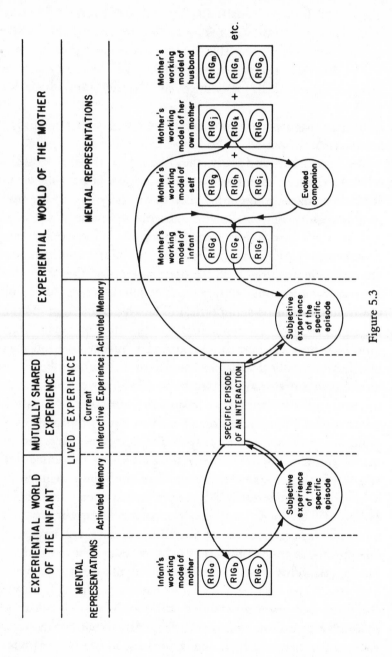

Figure 5.3

specific representation of how the mother's mother tended to meet the appeals for attention (of Joey's mother when she was a child) with disdain and aversion. This particular aspect of the mother's mother becomes activated in the form of an evoked companion (a "ghost in the nursery," in Fraiberg's words, 1974). The evoked companion then plays a role in determining the choice of RIG_c to be evoked within the mother's working model of her own infant, Joey. The generalized interaction represented in RIG_c might be something like: Joey is always making unwanted, unreasonable demands for attention that are unpleasant. The evocation of the particular RIG_c will largely determine the mother's subjective experience of Joey's present appeal for attention.

In a similar fashion, the infant is forming a different subjective experience, from his past history, of the ongoing specific episode. It is in this way that the observable interactive event acts as a bridge between the two subjective worlds of infant and mother. In principal, this formulation is no different from that used in a global way by most psychodynamically-oriented clinicians. However, because it is conceptualized with more specificity and implies various discrete hierarchically arranged units and processes it may prove helpful in advancing our thinking about how maternal fantasies and attributions can influence not only the observable interaction but ultimately the shape of the infant's fantasies and attributions. It may also prove helpful in understanding how therapeutic interventions may operate to alter the parent's view of what her infant is doing and who that infant is. Further exploration of this enormous area is beyond the scope of this book, but active efforts in this direction are underway.[7]

We have attempted to retrieve what was missing in the last chapter, namely, the very social nature and presumably social subjective experience of the infant in the domain of core relatedness. There is one final issue to consider, which extends the social nature of the infant's experience even further.

7. Dr. Cramer and I are currently studying the interplay between the levels of observable interaction and maternal fantasies as well as the impact of intervention on both. (See B. Cramer and D. Stern, "A bridge between minds: How do the mother's and infant's subjective worlds meet?" [In preparation, to be presented at the World Association of Infant Psychiatry and Allied Professions, Stockholm, August 1986].) The above schematization was greatly contributed to by Dr. Cramer's group in Geneva.

Self-Regulating Experiences with Inanimate Things

Self-regulating experiences with things that have become personified can also occur at this age and level of relatedness. Such events fall at an early point on the developmental line that later includes transitional objects (like security blankets, which stand for and can be freely substituted for persons) and even later the larger realm of transitional phenomena embracing the worlds of art, as Winnicott (1971) has taught us.

During this period the mother very often enters into the infant's play by lending some things animate properties. She manipulates toys so that they swoop in and out and speak and tickle. They take on the organic rhythms and feelings of force, that is, the vitality affects of persons. And they elicit in the infant feeling states that are generally only elicited by persons. Both while and immediately after the mother imbues a toy with the actions, motions, vitality affects, and other invariant attributes of persons, the infant's interest in the toy is heightened. It is one of mother's main ways of maintaining the general flow of the infant's play with things. Once she has so imbued an object and withdraws, the infant is likely to continue to explore it alone, so long as it has the afterglow of personification. It has become, for the moment, a self-regulating person-thing, because like a self-regulating other it can dramatically alter experience of self.[8]

Well before the age of six months, infants appear to be able to discriminate animate from inanimate—that is, persons from things (Sherrod 1981). This means that they have identified the invariants that generally specify one or the other. Given this situation, a person-

---

8. We will encounter this again when the child starts to learn words, for a word can also become a personified thing. Fernald and Mazzie (1983) have shown that when a mother teaches a fourteen-month-old child the names of things, she uses a predictable strategy. When she wishes to mark a new or novel word in contrast to an old or familiar one, she does so by marking it with increased and exaggerated pitch contours, using both sharp pitch rises and rise-fall contours. Fernald points out that these marked pitch contours are intrinsically attention-getting, but she also implies that there is more to it than that. The most qualitatively special things to infants are the social behaviors of persons that are eliciting of and expressive of human vitality affects and regular emotions. When the mother intonationally marks a word, she is not simply raising the infant's attention nonspecifically; she is imbuing one particular word with human magic by making it a person-thing for the moment.

performed-thing will be viewed by the infant as some form of composite entity, a thing that has taken on some of the characteristics of a person. It has some of the invariant properties of both. The infant maintains an intact sense of things versus persons. The wonder of a personified thing lies in a successful constructionistic effort. It, too, is a success of integration, not a failure of differentiation.

At this point in the infant's development, a personified thing is a short-lived self-regulating person-thing. It is different, in several respects, from Winnicott's transitional objects: (1) the transitional object appears developmentally later; (2) the transitional object involves symbolic thinking, while the person-thing can be accounted for by episodic memory; (3) the existence of the transitional object, Winnicott assumed, implies some remaining lack of (or regression toward) self/other undifferentiation, while a personified thing does not.

The phenomena of self-regulating others and personified things indicate the degree to which the subjective world of infants is deeply social. They experience a sense of a core self and other, and along with these, they experience a pervasive sense of self being with other in multiple forms. All of these forms of being-with are active constructions. They will grow and become elaborated in the course of development, a process that results in the progressive socializing of experience.

Chapter 6

The Sense of a Subjective Self: I. Overview

THE NEXT QUANTUM LEAP in the sense of self occurs when the infant discovers that he or she has a mind and that other people have minds as well. Between the seventh and ninth month of life, infants gradually come upon the momentous realization that inner subjective experiences, the "subject matter" of the mind, are potentially shareable with someone else. The subject matter at this point in development can be as simple and important as an intention to act ("I want that cookie"), a feeling state ("This is exciting"), or a focus of attention ("Look at that toy"). This discovery amounts to the acquisition of a "theory" of separate minds. Only when infants can sense that others distinct from themselves can hold or entertain a mental state that is similar to one they sense themselves to be holding is the sharing of subjective experience or intersubjectivity possible (Trevarthan and Hubley 1978). The infant must arrive at a theory not only of separate minds but of "interfaceable separate minds" (Bretherton and Bates 1979; Bretherton et al. 1981). It is not, of course, a full-blown theory. It is rather a working notion that says something like, what is going on in my mind may be similar enough to what is going on in your mind that we can somehow communicate this (without words) and thereby experience intersubjectivity. For such an experience to occur, there must be some shared framework of meaning and means of communication such as gesture, posture, or facial expression.

When it does occur, the interpersonal action has moved, in part, from overt actions and responses to the internal subjective states that lie behind the overt behaviors. This shift gives the infant a different "presence" and social "feel." Parents generally begin to treat the infant differently and address themselves more to the subjective domain of experience. This sense of the self and other is quite different from what was possible in the domain of core-relatedness. Infants now have a new organizing subjective perspective about their social lives. The potential properties of a self and of an other have been greatly expanded. Selves and others now include inner or subjective states of experience in addition to the overt behaviors and direct sensations that marked the core self and other. With this expansion in the nature of the sensed self, the capacity for relatedness and the subject matter with which it is concerned catapult the infant into a new *domain of intersubjective relatedness*. A new organizing subjective perspective about the self emerges.

What relation does this new perspective bear to the already present sense of a core self? Intersubjective relatedness is built on the foundation of core-relatedness. Core-relatedness, with its establishment of the physical and sensory distinctions of self and other, is the necessary precondition, since the possibility of sharing subjective experiences has no meaning unless it is a transaction that occurs against the surety of a physically distinct and separate self and other. While intersubjective relatedness transforms the interpersonal world, however, core-relatedness continues. Intersubjective relatedness does not displace it; nothing ever will. It is the existential bedrock of interpersonal relations. When the domain of intersubjective relatedness is added, core-relatedness and intersubjective relatedness coexist and interact. Each domain affects the experience of the other.

When this leap in the sense of self occurs, how does the interpersonal world appear to be different? Empathy on the part of the caregiver now becomes a different experience. It is one thing for a younger infant to respond to the overt behavior that reflects a mother's empathy, such as a soothing behavior at the right moment. In the younger infant the empathic *process* itself goes unnoticed, and only the empathic *response* is registered. It is quite another thing for the infant to sense that an empathic process bridging the two minds has been created. The caregiver's empathy, that process crucial to the infant's development, now becomes a direct subject of the infant's experience.

At this stage, for the first time, one can attribute to the infant the capacity for psychic intimacy—the openness to disclosure, the permeability or interpenetrability that occurs between two people (Hinde 1979). Psychic intimacy as well as physical intimacy is now possible. The desire to know and be known in this sense of mutually revealing subjective experience is great. In fact, it can be a powerful motive and can be felt as a need-state. (The refusal to be known psychically can also be experienced with great power.)

Finally, with the advent of intersubjectivity, the parents' socialization of the infant's subjective experience comes to be at issue. Is subjective experience to be shared? How much of it is to be shared? What kinds of subjective experience are to be shared? What are the consequences of sharing and not sharing? Once the infant gets the first glimpse of the intersubjective domain and the parents realize this, they must begin to deal with these issues. What is ultimately at stake is nothing less than discovering what part of the private world of inner experience is shareable and what part falls outside the pale of commonly recognized human experiences. At one end is psychic human membership, at the other psychic isolation.

The Background of the Focus on Intersubjectivity

Given the far-reaching consequences of this quantum leap in the sense of self, how did it happen that we have been so slow to come upon the infant's discovery of intersubjective relatedness? Historically, several streams of inquiry flowed together to produce the recognition of this major developmental step. Philosophy has long dealt with the issue of separate minds. The necessity of assuming a developmental point when infants acquired a theory or working sense of separate minds is not alien to philosophical inquiry and, in fact, was often tacitly assumed (Habermas 1972; Hamlyn 1974; MacMurray 1961; Cavell 1984). Psychology, on the other hand, has been slower to deal with this issue in these terms, largely because the study of the development of subjective experience with persons, in comparison with the study of the development of knowledge of things, has been relatively neglected in recent academic psychology. Only now is the pendulum starting to swing back the other way, and pioneers such as Baldwin (1902), who firmly designated subjective experience of the self and other as the starting units for a developmental psychology, are being rediscovered in this country, as is Wallon (1949) in Europe.

Psychoanalysis has always been intensely concerned with the subjective experience of individuals. Except in the very special case of therapeutic empathy, however, it has not conceptualized intersubjective experience as a dyadic event, and this conceptualization is necessary to a generic view of intersubjectivity. It is also possible that the dominance of separation/individuation theory to explain the life period under discussion acted as an obstacle to a fuller appreciation of the role of intersubjectivity.

To be more specific on this point, ego psychoanalytic theory has viewed the period after seven to nine months as the time of emerging more fully ("hatching" is the metaphor) from the undifferentiated and fused state that preceded it. This phase was predominantly devoted to establishing a separate and individuated self, to dissolving merger experiences, and to forming a more autonomous self that could interact with a more separated other. Given this view of the major life task of this period, it is not surprising that the theory failed to notice that the appearance of intersubjective relatedness permitted, for the first time, the creation of mutually held mental states and allowed for the reality-based joining (even merging) of inner experience. Paradoxically, it is only with the advent of intersubjectivity that anything like the joining of subjective psychic experience can actually occur. And this is indeed what the leap to an intersubjective sense of self and other makes possible, just at the developmental moment when traditional theory had the tide beginning to flow the other way. In the present view, both separation/individuation and new forms of experiencing union (or being-with) emerge equally out of the same experience of intersubjectivity.[1]

1. The point is not to exchange symbiosis for intersubjectivity and reverse the order of developmental tasks. The point is that intersubjectivity is equally crucial for creating experiences of being with a mentally similar other and for furthering individuation and autonomy, just as core-relatedness is equally crucial for both physical autonomy and togetherness.

In spite of a general disregard of intersubjective experience as a dyadic phenomenon, theorists have regularly appeared, often just outside of the mainstream, who have held positions receptive to the concept of intersubjectivity or subjective relatedness. Vygotsky's notion of the "intermental" (1962), Fairbairn's of the infant's innate interpersonal relatedness (1949), and MacMurray's of the field of the personal (1961) as well as Sullivan's of the interpersonal field (1953), are influential examples. It was against this background that the recent findings of the developmentalists acted to bring the developmental leap of intersubjectivity into its present sharp focus. It is not surprising that these developmentalists were largely interested either in the role of intentionality in the mother-infant interaction or in how infants acquire language. Both routes would ultimately lead to the issue of intersubjectivity and its underlying assumptions, which the philosophers had long been dealing with.

The Evidence for Intersubjective Relatedness

What, then, is the evidence for the appearance of intersubjective relatedness at seven to nine months? Trevarthan and Hubley (1978) have provided a definition of intersubjectivity that can be operationalized: "a deliberately sought sharing of experiences about events and things." What subjective experiences does the infant give evidence of sharing or, at least, expecting the mother to share?

Recall that infants at this point in development are still preverbal. The subjective experiences that they can share must be of a kind that do not require translation into language. Three mental states that are of great relevance to the interpersonal world and yet do not require language come to mind. These are sharing joint attention, sharing intentions, and sharing affective states. What behaviors do infants show to suggest that they can conduct or appreciate these sharings?

128

SHARING THE FOCUS OF ATTENTION

The gesture of pointing and the act of following another's line of vision are among the first overt acts that permit inferences about the sharing of attention, or the establishing of joint attention. Mothers point and infants point. Let us start with the mother's pointing. For her pointing to work, the infant must know to stop looking at the pointing hand itself and look in the direction it indicates, to the target. For a long time it was believed that infants could not do this until well into their second year because they could not escape their egocentric position. But Murphy and Messer (1977) showed that nine-month-olds do indeed detach their gaze from the pointing hand and follow the imaginary line to the target. "What has been mastered at this stage is a procedure for homing in on the attentional focus of another. It is a disclosure and discovery routine . . . highly generative within the limited world inhabited by the infant in the sense that it is not limited to specific kinds of objects. It has, moreover, equipped the child with a technique for transcending egocentrism, for insofar as he can appreciate another's line of regard and decipher their marking intentions, he has plainly achieved a basis for what Piaget has called decentration, using a coordinate system for the world other than the one of which he is the center" (Bruner 1977, 276). Earlier than nine months, infants show a preliminary form of this discovery procedure: they follow the mother's line of vision when she turns her head (Scaife and Bruner 1975), just as the mother follows the infant's line of vision (Collis and Schaffer 1975).

So far, we have seen only a routine or procedure for discovering another's attentional focus. Infants of nine months, however, do more than that. They not only visually follow the direction of the point but, after reaching the target, look back at the mother and appear to use the feedback from her face to confirm that they have arrived at the intended target. This is now more than a discovery procedure. It is a deliberate attempt to validate whether the joint attention has been achieved, that is, whether the focus of attention is being shared, although the infant is not self-aware of these operations.

Similarly, infants begin to point at about nine months of age, though they do so less frequently than mothers do. When they do, their gaze alternates between the target and the mother's face, as when she is pointing to see if she has joined in to share the attentional focus.[2] It seems reasonable to assume that, even prior to pointing, the infant's beginning capacity to move about, to crawl or cruise, is crucial in discovering alternative perspectives as is necessary for joint attention. In moving about, the infant continually alters the perspective held on some known stationary sight. Perhaps this initial acceptance of serially different perspectives is a necessary precursor to the more generic "realization" that others can be using a different coordinate system from the infant's own.

These observations lead one to infer that by nine months infants have some sense that they can have a particular attentional focus, that mother can also have a particular attentional focus, that these two mental states can be similar or not, and that if they are not, they can be brought into alignment and shared. *Inter-attentionality* becomes a reality.

SHARING INTENTIONS

Researchers interested in infants' language acquisition have naturally been drawn to look at the most immediate origins of language use. These origins include the gestures, postures, actions, and nonverbal vocalizations that infants display just prior to and presumably as a precursor to language. Such protolinguistic forms have been examined closely by a number of researchers, all of whom agree in one way or another that beginning at about nine months the infant intends to communicate (Bloom 1973, 1983; Brown 1973; Bruner 1975, 1977, 1981; Dore 1975, 1979; Halliday 1975; Bates 1976, 1979; Ninio and Bruner 1977; Shields 1978; Bates et al. 1979; Bretherton and Bates 1979; Harding and Golinkoff 1979; Trevarthan 1980; Harding 1982). The intention to communicate is different from the intention simply to influence another person. Bates (1979) provides a working definition of intentional communication that we can use:

> Intentional communication is signaling behavior in which the sender is aware, a priori, of the effect that the signal will have on his listener, and he persists in that behavior until the effect is obtained or failure is clearly indicated. The behavioral evidence that permits us to infer the

2. Pointing is thought to originate in reaching, which gradually gets converted into a gesture (Bower 1974; Trevarthan 1974; Vygotsky 1966). In reaching, prior to age nine months, the child does not check back to mother's face; after nine months, in reaching that is more gesture than action, the infant does.

presence of communicative intentions includes (a) alternations in eye gaze contact between the goal and the intended listeners, (b) augmentations, additions, and substitution of signals until the goal has been obtained, and (c) changes in the form of the signal towards abbreviated and/or exaggerated patterns that are appropriate only for achieving a communicative goal (p. 36).

The most straightforward and common examples of intentional communication are protolinguistic forms of requesting. For example, the mother is holding something the infant wants—say, a cookie. The infant reaches out a hand, palm up towards mother, and while making grasping movements and looking back and forth between hand and mother's face intones, "Eh! Eh!" with an imperative prosody (Dore 1975).[3] These acts, which are directed at a referent person, imply that the infant attributes an internal mental state to that person—namely, comprehension of the infant's intention and the capacity to intend to satisfy that intention. Intentions have become shareable experiences. *Interintentionality* becomes a reality. Once again, it need not be self-aware.

Soon after nine months of age, the beginning of jokes and teasing on the infant's part can be seen. Dunn has observed the interactions between older and younger siblings and has richly described many subtle events between them that imply that they have shared moments of intersubjectivity. For instance, a three-year-old and a one-year-old suddenly burst into laughter over a private joke for which no one else can find the eliciting cause. Similar eruptions of teasing episodes occur that also remain opaque to adult comprehension (Dunn 1982; Dunn and Kendrick 1979, 1982). Such events require the attribution of shareable mental states that involve intentions and expectations. You can't tease other people unless you can correctly guess what is "in their minds" and make them suffer or laugh because of your knowing.

SHARING AFFECTIVE STATES

Can infants also attribute shareable affective states to their social partners? A group of researchers (Emde et al. 1978; Klinert 1978;

3. This can rapidly become a "give and take" game, as commented on by Spitz (1965) and Piaget (1954). For a list of related examples see Trevarthan and Hubley (1978) and Bretherton et al. (1981).

Campos and Stenberg 1980; Emde and Sorce 1983; Klinert et al. 1983) have described a phenomenon they call social referencing.

The year-old infants are placed in a situation bound to create uncertainty, usually ambivalence between approach and withdrawal. The infant may be lured with an attractive toy to crawl across a "visual cliff" (an apparent drop-off, which is mildly frightening at one year of age or so) or may be approached by an unusual but highly stimulating object such as a bleeping, flashing robot like R2D2 from *Star Wars*. When the infants encounter these situations and give evidence of uncertainty, they look towards mother to read her face for its affective content, essentially to see what they should feel, to get a second appraisal to help resolve their uncertainty. If the mother has been instructed to show facial pleasure by smiling, the infant crosses the visual cliff. If the mother has been instructed to show facial fear, the infant turns back from the "cliff," retreats, and perhaps becomes upset. Similarly, if the mother smiles at the robot, the infant will too. If she shows fear, the infant will become more wary. The point for our purposes is that infants would not check with the mother in this fashion unless they attributed to her the capacity to have and to signal an affect that has relevance to their own actual or potential feeling states.

Recent preliminary findings in our laboratory (MacKain et al. 1985) suggest that infants at about nine months notice the congruence between their own affective state and the affect expression seen on someone's face. If infants are made sad and upset by several minutes' separation from mother (this is the age of acute separation reactions), as soon as they are reunited with her they stop being upset but remain solemn and are judged by mother and experimenters still to be sadder than usual. If then, right after the reunion when they are still sad, the infants are shown a happy face and a sad face, they prefer to look at the sad face. This does not happen if the infants are either made to laugh first or had not been separated in the first place. One conclusion is that the infant somehow makes a match between the feeling state as experienced within and as seen "on" or "in" another, a match that we can call *interaffectivity*.

Interaffectivity may be the first, most pervasive, and most immediately important form of sharing subjective experiences. Demos (1980, 1982a), Thoman and Acebo (1983), Tronick (1979), and others, as well as psychoanalysts, propose that early in life affects are both the primary *medium* and the primary *subject* of communication. This is in accord with our observations. And at nine to twelve months, when the infant has begun to share actions and intentions about objects and to exchange propositions in prelinguistic form, affective exchange is still the predominant mode and substance of communications with mother. It is for this reason that the sharing of affective states merits primary emphasis in our views of infants of these ages. Most protolinguistic exchanges involving intentions and objects are at the same time affective exchanges. (When the baby for the first time says "ba-a" and points to the ball, the people around respond with delight and excitement.) The two go on simultaneously, and findings that define a given event as primarily linguistic or primarily affective depend on perspective. However, the infant who is just learning the discursive mode appears to be far more expert in the domain of affect exchange. In a similar vein, Trevarthan and Hubley (1978) have commented that the sharing of affective moods and states appears before the sharing of mental states that reference objects, that is, things outside of the dyad. It seems clear that the sharing of affective states is of paramount importance during the first part of intersubjective relatedness, so much so that the next chapter will be devoted to a different view of the intersubjective sharing of feeling states.

The Nature of the Leap to Intersubjective Relatedness

Why does the infant suddenly adopt an organizing subjective perspective about self and others that opens the door to intersubjectivity? Is this quantum leap simply the result of a newly emergent, specific capacity or skill? Or does it result from the experience of social interactions? Or is it the maturational unfolding of a major human need and motive state? Piaget (1954), Bruner (1975, 1977), Bates (1976, 1979), and others whose primary approach is cognitive or linguistic view this achievement mainly in terms of an acquired social skill; the infant discovers generative rules and procedures for interactions that ultimately lead to the discovery of intersubjectivity. Trevarthan (1978) has called this a constructionist approach.

Shields (1978), Newson (1977), Vygotsky (1962), and others have understood this achievement more as the result of mother's entrance into "meaningful" exchanges, beginning at the infant's birth. She interprets all the infant's behaviors in terms of meanings; that is, she attributes meanings to them. She provides the semantic element, all by herself at first, and continues to bring the infant's behavior into her framework of created meanings. Gradually, as the infant is able, the framework of meaning becomes mutually created. This approach, based on social experience, might be called the approach of interpersonal meanings.

Many thinkers in France and Switzerland have independently approached the problem along similar lines and pushed the notion of maternal interpretation into richer clinical territory. They assert that mother's "meanings" reflect not only what she observes but also her fantasies about who the infant is and is to become. Intersubjectivity, for them, ultimately involves interfantasy. They have asked how the fantasies of the parent come to influence the infant's behavior and ultimately to shape the infant's own fantasies. This reciprocal fantasy interaction is a form of created interpersonal meaning at the covert level (Kreisler, Fair, and Soulé 1974; Kreisler and Cramer 1981; Cramer 1982, 1982b; Lebovici 1983; Pinol-Douriez 1983). The creation of such meanings has been called "interactions fantasmatique." Fraiberg et al. (1975) and Stern (1971) in the United States have also paid close attention to the relationship between maternal fantasy and overt behavior.

Trevarthan (1974, 1978) has stood relatively alone in maintaining that intersubjectivity is an innate, emergent human capacity. He points out that the other explanations for the appearance of intersubjectivity, especially the constructionist explanation, do not allow for any special awareness of humans or for the shared awareness that is so highly developed in humans. He sees this developmental leap as the "differentiation of a coherent field of intentionality" (Trevarthan and Hubley 1978, p. 213) and views intersubjectivity as a human capacity present in a primary form from the early months of life.[4]

4. In fact, what we are calling intersubjectivity Trevarthan calls "secondary intersubjectivity" (Trevarthan and Hubley 1978), the later differentiation of a uniquely human intersubjective function. Intersubjectivity does seem to be an emergent human capacity. However, it is not

All three viewpoints seem necessary for an adequate explanation of the emergence of intersubjectivity. Trevarthan is right that some special form of awareness must come into play at this point and that the capacity for it must unfold maturationally. And that special awareness is what we are calling an organizing subjective perspective. However, the capacity must have some tools to work with, and the constructivist approach has provided the tools in the form of rule structures, action formats, and discovery procedures. Finally, the capacity plus the tools would be operating in a vacuum without the addition of interpersonal meanings that are mutually created. All three taken together are required for a fuller account of intersubjective relatedness.

Once intersubjectivity has been tasted, so to speak, does it just remain as a capacity to be used or not, or as a perspective on self and other to be adopted or not? Or does it become a new psychological need, the need to share subjective experience?

We cannot cavalierly add to the list of basic psychological needs every time we come upon a new potentially autonomous capacity or need. The usual psychoanalytic solution to this problem, since the pioneering work of Hartmann, Kris, and Lowenstein (1946), is to call all such autonomously functioning capacities and need-like states "autonomous ego functions," rather than instincts or motivational systems. This label gives them their self-evident primary autonomous status but also puts them potentially at the service of the "basic" psychoanalytic needs, whose higher status is protected. (It is mainly in the area of infancy research that the presence and pervasiveness of newly recognized capacities and needs has become apparent and poses the problem.)

Up to a point, this solution of autonomous ego functions has proven extremely helpful and generative for the field. The question is, when does an autonomous ego function become of such magnitude that it is better conceived as a "basic need or motivational system?" Curiosity and stimulus seeking are good cases in point. These appear

---

meaningful to speak of primary intersubjectivity at three or four months of age, as Trevarthan does (1979). This can only refer to protoforms that lack the essential ingredients for being called intersubjectivity. Only Trevarthan's secondary stage is true intersubjectivity.

There is much reason to believe that other social animals, for example dogs, are also capable of intersubjectivity as the concept is used here.

to partake more of the quality of motivational systems than of mere autonomous ego functions.

What, then, about intersubjective relatedness? Are we to consider this another autonomous ego function? Or are we dealing with a primary psychobiological need? The answers to these questions are actually momentous for clinical theory. The more one conceives of intersubjective relatedness as a basic psychological need, the closer one refashions clinical theory toward the configurations suggested by Self psychologists and some existential psychologists.

From the perspective of infancy research, the question remains open. One consideration in this issue is to figure out what is so reinforcing about intersubjectivity. There is no question but that its reinforcing power can be related to achieving security needs or attachment goals. For instance, intersubjective successes can result in feelings of enhanced security. Similarly, minor failures in intersubjectivity can be interpreted, experienced, and acted upon as total ruptures in a relationship. This is often seen in therapy.

A parallel view is that an overriding human need develops for human-group-psychic-membership—that is, inclusion in the human group as a member with potentially shareable subjective experiences, in contrast to a nonmember whose subjective experiences are wholly unique, idiosyncratic, and nonshareable. The issue is basic. Opposite poles of this one dimension of psychic experience define different psychotic states. At one end is the sense of cosmic psychic isolation, alienation, and aloneness (the last person left on earth), and at the other end is the feeling of total psychic transparency, in which no single corner of potentially shareable experience can be kept private. The infant presumably begins to encounter this dimension of psychic experience somewhere in the middle, between the extreme poles, as most of us continue to do.[5]

Speaking teleologically, I assume that nature in the course of evolution created several ways to assure survival through group

5. The notion that the infant delegates omnipotence to the parent, imagining that the parent can always read the infant's mind, would predict that the infant could experience intersubjective experience like the psychotic at the total-transparency end of this dimension. This, however, would require a level of metacognition well beyond what is available at the age we are discussing. It is more likely that the infant starts in the middle, learning that some subjective states are shareable and others not.

membership in social species. Ethology and attachment theory have spelled out for us the behavior patterns that serve to assure those physical and psychological intermeshings of individuals that enhance survival. I suggest that nature has also provided the ways and means for any subjective intermeshings of individuals that would add survival value. And the survival value of intersubjectivity is potentially enormous.

There is no question that different societies could minimize or maximize this need for intersubjectivity. For instance, if a society were socially structured so that it was assumed that all members had essentially identical, inner subjective experiences, and if homogeneity of this aspect of felt life were stressed, there would be little need, and no societal pressure, to enhance the development of intersubjectivity. If on the other hand a society highly valued the existence and the sharing of individual differences at this level of experience (as ours does), then their development would be facilitated by that society.

Let us return to life as lived from moment to moment and examine more fully how affective experiences can enter the intersubjective domain, a phenomenon that I call *affect attunement.*

Chapter 7

The Sense of a Subjective Self: II. Affect Attunement

The Problem of Sharing Affective States

The sharing of affective states is the most pervasive and clinically germaine feature of intersubjective relatedness. This is especially true when the infant first enters this domain. Interaffectivity is mainly what is meant when clinicians speak of parental "mirroring" and "empathic responsiveness." Despite the importance of these events, it is not at all clear how they work. What are the acts and processes that let other people know that you are feeling something very like what they are feeling? How can you get "inside of" other people's subjective experience and then let them know that you have arrived there, without using words? After all, the infants we are talking about are only between nine and fifteen months old.

Imitation immediately comes to mind as a possible way one might show this. The mother might imitate the infant's facial expressions and gestures, and the baby would see her doing this. The problem with this solution is that the infant could only tell from the mother's imitation that mother got what the infant *did;* she would have reproduced the same overt behaviors, but she need not have had any similar inner experience. There is no reason why the infant should make the further assumption that mother also experienced the same feeling state that gave rise to the overt behavior.

For there to be an intersubjective exchange about affect, then, strict imitation alone won't do. In fact, several processes must take place. First, the parent must be able to read the infant's feeling state from the infant's overt behavior. Second, the parent must perform some behavior that is not a strict imitation but nonetheless corresponds in some way to the infant's overt behavior. Third, the infant must be able to read this corresponding parental response as having to do with the infant's own original feeling experience and not just imitating the infant's behavior. It is only in the presence of these three conditions that feeling states within one person can be knowable to another and that they can both sense, without using language, that the transaction has occurred.

To accomplish this transaction the mother must go beyond true imitations, which have been an enormous and important part of her social repertoire during the first six months or so of the infant's life (Moss 1973; Beebe 1973; Stern 1974b, 1977; Field 1977; Brazelton et al. 1979; Papoušek and Papoušek 1979; Trevarthan 1979; Francis et al. 1981; Uzgiris 1981, 1984; Kaye 1982; Malatesta and Izard 1982; Malatesta and Haviland 1983). Most of these investigators have described in detail how caregivers and infants mutually create the chains and sequences of reciprocal behaviors that make up social dialogues during the infant's first nine months. The Papoušeks describe this process in the vocal—in fact, musical—domain in great detail (1981). What is striking in these descriptions is that the mother is almost always working within the same modality as the infant. And in the leadings, followings, highlightings, and elaborations that make up her turn in the dialogue, she is generally performing close or loose imitations of the infant's immediate behavior. If the infant vocalizes, the mother vocalizes back. Similarly, if the infant makes a face, the mother makes a face. However, the dialogue does not remain a stereotypic boring sequence of repeats, back and forth, because the mother is constantly introducing modifying imitations (Kaye 1979; Uzgiris 1984) or providing a theme-and-variation format with slight changes in her contribution at each dialogic turn;

for example, her vocalization may be slightly different each time (Stern 1977).

When the infant is around nine months old, however, one begins to see the mother add a new dimension to her imitation-like behavior, a dimension that appears to be geared to the infant's new status as a potentially intersubjective partner. (It is not clear how mothers know this change has occurred in the infant; it seems to be part of their intuitive parental sense.) She begins to expand her behavior beyond true imitation into a new category of behavior we will call *affect attunement.*

The phenomenon of affect attunement is best shown by examples (Stern 1985). Affect attunement is often so embedded in other behaviors that relatively pure examples are hard to find, but the first five examples that follow are relatively unencumbered by other goings-on.

- A nine-month-old girl becomes very excited about a toy and reaches for it. As she grabs it, she lets out an exuberant "aaaah!" and looks at her mother. Her mother looks back, scrunches up her shoulders, and performs a terrific shimmy with her upper body, like a go-go dancer. The shimmy lasts only about as long as her daughter's "aaaah!" but is equally excited, joyful, and intense.
- A nine-month-old boy bangs his hand on a soft toy, at first in some anger but gradually with pleasure, exuberance, and humor. He sets up a steady rhythm. Mother falls into his rhythm and says, "kaaaaa-*bam,* kaaaaa-*bam,*" the *"bam"* falling on the stroke and the "kaaaaa" riding with the preparatory upswing and the suspenseful holding of his arm aloft before it falls.
- An eight-and-one-half-month-old boy reaches for a toy just beyond reach. Silently he stretches toward it, leaning and extending arms and fingers out fully. Still short of the toy, he tenses his body to squeeze out the extra inch he needs to reach it. At that moment, his mother says, "uuuuuh . . . uuuuuh!" with a crescendo of vocal effort, the expiration of air pushing against her tensed torso. The mother's accelerating vocal-respiratory effort matches the infant's accelerating physical effort.
- A ten-month-old girl accomplishes an amusing routine with mother and then looks at her. The girl opens up her face (her mouth opens, her eyes widen, her eyebrows rise) and then closes it back, in a series of changes whose contour can be represented by a smooth arch (⌒). Mother responds by intoning "Yeah," with a pitch line that rises and falls as the volume crescendos and decrescendos:

"Yãh." The mother's prosodic contour has matched the child's facial-kinetic contour.

A nine-month-old boy is sitting facing his mother. He has a rattle in his hand and is shaking it up and down with a display of interest and mild amusement. As mother watches, she begins to nod her head up and down, keeping a tight beat with her son's arm motions.

More often the attunement is so embedded in other actions and purposes that it is partially masked, as in the next example:

A ten-month-old girl finally gets a piece in a jig saw puzzle. She looks toward her mother, throws her head up in the air, and with a forceful arm flap raises herself partly off the ground in a flurry of exuberance. The mother says "YES, thatta girl." The "YES" is intoned with much stress. It has an explosive rise that echoes the girl's fling of gesture and posture.

One could easily argue that the "YES, thatta girl" functions as a routine response in the form of a positive reinforcer, and it certainly does do so. But why does the mother not just say "Yes, thatta girl"? Why does she need to add the intense intonation to "YES" that vocally matches the child's gestures? The "YES," I suggest, is an attunement embedded within a routine response.

The embedding of attunements is so common and most often so subtle that unless one is looking for it, or asking why any behavior is being performed exactly the way it is, the attunements will pass unnoticed (except, of course, that one will gather from them what we imagine to be "really" going on clinically). It is the embedded attunements that give much of the impression of the quality of the relationship.

Attunements have the following characteristics, which makes them ideal for accomplishing the intersubjective sharing of affect:

1. They give the impression that a kind of imitation has occurred. There is no faithful rendering of the infant's overt behavior, but some form of matching is going on.
2. The matching is largely cross-modal. That is, the channel or modality of expression used by the mother to match the infant's behavior is different from the channel or modality used by the infant. In the first example, the intensity level and duration of the girl's voice is matched by the mother's body movements. In the second example, features of the boy's arm movements are matched by features of the mother's voice.

3. What is being matched is not the other person's behavior *per se*, but rather some aspect of the behavior that reflects the person's feeling state. The ultimate reference for the match appears to be the feeling state (inferred or directly apprehended), not the external behavioral event. Thus the match appears to occur between the expressions of inner state. These expressions can differ in mode or form, but they are to some extent interchangeable as manifestations of a single, recognizable internal state. We appear to be dealing with behavior as expression rather than as sign or symbol, and the vehicles of transfer are metaphor and analogue.[1]

Affect attunement, then, is the performance of behaviors that express the quality of feeling of a shared affect state without imitating the exact behavioral expression of the inner state. If we could demonstrate subjective affect-sharing only with true imitations, we would be limited to flurries of rampant imitation. Our affectively responsive behavior would look ludicrous, maybe even robot-like.

The reason attunement behaviors are so important as separate phenomena is that true imitation does not permit the partners to refer to the internal state. It maintains the focus of attention upon the forms of the external behaviors. Attunement behaviors, on the other hand, recast the event and shift the focus of attention to what is behind the behavior, to the quality of feeling that is being shared. It is for the same reasons that imitation is the predominant way to teach external forms and attunement the predominant way to commune with or indicate sharing of internal states. Imitation renders form; attunement renders feeling. In actuality, however, there does not appear to be a true dichotomy between attunement and imitation; rather, they seem to occupy two ends of a spectrum.

Alternative Conceptualizations

One might well ask why I call this phenomenon affect attunement when there already exist several terms to encompass it. One reason is that these terms and their underlying concepts fail to capture the

---

1. Strictly speaking one could call this the imitation of selected features, in that one or two features of a behavior are chosen to be imitated while most other features are not so selected. The reason we have not chosen this term is that the imitated features are recast in a different form, creating the impression of referencing the inner state rather than the overt behavior.

phenomenon adequately. While the mother's attunings are often not even reasonably faithful imitations, the virtue of a loose definition of imitation can be argued. Kaye (1979) has pointed out that "modifying imitations" are intended to just miss the mark in order to maximize or minimize aspects of the original behavior. And Uzgiris refers to essentially the same issues with the terms "imitation" and "matching" (1984). Nonetheless, there is a limit beyond which fidelity cannot be stretched if "imitation" is still to keep its usual meaning.

A second problem is that of the representations necessary for imitation. "Deferred imitation," as meant by Piaget (1954), requires the capacity for acting on the basis of an internal representation of the original. The reproduction (or imitation) is guided by the blueprint provided by the internal representation. Piaget had in mind the *observed behaviors* as the referent which is represented. The nature of such representations is well conceptualized. But if the referent is the feeling state, how do we conceptualize its representation so that it can act as a blueprint? We are going to require a different notion of the nature of the representation that is operating, namely a representation of the feeling state, not its overt behavioral manifestation.

The terms "affect matching" or "affect contagion" have a similar appeal. These processes refer to the automatic induction of an affect in one person from seeing or hearing someone else's affect display. This process may well be a basic biological tendency among highly evolved social species, which becomes perfected in man (Malatesta and Izard 1982). The earliest affect contagion that has been demonstrated involves the human distress cry. Wolff (1969) found that two-month-old infants showed "infectious crying" when they heard tape recordings of their own distress cries. Simner (1971) and Sagi and Hoffman (1976) showed that contagious crying occurred in newborns. Newborns cried more to infant cries in general than to equally loud artificially produced sounds. Similarly, the contagious properties of the smile have been well documented in infancy, even though mechanisms for it may shift during development.

Affect matching with its probable basis in "motor mimicry" (Lipps 1906) cannot alone explain affect attunement, although it may well provide one of the underlying mechanisms on which that phenomenon is founded. By itself, affect matching, like imitation, explains only a reproduction of the original. It cannot account for the phenomenon of responding in different modes or with different forms of behavior, with the internal state as the referent.

"Intersubjectivity" as articulated by Trevarthan (1977, 1978, 1979, 1980) approaches the essence of the problem, although from a different direction. It concerns the mutual sharing of psychic states, but it refers mainly to intentions and motives rather than to qualities of feeling or affects. Its major concern is interintentionality, not interaffectivity. Intersubjectivity is an entirely adequate term and concept, but it is too inclusive for our purposes. Affect attunement is a particular form of intersubjectivity that requires some processes that are unique to it.

"Mirroring" and "echoing" represent the clinical terms and concepts that come closest to affect attunement. As terms, both run into the problem of fidelity to the original. "Mirroring" has the disadvantage of suggesting complete temporal synchrony. "Echoing," taken literally, at least avoids the temporal constraint. In spite of these semantic limitations, however, these concepts represent attempts to grapple with the issue of one person reflecting another's inner state. In this important respect, unlike imitation or contagion, they are appropriately concerned with the subjective state rather than the manifest behavior.

This meaning of reflecting inner state has been used mostly in clinical theories (Mahler et al. 1975; Kohut 1977; Lacan 1977), which have noted that reflecting back an infant's feeling state is important to the infant's developing knowledge of his or her own affectivity and sense of self. When used in this sense, however, "mirroring" implies that the mother is helping to create something within the infant that was only dimly or partially there until her reflection acted somehow to solidify its existence. This concept goes far beyond just participating in another's subjective experience. It involves changing the other by providing something the other did not have before or, if it was present, by consolidating it.

A second problem with mirroring as a term is the inconsistency and overinclusiveness of its usage. In clinical writings, it sometimes refers to the behavior itself—that is, to true imitation, a literal reflecting back, in the domain of core-relatedness—and sometimes to the sharing or alignment of internal states—in our terms, affect attunement in the domain of intersubjective relatedness. At still other times, it refers to verbal reinforcements or consensual validation at the level of verbal relatedness. "Mirroring" is thus commonly used to embrace three different processes. Moreover, it is not clear which subjective states are to be included in mirroring affects—intentions? motives? beliefs? ego functions? In short, while mirroring has focused upon the essence of the problem, the indeterminate usage has blurred what appear to be real differences in mechanism, form, and function.

Finally, there is "empathy." Is attunement sufficiently close to what is generally meant by empathy? No. The evidence indicates that attunements occur largely out of awareness and almost automatically. Empathy, on the other hand, involves the mediation of cognitive processes. What is generally called empathy consists of at least four distinct and probably sequential processes: (1) the resonance of feeling state; (2) the abstraction of empathic knowledge from the experience of emotional resonance; (3) the integration of abstracted empathic knowledge into an empathic response; and (4) a transient role identification. Cognitive processes such as these involved in the second and third events are crucial to empathy (Schaffer 1968; Hoffman 1978; Ornstein 1979; Basch 1983; Demos 1984). (Cognitive imaginings of what it must be like to be another person, however, are nothing more than elaborated acts of role taking and not empathy, unless they have been ignited by at least a spark of emotional resonance.) Affect attunement, then, shares with empathy the initial process of emotional resonance (Hoffman 1978); neither can occur without it. The work of many psychoanalytic thinkers concurs on this formulation (Basch 1983). But while affect attunement, like empathy, starts with an emotional resonance, it does something different with it. Attunement takes the experience of emotional resonance and automatically recasts that experience into another form of expression. Attunement thus need not proceed towards empathic knowledge or response. Attunement is a distinct form of affective transaction in its own right.

The Evidence for Attunement

What evidence exists for the phenomenon of attunement, and what kind of evidence could be developed to demonstrate it? The problem of demonstration boils down to this: the existence of an attunement is at first glance a clinical impression, perhaps an intuition. To operationalize this impression, it is necessary to identify those aspects of a person's behavior that could be matched without actually imitating them. Stern et al. (in press) reasoned that there were three general features of a behavior that could be matched (and thereby form the basis of an attunement) without rendering an imitation. These are intensity, timing, and shape. These three dimensions were then broken down into six more specific types of match:

1. *Absolute intensity.* The level of intensity of the mother's behavior is the same as that of the infant's, irrespective of the mode or form of the behavior. For instance, the loudness of a mother's vocalization might match the force of an abrupt arm movement performed by the infant.
2. *Intensity contour.* The changes of intensity over time are matched. The second example on page 140 provides a good instance of this type of match. The mother's vocal effort and the infant's physical effort both showed an acceleration in intensity, followed suddenly by an even quicker intensity deceleration phase.
3. *Temporal beat.* A regular pulsation in time is matched. The fifth example, on page 141, is a good example of a temporal beat match. The nodding of the mother's head and the infant's gesture conform to the same beat.
4. *Rhythm.* A pattern of pulsations of unequal stress is matched.
5. *Duration.* The time span of the behavior is matched. If the mother's and infant's behaviors last about the same time, a duration match has occurred. A duration match by itself is not considered to constitute a sufficient criterion for an attunement, however, because too many non-attunement, infant/mother response chains show duration matching.
6. *Shape.* Some spatial feature of a behavior that can be abstracted and rendered in a different act is matched. The fifth example, on page 141, provides an instance. The mother has borrowed the vertical shape of the infant's up-down arm motion and adapted it in her head motion. Shape does not mean the same form; that would be imitation.

The second step in examining the nature of affect attunements, once matching criteria were established, was to enlist the collaboration of mothers in answering a series of questions about their matchings. Why did she do what she did, the way she did it and when she did it? What did she think the baby felt at the moment that . . . ? Was she aware of her own behavior when she . . . ? What did she wish to accomplish . . . ?

Accordingly, mothers were first asked to play with their infants as they normally would at home. The play session took place in a pleasant observation room filled with some age-appropriate toys. The mother and infant were left alone for ten to fifteen minutes while their interaction was videotaped. Immediately afterwards, the mother and the experimenters watched a replay of the taped interaction. Many questions were then asked. The experimenters made every attempt to create a collaborative, easy, working atmosphere with the mothers, rather than an inquisitional or judgmental one. Most mothers felt that an alliance had been forged with the researchers. This "research-therapeutic alliance" is crucial to this kind of joint inquiry.

An important issue in the process was when to stop the taped flow of interaction and ask the questions. Entry criteria were set up to identify points at which to jump into the stream of interaction. The first such criterion was that the baby had made some affective expression—facial, vocal, gestural, or postural. The second was that the mother had responded in some observable way. And the third was that the baby had seen, heard, or felt her response. When an event meeting these criteria was viewed, the videotape was stopped and the questions were asked. The taped episode was replayed as often as necessary. The results of the experiments with ten mothers as participant-researchers and their infants aged eight to twelve months are reported elsewhere in detail (Stern et al., in press). The major findings that have relevance to the present discussion are summarized here.

1. In response to an infant expression of affect, maternal attunements were the most common maternal response (48 percent), followed by comments (33 percent), and imitations (19 percent). During play interactions attunements occurred at a rate of one every sixty-five seconds.

2. Most attunements occurred across sensory modes. If the infant's expression was vocal, the mother's attunement was likely to be gestural or facial, and vice versa. In 39 percent of the instances of attunement, the mothers used entirely different modalities from those used by the infant (cross-modal attunement). In 48 percent of the cases, the mothers used some modalities that were the same as those used by the infant (intramodal attunement) and some that were different. Thus 87 percent of the time, the mothers' attunements were partially, if not wholly, cross-modal.

3. Of the three aspects of behavior—intensity, timing, and shape—that a mother can use to accomplish an attunement, intensity matches were the most common, followed by timing matches and last by shape matches. In the majority of cases, more than one aspect of behavior was simultaneously matched. For instance, when the infant's up-and-down hand gesture was matched by the mother's head nodding up and down, both beat and shape were being matched. The percentages of all attunements that represented matchings of the various aspects are: intensity contour, 81 percent; duration, 69 percent; absolute intensity, 61 percent; shape, 47 percent; beat, 13 percent; and rhythm, 11 percent.

4. The largest single reason that mothers gave (or that we inferred) for performing an attunement was "to be with" the infant, "to share," "to participate in," "to join in." We have called these functions *interpersonal communion*. This group of reasons stands in contrast to the other kinds of reasons given: to respond, to jazz the baby up or to quiet, to restructure the interaction, to reinforce, to engage in a standard game. This later group can be lumped together as serving the function of communication rather than communion. Communication generally means to exchange or transmit information with the attempt to alter another's belief or action system. During many of these attunements the mother is doing none of these things. Communion means to share in another's experience with no attempt to change what that person is doing or believing. This idea captures far better the mother's behavior as seen by experimenters and by the mothers themselves.

5. Several variations on attunements occurred. In addition to *communing attunements*, true attunements in which the mother tried to match exactly the infant's internal state for the purpose of "being with" the baby, there were misattunements, which fell into two types. In *purposeful misattunement*, the mother "intentionally" over- or under-matched the infant's intensity, timing, or behavioral shape. The purpose of these misattunements was usually to increase or decrease the baby's level of activity or affect. The mother "slipped inside of" the infant's feeling state far enough to capture it, but she then misexpressed it enough to alter the infant's behavior but not enough

to break the sense of an attunement in process. Such purposeful misattunements were called *tuning*. There were also *nonpurposeful misattunements*. Either the mother incorrectly identified, to some extent, the quality and/or quantity of the infant's feeling state, or she was unable to find in herself the same internal state. These misattunements we called *true misattunements*.[2]

6. When mothers were shown the taped replay of their attunements, they judged themselves to have been entirely unaware of their behavior at the time of occurrence in 24 percent of cases; only partly aware of their behavior in 43 percent of cases; and fully aware of their behavior in 32 percent of cases.

Even in the 32 percent of cases where the mother said she was fully aware of her behavior, she was often referring to the desired consequences of her behavior more than to what she actually did. Thus the attunement *process* itself occurs largely unawares.

It is easy enough to determine experimentally that tunings and misattunements influence the infant: they usually result in some alteration or interruption of ongoing infant behavior. That is their purpose, and the result can be readily gauged. The situation with communing attunements is different. Most often after the mother has made such an attunement, the infant acts as if nothing special has happened. The infant's activity continues uninterrupted, and we are left with no evidence, only speculation, that the fact of attunement has "gotten in," taken hold, and had some psychic consequence. To get underneath this still surface, we chose the method of perturbing ongoing interactions and seeing what happens.

The approach of creating defined perturbations in naturalistic or seminaturalistic interaction is well established in infancy research. For example, the "still-face" procedure (Tronick et al. 1978) asks a mother or father to go "still-faced"—impassive and expressionless— in the middle of an interaction, creating a perturbation in the expected flow. Infants by three months of age react with mild upset and social withdrawal, alternating with attempts to re-engage the impassive partner. This kind of perturbation can be used with any and all parent/infant pairs. The perturbations of attunement, however, had to be tailored to a specific pair and aimed at a previously

---

2. The obvious clinical import of the characteristic and selective use of attunements, tuning, and misattunements in different affective contexts will be addressed in chapter 9.

identified and likely-to-recur attunement episode. No two pairs presented the same opportunity.

For each pair, the specific attunement episode chosen for perturbation was identified while the mother and researchers watched the replay of the videorecording. After discussing the structure of behaviors that made up the attunement episode, the researchers instructed the mothers in how to perturb the structure. The mothers then returned to the observation room, and when the appropriate context for the expectable attunement behavior arose, they performed the planned perturbation. Two examples will serve to illustrate the results.

In the videotape of the initial play period, a nine-month-old infant is seen crawling away from his mother and over to a new toy. While on his stomach, he grabs the toy and begins to bang and flail with it happily. His play is animated, as judged by his movements, breathing, and vocalizations. Mother then approaches him from behind, out of sight, and puts her hand on his bottom and gives it an animated jiggle side to side. The speed and intensity of her jiggle appear to match well the intensity and rate of the infant's arm movements and vocalizations, qualifying this as an attunement. The infant's response to her attunement is—nothing! He simply continues his play without missing a beat. Her jiggle has no overt effect, as though she had never acted. This attunement episode was fairly characteristic of this pair. The infant wandered from her and became involved in another toy, and she leaned over and jiggled his bottom, his leg, or his foot. This sequence was repeated several times.

For the first perturbation, the mother was instructed to do exactly the same as always, except that now she was purposely to "misjudge" her baby's level of joyful animation, to pretend that the baby was somewhat less excited than he appeared to be, and to jiggle accordingly. When the mother did jiggle somewhat more slowly and less intensely than she truly judged would make a good match, the baby quickly stopped playing and looked around at her, as if to say "What's going on?" This procedure was repeated, with the same result.

The second perturbation was in the opposite direction. The mother was to pretend that her baby was at a higher level of joyful animation and to jiggle accordingly. The results were the same: the infant noticed the discrepancy and stopped. The mother was then asked to go back to jiggling appropriately, and again the infant did *not* respond.[3]

One could argue that the jiggle, when performed within some band of speed/intensity, is simply a form of reinforcement, rather than a signal. There is no problem with this formulation except that it does not account for the fact that the acceptable band is determined by the relationship between the infant's and the mother's speed and level of intensity, not by the absolute level on the mother's part. And there is no problem with attunements also serving reinforcing functions. But simple reinforcement cannot explain away attunement. The two phenomena are undoubtedly embedded one within the other and serve different functions in the developing relationship. Interviews with the mother afterwards confirmed this dual function. She said that she did the regular attunement "to get into the playing with him," but she also said that she figured, in retrospect, that it probably "encouraged" him to continue.

In another example, the initial videotape shows an eleven-month-old going after an object with determination and excitement. He gets it and brings it to his mouth with much excitement and body tension. Mother says, "*Yeah, ya like that.*" The infant does not respond to her utterance. When the mother was asked to over-shoot or under-shoot the pitch contouring, rate, and stress patterning of her standard utterance, compared with the perceived excitement and tension of her infant, the infant took notice and looked at her, as if for further clarification.

Many more such individualized perturbations have been performed, all indicating that the infant does indeed have some sense of the extent of matching. Closeness of match, in itself, is an expectation under some circumstances, and its violation is meaningful.

It is clear that interpersonal communion, as created by attunement, will play an important role in the infant's coming to recognize that internal feeling states are forms of human experience that are shareable with other humans. The converse is also true: feeling states that are never attuned to will be experienced only alone, isolated

3. Note that each time a perturbation was attempted the infant was at a somewhat different level of excitation and the mother had to adjust her "misjudgment" to his current level. It is also notable that some mothers found misjudgments hard to execute. One said that it is like trying to pat your head and rub your stomach at the same time.

from the interpersonal context of shareable experience. What is at stake here is nothing less than the shape of and extent of the shareable inner universe.

Underlying Mechanisms for Attunement

For attunement to work, different behavioral expressions occurring in different forms and in different sensory modalities must somehow be interchangeable. If a certain gesture by the mother is to be "correspondent" with a certain kind of vocal exclamation by the infant, the two expressions must share some common currency that permits them to be transferred from one modality or form to another. That common currency consists of amodal properties.

There are some qualities or properties that are held in common by most or all of the modalities of perception. These include intensity, shape, time, motion, and number. Such qualities of perception can be abstracted by any sensory mode from the invariant properties of the stimulus world and then translated into other modalities of perception. For instance, a rhythm, such as "long short" (—— –), can be delivered in or abstracted from sight, audition, smell, touch, or taste. For this to occur, the rhythm must at some point exist in the mind in a form that is not inextricably bound to one particular way of perceiving it but is rather sufficiently abstract to be transportable across modalities. It is the existence of these abstract representations of amodal properties that permits us to experience a perceptually unified world.

From what has gone before, it is clear that infants can perceive the world amodally from early on and that they get better at it during maturation. This position has been strongly put forth by developmentalists such as Bower (1974), who states that from the earliest days of life, the infant forms and acts upon abstract representations of qualities of perception.

The qualities of experience that lend themselves to intermodal fluency, which will be of paramount interest to us here, are the ones that were determined to be the best criteria for defining attunements—namely, intensity, time, and shape. This intermodal fluency is the phenomenon in want of an explanatory mechanism. What, then, is the evidence that infants can perceive or experience intensity, time, and shape amodally?

INTENSITY

Level of intensity, as we have seen, was one of the qualities most frequently matched in designating attunements. Most often the match was between the intensity of an infant's physical behavior and the intensity of the mother's vocal behavior. Can an infant match levels of intensity across the visual and auditory modalities? Yes, and quite well, as indicated in the experiment described in chapter 3 in which three-week-old infants matched levels of loudness of sounds to levels of brightness of lights (Lewcowicz and Turkewitz 1980). The ability to perform audio-visual cross-modal matches of the absolute level of intensity appears to be a very early capacity.[4]

TIME

The temporal qualities of behavior were the second most commonly matched in performing attunements. Here too, as mentioned in chapter 3, infants appear to be well endowed with the capacity to match temporal patterns across modes. In fact, intensity level and timing may be the perceptual qualities that the infant is best able to represent modally, and at the earliest points in development.

SHAPE

Intensity and time are quantitative properties of stimulation or perception, in contrast to shape, which is qualitative. What is known about the infant's competence in the intermodal coordination of shape or configuration? The Meltzoff and Borton (1979) experiment described on pages 47–48 is an example par excellence of the transfer of the shape of a static object from the tactile mode to the visual mode. After this demonstration, it was logical to ask whether correspondences in kinetic shapes could also be made, and whether correspondences would also occur across vision and audition as well as across vision and touch. After all, most human behavior consists

4. This intermodal capacity for matching relative level of intensity does not directly address the capacity for matching intensity contours, the profiles of change in intensity over time. This was the other intensity criterion for attunement—in fact, the most common type of match. An intensity contour also involves time and is in some ways closer to shape as a quality than to intensity as a quantity.

of kinetic shapes—that is, configurations that change in time—and vocalizations are one of the most pervasive kinetic shapes involved in attunements. As the experiments of MacKain et al. (1983) and Kuhl and Meltzoff (1982) have shown, infants should have no trouble at all in making these cross-modal transformations (see chapter 3).

The Unity of the Senses

It thus appears that shape, intensity, and time can all be perceived amodally. And, indeed, philosophy, psychology, and art have a long history of designating shape, time, and intensity to be amodal qualities of experience (in psychological terms) or primary qualities of experience (in philosophical terms) (see Marks 1978). These issues have a long history, because what is at stake is the unity of the senses, which ultimately boils down to the knowledge or experience that the world as seen is the same world that is heard or felt.

Aristotle first postulated a doctrine of sensory correspondence, or a doctrine of the unity of the senses. His sixth sense, the common sense, was the sense that could apperceive the qualities of sensation that are primary (that is, amodal) in that they do not belong exclusively to any one sense alone, as color belongs to vision, but are shared by all the senses. Aristotle's list of primary qualities that could be extracted from any modality, represented in abstract form, and translated among all sense modes included intensity, motion, rest, unity, form, and number. Philosophers since have argued about which attributes of perception meet the requirements of primary qualities, but intensity, form, and time are usually included.

Psychologists were probably first drawn to the issue of the unity of the senses by the phenomenon of synesthesia, in which stimulation in a single sense evokes sensations that belong to a different modality of stimulation. The most common synesthesia is "colored hearing." Particular sounds, such as a trumpet, produce the visual image of a particular color, perhaps red, along with the auditory percept (see Marks [1978] for a review). The existence of synesthesia was only part of the allure of unity of the senses, however. The issue of intramodal equivalences or correspondences has always been of interest to students of perception, and the developmental psychologists have recently picked up the age-old trail. The problem is subsumed under what Marks calls the Doctrine of Equivalent Information, which states that different senses can inform about the same features of the external world. Much of the theoretical work of the Gibsons (1959, 1969, 1979), Piaget (1954), T. Bower (1974), and others addresses this issue.

Therapists are so familiar with this phenomenon that it is taken for granted as a way to communicate feelings about important perceptions. When a patient says, "I was so anxious and uptight about how she would greet me, but as soon as she spoke it was like the sun came out—I melted," we understand directly. How could most metaphors work without an underlying capacity for the transposition of amodal information?

Artists, especially poets, have taken the unity of the senses for granted. Most poetry could not work without the tacit assumption that cross-sensory analogies and metaphors are immediately apparent to everyone. Certain poets, such as the French Symbolists during the nineteenth century, elevated the fact of the cross-modal equivalence of information to a guiding principle of the poetic process.

There are odors fresh as the skin of an infant,
Sweet as flutes, green as any grass,
And others, corrupt, rich and triumphant.
(Baudelaire, *Correspondences,* 1857)

In just three lines, Baudelaire asks us to relate smells to experiences in the domains of touch, sound, color, sensuality, finance, and power. A similar preoccupation has visited the other arts.[5]

5. Around the turn of the twentieth century, visual artists and musicians engaged in innumerable experiments at symphonic light shows, using novel instruments such as color organs to express in one medium or perceptual modality the qualities rendered in another. Such cross-sensory attempts were also conducted in traditional media; an example is Mussorgsky's *Pictures at an Exhibition.*

When sound film became possible, the opportunities for intermingling and integrating the qualities of sound and vision became obvious and irresistible for pioneers in the new medium. Sergei Eisenstein's attempts to integrate the two media are perhaps best known because of his extensive writing about film-making (1957) and the success of his genius in intramodal integration. In his classic film *Alexander Nevsky,* Eisenstein worked closely with Prokofiev, the composer of the score. Together they matched the visual structure of each film frame with the auditory structure of the music being played during that shot; the battle scene is perhaps still the most careful and painstaking artistic exploration of the integration of sight and sound

The point of this discussion about the unity of the senses is that the capacities for identifying cross-modal equivalences that make for a perceptually unified world are the same capacities that permit the mother and infant to engage in affect attunement to achieve affective intersubjectivity.

What Inner State is Being Attuned to?

It appears that both forms of affects—discrete categorical affects such as sadness and joy as well as vitality affects such as explosions and fading—are attuned to. In fact, most attunements seem to occur with the vitality affects.

In chapter 3, we identified vitality affects as those dynamic, kinetic qualities of feeling that distinguish animate from inanimate and that correspond to the momentary changes in feeling states involved in the organic processes of being alive. We experience vitality affects as dynamic shifts or patterned changes within ourselves or others. One of the reasons we went to such efforts there to establish vitality affects as entities in their own right, distinct from what is usually meant by activation as well as from categories of affect, is that now they become essential to an understanding of attunement.

During an average mother-infant interaction, discrete affect displays occur only occasionally—perhaps every thirty to ninety seconds. Since this is so, affective tracking or attuning with another could not occur as a continuous process if it were limited to categorical affects. One cannot wait around for a discrete categorical affect display, such as a surprise expression, to occur in order to re-establish attunement. Attunement feels more like an unbroken process. It cannot await

---

ever attempted. The works of Walt Disney achieve their various effects through the same impact of sound-sight coordination. And dance is the ultimate example—in fact, the prototype.

At a more mundane level, the pervasiveness of our familiarity with the unity of the senses is seen in many games. One variant of the parlor game of Twenty Questions depends upon this familiarity. The person who is "it," thinks of some person. Everyone else has to guess that person's identity by asking for intra- and cross-modal correspondences; for example, "If the person were a vegetable, what vegetable would he be?" "What kind of drink would she be?" "What kind of sound?" "What smell?" "What kind of geometric shape?" "What surface would he feel like?" and so on.

discrete affect eruptions; it must be able to work with virtually all behavior. And that is one of the great advantages of the vitality affects. They are manifest in all behavior and can thus be an almost omnipresent subject of attunement. They concern *how* a behavior, *any* behavior, *all* behavior is performed, not *what* behavior is performed.

Vitality affects therefore must be added to affect categories as one of the kinds of subjective inner states that can be referenced in acts of attunement. Vitality is ideally suited to be the subject of attunements, because it is composed of the amodal qualities of intensity and time and because it resides in virtually any behavior one can perform and thus provide a continuously present (though changing) subject for attunement. Attunements can be made with the inner quality of feeling of how an infant reaches for a toy, holds a block, kicks a foot, or listens to a sound. Tracking and attuning with vitality affects permit one human to "be with" another in the sense of sharing likely inner experiences on an almost continuous basis. This is exactly our experience of feeling-connectedness, of being in attunement with another. It feels like an unbroken line. It seeks out the activation contour that is momentarily going on in any and every behavior and uses that contour to keep the thread of communion unbroken.

Communicating Vitality Affects: Art and Behavior

Both categorical and vitality affects, then, are the subject matter for attunement. One can imagine how a categorical affect display such as sadness, once seen, is directly felt by the viewer. Evolution and experience have teamed up to make that transposition of feeling from one to another comprehensible. But how and why can we automatically make these transpositions with vitality affects? We have identified time-intensity contours as one of the salient perceptual qualities that undergo the transformation and the way in which this process relies on capacities for amodal perception. But we still have not fully answered how we get from perceptions of others to feelings in ourselves, when there are no specific prewired programs operating, as there appear to be for the discrete categorical affects.

The problem can be restated as follows. We tend automatically to transpose perceptual qualities into feeling qualities, particularly when the qualities belong to another person's behavior. For instance, we may gather from someone's arm gesture the perceptual qualities of rapid acceleration, speed, and fullness of display. But we will *not* experience the gesture in terms of the perceptual qualities of timing, intensity, and shape; we will experience it directly as "forceful"— that is, in terms of a vitality affect.

How, then, do we get from intensity, timing, and shape to "forcefulness"? This is the question that lies at the heart of understanding one aspect of how art works, and perhaps a look at how the question has been approached in the domain of art may be helpful in understanding it in the domain of behavior.

Suzanne Langer (1967) has proposed a route for getting from perception to feeling. She suggests that, in works of art, the organization of elements seems to present an aspect of felt life. The feeling that is presented is in fact an apparition, an illusion, a virtual feeling. For instance, a two-dimensional painting creates the virtual feeling of three-dimensional space. What is more, virtual space can have the virtual properties of vastness, distance, advancing, receding, and so on. In a similar fashion, sculpture, an unmoving volume, can present virtual feelings of kinetic volume: leanings, liftings, and soarings. Music as an actual physical temporal event is one dimensional and homogeneous in time, yet it presents virtual time—that is, time as lived or experienced, rushing, tripping, drawn out, or suspenseful. Dance as actual effortful movement and gesture presents virtual "realms of power, a play of powers made visible" (Ghosh 1979, p. 69): explosions and implosions, restraint, meanderings, and effortlessness.

Is it possible that the activation contours (intensity in time) perceived in another's overt behavior become a virtual vitality affect when experienced in the self?

Spontaneous behaviors include conventionalized elements such as the configurations (the smiles and weeping) of the discrete categorical affects. These are analogous to conventionalized representational forms or iconic elements in painting, such as the Madonna and Child, except that their shared import comes about because of biological ritualization (by force of evolution), not by cultural convention, as in the case of the Madonna and Child.

The translation from perception to feeling in conventionalized forms (icons in art or discrete affect displays in spontaneous behavior) is the least interesting part of the problem, however. In both art and behavior, there is also the *rendering* of the conventional forms. In the case of the Madonna and Child, that might mean the exact treatment of the Madonna's robe and the background, how the colors contrast and harmonize, how the linear and planar tensions are resolved—in short, how the forms will be handled. This is the domain of style.[6] In spontaneous behavior, the counterpart to artistic style is the domain of vitality affects. As we have seen, these concern the manner in which conventionalized affect displays such as smiling and other highly fixed motor programs such as walking are performed. This is where the exact performance of the behavior, in terms of timing, intensity, and shape, can render multiple "stylistic" versions or vitality affects of the same sign, signal, or action.[7]

The translation, then, from perception to feeling in the case of style in art involves the transmutation from "veridical" perceptions (color harmonies, linear resolutions, and the like) into such virtual forms of feeling as calmness. The analogous translation from perception of another person's behavior to feelings involves the transmutation from the perception of timing, intensity, and shape via cross-modal fluency into felt vitality affects in ourselves. I am in no way making a case that art and spontaneous behavior are equivalent; I am simply pointing out some similarities that may be helpful in understanding how affect attunement works when the attunement is to a vitality affect.

6. In the manner in which the representational elements are rendered, a high degree of the conventionalization is a product of a particular historical, geographic, or cultural setting or even of momentary fashions. The same is true for behavior. Still, style and conventionalized form are distinguishable.

7. This is the area in which many of the dance or movement analysis pioneers have labored, for example, and which Kestenberg (1979) and Sossin (1979) have fruitfully applied to mother/infant interactions. A recent photography show (*Form and Emotion in Photography*. The Metropolitan Museum of Art, New York, March 1982) brought home the difference that vitality affects can make. Mark Berghash took six photographs of the same woman's face. He simply asked her to think about a subject and "get into it"; he then took a photograph. The six subjects were her mother, her father, her brother, her past self, her present self, her future self. Together, the six pictures were titled "Aspects of the True Self." In no photograph (except possibly one) did the woman display a recognizable or nameable categorical display; her face was largely neutral by behavioral display rules. But the "stylistic" differences spoke volumes. Each photograph was a captured vitality affect.

There is one crucial difference between art and behavior that highlights an important limitation in attunement. The apprehension of art (although not its creation) involves a certain kind of contemplative mode, which has long been an issue in aesthetics. Mrs. Canbell Fischer expresses the essence of this issue for our purposes: "My grasp of the essence of sadness ... comes not from moments in which I have been sad, but from moments when [through art] I have seen sadness before me released from entanglements with contingency" (quoted in Langer [1967], p. 88). But spontaneous behavior between persons is invariably and irreversibly entangled with contingencies at innumerable levels. There are two consequences of this reality. The first is that while art can deal with an idea or ideal, spontaneous behavior deals only with a particular instance of an idea; the particulars are defined by the "entanglements." The second issue is that certain "entanglements with contingency" may even make it impossible to attune. Can you attune with anger that is directed at you? Certainly you can experience the level of intensity and quality of feeling that is occurring in the other and that may be elicited in yourself. But it can then no longer be said that you are "sharing in" or "participating in" the other's anger; you are involved in your own. The entangling contingency of threat and harm places a barrier between the two separate experiences such that the notion of communion is no longer applicable. The range of attunement has some limitations in the contingent world of interpersonal reality.

It is inescapable that the infant and child first learn about vitality affects, or in Langer's term "forms of feeling," from their interactions with their own behavior and bodily processes and by watching, testing, and reacting to the social behaviors that impinge on and surround them. They must also learn or somehow arrive at the realization that there are transformational means for translating perceptions of external things into internal feelings, besides those for categorical affects. These transformations from perception to feeling are first learned with spontaneous social behaviors. It seems that only after many years of performing these transformations and building up a repertoire of vitality affects is a child ready to bring this experience to the domain of art as something that is externally perceived but transposed into felt experience.

Attunement is more fully explicable when social behavior is seen, at least in part, as a form of expressionism. The apprehension of some behavior as a form of expressionism makes attunement a precursor to the experience of art. But attunements have achieved something else of developmental significance.

Attunement as a Stepping Stone Toward Language

An attunement is a recasting, a restatement of a subjective state. It treats the subjective state as the referent and the overt behavior as one of several possible manifestations or expressions of the referent. For example, a level and quality of exuberance can be expressed as a unique vocalization, as a unique gesture, or as a unique facial display. Each manifestation has some degree of substitutability as a recognizable signifier of the same inner state. And thus attunement recasting behaviors by way of nonverbal metaphor and analogue. If one imagines a developmental progression from imitation through analogue and metaphor to symbols, this period of the formation of the sense of a subjective self provides the experience with analogue in the form of attunements, an essential step toward the use of symbols, to which we now turn.

Chapter 8

The Sense of a Verbal Self

DURING THE SECOND YEAR of the infant's life language emerges, and in the process the senses of self and other acquire new attributes. Now the self and the other have different and distinct personal world knowledge as well as a new medium of exchange with which to create shared meanings. A new organizing subjective perspective emerges and opens a new domain of relatedness. The possible ways of "being with" another increase enormously. At first glance, language appears to be a straightforward advantage for the augmentation of interpersonal experience. It makes parts of our known experience more shareable with others. In addition, it permits two people to create mutual experiences of meaning that had been unknown before and could never have existed until fashioned by words. It also finally permits the child to begin to construct a narrative of his own life. But in fact language is a double-edged sword. It also makes some parts of our experience less shareable with ourselves and with others. It drives a wedge between two simultaneous forms of interpersonal experience: as it is lived and as it is verbally represented. Experience in the domains of emergent, core- and intersubjective relatedness, which continue irrespective of language, can be embraced only very partially in the domain of verbal relatedness. And to the extent that events in the domain of verbal relatedness are held to be what has really happened, experiences in these other domains suffer an alienation. (They can become the nether domains of experience.) Language, then, causes a split in the experience of the self. It also moves relatedness onto the impersonal, abstract level intrinsic to language and away from the personal, immediate level intrinsic to the other domains of relatedness.

It will be necessary to follow both these lines of development—language as a new form of relatedness and language as a problem for the integration of self-experience and self-with-other experiences. We must somehow take into account these divergent directions that the emergence of a linguistic sense of self has created.

But first, let us see what capacities have developed in the infant that permit a new perspective on the self to emerge and revolutionize the possible ways that the self can be with another and with itself.

New Capacities Available in the Second Year

Toward the middle of the second year (at around fifteen to eighteen months), children begin to imagine or represent things in their minds in such a way that signs and symbols are now in use. Symbolic play and language now become possible. Children can conceive of and then refer to themselves as external or objective entities. They can communicate about things and persons who are no longer present. (All of these milestones bring Piaget's period of sensorimotor intelligence towards an end.)

These changes in world perspective are best illustrated by Piaget's concept of "deferred imitation" (1954). Deferred imitation captures the essence of the developmental changes needed to lead to the sharing of meanings. At about eighteen months, a child may observe someone perform a behavior that the child has never performed—say dial a telephone, or pretend to bottle-feed a doll, or pour milk into a cup—and later that day, or several days later, imitate the dialing, feeding, or pouring. For infants to be able to perform such simple delayed imitations, several capacities are necessary.

1. They must have developed a capacity to represent accurately things and events done by others that are not yet part of their own action schemas. They must be able to create a mental prototype or representation of what they have witnessed someone else do. Mental representations require some currency or form in which they "exist" or are "laid down" in the mind; visual images and language are the two that first come to mind. (To get around the developmental problem of specifying what form the representation is being processed in, Lichtenberg has called this capacity an "imagining" capacity (1983, p. 198). (See also Call [1980]; Golinkoff [1983].)
2. They must, of course, already have the physical capacity to perform the action in their repertoires of possible acts.
3. Since the imitation is delayed and being performed when the original model is no longer doing it, perhaps not even around, the representation must be encoded in long-term memory and must be retrieved with a minimum of external cues. The infants must have good recall or evocative memory for the entire representation.

Children have already acquired these three capacities prior to the age of eighteen months. It is the next two capacities that make the difference and truly mark the boundary.

4. To perform delayed imitations, infants must have two versions of the same reality available: the representation of the original act, as performed by the model, and their own actual execution of the act. Furthermore, they must be able to go back and forth between these two versions of reality and make adjustments of one or the other to accomplish a good imitation. This is what Piaget meant by "reversibility" in the coordination of a mental schema and a motor schema. (The infant's capacity for recognizing maternal attunements during intersubjective relatedness falls short of what is now being described. In attunements the infant senses whether two expressions of an internal state are equivalent or not but does not need to make any behavioral adjustments on the basis of these perceptions. Moreover, only short-term memory is required for the registration of attunement, since the match is almost immediate.)
5. Finally, infants must perceive a psychological relationship between themselves and the model who performs the original act, or they would not embark on the delayed imitation to begin with. They must have some way of representing themselves as similar to the model, such that they and the model could be in the same position relative to the act to be imitated (Kagan 1978). This requires some representation of self as an objective entity that can be seen from the outside as well as felt subjectively from the inside. The self has

become an objective category as well as a subjective experience (Lewis and Brooks-Gunn 1979; Kagan 1981).

What is most new in this revolution about sense of self is the child's ability to coordinate schemas existing in the mind with operations existing externally in actions or words. The three consequences of this ability that most alter the sense of self and consequently the possibilities for relatedness are the capacity to make the self the object of reflection, the capacity to engage in symbolic action such as play, and the acquisition of language. These consequences, which we will take up in turn, combine to make it possible for the infant to negotiate shared meaning with another about personal knowledge.

THE OBJECTIVE VIEW OF SELF

The evidence that children begin at this age to see themselves objectively is thoroughly argued by Lewis and Brooks-Gunn (1979), Kagan (1981), and Kaye (1982). The most telling points in this argument are infants' behavior in front of a mirror, their use of verbal labels (names and pronouns) to designate self, the establishment of core gender identity (an objective categorization of self), and acts of empathy.

Prior to the age of eighteen months, infants do not seem to know that what they are seeing in a mirror is their own reflection. After eighteen months, they do. This can be shown by surreptitiously marking infants' faces with rouge, so that they are unaware that the mark has been placed. When younger infants see their reflections, they point to the mirror and not to themselves. After the age of eighteen months or so, they touch the rouge on their own faces instead of just pointing to the mirror. They now know that they can be objectified, that is, represented in some form that exists outside of their subjectively felt selves (Amsterdam 1972; Lewis and Brooks-Gunn 1978). Lewis and Brooks-Gunn call this newly objectifiable self the "categorical self," in distinction to the "existential self." It might also be called the "objective self" as against the "subjective self," or the "conceptual self" as against the "experiential self" of the previous levels of relatedness.

In any event, at about the same time infants give many other evidences of being able to objectify self and act as though self were an external category that can be conceptualized. They now begin to use pronouns ("I," "me," "mine") to refer to self, and they sometimes even begin to use proper names.[1] It is also at about this time that gender identity begins to become fixed. Infants recognize that the self as an objective entity can be categorized with other objective entities, either boys or girls.

It is also beginning around this time that empathic acts are seen (Hoffman 1977, 1978; Zahn-Waxler and Radke-Yarrow 1979, 1982). To act empathically the infant must be able to imagine both self as an object who can be experienced by the other and the objectified other's subjective state. Hoffman provides a lovely example of a thirteen-month-old boy who could, at that age, only incompletely sort out whose person (self or other) was to be objectified and whose subjective experience was to be focused upon. The failures in this case are more instructive than the successes. This child characteristically sucked his thumb and pulled on his ear lobe when he was upset. Once he saw his father clearly upset. He went over to his father and pulled the father's ear lobe but sucked on his own thumb. The boy was truly caught halfway between subjective and objective relatedness, but the coming months would see him performing more fully formed acts of empathy.

THE CAPACITY FOR SYMBOLIC PLAY

Lichtenberg (1983) has pointed out how the new capacities for objectifying the self and for coordinating mental and action schemas permit infants to "think" about or "imagine" about their interpersonal life. The clinical work of Herzog that Lichtenberg relies on illustrates this. In a study of eighteen- to twenty-month-old boys whose fathers had recently separated from the family, Herzog (1980) describes the following vignette. An eighteen-month-old boy was miserable because his father had just moved out of the home. During a play session with dolls, the boy doll was sleeping in the same bed as the mother doll. (The mother did, in fact, have the boy sleep in her bed after

---

1. Pseudo–proper names may appear earlier than semantically controlled pronouns (Dore, personal communication, 1984). There is some question about how much the infant initially sees the name or pronoun as an unencumbered, objectified referent for the self and how much as a referent for a more complex set of situational conditions involving caregiver and self in some activity: "Lucy don't do that!" In any event, the objectification process is well begun.

the father left.) The child got very upset at the dolls' sleeping arrangement. Herzog tried to calm the boy by having the mother doll comfort the boy doll. This did not work. Herzog then brought a daddy doll into the scene. The child first put the daddy doll in bed next to the boy doll. But this solution did not satisfy the child. The child then made the daddy doll put the boy doll in a separate bed and then get into bed with the mother doll. The child then said, "All better now" (Herzog 1980, p. 224). The child had to be juggling three versions of family reality: what he knew to be true at home, what he wished and remembered was once true at home, and what he saw as being enacted in the doll family. Using these three representations, he manipulated the signifying representation (the dolls) to realize the wished-for representation of family life and to repair symbolically the actual situation.

With this new capacity for objectifying the self and coordinating different mental and actional schemas, infants have transcended immediate experience. They now have the psychic mechanisms and operations to share their interpersonal world knowledge and experience, as well as to work on it in imagination or reality. The advance is enormous.

From the point of view of psychodynamic theories, something momentous has happened here. For the first time, the infant can now entertain and maintain a formed wish of how reality ought to be, contrary to fact. Furthermore, this wish can rely on memories and can exist in mental representation buffered in large part from the momentary press of psychophysiological needs. It can carry on an existence like a structure. This is the stuff of dynamic conflict. It reaches far beyond the real or potential distortions in perception due to immaturity or to the influence of "need state" or affect seen at earlier levels of relatedness. Interpersonal interaction can now involve past memories, present realities, and expectations of the future based solely on the past. But when expectations are based on a selective portion of the past, we end up with wishes, as in the case of Herzog's patient.

All these interpersonal goings-on can now take place verbally, or at least they will be reportable to the self and others verbally. The already existing knowledge of interpersonal transactions (real, wished for, and remembered) that involves objectifiable selves and others can be translated into words. When that happens, mutually shared meaning becomes possible and the quantum leap in relatedness occurs.[2]

THE USE OF LANGUAGE

By the time babies start to talk they have already acquired a great deal of world knowledge, not only about how inanimate things work and how their own bodies work but also about how social interactions go. The boy in Herzog's example cannot yet tell us verbally exactly what he wants and doesn't want, but he can enact what he knows and wishes with considerable precision. Similarly, children can point to the rouge on their own noses when they see it in a mirror before they can say "me," "mine," or "nose." The point is simply that there is a stretch of time in which rich experiential knowledge "in there" is accumulated, which somehow will later get assembled (although not totally) with a verbal code, language. And at the same time, much new experience will emerge along with the verbalization of the experience.

Such statements seem self-evident, yet until the 1970s most of the work on children's language acquisition was either concerned more with language itself, not experience, or focused on the child's innate mental devices and operations for making sense of language as a formal system, as in the work of Chomsky. There have also been fascinating and invaluable discoveries about the infant's perception of speech sounds, but these are largely outside the scope of this book.

It was mainly the seminal works of Bloom (1973), Brown (1973), Dore (1975, 1979), Greenfield and Smith (1976), and Bruner (1977) that insisted that world knowledge of interpersonal events was the essential key to unlocking the mysteries of language acquisition. As Bruner (1983) put it, a "new functionalism began to temper the formalism of the previous decades" (p. 8). Nonetheless, the words and structures of language have more than a one-to-one relationship to things and events in real experience. Words have an existence, a

---

2. The present description implies that concepts come first and that words are then attached, or that experiences established earlier get translated into words. Much current thinking suggests that felt-experience and words as an expression of felt-experience coemerge. The present argument does not depend upon this issue, which is crucial to the conception of language development *per se*.

life of their own that permits language to transcend lived experience and to be generative.

How world knowledge and language are assembled from the beginning of language acquisition remains at the cutting edge of experimental studies of child language in the interpersonal context (Golinkoff 1983; Brunner 1983). This issue has resurfaced simultaneously with a growing interest in the kinds of world knowledge and language structures our theories really look at and the kinds of interactions between experience and language we are imagining take place (Glick 1983). These considerations are necessary to our discussion because the essence of the question is how language may change the sense of self and what the acquisition of language, and all that it implies, makes possible between self and others that was not possible before. Since our subject is interpersonal relatedness rather than the equally enormous subject of language acquisition, we will very selectively draw on notions that have particular clinical relevance because they take into account the interpersonal motivational or affective context of language learning.

Michael Holquist (1982) suggests that the problem of different views of understanding language and its acquisition can be approached by asking who "owns" meanings. He defines three major positions. In Personalism, *I* own meaning. This view is deeply rooted in the western humanist tradition of the individual as unique. In contrast, a second view, more likely to be found in departments of comparative literature, holds that *no one* owns meaning. It exists out there in the culture. Neither of these views is very hospitable to our concerns, since it is hard to see how interpersonal events can influence the sharing or joint ownership of meaning in either case. However, Holquist defines a third view, which he calls Dialogism. In this view, *we* own meaning, or "if we do not own it, we may, at least, *rent* meaning" (p. 3). It is this third view that opens the door wide for interpersonal happenings to play a role, and it is from this perspective that the works of several students of language are of such interest.

The Effects of Language on Self-Other Relatedness: New Ways of "Being-With"

Vygotsky (1962) maintained that the problem of understanding language acquisition was, stated oversimply, how do mutually negotiated meanings (*we* meanings) "get in" to the child's mind? As Glick (1983) puts it, "The underlying conceptual problem is the *relationship* that exists between socialized systems of mediation (provided mainly by parents) and the individual's (infant's) reconstruction of these in an interior, and perhaps not fully socialized, way" (p. 16). The problem of language acquisition has become an interpersonal problem. Meaning, in the sense of the linkage between world knowledge (or thought) and words, is no longer a given that is obvious from the beginning. It is something to be negotiated between the parent and child. The exact relationship between thought and word "is not a thing, but a process, a continual movement back and forth from thought to word and from word to thought" (Vygotsky 1962, p. 125). Meaning results from interpersonal negotiations involving what can be agreed upon as shared. And such mutually negotiated meanings (the relation of thought to word) grow, change, develop and are struggled over by two people and thus ultimately owned by *us*.

This view leaves a great deal of room for the emergence of meanings that are unique to the dyad or to the individual.[3] "Good girl," "bad girl," "naughty boy," "happy," "upset," "tired," and a host of other such value and internal-state words will continue (often throughout life) to have the meanings uniquely negotiated between one parent and one child during the early years of assembling world knowledge and language. Only when the child begins to engage in an interpersonal dialectic with other socializing mediators such as peers can these meanings undergo further change. At that stage, new mutually negotiated *we* meanings emerge.

This process of the mutual negotiations of meaning actually applies to all meanings—"dog," "red," "boy," and so on—but it becomes most interesting and less socially constrained with internal state words. (There may be a difference between children in their interest

---

3. An extreme example is the "private speech" of twins.

in verbalizing things versus internal states. See Bretherton et al. [1981]; Nelson [1973]; and Clarke-Stewart [1973] for differences between individual styles and sexes.) When daddy says "good girl," the words are assembled with a set of experiences and thoughts that is different from the set assembled with mother's words "good girl." Two meanings, two relations coexist. And, the difference in the two meanings can become a potent source of difficulty in solidifying an identity or self-concept. The two diverse sets of experiences and thoughts are supposed to be congruent because they are claimed by the same words, "good girl." In the learning of language, we act overtly as though meaning lies either inside the self or somewhere out there belonging to anyone and meaning the same to all. This obscures the covert, unique *we* meanings. They become very hard to isolate and rediscover; much of the task of psychotherapy lies in doing so.

Dore has carried the notion of *we* meanings and negotiated shared meanings further in a manner that has implications for interpersonal theories. In the matter of the child's motivation to talk to begin with, Dore believes that infants talk, in part, to re-establish "being-with" experiences (in my terms) or to re-establish the "personal order" (MacMurray 1961). Dore (1985) describes it as follows:

> At this critical period of the child's life (. . . when he begins to walk and talk), his mother . . . reorients him away from the personal order with her, and towards a social order. In other words, whereas their previous interactions were primarily spontaneous, playful, and relatively unorganized for the sake of being together, the mother now begins to require him to organize his action for practical, social purposes: to act on his own (getting his own ball), to fulfill role functions (feeding himself), to behave well by social standards (not throwing his glass), and so on. This induces in the child the fear of having to perform in terms of non-personal standards (towards a social order) which orients away from the personal order of infancy. (p. 15)

It is in this context of pressure to maintain the new social order that the infant is motivated by the need and desire to re-establish the personal order with mother (Dore 1985). Dore is quick to point out that motivation alone, of this sort or any other, is not sufficient to explain the appearance of language. From our point of view, however, it adds an interpersonal motive (tenable but unproven) to the interpersonal process already pointed out by Vygotsky.

One of the major imports of this dialogic view of language is that the very process of learning to speak is recast in terms of forming shared experiences, of re-establishing the "personal order," of creating a new type of "being-with" between adult and child. Just as the being-with experiences of intersubjective relatedness required the sense of two subjectivities in alignment—a sharing of inner experience of state—so too, at this new level of verbal relatedness, the infant and mother create a being-with experience using verbal symbols—a sharing of mutually created meanings about personal experience.

The acquisition of language has traditionally been seen as a major step in the achievement of separation and individuation, next only to acquiring locomotion. The present view asserts that the opposite is equally true, that the acquisition of language is potent in the service of union and togetherness. In fact, every word learned is the by-product of uniting two mentalities in a common symbol system, a forging of shared meaning. With each word, children solidify their mental commonality with the parent and later with the other members of the language culture, when they discover that their personal experiential knowledge is part of a larger experience of knowledge, that they are unified with others in a common culture base.

Dore has offered the interesting speculation that language acts in the beginning as a form of "transitional phenomenon." To speak in Winnicott's terms, the word is in a way "discovered" or "created" by the infant, in that the thought or knowledge is already in mind, ready to be linked up with the word. The word is given to the infant from the outside, by mother, but there exists a thought for it to be given to. In this sense the word, as a transitional phenomenon, does not truly belong to the self, nor does it truly belong to the other. It occupies a midway position between the infant's subjectivity and the mother's objectivity. It is "rented" by "us," as Holquist puts it. It is in this deeper sense that language is a union experience, permitting a new level of mental relatedness through shared meaning.

The notion of language as a "transitional object" seems at first glance somewhat fanciful. However, observed evidence makes it seem very real. Katherine Nelson has recorded "crib talk" of a girl before and after her second birthday. Routinely, the infant's father put her to bed. As part of the putting-to-bed ritual, they held a dialogue in which the father went over some of the things that had happened that day and discussed what was planned for the next day. The girl participated actively in this dialogue and at the same time went through many obvious and subtle maneuvers to keep daddy present and talking, to prolong the ritual. She would plead, fuss-cry, insist, cajole, and devise new questions for him, intoned ingenuously. But when he finally said "good night" and left, her voice changed dramatically into a more matter of fact, narrative tone and her monologue began, a soliloquy.

Nelson gathered a small group consisting of herself, Jerome Bruner, John Dore, Carol Feldman, Rita Watson, and me. We met monthly for a year to examine how this child conducted both the dialogue with her father and the monologue after he left. The important features of her monologues were her practice and discovery of word usage. She could be seen to struggle with finding the right linguistic forms to contain her thoughts and knowledge of events. At times, one could see her moving closer and closer, with successive trials, to a more satisfying verbal rendition of her thinking. But even more striking, for the point at hand, is that it was like watching "internalization" happen right before our eyes and ears. After father left, she appeared to be constantly under the threat of feeling alone and distressed. (A younger brother had been born about this time.) To keep herself controlled emotionally, she repeated in her soliloquy topics that had been part of the dialogue with father. Sometimes she seemed to intone in his voice or to recreate something like the previous dialogue with him, in order to reactivate his presence and carry it with her toward the abyss of sleep. This, of course, was not the only purpose that her monologue served (she was also practicing language!), but it certainly felt as though she were also engaged in a "transitional phenomenon," in Winnicott's sense.

Language, then, provides a new way of being related to others (who may be present or absent) by sharing personal world knowledge with them, coming together in the domain of verbal relatedness. These comings-together permit the old and persistent life issues of attachment, autonomy, separation, intimacy, and so on to be re-encountered on the previously unavailable plane of relatedness through shared meaning of personal knowledge. But language is not primarily another means for individuation, nor is it primarily another means for creating togetherness. It is rather the means for achieving the next developmental level of relatedness, in which all existential life issues will again be played out.

The advent of language ultimately brings about the ability to narrate one's own life story with all the potential that holds for changing how one views oneself. The making of a narrative is not the same as any other kind of thinking or talking. It appears to involve a different mode of thought from problem solving or pure description. It involves thinking in terms of persons who act as agents with intentions and goals that unfold in some causal sequence with a beginning, middle, and end. (Narrative-making may prove to be a universal human phenomenon reflecting the design of the human mind.) This is a new and exciting area of research in which it is not yet clear how, why or when children construct (or co-construct with a parent) narratives that begin to form the autobiographical history that ultimately evolves into the life story a patient may first present to a therapist. The domain of verbal relatedness might, in fact, be best subdivided into a sense of a categorical self that objectifies and labels, and of a narrated self that weaves into a story elements from other senses of the self (agency, intentions, causes, goals, and so on).

The Other Edge of the Sword: The Alienating Effect of Language on Self-Experience and Togetherness

This new level of relatedness does not eclipse the levels of core-relatedness and intersubjective relatedness, which continue as ongoing forms of interpersonal experience. It does, however, have the capacity to recast and transform some of the experiences of core- and intersubjective relatedness, so that they lead two lives—their original life as nonverbal experience and a life as the verbalized version of that experience. As Werner and Kaplan (1963) suggest, language grabs hold of a piece of the conglomerate of feeling, sensation, perception, and cognition that constitutes global nonverbal experience. The piece that language takes hold of is transformed by the process of language-making and becomes an experience separate from the original global experience.[4]

Several different relationships can exist between the nonverbal global experience and that part of it that has been transformed into words. At times, the piece that language separates out is quintessential and captures the whole experience beautifully. Language is generally thought to function in this "ideal" way, but in fact it rarely does, and we will have the least to say about this. At other times, the language version and the globally experienced version do not coexist well. The global experience may be fractured or simply poorly represented, in which case it wanders off to lead a misnamed and poorly understood existence. And finally, some global experiences at the level of core- and intersubjective relatedness (such as the very sense of a core self) do not permit language sufficient entry to separate out a piece for linguistic transformation. Such experiences then simply continue underground, nonverbalized, to lead an unnamed (and, to that extent only, unknown) but nonetheless very real existence. (Unusual efforts such as psychoanalysis of poetry or fiction can sometimes claim some of this territory for language, but not in the usual linguistic sense. And this is what gives such power to these processes.)

Specific examples of particular experiences will illustrate this general issue of divergence between world knowledge and words. The notion of divergence, or slippage, between world knowledge and word knowledge is well known as it concerns knowledge of the physical world. Bower (1978) provides an excellent example of it. When a child is shown a lump of clay first rolled long and thin and then made into a fat ball, the child will claim that the ball version of the same amount of clay is heavier. According to the verbal account, the child does not have conservation of volume and weight. One would therefore expect that if the child is handed the two balls, first the thin one and then the fat one, the child's arm would rise up when it received the fat ball, since it was expected to be heavier and the muscles of the arm should be tensed to compensate for the difference. But a high-speed film shows that the arm does not move up. Bower concludes that the child's body, at the sensorimotor level,

4. We are not concerned here with the experiences that are created *de novo* by language. Some might claim that all experience rendered linguistically is experience *de novo,* but this position is not being assumed here.

has already achieved conservation of weight and volume, even though verbally the child seems to have lost or never to have had this capacity. Similar phenomena occur in domains that concern interpersonal world knowledge more directly.

The infant's capacity for amodal perception has loomed large in this overall account. The abilities to sense a core self and other and to sense intersubjective relatedness through attunement have depended in part on amodal capacities. What might happen to the experience of amodal perception when language is applied to it?

Suppose we are considering a child's perception of a patch of yellow sunlight on the wall. The infant will experience the intensity, warmth, shape, brightness, pleasure, and other amodal aspects of the patch. The fact that it is yellow light is not of primary or, for that matter, of any importance. While looking at the patch and feeling-perceiving it (à la Werner), the child is engaged in a global experience resonant with a mix of all the amodal properties, the primary perceptual qualities, of the patch of light—its intensity, warmth, and so on. To maintain this highly flexible and omni-dimensional perspective on the patch, the infant must remain blind to those particular properties (secondary and tertiary perceptual qualities, such as color) that specify the sensory channel through which the patch is being experienced. The child must not notice or be made aware that it is a visual experience. Yet that is exactly what language will force the child to do. Someone will enter the room and say, "Oh, *look* at the *yellow* sun*light!*" Words in this case separate out precisely those properties that anchor the experience to a single modality of sensation. By binding it to words, they isolate the experience from the amodal flux in which it was originally experienced. Language can thus fracture amodal global experience. A discontinuity in experience is introduced.

What probably happens in development is that the language version "yellow sunlight" of such perceptual experiences becomes the official version, and the amodal version goes underground and can only resurface when conditions suppress or outweigh the dominance of the linguistic version. Such conditions might include certain contemplative states, certain emotional states, and the perception of certain works of art that are designed to evoke experiences defying verbal categorization. Again, works of the symbolist poets serve as an example of the latter. The paradox that language can evoke experience that transcends words is perhaps the highest tribute to the power of language. But those are words in poetic use. The words in our daily lives more often do the opposite and either fracture amodal global experience or send it underground.

In this area, then, the advent of language is a very mixed blessing to the child. What begins to be lost (or made latent) is enormous; what begins to be gained is also enormous. The infant gains entrance into a wider cultural membership, but at the risk of losing the force and wholeness of original experience.

The verbal rendering of specific instances of life-as-lived presents a similar problem. Recall that in earlier chapters we distinguished *specific episodes* of life-as-lived (for example, "that one time when Mommy put me to bed to go to sleep, but she was distraught and only going through the motions of the bedtime ritual and I was overtired, and she couldn't help me push through that familiar barrier into sleep") and *generalized episodes* ("what happens when Mommy puts me down to sleep"). It is only the generalized ritual that is nameable as "bedtime." No specific instance has a name. Words apply to classes of things ("dog," "tree," "run," and so on). That is where they are most powerful as tools. The generalized episode is some kind of average of similar events. It is a prototype of a class of events-as-lived (generalized interactions [RIGs]): going to bed, eating dinner, bathtime, dressing, walk with Mommy, play with Daddy, peek-a-boo. And words get assembled with experiences of life-as-lived at this generalized level of the prototypic episode. Specific episodes fall through the linguistic sieve and cannot be referenced verbally until the child is very advanced in language, and sometimes never. We see evidence of this all the time in children's frustration at their failures to communicate what seems obvious to them. The child may have to repeat a word several times ("eat!") before the parent figures out what specific instance (which food) of the general class (of edible things) the infant has in mind and expects the adult to produce.

In the clinical literature, such phenomena have often been ascribed to children's belief in or wish for adults' omniscience and omnipotence. In contrast to that view, I suggest that such misunderstandings are not based on the child's notion that the mother knows what is in her child's mind to begin with. They are true misunderstandings about meaning. To the infant who says "eat," that means a specific edible thing. It requires only understanding, not mind-reading. The mother's misunderstanding serves to teach the child that the child's specific meaning is only a subset of her possible meanings. It is in this way that mutual meanings get negotiated. In such cases, we are observing the infant and mother struggling together with the peculiar nature of language and meaning. We are not observing ruptures and repairs in the infant's sense of an omniscient parent. The passions, pleasures, and frustrations seem to come more from the success and failure of mental togetherness at the levels of shared meaning, which the infant is motivated toward, not from anxiety at the loss of delegated omnipotence and/or from the good feeling of security when omnipotence is re-established. The misunderstandings simply motivate the infant to learn language better. They do not seriously rupture the child's sense of competence.

There may be more opportunities for such frustrations at the outset of language learning, because at the levels of core- and intersubjective relatedness the mother and infant have had a good deal of time to work out a nonverbal interactive system for relating. Negotiating shared meanings necessarily invokes much failing. To an infant who at prior levels has become accustomed to smoother transactions with mother concerning the import and intent of their mutual behaviors, this may be particularly frustrating.

Our point in demonstrating the many ways that language is inadequate to the task of communicating about specific lived-experience is not to minimize the import of language at all. Rather, it is to identify the forms of slippage between personal world knowledge and official or socialized world knowledge as encoded in language, because the slippage between these two is one of the main ways in which reality and fantasy can begin to diverge. The very nature of language, as a specifier of the sensory modality in use (in contrast to amodal nonspecification) and as a specifier of the generalized episode instead of the specific instance, assures that there will be points of slippage.

There are other points of slippage that should be noted. One of these is in the verbal accounts of internal states. Affect as a form of personal knowledge is very hard to put into words and communicate. Words to label internal states are not among the first to be used by children, even though children have presumably had long familiarity with the internal states (Bretherton et al. 1981). It is easier to label the categories of affective states (happy, sad) than the dimensional features (how happy, how sad). One problem is that the dimensional features of affect are gradient features (a little happy, very happy), while categorical features are not (happy versus not happy). Language is the ideal medium to deal with categorical information—that is partly what naming is all about—but it is at a great disadvantage in dealing with an analogue system, such as fullness of display, in ethological terms, which is geared to express gradient information. And it is the gradient information that may carry the most decisive information in everyday interpersonal communications.

The well-worn joke about the two psychiatrists passing on the sidewalk provides an illustration. They say "hello" and smile as they pass, and then each thinks to himself, "I wonder what he meant by that?" We can untrivialize this story by discussing it in terms of its categorical and gradient information. To begin with, greeting behaviors are conventionalized emotional responses containing elements from the Darwinian categories of surprise and happiness. As soon as one becomes aware that a greeting response will be initiated or responded to, one must tune in to the subtle but inevitable social cues that will be carried in the gradient features of the greeting. A number of factors will influence the gradient features and how each greeter will assess the greeting received: the nature of the relationship between the two greeters, the state of the relationship since their last meeting, the amount of time since they last met, their sexes, their cultural norms, and so on. In accordance with each participant's assessments of these factors, they expect each other to say a "hello" of a roughly specific volume, gusto, and intonational richness and to raise their eyebrows, widen their eyes, and open their smiles to a roughly expected height, width, and duration of display. Any significant variance from these expectations will occasion the question, "I wonder what he meant by that?" Each responder or recipient of the greeting will also be in the active position of gauging exactly how to adjust the delivery of his or her own greeting (Stern et al. 1983).

In this example, the work of interpreting the other person's behavior did not reside in the category of the signal. In fact, it did not even lie, as I have been implying, in the gradient features of the signal as performed. It lay in the discrepancy between the way the gradient features were actually performed and the way they were expected to be performed, given the context. The work of interpretation thus consists of measuring the distance between an imaginary performance (perhaps never before even seen in reality) and an actual performance of gradient features.

There is no reason why the situation should be much different for the child. The infant who hears mother say "Hi, honey" in an unaccustomed way would sense, but would not think to say, "You did not say it right." But the child would be wrong. What mother said, in linguistic fact, is right, but she did not act it (mean it) right. What is said and what is meant have a complicated relationship in the interpersonal domain.

When two messages, usually verbal and nonverbal, clash in the extreme, it has been called a "double-bind message" (Bateson et al. 1956). It is usually the case that the nonverbal message is the one that is meant, and the verbal message is the one of "record." The "on-record" message is the one we are officially accountable for.

Several authors, such as Scherer (1979) and Labov and Fanshel (1977), have pointed out that some of our communications are deniable, while others we are held accountable for. Gradient information is more easily denied. These different signals are going on simultaneously in various communicative channels. Furthermore, for the greatest flexibility and maneuverability of communication it is necessary to have this kind of mix (Garfinkel 1967). Labov and Fanshel (1977) describe this necessity very well in discussing intonational signals; for our purposes, their point applies equally well to other nonverbal behaviors:

> The lack of clarity or discreteness in the intonational signal is not an unfortunate limitation of this channel, but an essential and important aspect of it. Speakers need a form of communication which is deniable. It is advantageous for them to express hostility, challenge the competence of others, or express friendliness and affection in a way that can be denied if they are explicitly held to account for it. If there were not such a deniable channel of communication and intonation contours became so well recognized and explicit that people were accountable for their intonations, then some other mode of deniable communication would indoubtedly develop. (p. 46)

The surest way to keep a channel deniable is to prevent it from becoming a part of the formal language system. In learning a new word, a baby isolates an experience for clear identification and at the same time becomes accountable to mother for that word.)

This line of argument suggests that in a multi-channel communicative system there will exist constant environmental or cultural pressure to keep some signals more resistant to explicit accountable encoding than others, so that they will remain deniable. Because language is so good at communicating what, rather than how, something happened, the verbal message invariably becomes the accountable one. A year-old-boy was angry at his mother and in a fit of temper, while not looking at her, yelled, "Aaaaah!" and brought his fist down hard on a puzzle. Mother said, "Don't you yell at your mother." She would have been very unlikely to say, "Don't you bring your fist down like that at your mother." Neither message, the verbal one nor the nonverbal one, was more closely directed at her than the other. One is accountable very early for what one says, and this child is being prepared for that by making his vocalizations rather than his gestures the accountable act.

One of the consequences of this inevitable division into the accountable and the deniable is that what is deniable to others becomes more and more deniable to oneself. The path into the unconscious (both topographic and potentially dynamic) is being well laid by language. Prior to language, all of one's behaviors have equal status as far as "ownership" is concerned. With the advent of language, some behaviors now have a privileged status with regard to one having to own them. The many messages in many channels are being fragmented by language into a hierarchy of accountability/deniability.

There is another type of slippage between experience and words that deserves mention. Some experiences of self, such as continuity of coherence, the "going on being" of a physically integrated, nonfragmented self, fall into a category something like your heartbeat or regular breathing. Such experiences rarely require the notice needed to be verbally encoded. Yet periodically some transient sense of this experience is revealed, for some inexplicable reason or via psychopathology, with the breathtaking effect of sudden realization that your existential and verbal selves can be light years apart, that the self is unavoidably divided by language.

Many experiences of self-with-other fall into this unverbalized category; mutually gazing into one another's eyes without speaking qualifies. So does the sense of another person's characteristic vitality affects—the individual subtleties of physical style, which are also experienced as the child experiences a patch of sunlight. All such experiences are ineluctable, with the consequence of further distancing personal knowledge as experienced as word or thought. (It is little wonder we need art so badly to bridge these gaps in ourselves.)

A final issue involves the relation between life as experienced and as retold. How much the act of making an autobiographical narrative reflects or necessarily alters the lived experiences that become the personal story is an open question.

Infants' initial interpersonal knowledge is mainly unshareable, amodal, instance-specific, and attuned to nonverbal behaviors in which no one channel of communication has priviledged status with regard to accountability or ownership. Language changes all of that. With its emergence, infants become estranged from direct contact with their own personal experience. Language forces a space between interpersonal experience as lived and as represented. And it is exactly across this space that the connections and associations that constitute neurotic behavior may form. But also with language, infants for the first time can share their personal experience of the world with others, including "being with" others in intimacy, isolation, loneliness, fear, awe, and love.

Finally, with the advent of language and symbolic thinking, children now have the tools to distort and transcend reality. They can create expectations contrary to past experience. They can elaborate a wish contrary to present fact. They can represent someone or something in terms of symbolically associated attributes (for example, bad experiences with mother) that in reality were never experienced all together at any one time but that can be pulled together from isolated episodes into a symbolic representation (the "bad mother" or "incompetent me"). These symbolic condensations finally make possible the distortion of reality and provide the soil for neurotic constructs. Prior to this linguistic ability, infants are confined to reflect the impress of reality. They can now transcend that, for good or ill.

PART III

SOME CLINICAL IMPLICATIONS

Chapter 9

The "Observed Infant" as Seen with a Clinical Eye

BY SHIFTING the focus from different clinical developmental tasks, such as trust and autonomy, to different senses of the self as explanations of the major changes in the social organization of the infant, we have made it possible to examine different kinds of sensitive periods in early development. Since the major developmental shifts now involve the emergence of new senses of the self, the formative period for each sense of self can be considered sensitive. How critical these formative periods for each sense of the self will ultimately prove to be remains an open empirical issue. The weight of evidence from the neurological and ethological viewpoints, however, argues that the initial period of formation will prove relatively more sensitive than subsequent periods for later functioning (Hofer 1980).

In this chapter we will identify some of the patterns that are seen during the emergence of each sense of self, and we will speculate on how the initial form in which they are established may be critical for later functioning. First, however, several caveats are required.

When the development of an infant is observed with a clinical eye one sees almost no pathology, unless a preselected high-risk group has been chosen. Instead, there are characteristic patterns and some variant patterns, but there is very little basis for believing that any deviations from the norm are going to result in later pathology. When there are deviations, it is the relationship with the caregivers and not the infant alone that appears deviant. Often it is not even clear which variations are the most likely precursors of later pathology. And at each successive age, everything seems different, yet everything feels exactly the same, clinically. This is the paradox of continuity/discontinuity that fascinates and plagues the prospective view of development.

We have videotaped many mother/infant pairs at two, four, six, nine, eighteen, twenty-four, and thirty-six months, either at home or in the laboratory. Whenever we show a complete longitudinal series of tapes of one pair (shown in order, either forward or backward) to a group of students, whether new or experienced, they are forcibly struck by the sense that the two individuals are conducting their interpersonal business in a similar and recognizable fashion throughout. The same issues seem to get handled in the same general ways, although with different behaviors at different ages. The "feel" and even the subject matter of the interaction around these clinical issues is continuous, while the infant as a social person seems to be differently organized at each point.[1]

These impressions are one of the main reasons that we have shifted the focus from developmental tasks to senses of the self. Our emphasis, then, will be on the establishment of patterns of self-experience within each domain of senses of self that appear to have some clinical relevance for later functioning.

The problems of finding continuity of pattern and relating it to potential pathology are very real. These problems are beautifully exemplified in the recent history of attachment research. Initially, attachment was viewed as a specific developmental task of a particular life phase (Bowlby 1958, 1960; Ainsworth 1969). It became apparent that "quality of relatedness"—that is, attachment—extends beyond

---

1. This sense of continuity is reinforced by the fact that the people look the same physically from one time point to another. However, we find that during the first year after the infant's birth a large number of mothers go through a great number of drastic changes in hair style as they seek out their new identity, and they in fact look quite different from visit to visit.

the initial mother/infant bond and develops throughout childhood, applying to peers as well as to mother. In fact, it is a life-span issue. The question was how to discover the continuity in patterns of attachment. When one measured attachment with molecular behaviors such as gazes, vocalizations, proxemics, and so on, there appeared to be little continuity in quality of attachment from one age to another. It was only when researchers fell back on (or moved toward) a more global and qualitative summary measure of attachment such as the type of infant attachment—secure (type B), anxious/avoidant (type A), and anxious/resistant (type C) (Ainsworth et al. 1978)—that progress in the study of continuity could be made. Note that the summary measure of types of attachment yielded styles or patterns of attachment, not strength or goodness of attachment. Once this summary measure of patterns of attachment was available, researchers went on to show that type of attachment at twelve months correlated well with later patterns of relating.[2]

Indeed, it appears that quality of relationship at one year is an excellent predictor of quality of relating in various other ways up through five years, with the advantage to the securely attached infant compared with the resistantly or avoidantly attached infant. It has been suggested that the anxious attachment patterns at twelve months are predictive of psychopathology at age six in boys (Lewis et al., in press).

It would appear that resistant or avoidant attachment, which occurs in about 12 percent and 20 percent of middle-class U.S. samples, might be an indicator of later clinical problems. However, a caveat can be found in cross-cultural research. While data from a South German sample reflected U.S. norms, a North German sample had a preponderance of avoidant attachment (Grossmann and Grossmann, in press), and many Japanese children (37 percent) showed resistant attachment (Miyake, Chen, and Campos, in press). In this light, can type of attachment be considered a precursor to pathology? If so, it is quite culture-bound. More likely it is simply a style of conducting a motivational-clinical issue which may be a good nonspecific

---

2. The type of attachment shown at twelve months predicts: (1) type of attachment at eighteen months (Waters 1978; Main and Weston 1981); (2) frustratability, persistence, cooperativeness, and task enthusiasm at twenty-four months (Main 1977; Matas, Arend, and Sroufe 1978); (3) social competence of preschoolers (Lieberman 1977; Easterbrook and Lamb 1979; Waters, Wipman, and Sroufe 1979); and (4) self-esteem, empathy, and classroom deportment (Sroufe 1983).

indicator of general success in adaptation to life, however life is found (Sroufe and Rutter 1984; Garmenzy and Rutter 1983; Cicchetti and Schneider-Rosen, in press). But indicators of general adaptation are not precursors. Their relationship to later behavior is too non-specific and indirect.

In this chapter, we will confine the discussion to patterns of self-experience that are of potential clinical relevance and are best conceptualized in terms of the different domains of sense of self.

Constitutional Differences and Emergent Relatedness

The capacities that permit the infant to yoke his diverse experiences of the social world are to an enormous extent constitutionally—that is, genetically—determined. Either they are present right away or they unfold on an innate timetable, given an intact central nervous system and an intact environment. For the immediate future, the study of individual differences of these capacities may prove to be the most fruitful area of clinical research on the development of psychopathology in the very young. Whenever new capacities are identified, especially those needed in social perception and competence, they naturally become the focus of intense scrutiny, speculation, and hope. The hope is that the earliest deviation in social and intellectual functioning will be traceable to abnormalities in these capacities. If so, we would have an understanding of the underlying mechanisms that would help explain the emergence of pervasive developmental disorder, autism, later learning disabilities, attention deficit, characterological differences, and various problems in social conduct and competence. Discrete therapeutic strategies would also be more obvious.

Let us look briefly at some possible clinical ramifications of deficits in these capacities. The capacity to transfer information from one modality to another is so central to integrating perceptual experience that the potential problems resulting from a deficit are almost limitless. One of the first to leap to mind is learning disabilities, since so much learning calls for a transposition of information from one sensory mode to another, especially back and forth between vision and audition. And indeed, Rose et al. (1979) now have suggestive evidence that learning-disabled children may be abnormal in specific cross-modal transfer capacities. Infants could also be socially and emotionally disabled by such deficits; intermodal fluency greatly facilitates the apprehension of the social behavior of other persons as well as the integrated actions, sensations, affects, and so on of one's own self. These findings are still too new for one to have any idea, as yet, of the limits of their psychopathological relevance.

In a different vein, the perennial search for early predictors of later general intelligence seems to have been revived by promising results that show the extent to which the infant's capacities for long-term recognition memory and other information-processing feats predict later intellectual functioning (Caron and Caron 1981; Fagan and Singer 1983). The study of episodic memory in infancy has only just begun.

Ever since the work of Thomas et al. (1970) on temperamental differences and the emphasis of Escalona (1968) on the importance of the "fit" between maternal and infant temperaments, it has been clear that all considerations of interaction from the clinical point of view must take temperament into full account. Clinically, most practitioners find it absolutely essential to keep issues of temperament and fit in mind. In spite of this, researchers have to date been fairly unsuccessful in documenting the continuity of temperamental differences in infancy when they are viewed prospectively. (See Sroufe [in press] for a discussion of the problems of considering temperamental determinants outside of a relational perspective.) Nonetheless, it is worth speculating about how a temperamental difference in something such as tolerance for stimulation might be viewed clinically.

Individual differences in infants' tolerance for stimulation or the capacity to regulate arousal may have relevance to issues such as later anxiety disorders, which have a significant constitutional component. One can think of the relationship between absolute stimulation and arousal or excitation in several different ways, only one of which is shown in figure 9.1,[3] as an example. The asterisks mark individually

3. For any one child, there is no one, single curve; rather, there is a family of curves. For example, if the mother stays at home all day and the father has a quick bout of interaction with the baby in the evening after work, he usually does so at a higher level of stimulus intensity than what has been going on all day with mother. His games will be more explosive,

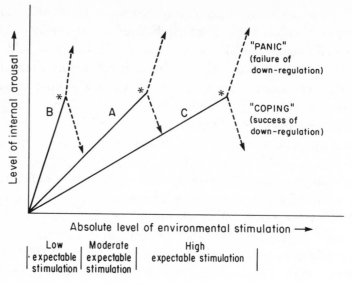

Figure 9.1

characteristic points at which the infant's capacity to cope with the stimulation level is about to be exceeded. At this point the child must down-regulate the level by dampening or terminating stimulus input through some coping maneuver, or the threshold for coping will be exceeded and the infant will experience something like panic. Assume that line A represents a normal curve. Suppose a baby had a characteristic curve like that shown in line B. The stimulation of normal daily events would exceed the infant's coping capacity and trigger anxiety episodes. Because the thresholds for external stimulation are set so low, it would look as though the anxiety attacks were spontaneous—that is, internally caused, as Klein (1982) suggests—when in fact they were simply promiscuously triggered by expectable, everyday stimulation arising from almost anywhere. In this regard, Brazelton's (1982) descriptions of the low stimulation tolerance of small-for-gestational-age infants may prove relevant.

There may also prove to be different thresholds of tolerance for different *kinds* of stimulation. It has long been suggested that autistic

---

with more throwing in the air and vigorous touching and kinesthetic stimulations. What is interesting is that the infant seems to expect and even want this higher level of excitement; the baby tolerates and even seeks higher levels of arousal and intensities of stimulation in the coming-home situation (Yogman 1982). If the father is a house-husband and mother goes to work, the parents reverse patterns and the two curves tend to switch. Still, each may have a characteristic limit.

children may have an extremely low tolerance for human stimulation (especially gaze), but not for nonhuman stimulation (Hutt and Ounsted 1966). Similarly, some people are predominantly aural or visual or tactile, and many investigators have proposed different sensitivities to stimulation in different modalities as a cause for mismatch in the regulation of arousal between mothers and infants (Greenspan 1981). Or again, the nature of the coping operation characteristically used may show wide individual differences, resulting in various pictures, such as shyness, avoidance, or vigilance.

While the potential of amodal and other constitutional capacities for the understanding of later psychopathology is great, it remains largely unresearched and fraught with many problems. First, there is the problem of specificity. We do not yet know if it is possible to have a severe disfunction in any one or two of these capacities without having disfunctions in almost all of them. Second, the relationship between severity of defect in these capacities and functional social behavior is unknown. Suppose something went drastically wrong with many of these capacities. What might result? In the most extreme case, one would predict pervasive developmental disorders (mental retardation with autistic features). Neither a core self nor a core other could be fully constituted, and social relatedness would be massively compromised. Unity of the senses would gel slowly, if at all, through experience. Causal relations would go largely undetected. The perceptual world would be disorganized and partially unconstructable. Memory would be limited, so that continuity of experience would be minimal. All transactions with the inanimate world as well as with the human world would be grossly compromised. The disorder would indeed be pervasive—so pervasive that it would be difficult or impossible to sort out which specific defects contributed to which specific disorders in function. And if a sense of a core self could not form, there would be no basis from which to form a sense of a subjective self, and so on.

Less drastic defects in these capacities could be the precursors of a spectrum of outcomes, from serious illness through subtle personal oddities, including differences in interpersonal, cognitive, or perceptual style. There is much new information that is very promising for later clinical issues. Now is the time to begin to evaluate its true clinical import. In particular, studies in individual differences with longitudinal follow-up are needed. Whatever the results, this early period of life will never again look the same clinically.

So far, this discussion has not directly concerned the infant's emergent sense of self. Since these capacities are the very ones involved in creating emergent experiences, however, the sense of the emergent self would be profoundly affected by deficits in any of these capacities. In the following sections we will focus more centrally on the clinical implications for the different senses of self. These will clearly have more relevance for the more characterological or neurotic features of pathology in contrast to the Axis I diagnostic categories of the *Diagnostic and Statistical Manual of Mental Disorders* (*DSM-III*).

Core-Relatedness

When watching an infant, can one get a clinical impression of future dangers to the core sense of self? Clinical vignettes will serve best to answer this question. The regulation of excitation, arousal, activation, stimulation, and tension are the aspects of self that clinicians focus on most in evaluating the health-promoting nature of the parent-infant relationship during the first half-year of life. Our major concern here, therefore, will be on the contouring of excitation as it is mutually performed by infant and parent.

Two statements first. There is no such thing as a perfect mutual contouring of excitation, either all the time or even for a short time. Interaction does not work that way. Constant failures of stimulation, overshooting, and under-shooting are built into the dynamic nature of an interaction. The goal or set point is always changing. These over- and under-shootings make up the ordinary repeating interactive patterns. Secondly, we are operating on assumptions, stated before, that the representational world is constituted mainly from the ordinary events of life, not from the exceptional ones. Exceptional moments are probably no more than superb yet slightly atypical examples of the ordinary. One can only address characteristic "misfittings" and their likely consequences.

EXPECTABLE AND TOLERABLE OVERSTIMULATION IN THE DOMAIN
OF CORE-RELATEDNESS

Eric is a somewhat bland infant compared with his more affectively intense mother, but both are perfectly normal. His mother constantly likes to see him more excited, more expressive and demonstrative about feelings, and more avidly curious about the world. When Eric does show some excitement about something, his mother adroitly joins in and encourages, even intensifies, the experience a little— usually successfully, so that Eric experiences a higher level of excitement than he would alone. The cajoling, exaggerating, slightly overresponsive, eliciting behavior that she characteristically performs are in fact usually very enjoyable to Eric. Her behavior does not create a gross mismatch, but rather a small one. His tolerance for stimulation can encompass it, but at a level of excitement that he would not reach by his own efforts. It would not be accurate to call her controlling or intrusive. She does not try to disrupt or redirect his experience on the basis of her own needs or insensitivities. Rather, she is trying to augment the range of his experiences (granted, for her own reasons and in accord with her own temperamental type). It is a very common experience for any mother to try to expand her infant's tolerance for excitement or arousal and generally stretch her infant's world ("Did you realize that this old rattle could be that fascinating?"). It is no more than working in the infant's zone of proximal (affective) development, the place just beyond where he is and that he is developing toward.

What made the "constructive" mismatches more obvious in this case was the discrepancy in "temperamental" types between mother and son. But that only highlighted the situation. A mother of a temperament identical to her child's would have to act similarly at times to work in her infant's zone of proximal affective development.

In any event, Eric's self-experience of higher-than-usual excitement is, in fact, largely achieved and regulated by his mother's behavior. His experience of his own higher levels of excitement occurs only in the lived episodes in which her augmenting antics are a crucial attribute. She thus becomes for him a self-excitement-regulating other. Eric's self-experience of high positive excitement never occurs unless mother is there participating in it. Specific episodes coalesce to form a RIG. And the activated RIG takes the form of an evoked companion, the experience of whom can be captured by questions like: "What is it like to be with mother when I feel this way in myself? or, "How do I feel in myself when I am with mother?"

Now suppose Eric is alone or with another person. And by himself, he begins to exceed the level of positive excitement that is usual for him when he is not with his mother. (Maturation and development are proceeding rapidly day by day, making this experience frequent and inevitable.) He begins to "feel this way," that is, to reach a certain higher level of excitement. "Feeling this way" is one of the attributes of the RIG, the other indivisible attribute of which is mother's encouraging, experience-augmenting performance. Beginning to "feel this way" will serve as the attribute that unconsciously recalls to mind the evoked companion. (A representation has been reactivated.) Eric then experiences a fantasied being with mother. In some sense, she is functionally "there," and that helps him to stretch the level of excitement he has created for himself. The evoked companion as a self-regulating other is promoting development. There is no distortion of reality. Everything is reality-based. Let us now look at other RIGs, evoked companions, and their influence on development.

FORMS OF INTOLERABLE OVERSTIMULATION IN THE DOMAIN OF CORE-RELATEDNESS

The experience of overstimulation for the infant can only be understood in terms of what happens next, since that becomes part of the lived episode. It must be understood that by the age of three months or so, the infant's immediate response to overstimulation (short of excessive overstimulation) is *not* to cry and fall apart but rather to try to deal with it. After all, "it" is elicited by mother's or father's behavior, in an interaction for which the infant has a repertoire of regulating maneuvers. Coping and defensive operations form in the small space between the upper threshold of the infant's stimulation tolerance and final crying. This space is the growing and testing ground of adaptive maneuvers. And their performance becomes part of the lived experience of overstimulation.

In the case of Stevie, an overstimulating, controlling mother regularly forced the face-to-face interaction into a "game of chase and dodge," well described by Beebe and Stern (1977). In essence, when the mother overstimulated him, Stevie would avert his head to the side. Mother would respond to this dodge by chasing him with her face and escalating the stimulus level of her behavior to capture his attention. He would then execute another dodge, swinging his face away to the opposite side. Mother would follow his head with hers, still trying to maintain the vis-à-vis engagement at the level she wanted. Finally, if he was unable to avoid her gaze, Stevie would become more upset and end up crying. More often than not, however, his aversions were successful and mother would get the message long before he cried. This example is extreme, but the general pattern in milder form has been described over and over (Stern 1971, 1977; Beebe and Sloate 1982).

This kind of intrusive overstimulating behavior on the part of the mother can arise from many causes: hostility, need for control, insensitivity, or an unusual sensitivity to rejection such that mother interprets each infant head aversion as a "microrejection" and attempts to repair and undo it (Stern 1977). Whatever the reason for his mother's behavior, Stevie experiences the following RIG: a high level of arousal, maternal behavior that tends to push him beyond his tolerable limits, the need to self-regulate downward, and the (usually) successful self-regulation by persistent aversions. In Stevie's case, when he is experiencing the higher levels of excitement, his mother has become a different kind of evoked companion, a self-disregulating other.

Now let us suppose that Stevie is alone or with another person, and he begins to approach his upper level of tolerable stimulation, to "feel a certain way." Feeling that certain way will activate the RIG. Like Eric, he will experience an evoked being-with-mother, but in his case it is a disregulating union with mother that will result in his execution of potentially maladaptive behavior. He will unnecessarily avoid stimulation that threatens to exceed or has just exceeded his tolerance. If he is with someone else, he misses or does not stay open to the adjustments on the other's part that would permit him either to stay engaged or to re-engage. From observation of many infants such as Stevie, it is clear that they generalize their experience, so that they are relatively overavoidant with new persons. When they are alone, one of two things seems to happen. They cut short their potential positive excitement, most likely by activating a disregulating mother as the evoked companion, or they show freer access to their own pleasurable excitement and can even wallow in it, as if they inhibited or somehow prevented the activation of the RIG.[4]

We do not know why some infants seem able to regulate their excitement so much more successfully when alone than when interacting with a disregulating parent. Whether we are talking about inhibited evoked companions or selective generalization, it would appear that those children who are more successful at escaping the evoked presence of a problematic parent when alone gain the advantage of being able to utilize more of themselves. At the same time, they are dealt the disadvantage of living more alone in the world.

Molly and her mother illustrate a different form of intolerable overstimulation. Molly's mother was very controlling. She had to design, initiate, direct, and terminate all agendas. She determined which toy Molly should play with, how Molly was to play with it ("Shake it up and down—don't roll it on the floor"), when Molly was done playing with it, and what to do next ("Oh, here is Dressy Bessy. Look!"). The mother overcontrolled the interaction to such an extent that it was often hard to trace the natural crescendo and decrescendo of Molly's own interest and excitement. It was so frequently derailed or interrupted that it could hardly be said to trace its own course. This is an extreme form of disregulation of excitation. (Most experienced viewers who watch these televised interactions between Molly and her mother find themselves getting a tense feeling most often described as a knot in the stomach and slowly realize how enraged they are becoming. There is a co-opting of the child's self-regulating abilities that makes those who identify with Molly feel impotent and infuriated.)

Molly found an adaptation. She gradually became more compliant. Instead of actively avoiding or opposing these intrusions, she became one of those enigmatic gazers into space. She could stare through you, her eyes focused somewhere at infinity and her facial expressions opaque enough to be just uninterpretable, and at the same time remain in good contingent contact and by and large do what she was invited or told to do. Watching her over the months was like

---

4. All of these vignettes can also be explained in terms of traditional learning theory, generalization, and selective generalizations. However, these permit no account of the infant's subjective experience of performing these overt behaviors.

watching her self-regulation of excitement slip away. She appeared to let herself ride the stop-and-start course of arousal flow dictated by her mother. In fact, she seemed to have given up on the whole idea of self-regulation of this part of herself. When playing alone she did not recover it, remaining somewhat aloof from exciting engagements with things. This general dampening of her affectivity continued beyond this phase of development and was still apparent at age three years. She seems to have learned that excitement is not something that is equally regulated by two people—the self and the self-regulating other—but that it is mainly the self-regulating other who does all the regulating. (At some point in her development, anger, oppositionalism, hostility, and the like will be sorely needed to rescue her.)

FORMS OF INTOLERABLE UNDERSTIMULATION IN THE DOMAIN OF CORE-RELATEDNESS

Susie's mother was depressed, preoccupied with a recent divorce. She in fact had not wanted Susie to begin with except to hold the marriage together. She already had an older daughter, who was her favorite. Susie was a normally spunky infant, well endowed with all the capacities to appeal to and elicit social behavior from any willing adult, plus a lot of persistence to keep trying at the faintest hint of success. In spite of this, she was generally unsuccessful in getting her mother to join in for long. More important, she could not get her mother to spark enough so that the mother ever took over the up-regulation of excitation. The mother did not actually take control over the down-regulation of excitation, but her lack of responsivity acted as a drag on Susie's attempts to up-regulate.

What is happening in this situation? Suppose that the mother were completely unresponsive and unmoveable, essentially not there, and Susie were left to her own devices to experience and regulate her own excitement (a variant of the situation that once prevailed for institutionalized babies). During the period of forming a sense of a core self, she could only experience a narrow band of pleasurable arousal, because it is only stimuli provided by the unique social behavior of adults towards infants that can, so to speak, blast the infant into the next orbit of positive excitation. The infant would be left without a certain range of experience. The actual and fantasied experiences with a self-regulating other are essential for encountering the normally expected range of self-experiences, and without the other's presence and responsive behavior, the full range simply does not develop. There is a maturational failure, a "self-regulating-other–deficiency disease." This is just another way of stating that only a selected portion of the whole spectrum of self-experiences of excitation may get exercized during this period resulting in a permanent influence during this sensitive period upon what experiences become part of the sense of a core self.

This is not exactly Susie's situation, but it is close to the situation that obtains when her experiences with her mother are particularly barren. Susie is persistent, however, and she is drawn on to be persistent because she is sometimes moderately successful and occasionally very successful. When she is, she experiences a much higher than ordinary sense of pleasurable excitement. What happens, then, is that she has to work hard to get mother to ignite and thereby sends herself the rest of the way. Susie's experience with self-excitement-regulating other forms a very different RIG from that of the other children. She does not expect and accept experiences of being with the self-excitement-regulating other, as Eric does. Nor does she need to dread them, as Stevie does, or tune them out, as Molly does.

She must actively strive and perform to set her mother into motion to create the being-with experiences she needs. This interactive pattern based on a specific RIG has remained characteristic of Susie for the first three years, and one can readily imagine its continuing and gathering in more and more aspects of the interpersonal world. She is already a "Miss Sparkle Plenty" and precociously charming. Her behavior lends support to the idea that we may be dealing with sensitive periods that put a stamp on the future.

Susie's is only one adaptive solution to a prevailing but not complete understimulation. Some infants, endowed with less persistence and spark, follow a depressive. rather than a performance-oriented route.[5]

So far, we have discussed only the regulation of pleasurable excitement and the role of the other in that regulation. The issues

5. We have not pursued the developmental fate of each of the described RIGS. There are two reasons for this. We have not had the opportunity to conduct the needed longitudinal observations, and until recently we have not known in what forms to look for continuity at the next level of relatedness.

involved would be the same if we were discussing the regulation of security, curiosity/exploration, attention, and so on. Readers can trace from their own clinical experiences the line of development of those diverse self-regulating others and the RIGs they lend to.

Can potential problems in the formation of a sense of a core self be seen in these disregulations of contours of excitation? Does one see what look like possible precursors to "self pathology"? Is the period from two to six months a sensitive one for the formation of a sense of a core self?

These questions can only be answered in terms of how one conceptualizes a sense of a core self. The sense of core self, as a composite of the four self-invariants (agency, coherence, affectivity, and continuity), is always in flux. It is being built up, maintained, eroded, rebuilt, and dissolved, and all these things go on simultaneously. The sense of self at any moment, then, is the network of the many forming and dissolving dynamic processes. It is the experience of an equilibrium.

On one side, there are two general kinds of experiences that act continually to form or reconstitute these senses of self. There are the many events (such as deciding to sit up and doing so) that come and go and provide phasic perceptions that act to form and reform the sense of self. And there are the almost constant unattended events (remaining sitting up, with all the constant but out-of-awareness readjustments of antigravity and postural muscle tone) that provide tonic perception acting to maintain the sense of self. On the other side are all the influences that disrupt the organized perception of self: overstimulation, situations that disrupt the flow of tonic perceptions that maintain the sense of self (being thrown too high in the air with too long a fall); experiences of self/other similarity that confound the self/other boundary cues; maternal understimulation that reduces certain tonic and phasic self-experiences. The question of later clinical consequences boils down to whether the prevailing dynamic equilibrium of the sense of a core self, when the sense of a core self is first forming, influences the later sense of self.

The sense of a core self, since it is a dynamic equilibrium, is always in potential jeopardy. And indeed, it is a common life event to experience and/or fear major perturbations in the sense of a core self. Winnicott has made a list of what he calls the "primitive agonies" or "unthinkable anxieties" to which children are heir.

These are "going to pieces," "having no relation to the body," "having no orientation," "falling forever," "not going on being," and "complete isolation because of there being no means of communication" (Winnicott 1958, 1960, 1965, 1971). Such anxieties seem to be fairly ubiquitous in older children. They are common material for the fears, nightmares, favorite stories, and fairy tales of children. As adults, are any of us totally free of such fears, either waking or dreaming? In more severe form, they make up psychotic pathological experiences of fragmentation (ruptures of coherence), paralysis of action and/or will (ruptures of agency), annihilation (ruptures of continuity), and dissociation (ruptures in ownership of affectivity).

The infant, then, like everyone else, experiences the sense of a core self as having a fluctuating dynamic status. This is the normal state of existence. As one gets older, however, the forces of maintenance are so predominant that severe disequilibriums are infrequently felt under normal conditions, and then usually only as a hint or cue or "signal."

This picture leaves much room for individual differences in the prevailing dynamic equilibrium experienced by any one individual. And it is the prevailing dynamic equilibrium that may get established as a characteristic pattern during this early period. The question is not, then, does a sense of agency, coherence, affectivity, or continuity get established once and for all during this period? Nor is the question whether the sense of a core self gets established well or poorly. What seems to get established are some of the properties of the dynamic equilibrium that determines the sense of a core self.

In clinical terms, some patients have a relatively well-formed sense of a core self, which is stable but requires an enormous amount of maintaining input, in the form of both tonic and phasic contributions from others. When that input fails, the sense of self falls apart. Others have a less well-formed sense of self which, while equally stable, requires much less maintenance. And still others are most characterized by the great lability of this sense of self that cannot be fully explained by changes in maintaining input.

It is likely that these aspects of a sense of a core self receive a characteristic impress during the initial period of formation of the sense of a core self; the earlier in formation, the more lasting the likely influence. However, the sense of a core self does not stop forming, so there is much time after the initial phase of formation to provide compensatory influences. In any event the early formation of these three parameters of the core sense of self (degree of formation, maintenance needs, and lability) says more about the nature of the sense of self and less about the ultimate severity of any potential pathology.

In keeping with the focus on the infant's likely subjective experience, nothing has yet been said about how the infant might experience disequilibrations in the dynamic sense of a core self. Do infants experience anxiety as the (momentary and partial) dissolution of the sense of a core self, as adults generally do?

It is likely that in the domain of core-relatedness infants do not experience "unthinkable anxieties" about *potential* disruptions in the sense of a core self, but they may experience "primitive agonies" about *actual* disruptions. It is reasonable to assume that infants do not experience anxieties about these matters until later, because anxieties are ultimately fears, and fear is generally thought not to emerge as a full emotion until the second half of the first year of life (Lewis and Rosenblum 1978). Fear is not even seen as a facial display until after six months (Cicchetti and Sroufe 1978). Also, fear in the form of anxiety results from the cognitive appraisal of an immediate future, and the ability to anticipate an immediate future does not appear to be sufficiently present until after the age of six months or so.

The infant, then, should be left free of anxieties about the core self, at least during the short period during which this sense is first being formed. But how about "primitive agonies"? Assume that "primitive agonies" are some form of nonlocalizable distress that relies on *affect appraisals* of a situation, rather than *cognitive appraisals.* Affect appraisals ("Is it pleasurable or unpleasurable?" "Is it to be approached or avoided?") are presumed to be more primitive than cognitive appraisals. In other words, they are potentially independent of and developmentally prior to the cognitive appraising processes. Affect appraisals are therefore presumably operating prior to the emergence of fears and anxieties. They appraise the present.

Affect appraisal usually refers to the perception of external stimuli (a sweet or a bitter taste, a sudden loud voice, and so on), and the consequences of these appraisals are pleasures, unpleasures, approaches, or withdrawals (see Scheirla 1965). Other affect appraisals refer to the perception of internal stimuli specific to physiologic need states (hunger, thirst, physical comfort, oxygen). There is also a third source of affect appraisals, made up of the many interpersonal goal states that the young human is designed to achieve or maintain, which are ultimately necessary for species survival but do not involve physiological needs. These are the needs for specific social and self organizations (Bowlby 1969). We can add to these the need to organize perceptions such that a core sense of self agency, cohesion, affectivity, and continuity results. These, too, are essential for survival in a social world.

When there is a negative affect appraisal about the self required to meet those social and self-organizational goal states, what is felt? And what name can be given to this feeling? "Primitive agonies" is a good choice. It is meant to imply a nonlocalizable distress that does not attach to physiological state. (Physiological distress is better captured by Mahler's term "organismic distress . . . that forerunner of anxiety proper" [1968, p. 13].) "Primitive agonies" is specifically meant to capture failures in the ongoing functions needed to maintain essential social or interpersonal states. Borrowing from Winnicott, then, we can use it to describe this category of infant life experience.

The infant should experience "primitive agonies" whenever temporary and partial dissolutions of the sense of a core self occur. Furthermore, these agonies should occur during the period of core-relatedness well before cognitive appraisals of the exact same events add anxiety to the experience of agony, after about six months.

These considerations add a fourth property to the prevailing dynamic equilibrium that gets established: the presence or absence— or better, the dosage—of agony that characteristically accompanies the maintenance of a sense of a core self. This, too, can be carried forward in time as a characteristic feature of experience.

THE ISSUE OF PSYCHOPATHOLOGY DURING CORE-RELATEDNESS

During the formative phase of the domain of core-relatedness, an infant can readily present clinical problems. These are usually presented as sleep or eating problems. They are not signs or symptoms of any intrapsychic conflict within the infant, however. They are the accurate reflection of an ongoing interactive reality, manifestations of a problematic interpersonal exchange, not psychopathology of a psychodynamic nature.

In fact, at these early ages there are no mental disorders in infants, only in the relationships in which infants participate. (Mental retardation, Down's syndrome, and autism represent partial exceptions.)

One of the most common examples is sleeping problems. Usually the infant will not go to sleep, keeps crying until the mother returns to the bedside, sputters along until she has reenacted her put-down-to-sleep ritual, may or may not get some milk or water, and then cries again after she leaves for the third or fifth time. The infant's behavior in this situation is not a sign or symptom in the usual sense. Given the uncertain and unclear limit-setting by the mother, the natural fears of being alone or in the dark, the reinforcement of the behavior, and so on, the infant is acting in a manner concordant with current reality. In the vast majority of such common cases, there is nothing wrong with the infant per se. The behavior is simply a characteristic, predictable pattern that has become a family problem.

Intersubjective Relatedness

The clinical issues at stake during the formation of intersubjective relatedness are the same as those encountered during the formation of core-relatedness. But now the focus shifts from the regulation of behaviorally overt self-experience by the other to the sharing of subjective experience between self and other and the influencing of one another's subjective experience. To begin with sharing, can you share your inner experience with an other at all? And can others share their inner experience with you? If you both can share some subjective experiences, which ones are shareable and which are not? What is the fate of experiences that are not shareable? What is the fate of experiences that are shareable? And finally, what are some of the possible interpersonal consequences of sharing?

We stated that the focus shifts from regulating experiences to sharing them. This is true only to the extent that intersubjective sharing can now begin—not that the mutual regulation of experience stops—to give way to this new form. Now they can proceed together.

The following patterns with clinical relevance are describable in this domain.

NON-ATTUNEMENT: UNSHAREABILITY OF SUBJECTIVE EXPERIENCE

It is hard to imagine a situation in which there is no interaffective sharing. In its extreme form it is probably only encountered in severe psychosis or among normal persons in science-fiction plots in which the hero is the only human among robots or an alien species whose inner experiences are impenetrable. This fictional situation is particularly apt, because the human and the aliens can have physical relatedness (if the aliens are attractive enough) and can even communicate about external matters. But if affective subjectivity is impossible, a cosmic loneliness ensues in the hero. Milder versions of this state of affairs occur in character disorders and neuroses. But in these conditions there is the wish for, or illusion of, or bungled attempts at, possible intersubjective sharing. In the psychotic or science-fiction situation, no possibility of affective intersubjectivity exists a priori.

The extreme condition of lack of interaffective sharing might apply to the institutionalized infants described decades ago or to a mother sufficiently depressed or psychotic that she is judged as no longer able to care adequately for her baby. What follows is a description of the last-mentioned situation and is intended to illustrate how nonshareability of inner experience can occur and at the same time not scream out as a clinical fact.

A twenty-nine-year-old divorced mother was admitted to the psychiatric ward of a community hospital because of decompensation of her chronic paranoid schizophrenic condition. She had had two previous hospitalizations and had been maintained on antipsychotic medication. She had a ten-month-old daughter, who was rooming on the pediatric ward. The child was kept there because no extended family was available to take her and because some of the psychiatric ward staff did not think she was safe with her mother. Others felt that the baby was safe and urged that she be returned to the mother and live on the ward around the clock with her, instead of having just two supervised visits daily. Those who wanted separation thought that the mother's overconcern for the child's safety and her fear that someone or something might hurt the girl were ominous projections indicating hostile destructive wishes of her own. Those who wanted the girl to live on the ward felt that the projections were less of a threat than the real distress experienced by mother and child because of the separation.

The mother was usually quite compensated and could pull herself together. She was not overtly psychotic. Rather, she was secretive and unrevealing of her thoughts. She cared for the baby adequately and had been doing so for the ten months prior to admission. The baby was healthy. The entire ward staff felt that the mother was extremely overidentified with her daughter and that there was a symbiotic loss of boundaries, with the mother melting into the child. We—Lynn Hofer, Wendy Haft, John Dore, and I—were called in to help resolve the stalemate on the ward.

When we first observed the baby arriving for one of her visits, the child was asleep. The mother gently took her sleeping baby and began to lay her on the bed so she would stay asleep. The mother did this with enormous concentration that left us closed out. After she had ever-so-slowly eased the baby's head onto the bed, she took one of the baby's arms, which was awkwardly positioned, and with her two hands carefully guided it to a feather-like landing on the bed, as though the arm were made of eggshells and the bed made of marble. She poured herself into this activity with complete and total participation of her body and preoccupation of her mind. Once that was done, she turned to us and picked up the interrupted topic of conversation in a normal manner. It was incidents like this that made the staff feel that she was overidentified, had a loss of boundaries, was reacting against harmful impulses within herself, and at the same time was a competent caregiver—so far.

The mother also felt that she had some unspecified insecurities about her caregiving and about being overidentified with the child. With the promise of trying to help her in that area, we asked her to collaborate with us in our data collection and scoring technique for evaluating attunement as described in chapter 7.[6]

6. It is a common procedure in our laboratory to have a mother with some complaint, problem, or question about her caregiving first try to recreate for us "naturally" the events or situation in question while being videotaped and then to conduct the interview with the videotape to refer to as the focus. Routine consultation procedure and the data collection procedure for the attunement observation were therefore basically the same. We find that in

What emerged from this procedure was that of all the mothers we had ever observed, this mother was the *least* attuned. In the course of two observations on different days, she performed no behaviors that met our criteria for affect attunement. (They usually occur once a minute, using strict criteria.) Yet at the same time she was attentive to the baby, overly so; she hovered to make sure that no harm befell her, tried to anticipate all her needs, and was totally absorbed by these tasks.

When this became apparent, we commented to her that she seemed so attentive to potential sources of danger for her daughter that she seemed unable to share in her daughter's experiences. We did this by asking her about several instances when she had been protective without apparent external reason and also about several instances when she had missed responding to a particular expression or other behavior by the girl, opportunities for real engagement. Gradually, over four visits (she had two such sessions alone with Lynn Hofer), she revealed to us that she was almost exclusively attentive to the external environment and not to her daughter. She concerned herself with the hard edges of the desk, the sharp things on the floor, and the sounds from outside. If the horn that she had just heard beeping, beeped a second time, she would alter what she was doing with the baby at the moment. If it did not beep again, she would continue doing what she was doing and await some other external signs, all of which were nonspecific to her and open to her interpretation. Because of her preoccupation with trying to both read and control the external world impinging on her baby, she remained unavailable to enter into the baby's experiences and share them. The mother was aware of this. The baby had presumably become accustomed to the shifting of the mother's interactional tack. She seemed to have adapted passively, falling in with the mother's new direction of activity when it shifted. This compliance on the baby's part, along with the mother's rapt attention, made the interactions look far more harmonious and in accord than they in fact were.

This mother was partially in touch with her baby at the level of core-relatedness, but entirely out of touch at the level of intersubjective

---

dealing with nonverbal events, such as occur between parent and infant, it is often hard for the parent to verbalize a problem without a concrete instance to refer to. Lebovici (1983) has also commented on the power of video to evoke emotion and memory in a therapeutic situation.

relatedness. She provided the girl with no experiences of intersubjectivity. The initial impression of excessive intimacy was a partial illusion. The mother was in communion with her own delusions and unable to break away to "be with" her child.

This vignette is remarkable on several scores. It illustrates the almost complete lack of attunement that is possible even while physical and physiological needs are being met. It implies that most observers of human behavior (including the ward staff and us, initially) so expect attuning behaviors to be embedded in other communicative or caregiving behaviors that we tend to assume their presence and may read them in even when they are not there. (Recall the initial impression of this mother's behavior.) Finally, it illustrates one way that an infant can temporarily adapt to the absence of intersubjective relatedness—namely, to become very compliant at the level of core-relatedness. The future of such an adaptation would ultimately be disastrous for the child, if the mother could not change and if no others were available to open up the intersubjective world. We would anticipate a pervasive feeling of aloneness—not loneliness, because the child would never have experienced the presence and then loss of subjective sharing. It would probably be hard for such a child at an older age not to get some hint that things were going on between other people about which she had only a glimpse but no real experience. Then she would truly experience an ego-alien aloneness and would probably fear the possibility of such a form of intimacy. If, however, she never got to know that she didn't know, she would experience an ego-syntonic, acceptable, chronic isolation at the level of intersubjective relatedness.[7]

SELECTIVE ATTUNEMENTS

Selective attunement is one of the most potent ways that a parent can shape the development of a child's subjective and interpersonal life. It helps us account for "the infant becoming the child of his particular mother" (Lichtenstein 1961). Attunements are also one of the main vehicles for the influence of parents' fantasies about their

7. For the sake of readers who want more closure on such case material, the mother did gain some insight from working in this way with us for two weeks and began to show the ability either not to attend to or, at least, not to get fully captured by her delusions and illusions and to enter more, but still not fully, into the child's subjective world. She was discharged and lost to follow-up before we could evaluate these beginnings any further.

infants. In essence, attunement permits the parents to convey to the infant what is shareable, that is, which subjective experiences are within and which are beyond the pale of mutual consideration and acceptance. Through the selective use of attunement, the parents' intersubjective responsivity acts as a template to shape and create corresponding intrapsychic experiences in the child. It is in this way that the parents' desires, fears, prohibitions, and fantasies contour the psychic experiences of the child.

The communicative power of selective attunement reaches to almost all forms of experience. It determines which overt behaviors fall inside or outside the pale (Is it "all right"—within the intersubjective pale—to bang toys hard and noisy? to masturbate? to get real dirty?). It includes preferences for people (Is it all right to find delight in Aunt Ronnie but not in Aunt Lucy, who then says, "My nephew just doesn't take to me"?). And it includes degrees or types of internal states (joy, sadness, delight) that can occur with another person. It is these internal states rather than overt activities *per se* that we will focus on most, since they have generally been less emphasized in this context.

In a sense, parents have to make a choice, mostly out of awareness, about what to attune to, given that the infant provides almost every kind of feeling state, covering a wide range of affects, a full spectrum of the gradations of activation, and many vitality affects. This process of creating an intergenerational template is part of ordinary everyday transactions. It has an almost infinite number of opportunities to develop, some taken, some missed. The process does not divide the world sharply into black and white but rather into many shades of gray. An example from the experience of "enthusiasm" and its opposite will illustrate.

Molly's mother very much valued and sometimes appeared to overvalue "enthusiasm" in Molly. This was lucky in that Molly seemed to be well endowed with it. Together, they most characteristically made attunements when Molly was in the throes of a bout of enthusiasm. This is easy enough to do, since such moments are of enormous appeal and the explosive behavioral manifestations of infant enthusiasm are most contagious. The mother also made attunements with Molly's lower states of interest, arousal, and engagement with the world, but less consistently so. These lower states were not selected out and left totally unattuned; they simply received relatively and absolutely less attunement.[8]

One could argue that parental attunement with states of enthusiasm could only be a good thing. When it is relatively selective, however, the infant accurately perceives not only that these states have special status for the parent but that they may be one of the few ways of achieving intersubjective union. With Molly, one could begin to see a certain phoniness creep into her use of enthusiasm. The center of gravity was shifting from inside to outside, and the beginning of a particular aspect of "false self" formation could be detected. Her natural assets had joined forces with parental selective attunement, probably to his later disadvantage.

The situation with Annie was quite different. She was equally well endowed with enthusiasm, but her mother more characteristically attuned when her bubble of enthusiasm had just broken, when the gods had left. This mother made relatively more of an intersubjective alliance with the depleted Annie than with the filled-up Annie ("Oh, that's all right, honey." "That is hard, isn't it?"). The mother did this partly to soothe and comfort but also to buoy her up in a different form of intersubjective union, which we might call "*ex*thusiasm." Annie's mother was in fact more comfortable with a subjective partnership in exthusiasm than in enthusiasm. The latter seemed more dangerous to her.

For an infant to be a subjective partner only in enthusiasm will place the more depressive-like states of exthusiasm outside the pale of shareable personal experience. And, on the other hand, to be a partner only in exthusiasm will place the positively exciting states of enthusiasm outside of shareable personal experience.

In being themselves, parents inevitably exert some degree of selective bias in their attunement behaviors, and in doing so they create a template for the infant's shareable interpersonal world. This applies to all internal states; enthusiasm and exthusiasm are only examples.

8. Attunement with states of enthusiasm would certainly promote what are considered to be desirable and healthy feelings of omnipotence and grandiosity. In this light, the linguistic roots of the word "enthusiasm" are of interest. It literally means to have a god enter into one, to be imbued with his or her spirit or presence. This idea raises the question of whether enthusiasm is in fact possible without the infusion of someone else's real or fantasied spirit— an other's subjective experience—into one's feeling state. How different is this from the earlier formulation of an evoked companion?

And this is clearly how the "false self" can begin—by utilizing that portion of inner experience that can achieve intersubjective acceptance with the inner experience of an other, at the expense of the remaining, equally legitimate, portions of inner experience. The notions of the "false self" (Winnicott 1960), or of alienating interpersonal events that create the "not me" experiences of Sullivan (1953), or of the disavowal or repression of one's own experience (see Basch 1983) are all future elaborations of what we are discussing. We are describing the first step in that process, the exclusion from intersubjective sharing of certain experiences. Whatever happens next, whether the experience excluded from the interpersonal sphere becomes a part of the "false self" or a "not me" phenomenon, whether it is simply relegated out of consciousness, one way or another, or whether it remains a private but accessible part of self, the beginning lies here.

Similarly, the use of selective attunements continues to be seen throughout childhood, acting in the fashion described but for developmentally changing purposes. For instance, in considering the earliest masturbation practices of children (see Galenson and Roiphe 1974), how may prohibition or the ultimate need for disavowal or repression get transmitted? In discussing the potential clinical impact of selective attunement, Michael Basch put the case clearly:

> How, to use Freudian terminology, could the superego of the parents be conveyed so exquisitely accurately to the infant and young child? Take, for example, masturbatory practices ... How, if the parents are psychologically enlightened and determined not to either shame the child or make it feel guilty for those activities, does it get the idea that these activities are beyond the pale of acceptance? Although the parents may say nothing to the child in the way of criticism or censure, they do not share the activity through cross-modal attunement, and that sends the message loud and clear. (Basch, personal communication, 28 September 1983)

The clinical processes I have just described have usually been discussed in terms of mirroring. I maintain that mirroring is really three different interpersonal processes, each having an age-specific use: appropriate responsivity and regulation (during core-relatedness); attunement (during intersubjective relatedness); and reinforcement shaping and consensual validation (during verbal relatedness). Taken together, these are what is usually meant by mirroring.

Before leaving the subject of selective attunement, we should note that as we move from core-relatedness to intersubjective relatedness, we can now begin to see separate continuous lines of development for separate internal states. The same phenomena (enthusiasm, for example) are seen to be under similar developmental pressures from the self-regulating other and from the subjective state-sharing other that is, from the mother, in different domains of relatedness. The self-regulating other acts with her physical presence, the state-sharing other acts with her mental presence—but both act in concert over time to create characteristic patterns that may last a lifetime.

Misattunement and Tuning

Misattunements and tunings are yet another way in which the parent's behavior (and the desires, fantasies, and wishes behind that behavior) act as a template to shape and create corresponding intrapsychic experiences in the child. Misattunement and tuning are difficult to isolate and define for research purposes, but they are clinically quite recognizable. The reason why misattunements are troublesome is that they fall somewhere between a communing (well-matching) attunement and a maternal comment (that is, an affectively nonmatching response). They fall closer towards attunements; in fact, their main feature is that they come close enough to true attunements to gain entry into that class of event. But they then just miss achieving a good match, and it is the amount that they miss by that packs the wallop.

Sam's mother was observed characteristically to just undermatch the affective behaviors of her ten-month-old son. For instance, when he evidenced some affect and looked to her with a bright face and some excited arm-flapping, she responded with a good, solid, "Yes, honey" that, in its absolute level of activation, fell just short of his arm-flapping and face-brightness. Such behavior on her part was all the more striking because she was a highly animated, vivacious person.

In our usual fashion, we asked her our routine questions—why she did what she did when she did it the way she did it—for each such interchange. Her answers to the first questions—why, what, and when—were quite expected and unremarkable. When we asked her why she did it the way she did it, more was revealed. In particular, when asked if she had intended to match the infant's level of enthusiasm in her response to him, she said "no." She was vaguely aware of the fact that she frequently undermatched him. When asked why, she struggled toward verbalizing that if she were to match him—not even overmatch, but just match him—he would tend to focus more on her behavior than on his own; it might shift the initiative over from him to her. She felt that he tended to lose his initiative if she joined in fully and equally and shared with him. When asked what was wrong if the initiative passed over to her some of the time, she paused and finally said that she felt he was a little on the passive side and tended to let the initiative slip to her, which she prevented by undermatching.

When the mother was asked what was wrong with the child's being relatively more passive or less initiatory than she at this life phase, she revealed that she thought he was too much like his father, who was too passive and low-keyed. She was the initiator, the spark plug in the family. She was the one who infused enthusiasm into the marriage, decided what to eat, whether to go to the movies, when to make love. And she did not want her son to grow up to be like his father in these ways.

Both mother and we were surprised to find that this one piece of behavior, purposeful slight misattunements, carried such weight and had become a cornerstone of her upbringing strategy and fantasy. Actually, it should not have been surprising. After all, there has to be some way in which attitudes, plans, and fantasies get transposed into palpable interactive behavior to achieve their ultimate aim. We happened to uncover one such point of transposition. Attunement and misattunement exist at the interface between attitude or fantasy and behavior, and their importance lies in their capacity to translate between the two.

One of the fascinating paradoxes about her strategy is that left alone, it would do exactly the opposite of what she intended. Her underattunements would tend to create a lower-keyed child who was less inclined to share his spunk. The mother would inadvertently have contributed to making the son more like the father, rather than different from him. The lines of "generational influences" are often not straight.

Clearly, misattunements are not attempts at communion, straightforward participation in experience. They are covert attempts to change the infant's behavior and experience. What, then, might the experience of maternal misattunement be like from the infant's viewpoint? We speculate as follows. Sometimes the infant seems to treat such events as if they were not even in the class of attunement and are like any other nonattuning response. In such cases, the misattunement simply fails. It is not close enough to a communing attunement to gain entrance. "Successful" misattunements must feel as though the mother has somehow slipped inside of the infant subjectively and set up the illusion of sharing, but not the actual sense of sharing. She has appeared to get into the infant's experience but has ended up somewhere else, a little way off. The infant sometimes moves to where she "is," to close the gap and establish (or re-establish) a good match. The misattunement then has been successful in altering the infant's behavior and experience in the direction the mother wanted.

This is a very common and necessary technique, but if it is used excessively or selectively for certain types of experiences it may throw open to question the infant's sense of and evaluation of his or her own internal states or those of the other. It also reveals some of the potential dangers of the whole realm of selective attunements and misattunements. Intersubjectivity and attunement, like most potent things, can be a mixed blessing.

Misattunements can be used not only to alter an infant's experience but to steal it, resulting in "emotional theft." There are dangers to letting someone inside your subjective experience, even at these young ages. The mother may attune to the infant's state, establishing a shared experience, and then change that experience so that it is lost to the child. For instance, the baby takes a doll and starts to chew on its shoes with gusto. The mother makes a number of attunements to his expressions of pleasure, enough so that she is seen as a mutually ratified member of the ongoing experience. This membership gives her the entrée to take the doll from the baby. Once she has the doll she hugs it, in a way that breaks the previously established chewing experience. The baby is left hanging. Her act is actually a prohibitive or preventive act to stop the infant from mouthing, and also a teaching act: dolls are to be hugged, not chewed. The prohibition or didactic act is not accomplished straight-forwardly, however. She does not simply prohibit or teach. She slips inside the infant's experience by way of attunement and then steals the affective experience away from the child.

This type of exchange can happen in many ways, and it is not always an actual object-experience that is lost. For instance, a parent can make an attunement with the infant's ongoing state and then gradually tune up or vary her behavior to a point where the infant can no longer follow. The infant is left with the initial experience ebbing away, watching the parent go on with yet another variation of the infant's own original experience.

These simple examples, which are not uncommon, are intriguing, because one of their main features for the infant is the danger in permitting the intersubjective sharing of experience, namely that intersubjective sharing can result in loss. This is likely to be the point of origin of the long developmental line that later results in older children's need for lying, secrets, and evasions, to keep their own subjective experiences intact.

When viewing the ways attunement can be used, for good or ill, one might get the impression that dangers lurk everywhere, but that is no more true here than in any other form of human activity. After all, parents, at best, are only "good enough." That leaves room, on both sides of the optimal, for the infant to learn the necessary realities about attunement—that it is a key that unlocks the intersub-jective doors between people; and that it can be used both to enrich one's mental life, by a partial union with an other, and to impoverish one's mental life, by bending or appropriating some part of one's inner experience.

AUTHENTICITY OR SINCERITY

At the level of intersubjective relatedness, the authenticity of the parent's behavior looms as an issue of great magnitude. This is obviously true for the formation of psychopathology, but it is also true for normal development.

The issue is not authentic versus unauthentic. There is a spectrum, not a dichotomy. The issue is, how authentic? Because of the natural asymmetries in the mother/infant relationship, in their knowledge, skills, plans, and so on, much of the time the mother is conducting several agendas of her own simultaneously, while the infant can only entertain and participate in one of these. Some of these multiple agendas have already been alluded to; the aim of Sam's mother of playing with her infant but not letting him become "passive" is one example. Then there are a host of more mundane multiple agendas: encouraging play with an object while directing the infant how to and how not to play with it; directing an infant's attention away from something relatively dangerous to something safe, as though the whole event were really only a game; wanting to show off the baby's responsivity or precocity, without appearing to; letting an exciting game proceed, but with one foot on the brakes as the baby starts to show the first signs of fatigue or overload. All these situations may necessarily involve some blend of sincere and insincere behaviors.

The pervasiveness of this issue became apparent when we tried to observe how a mother prohibits her infant. During this research project, we learned most from its problems and our failures. Three of us formed a team that we thought was well suited to the task of determining how a mother goes about prohibiting an infant at various ages. John Dore was expert at analyzing speech acts and covered the domain of the pragmatics and semantics of what mother said. Helen Marwick was expert in voice quality analysis and covered the domain of the paralinguistic messages of the mother. I had the responsibility of analyzing the facial, postural, and gestural maternal behaviors.

Our first problem came in defining an act of prohibition. Dore laid out what seemed appropriate linguistic and speech act criteria for prohibitives, but they did not work. Sometimes the mother would say, "Don't do that," an excellent prohibitive from the linguistic viewpoint, but she would say it in the sweetest, most playful voice and with a smile. Was that a prohibitive? At other times she would say just the baby's name or ask, "Do you want to do that?" and we would all agree, from her tone of voice and facial expression, that it served as a prohibitive, although it was not one linguistically. We ended up not being able to define in linguistic terms the very act we wished to study.

We therefore decided to switch tactics. We picked a mother who we knew hated to see her infant mouthing or sucking on anything and invariably tried to prohibit this behavior. We would study all interchanges that took place when the mother saw the infant mouthing or bringing something to his mouth. We were now no longer studying "prohibitives" but rather maternal responses to infant behaviors that were a priori designated "prohibitable." The subject of study became "prohibitables," not "prohibitives."

We categorized her behavior according to the different channels in which it occurred, realizing that mixed messages across channels would be the rule. The maternal communicative channels analyzed were: linguistic (pragmatic and semantic), paralinguistic (larangeal tension, pitch contour, absolute pitch, loudness, stress, nasality, creek, and whisper), facial (category of affect and fullness of display), gestural, positional, and proxemic. We also gave each behavior a subjective rating of our impression of her seriousness or authenticity and aim.

Our overall impression was that the mother sent out the "authentic" prohibition in one or more channels and then used the other channels to modify, contradict, or support the prohibitive message or to send out a competing "authentic" message. The situation was very similar to that so beautifully described by Labov and Fanshel (1977) in their analysis of the multiple messages sent via the different channels during a psychotherapy hour. We had expected adults to be able to deal with this level of complexity, but we did not foresee that infants too, almost from the beginning, have to learn to decipher mixed messages. To put the situation more strongly, the infant's very acquisition of communicative skill emerges in a complex medium, and this fact must have some impact on how the signal system is learned.

It was clear that when the mother was maximally serious and authentic—for instance, when the infant was about to play with an electric wall plug—all of her behaviors in all of the communicative channels lined up exactly as one would predict for a prohibition, and there were no competing, contradicting, or modifying signals. She yelled, "No!" with great vocal tension, flat pitch, great stress, full facial display, and a rush forward. Such behaviors stopped the infant short. It was thus clear that the infant was given occasional opportunities to see a pure array of prohibitives assembled. Most of the time, however, this was far from the case.

The question of how the infant reads the seriousness of the mother's diverse simultaneous behaviors may miss a major point. It assumes that there is *a* way to read them. It treats them as signals to be decoded, signals that have an absolute meaning. What is missed in this approach is that these behaviors are put out as part of a progressive negotiating process. Any one set of behaviors does not *in itself* have a knowable signal value, but only an approximate one, with built-in ambiguity. The more precise signal value is determined by what went before, in what direction the negotiation is tending, and other factors. Separate moves have limited meaning alone; they derive specific meanings in the context of the whole sequence.

This is a different way of viewing the problem of interpersonal signal interpretation and, more specifically, the problem of determining the degree of authenticity of someone's behavior. The situation is analogous to what is called the sincerity or felicity conditions in speech act theory, the essence of which is how much a speaker intends and expects an utterance to be taken as fully meant (Austin 1962; Searle 1969). What the infant is learning in these situations is to recognize the sincerity conditions of nonverbal behaviors. Since the term *sincerity condition* applies to speech acts, we will refer to *authenticity conditions.* It is crucial for the infant to learn what constitute the authenticity conditions for any interpersonal transaction.

UNAUTHENTIC ATTUNEMENTS

Attuning behavior can be quite good even when your heart isn't in it. And as every parent knows, your heart can't always be in it, for all of the obvious reasons from fatigue through competing agendas to external preoccupations that fluctuate from day to day. Going through the motions is an expectable part of everyday parental experience. Attunements, then, vary along the dimension of authenticity, as well as of goodness of match. And the infant would do well to start learning this, too. One of the great advantages of interpersonal conventions or standards is that by being varied along the authenticity dimension they can achieve infinitely more signal potential. (Recall the "hello" of the two psychiatrists meeting on the street in chapter 8.)

As observers, we do not have much trouble determining how authentic any given attunement is. The more obviously unauthentic attempts at attunement end up as misattunements. Unlike most misattunements, however, they do not have a characteristic covert intent. They are more like unsystematic failures at communion than like potential successes at systematically altering the infant's behavior in a known way. There is no consistent pattern, and mother is experienced as less consistent.

The difference between purposeful (covert or unconscious) misattunements and unauthenticity is like the difference between "magnetic north" which is not really at the top of the world and systematically distorts the compass reading of true north, and local magnetic interferences that cause a compass to behave erratically and jump all over the place. To the extent that communing attunements are the ultimate reference point (true north) for measuring affective intersubjectivity, misattunements are a systematic distortion (magnetic north) but gross unauthenticity leaves one without a working interpersonal compass for intersubjective relatedness.

So far in our research, the more subtle unauthenticities in attunements have escaped our ability to analyze them. It is not simply a matter of attuning well in one modality and poorly in another, although that is true of most people. It has more to do with slight violations in expectation of the profile of attunement. We do not know the extent of infants' abilities to pick up these subtle unauthenticities, but to the extent that they can discriminate them it would be like having an only slightly fluky interpersonal compass. Intersubjectivity would still rest on a shaky set of coordinates; it would not have the certainty of dead reckoning. This entire area of the negotiation, rather than the signaling, of the status of intersubjectivity and the emergence of the infant's ability to gauge authenticity conditions needs much more actual observation and theoretical attention.

OVERATTUNEMENT

Occasionally, we have seen a mother who appears to overattune. This is a form of "psychic hovering" that is usually accompanied by physical hovering. The mother is so overidentified with her child that she seems to want to crawl inside of the infant's every experience. If any such mother were a perfect and invariable attuner, if she never missed any opportunity to attune and hit each one exactly right (which is of course impossible), the infant might have the feeling of sharing a single dual mentality with the mother, similar to that proposed by "normal symbiosis," while still having a separate and distinct core boundary not proposed in normal symbiosis. Or, because of the continued presence of a sense of a core self and other, the child in this imaginary situation might have the sense of a transparent subjectivity and an omniscient mother. Mothers, even overattuners, do not attune with the vast majority of infant experiences, however, and even when they do they achieve only relative success. The infant learns that subjectivity is potentially permeable but not transparent and that mother can reach toward it but not automatically divine it. Overattunement is the psychic counterpart of physical intrusiveness, but it can never steal the infant's individual subjective experience; luckily, the process is too inefficient. This assures constant differentiation of self from other at the subjective level. Maternal psychic hovering, when complied with on the infant's part, may slow down the infant's moves toward independence, but it does not interfere with "individuation."

THE CLINICAL POSITION OF INTERSUBJECTIVITY AND EMPATHY

Intersubjectivity has currently become a cardinal issue in psychotherapy as viewed from the perspective of Self Psychology. The patient-therapist "system" is seen either implicitly (Kohut 1971, 1977, 1983) or explicitly as an "intersection of two subjectivities— that of the patient and that of the analyst ... [in which] ... psychoanalysis is pictured ... as a science of the intersubjective" (Stolerow, Brandhoft, and Atwood 1983, p. 117–18). Seen in this light, the parent-infant "system" and the therapist-patient "system" appear to have parallels. For instance, "negative therapeutic reactions" refer to those paradoxical clinical situations in which an interpretation that is given to a patient makes the patient worse rather than better, in spite of the fact that all current and subsequent evidence supports the correctness of the interpretation. Stolerow, Brandhoft, and Atwood (1983) explain these reactions in terms of "intersubjective disjunctions" (p. 121), rather than as masochism, resistance, unconscious envy, or other defensive maneuvers, or simply poor timing, which are the traditional explanations. An "intersubjective disjunction" appears to be analogous to a misattunement. More broadly, "empathic failures" (of which the "negative therapeutic reactions" resulting from "intersubjective disjunction" are only an instance) and "empathic successes" are the cardinal therapeutic processes of Self Psychology (Kohut 1977, in press; Ornstein 1979; Schwaber 1980a, 1980b, 1981). These appear to be analogous to the spectrum of nonattunements, misattunements, selective attunements, and communing attunements.

I wish to inject some caution in drawing these analogies too closely, however. What is meant by the therapeutic use of empathy is enormously complex from our point of view. It involves an integration of features that include what we are calling core-, intersubjective, and verbal relatedness as well as what Schafer (1968) has called "generative empathy" and Basch (1983) has called "mature empathy." Attunement, functioning at the level of intersubjective relatedness prior to the advent of verbal relatedness, is thus a necessary precursor to one of the components of therapeutic empathy, but that is not the same as an analogous relationship. The two do have some important similarities in function, especially the mutual influence of one person's subjective state upon that of another, but attunement between mother and infant and empathy between therapist and patient are operating at different levels of complexity, in different realms, and for ultimately different purposes.

There is a related issue. Self Psychology has suggested that it is the failures in maternal empathy in the beginning of life that later are responsible for the deficits and weaknesses in self-cohesion that are manifest as borderline disorders. Once again, on the basis of these similarities, it is tempting to point the finger at the level of intersubjective relatedness as the "critical" or "sensitive" period for the origin of empathy-related failures in self development. And such may prove to be the case. But while the normal or abnormal developmental line for the cohesive self—or self-concept, as designated in Self Psychology—receives invaluable structuring at the level of intersubjective relatedness, so did it at the level of core-relatedness, and so will it at the level of verbal relatedness. The similarities and close relationship between attunement and empathy should not bias us toward attributing undue importance to the level of intersubjective relatedness, compared with other levels, in the clinical issue of sense of self development. Its appropriate importance is sufficiently obvious.

SOCIAL REFERENCING AND INFLUENCING THE INFANT'S AFFECTIVE EXPERIENCE

A group of researchers in Denver has identified a phenomenon occurring around the same time as affect attunement which they call *social referencing* (Emde et al. 1978; Klinert 1978; Campos and

Stenberg 1980; Emde and Sorce 1983; Klinert et al. 1983). The prototype situation has already been described, in chapter 6. A year-old infant is lured across an apparent visual cliff by an attractive toy and a smiling mother. On reaching the apparent drop-off, the child stops and appraises the dangers versus the desirability of crossing over. Placed in this position of uncertainty, the infant invariably looks up at the mother to read her face and get a secondary appraisal. If she smiles, the infant crosses over, but if she looks frightened, the infant retreats and gets upset ("It is not O.K."). The mother's affective state determines or modifies the infant's affective state.

One could argue that the infant is not only looking at mother for an appraisal, a fairly cognitive view, but is also looking to see which of the infant's own conflicted feeling states is being matched or attuned to. After all, in this situation the infant's position is not simply one of cognitive uncertainty but of affective ambivalence between fear at the visual drop—an innate fear—and pleasure in exploration. The infant seeks mother to resolve the ambivalence by attuning with one emotion and not the other, thereby tipping the scales. These two interpretations are complementary, not contradictory. The processes they describe are simultaneously in operation much of the time.

This same group of researchers points out that it is possible for the mother to influence the infant's affective state to the extent of instilling a new affect that was not part of the infant's original experience. To demonstrate this they have utilized a variety of situations that, unlike the visual cliff, do not elicit and rely on an affective conflict: collapsing castles, and staged accidents, for example. In these situations, mothers can successfully signal what an infant is to feel, but the infant's looking for an affective match cannot be called upon as an explanation.

A very common example of mother's influencing or even deter-mining what a child will feel occurs when the child falls down and starts to cry. If the mother quickly moves into a fun-surprise mode, "Oh, what an interesting and funny thing just happened to you," the infant is likely to switch gears into a gleeful state. One might conclude that the mother brought the infant from one feeling state to an entirely different one. However, the mother's maneuver would never have worked if the level of arousal she showed in her fun-filled surprise had not matched the infant's initial level of negatively toned arousal. Some degree of attunement may have been necessary to permit a successful social referencing.

In any event the signalling of affect states adds another dimension to the one described for attunement and has equally important clinical implications. For instance, how might a mother make an infant feel some kind of badness about a neutral event without resorting to punishment or explanations? If we return to the study on prohibitions in light of the work on social referencing, the answer seems simpler. Let us assume that mouthing—teething on objects during the nine- to twelve-month period—is an experience made up of some pleasure and some pain for the infant and is morally neutral for most mothers these days. We have observed mothers who find the mouthing of objects disgusting, for intrapsychic reasons unrelated to cleanliness and health. Such mothers can instill a feeling of disgust by signaling disgust whenever the infant references her during a mouthing. One mother consistently flashed a disgusted facial display and said, "Yuuuck! That's icky—yuuuck!" while wrinkling up her nose. This began to serve as an effective prohibition, and the infant occasionally stopped mouthing an object and put it down while intoning a "yuuuck"-like noise and wrinkling up his nose in disgust. The mother had successfully introduced a "badness"-tinged feeling quality into the infant's total affective experience of mouthing.

In a similar fashion, another mother used "depressive-signals" just as the previous mother used "disgust-signals." Whenever her son did something maladroit, as is expectable in a one-year-old, so that something got knocked over or a toy was disarranged, the mother would let out a multi-modal depressive signal. This consisted of long expirations, falling intonations, slightly collapsing postures, furrowing the brows, tilting and drooping the head, and "Oh, Johnnys" that could be interpreted as "Look what you've done to your mother again," if not "What a tragedy that your clumsiness with that toy train has caused the death of another dozen people."

Gradually, Johnny's exuberant exploratory freedom became more circumspect. His mother too had brought an alien affective experience into an otherwise neutral or positive activity. She may also have succeeded in making it part of the infant's own affective experience during that activity, which then became a quite different kind of lived experience, to be recorded as a quite different kind of prototypic episodic memory, available to influence the future.

Social referencing and affect attunement are deeply complementary processes. Social referencing permits the mother to determine and alter to some extent what the infant actually experiences. It has real limitations, however, in that the mother can only tune the infant's subjective experience; she cannot create it wholly. And affect attunement permits the infant to know if what he or she experiences is shared by the mother and thus falls into the realm of the shareable. Selective attunement helps tune the infant's subjective experience by accentuating parts of that experience at the expense of others.

PSYCHOPATHOLOGY DURING THE FORMATIVE PERIOD OF
INTERSUBJECTIVE RELATEDNESS

Three different forms of potential psychopathology are visible during the period beginning at seven to nine months and ending at about eighteen months: neurotic-like signs and symptoms; characterological malformations; and self pathology.

Potential characterological and self pathological malformations have already been alluded to. These are readily explicable on the basis of an infant's accurately perceiving the interpersonal reality created by the primary caregiver and making some adaptive coping response to that reality, which then becomes habitual. Examples are the girl mentioned on pages 197–98, who really did have to "sparkle plenty" to get mother to respond to her, and the two other little girls, Annie and Molly, who were being forced by the different attuning responses of their mothers to make exthusiasm rather than enthusiasm the socially sanctioned predominant experience of self. These kinds of adaptations can become maladaptive, and in that sense pathological, when they are used in new contexts and with new people, so that the infant's own patterns are no longer responsive to the new realities. The problem is one of overgeneralization and/or of experiencing one's self not simply as using one form of adaptation but being defined by and limited to it. This is the most common situation of "disorder" seen at this point in development, and it appears to be relevant for the developmental psychopathology of relatively stable individual differences of the kind that are usually meant by character traits or personality types, or adaptive styles—that is, the Axis II disorders from the *DSM-III* phenomenology. They may also have the fixity of patterns first established during a sensitive period.

There are some circumstances, however, in which it looks as though the infant, by a year of age, has elaborated a neurotic-like sign and symptom. These signs and symptoms are particularly interesting, because they may require different explanatory models from those of overgeneralization and delimited senses of the self. The most common example is "one-year phobias," those inexplicably strong fears that otherwise unfearful infants develop toward one particular thing, such as vacuum cleaners. Such phobias can be explained on the basis of having been frightened by the thing on one or more occasions (and vacuum cleaners are universally frightening when they start up unexpectedly, because of the rapid acceleration in loudness). An association has been made between the sight and the fearful experience, or an episodic memory is retrieved by the visual sight alone. Why the fear persists despite many opportunities for extinction and/or many opportunities to form other, unfearful lived episodes with the vacuum cleaner is not obvious. These phobias are not quite neurotic, because the infant's signs and symptoms are unelaborated compared with the original fear response that the vacuum cleaner probably elicited the first time it scared the infant. No condensation, displacement, or other elaborations are involved in the "symptom."

In contrast, it is possible to see an infant prior to age twelve months elaborate a symptom or sign that has many of the characteristics of a neurotic symptom, especially the condensation and displacement of diverse experiences into one particular object. For instance, Bertrand Cramer and his colleagues at Service de Guidance Infantile in Geneva presented the following case (a fairly common one in a clinic that deals with infant and family problems during the first years of life). A young Italian couple living in Geneva were referred because their nine-month-old daughter had general feeding problems, with a moderate but subclinical failure-to-thrive (weight was in the 25th percentile). The most remarkable feature of the child's behavior was that she would manifest violent negative reactions to the bottle, but to nothing else. It was not necessary to try to feed her with it to trigger the reactions; they could be triggered by handing the bottle to her or simply having it in sight. Her response was a mix of different behaviors. She would have a tantrum and at the same time show fear (shrinking back) and anger (throwing the bottle away). What was most convincing was that she acted as though the bottle itself contained the qualities that made her fearful, anxious, and angry. The strong impression was not that the bottle simply evoked or recalled unpleasant experiences, but that the bottle had come to represent them.

These were the major known facts bearing on this symptom:

1. The couple had been living together for years but chose not to marry, nor had they plans to do so. It was felt by all of us who witnessed the intake interview (via videotape) that the future of the marital relationship was at issue. The child represented the most binding reality that made the parents a couple. The major clinical questions one wished to ask the father and mother were: How can your relationship continue to grow? How can it best be nourished? What kind of nourishment will be best for it? And which of you will provide what portion? The parents did covertly struggle as to which one of them was to feed the baby what, and when. From the clinical perspective it seemed reasonable to infer that the infant's feeding problems had become the focus for, and somehow reflected, this overall family problem.
2. The mother had been brought up by a cold, nongiving mother. She had written her own mother off when she left Italy. She seemed to have insecurities about her own caregiving abilities and was unsure about her ability to feed the baby appropriately and well.
3. The father's mother had been the most powerful figure in his family. He admired her power and even held it in awe, but he did not experience it as always benign. So the father, too, had dynamic reasons to be ambivalent about women, about his "wife" in her feeding role, and about his own identification with his strong mother when feeding the baby.

All together, there is a current dynamic issue concerning the marriage that fuels the feeding problem. And each parent brings a past history of conflicts that contributes to the present situation. The problem is multiply determined such that it was never fully resolved who was to feed the baby, what, and when, with what degrees of confidence, with what consequences for the "marital" relationship, and with what fantasied meanings to the parents as to their identities.

Somehow—and this is the crucial part—for this infant these intrapsychic phenomena and their overt manifestations in behavior appeared to take as their final common path the form of the bottle. She could have simply become a poor eater or a compliant good one, but instead she elaborated a symptom.

The bottle in this symptom does not symbolize the various conflicts surrounding feeding. It is not at all an arbitrary signifier. It does seem to act as an object representing the many conflicts. How this could happen might best be understood in terms of the dynamic episodic memory model. Some of the prototypic episodes (RIGs), of which the bottle is always an attribute, invoke anger or tentativeness in the mother alone; others involve anger or tentativeness in the father alone; others include tension between the parents felt by the girl; others include intrusive overfeedings and felt anger on the child's part; still others contain signals of depression from either parent, with corresponding feelings in the child; and some involve disruptions in the smooth flow of the caregiving routine. If the girl is capable of reindexing, so to speak, these various troublesome prototypic interaction episodes (RIGs) in terms of their invariant attributes, she comes upon the bottle as that which best represents her various sources and forms of agony. The bottle no longer represents one single form of lived experience. It serves to bring together and condense diverse forms of lived experience. And in that sense it serves as a "neurotic signal" that transcends any single experienced reality. It is in this fashion that neurotic symptoms can form in advance of a true capacity for symbolization.

Verbal Relatedness

Paradoxically, while language vastly extends our grasp on reality, it can also provide the mechanism for the distortion of reality as experienced. As we have seen, language can force apart interpersonal self-experience as lived and as verbally represented. The "false self," "not-me experiences," the extent of disavowal and splitting of direct experience, and those experiences that are simply always kept private will all be further determined by the way the divisions between experience as lived and experience as represented in language are created and repaired. It is for this reason that so much of what is clinically important when language emerges is invisible and silent. It includes everything that is not expressed verbally and involves the choices about what is being left unspoken as well as what is being said. How can one best think about the situation in which there is a lived-experience version (in episodic memory) and a verbally represented version (in semantic memory)? Basch (1983) has provided a helpful clarification. He points out that in *repression*, the path from lived experience to its representation in language is blocked. (The felt experience of a parent's death cannot be translated into the verbal form necessary for conscious attention.) On the other hand, in *disavowal* the path from language representation to the lived, felt experience of those represented events is blocked. (One recognizes the reality of the semantic version that the parent is factually dead, but this recognition does not lead to the felt, affective experiences attached to that fact. These are disavowed.) In *denial*, there is a distortion of the perception itself ("My parents are not dead"). In disavowal only the emotional-personal significance of the perception is repudiated. There is a splitting of experience in which two different versions of reality are kept apart.

Using this terminology, one can approach the various relationships between the two versions of reality. In the creation of a "false self" and a "true self," personal experience of the self becomes split into two types. Some self-experiences are selected and enhanced because they meet the needs and wishes of someone else (the false self), regardless of the fact that they may diverge from the self-experiences that are more closely determined by "internal design" (the true self). We have seen how this process of splitting begins during core-relatedness and is greatly furthered during intersubjective relatedness through the use of selective attunement, misattunement, and nonattunement on the part of the parent. What happens at the level of verbal relatedness is that language becomes available to ratify the split and confer the privileged status of verbal representation upon the false self. ("Aren't you being gentle with the teddy bear! Sally's always so gentle." Or "Isn't this exciting! We're having such a wonderful time." Or "That thing is not so interesting, is it? But look at this one.")

Gradually, with the cooperation between the parent and the child, the false self becomes established as a semantic construction made of linguistic propositions about who one is and what one does and experiences. The true self becomes a conglomerate of disavowed experiences of self which cannot be linguistically encoded. Disavowal can only occur when the infant is able to treat the previously present

227

core distinctions between self and other on a symbolic level. It requires a *concept* of self which can be held outside of immediate experience for reflection and in which experiences or attributes can be assigned personal meaning and affective significance. That is, disavowal separates the true personal, emotional meaning from the linguistic statement of what is reality. Since language provides the major vehicle for relating knowledge of the self to the self, the disavowal experiences are less able than other experiences to inform self-knowledge, and they remain less integrated because they are cut off from the organizing power existing in language.

For the first time we can speak of self-deception and distortion of reality on the part of the infant. The discrepancies with reality, however, are more acts of omission than acts of commission. There is not yet the active distortion of perception or meaning under the influence of a wish. ("There is too a penis on that little girl, it's just very small still—or there used to be one.") Instead there is a splitting into two equally "real" experiences, but only one of them is given full weight.

What is the pressure or motive that activates disavowal to keep the true and false selves separated? Primarily, it is the need for experiences of being with the other. It is only in the domain of false self that the infant is able to experience the communion of subjective sharing and the consensual validation of personal knowledge. In the domain of the true self, the mother holds herself unavailable, acting, in fact, as if it did not exist.

The development of the "domain of the private" (that which one will not share, and which may not even occur to one to share, with another) is related to the development of a false self. The domain of the private stands somewhere between the true disavowed self and the false or social self, but the private self has never been disavowed. It consists of self-experiences that have not been attuned with, shared, or reinforced but that when manifested would *not* have caused parental withdrawal. These private self-experiences do not cause interpersonal disengagement, nor do they provide a route to experiences of being-with. The infant learns simply that they are not part of what one shares, and they do not need to be disavowed. These private experiences have access to language and can become well known to the self and undergo more integration than the disavowed self-experiences.

The notion of a private self as distinct from a true but disavowed self is essential, because there is enormous individual and cultural variability in what constitutes self-experience that is to be shared and that which is not to be shared. Some of these differences are the result of different social pressures for disavowal, but some are not. They are conventions observed without imperative.

Because the domain of the private lacks the mechanism of disavowal for maintaining its position, this domain is the most changeable through experience. Much of growing up, learning to love, and learning to protect one's self realistically involves shifting the boundary lines of the domain of the private.

Implications of present or impending character pathology have become attached to the terms "true self" and "false self." Winnicott did not originally intend this. I believe he intended to imply that some splitting into true and false self was inevitable, given the imperfect nature of our interpersonal partners. Perhaps, then, we should adopt a different terminology and divide developing self-experiences into three categories: the "social self," the "private self," and the "disavowed self." The issue of how "true" or "false" the selves are or how much any of them hurts or suffers is a clinical issue of great complexity, but it is a clinical issue and not one of development *per se*. And the degree to which any of these selves has developed closest to the rhumb line of "internal design" is an issue to be debated after the direction of a whole life can be viewed (Kohut 1977). Perhaps it can never be known.

The fact that language is powerful in defining self to the self and that parents play a large role in this definition does not mean that an infant can readily be "bent out of shape" by those forces and become totally the creation of others' wishes and plans. The socialization process, for good or ill, has limits imposed by the biology of the infant. There are directions and degrees to which the child cannot be bent without the emergence of the disavowed self, which then makes claims on linguistic ratification.

We have so far delineated three domains of self-experience, the social, the private, and the disavowed. There is a fourth, the "not me" experience. Sullivan speculated that some self-experiences, such as masturbation, can become so tinged with resonant anxiety, set up in the infant but originating in the parent, that the experience could not be assimilated or integrated into the rest of self-experience.

Alternatively, if the experience is already partially integrated, the force of anxiety would dis-integrate it—dislodge it, so to speak—from its place within the organized experience of self. Clinical phenomena fitting this description are certainly known in older persons. Could it happen or begin in infancy, as Sullivan suggests? It all depends on the disintegrating or integration-inhibiting effect of anxiety or other extremely disruptive feeling states.

What is likely to happen is that the original disintegration or nonintegration occurs at the level of core-relatedness, so that the "not me" experience is not included in or gets dislodged from the sense of a core self. When this situation is enacted at the level of verbal relatedness, we have a part of self that is truly repressed, not disavowed. It has no access to language and thus cannot get in touch with the private or social self, or even the disavowed self.

We have only just begun to touch upon the clinical implications of language acquisition. Still to come in the child's development are the active ability to distort perceptions and meaning through defense and all the other variations on reality made possible by a truly symbolic vehicle such as language. However, these are rarely observed until after the age of two years and therefore are beyond the scope of this book. We stop our account at the earlier stages of language development, where the infant remains a relatively faithful recorder of reality and all deviations from the normal are close to the accurate reflections of the impress of interpersonal reality.

Chapter 10

Some Implications for the Theories Behind Therapeutic Reconstructions

THE CONCERN in this chapter is with the theories about development that operate in the therapist's mind and that therefore influence the creation of the reconstructed "clinical infant." These theories will be examined in the light of new knowledge about the "observed infant" and the development of the different domains of sense of self.

It is important to recall that an assessment of clinical theory from the perspective of direct infant observation says nothing about the validity of clinical theories as therapeutic constructs. Nor can it say much about the same theories as they apply to children past infancy, when symbolic functions are more in place. (We have suggested before that psychoanalytic developmental theory may make a better fit with direct observations during childhood than with observations during infancy.) What such an assessment can do is to measure and describe the distance between the two views, so that the tension between the two, when clarified can operate as a corrective to both.

Knowledge of the observed infant seems to have the greatest

potential impact on a number of theoretical issues at the level of metapsychology. They will be addressed by issue, in loose chronological order rather than by school of thought.

The Stimulus Barrier, the Early Handling of Stimulation and Excitation, and the Notion of a Normal Autistic Phase

It is a traditional psychoanalytic notion that during the first months of life, the infant is protected from external stimuli by a stimulus barrier, a "protective shield against stimuli" (Freud 1920). As described by Freud, this barrier was of intrinsic biological origin, in the form of heightened sensory thresholds except to internal stimuli. It was postulated that the infant was unable to handle stimulation that broke through the shield. There has been an active dialogue as to whether the stimulus barrier at some point came under some control of the infant, as an antecedent of ego defensive operations, or whether it remained as an essentially passive mechanism (Benjamin 1965; Gediman 1971; Esman 1983). Giving the infant more active control of the barrier altered the view of the concept somewhat.

An irrevocable change in our view of the stimulus barrier concept came with Wolff's (1966) description of the recurring states of consciousness that infants go through, beginning with neonates. The most important state, for this issue, is alert inactivity, the "window" during which questions can be posed to infants and answers given, as we saw in chapter 3. In this state the infant is quiet and not moving but has eyes and ears trained on the external world. It is not simply a passively receptive state; the infant is actively—in fact, avidly—taking it all in. If a stimulus barrier exists, either its threshold sinks to zero at times or the infant periodically reaches through it.

At the first International Conference of Infant Psychiatry in 1981, Eric Erikson was invited to give a special address. He told the audience that in preparation for his talk, he thought he had better go look closely at a newborn, for it had been a while since he had done so. So he went to a nursery for newborns, and the strongest impression he carried away was of the infants' eyes. He described the infants' gaze as "fierce" in their avidness to take the world in.

For parents who are at the other end of this fierce gaze, it is a compelling experience.[1]

It is true that the young infant's tolerance for stimulation, even during alert inactivity, is far less at one week or one month of age than it will be months or years later. But the very young infant, like anyone else, has optimal levels of stimulation, below which stimulation will be sought and above which stimulation will be avoided. As we saw in chapter 4, this is a general rule of infant interaction with stimuli (Kessen et al. 1970), and it has been amply described in the social interactive setting (Stechler and Carpenter 1967; Brazelton et al. 1974; Stern 1974b, 1977). What is different about the "stimulus barrier" period, then, is only the levels of stimulation and the durations of engagement with external stimulation that are acceptable or tolerable. There is no basic difference in the active regulatory engagement that the infant makes with the external environment. And this is the most telling point.

The infant engages in the same kind of active regulatory traffic with the external world as does anyone at any age. Different people or different psychiatric illnesses can be described as having different thresholds, set at characteristically higher or lower levels for tolerable amounts of stimulation and for tolerable durations of exposure. The relationship of the infant to external stimulation is *qualitatively* the same throughout the life span.

The stimulus barrier is a pivotal concept, because it is an instance, in the case of infancy, of Freud's pleasure principle and constancy principle (1920). In this view, the buildup of internal excitation is experienced as unpleasure, and one of the major roles of the entire mental apparatus is to discharge energy or excitation, so that the level of excitation within the psychic system is always minimized. Since in the eyes of classical psychoanalysis the infant does not have sufficient (if any) mental apparatuses for discharging the excitation that the outside world might impose in large quantities, the stimulus barrier is required to save the day. Actually, what is really at fault in the classical view of the stimulus barrier is not so much the idea itself. After all, infants' tolerance levels are limited, and they change,

1. Klaus and Kennel (1976) have remarked on the long periods of visual alertness that follow a nonmedicated birth and have allotted to the infant's gaze a role in bonding the parent to the infant. Bowlby (1969) has viewed the same event as playing a role in the other direction, bonding the infant to the parent.

perhaps even in quantum leaps. The problem is with the basic assumption that required the presence of the barrier to begin with. As we have seen in chapters 3 and 4, the infant does have the capacities to deal with the world of external stimulation, granted with some help from mother. Clearly, the complex of reasoning that resulted in the notion of a stimulus barrier, and that notion itself, should simply be discarded. Esman (1983), Lichtenberg (1981, 1983), and others all arrive at a similar conclusion and argue for major revision.

The basic reasoning that compelled the construction of the stimulus barrier is also at the foundation of the notion of an initial phase of "normal autism" to describe the infant's social interactions from birth through the second month of life (Mahler 1969; Mahler, Bergman, and Pine 1975). The idea of normal autism as an expectable phase of life has more immediate clinical implications, however, since it has been conceived as a developmental point at which fixation can occur and to which regression can lead back. The status of such a phase in light of new information is therefore no small matter for clinical theory.

If by autism we mean a primary lack of interest in and registration of external stimuli, in particular of human stimuli, then the recent data indicate that the infant is never "autistic." Infants are deeply engaged in and related to social stimuli. Even if they could not tell human from nonhuman stimuli, as some suggest, they are still avidly involved with both kinds, albeit indiscriminately. In autism there is a generally selective lack of interest in or avoidance of human stimuli. That is never the case with normal infants. It is true that the infant becomes more social, but that is not the same as becoming less autistic. The infant never was autistic and cannot become less so. The process is rather the continuous unfolding of an intrinsically determined social nature.

Another problem with the "normal autistic" phase is that it is anchored by name, and partially by concept, with a condition that is pathological and that does not occur until later in development. This normal phase is thus referenced pathomorphically and retrospectively. These problems have been adequately commented on by others (Peterfreund 1978; Milton Klein 1980). (Dr. Mahler herself is well aware of the general problems of pathomorphic definitions and hoped to avoid some of them by speaking of "*normal* autism." She is also aware of many of the recent findings of infancy research and has somewhat modified her conceptualization of the normal autistic phase to accommodate these findings. In a recent discussion, she suggested that this initial phase might well have been called "awakening," which is very close to "emergence," as it has been called here [Mahler, personal communication, 1983].) In contrast to the concept of normal autism, the concept of emergent relatedness assumes that the infant from the moment of birth is deeply social in the sense of being designed to engage in and find uniquely salient interactions with other humans.

Orality

It may be a surprise for a clinical theorist to find himself or herself this far into a book on infancy without having encountered a single word about the special importance of the mouth for relatedness or as an organizing focus of a developmental phase. There are several reasons for this omission. The current methods of infancy research have been most readily adapted to vision and audition, the distance receptors. The notion of the mouth as specially endowed as an erotogenic zone, in the strict sense that Freud and later Erikson meant, has not borne up in general observation or in attempts to operationalize the concept of erotogenic zones as developmental realities. There has been a general historical trend toward seeing early relatedness of one kind or another as a primary goal in itself, one which does not need to grow out of or lean upon physiological needs and therefore is not secondary to some more primary physiological goal such as hunger (Bowlby 1958).

Even if one wishes to speak of orality as a mode of interaction rather than as an anatomical locus of charged action (Erikson 1950), the same questions about the special status of the mouth arise. Erikson focused on the interactional mode of "incorporation," which was a primitive form of internalization by way of the mouth. Adhering to Freud's timetable for erotogenic zones, he made the mouth the primary organ for initially conducting the crucial business of internalization. And the initial internalizations became tightly associated, in dynamically oriented thinking, with oral activity or fantasy. The current data show the infant to be at least equally engaged in visual and auditory "incorporation." It is striking that when Erikson revisited newborn babies in 1981, he was most impressed with their *visual* taking in of the world. Had that been his impression thirty years earlier, early internalization might have become more closely associated with visual activity. That too would have been a mistake. Erikson's internalization is little different from Piaget's assimilation/accommodation, and it is the domain of all modalities and all sensible body parts. No organ or mode appears to have special status with regard to it.

The recent evidence for cross-sensory coordination of information (amodal perception) highlights this point. The lack of emphasis on the mouth in engaging the world, compared with the eyes and ears, is partially to redress the previous imbalance of emphasis, not to mitigate the contribution of the mouth.

What about the role of feeding—the consummatory act and the concomitant feelings of satiation? How are they to be conceptualized during a period of emergent relatedness? The feelings of satiation in association with the perception of a person or a part of a person are unquestionably important, and we have dealt with them in part already.

Feeding is a vital activity for emergent relatedness for many reasons. It is one of the first major recurrent social activities, an occasion that repeatedly brings parent and infant into intimate face-to-face contact, during which the infant cycles through various states, including alert inactivity. (The newborn sees things best at a distance of about ten inches—the usual distance from a mother's eyes to the eyes of an infant positioned at the breast.) The feeding activity thus assures that the infant, when in an appropriate state to be attentive and attracted to stimulation, will be offered an engagement at appropriate distances with a full array of human stimulation, in the form of the parental social behavior that generally accompanies the feeding activities.

None of this so far has anything directly to do with eating or consummatory acts, although these are what brought the social occasion into being. What, then, about the fact and feelings of hunger and satiation? The role and place of the hunger-satiation experience has loomed very large as a metaphor for much theory-building. Its importance is unquestionable in the light of both common observation and the prevalence of oral symptomatology and fantasy in many clinical circumstances. A relativistic perspective is instructive, however. Much evidence about the feeding patterns of existent primitive societies and historical evidence on patterns in preindustrial societies suggest that throughout most of human history, infants were fed very frequently, on the slightest demand—as often as twice an hour. Since most infants were carried about with the mother, against her body, she would sense the infant getting even slightly restless and would initiate short and frequent feedings, maybe just a few sips to keep the level of activation low (DeVore and Konnor 1974).[2]

The import of this perspective is that the drama of feeding today is in part the product of our system of creating a great deal of stimulation and activation in the form of hunger build-up, followed by a steep fall-off of activation. Satiation becomes a phenomenon of intensity and drama equal to that of hunger, but in the opposite direction. It may well be that constant experience with exaggerated peaks and valleys of motivational and affective intensity is an adaptive advantage for the infant who is to enter the faster, more stimulating modern world. That question is beyond the scope of this book however. What is within our immediate scope is the question of how the perception of human stimuli will be affected by the experience of hunger and satiation. We have almost no evidence about the infant's capacity to take in external stimulation or to engage in any of the perceptual processes during the high activation states of distressful hunger or the very low activation states of somnolent satiation. Current methods of experimentation have not permitted access to these states. A discussion of infant sensibilities, and specifically of the ability to register events in states of very high and low excitation, will be addressed later in this chapter.

---

2. Among mammals one can predict the frequency of feeding for any species from the ratio of fat, protein, and carbohydrates in the milk. On the basis of the composition of human milk, human newborns should be fed every twenty to thirty minutes, as was once the custom, rather than every three or four hours, as is present practice (Klaus and Kennell 1976).

Instincts: Id and Ego

The actual observation of infants has caused a curious turnaround. One would expect, as Freud originally postulated, that in very young humans, the id would be pervasively evident and the ego barely present at all. Also, the pleasure principle (guiding the id) would precede, or at least strongly dominate, the reality principle (guiding the just-forming ego) in the first months of life.

The observed infant presents a different picture, however. Besides the regulation of hunger and sleep (no small dismissal), one is struck most by the functions that could have been called "ego-instincts" in the past—that is, the preemptive, stereotypic patterns of exploration, curiosity, perceptual preferences, search for cognitive novelty, pleasure in mastery, even attachment, that unfold developmentally.

By presenting us with a plethora of motivational systems that operate early, appear separable, and are backed by some imperative, the infant faces us again and in a new way with the longstanding arguments about the distinctions between id instincts and ego instincts. There are three related issues here. The first concerns the id instincts alone. Has classical libido theory, in assuming one or two basic drives that shift developmentally from one erotogenic zone to another and have a variety of viscissitudes during development, been helpful in viewing an actual infant? The consensus is no. The classical view of instinct has proven unoperationalizable and has not been of great heuristic value for the observed infant. Also, while there is no question that we need a concept of motivation, it clearly will have to be reconceptualized in terms of many discrete, but interrelated, motivational systems such as attachment, competence-mastery, curiosity and others. It is of no help to imagine that all of these are derivatives of a single unitary motivational system. In fact, what is now most needed is to understand how these motivational systems emerge and interrelate and which ones have higher or lower hierarchical standing during what conditions at what ages. The pursuit of such questions will be hampered if these motivational systems are assumed a priori to be derivatives of one or two basic, less definable instincts rather than more definable separate phenomena.

The second issue concerns "ego instincts." Infants have surprised us with their rich repertoire of immediately available or emergent mental functions: memory, perception, amodal representation, specification of invariants, and so on. The concept of autonomous ego functions went some way in resolving the longstanding problem of what to do about "ego instincts" as known in the 1950s, but it is nowhere near inclusive enough to contain all that we know in the 1980s. Because it is no longer reasonable to think in terms of the general drives of eros and thanatos, at least when encountering the infant as observed, the "autonomous" in autonomous ego function has lost much of its meaning. An adult patient can certainly use perception uncolored by dynamic conflict, but for an infant the act of perception has its own motive force and invariably creates pleasure or unpleasure. Until we can form a clearer picture of the separate motivational systems involved, the notion of "autonomous function" in an observed infant may only obfuscate the issue.

The third related issue is the classical developmental postulate that the id and the pleasure principle precede the ego and the reality principle. More recent evidence suggests that this proposed developmental sequence was theoretical and arbitrary. The evidence weighs far more on the side of a simultaneous dialectic between a pleasure principle and reality principle, an id and an ego, all operating from the beginning of life. Ego psychologists have come to accept that the pleasure principle works within the context of the reality principle from the beginning, and vice versa. The suggestion of Glover (1945) that ego nuclei are present from the start and Hartmann's (1958) description on an undifferentiated matrix of ego and id attest to this shift in ego psychology, towards a greater appreciation of the presence of ego functioning in young infants.

The observational findings of the past decade have reinforced this shift in thinking and perhaps moved it further, in the sense that these "ego" functions are now seen as discrete and rather highly developed functions that go well beyond both ego nuclei and an undifferentiated matrix. It seems apparent that the ability of infants to deal with reality has to be considered on a par with the ability to deal with hedonics and that ego formation is better differentiated and functioning that Glover or Hartman could have known. Furthermore, many of the corollaries that flowed from the basic assumption of id before ego, such as the idea that primary process (autistic) thinking precedes secondary process (reality or socialized) thinking, were also arbitrary. Vygotsky (1962), for example, makes a potent developmental case that secondary process thinking develops first. He further points out that Piaget borrowed the same assumption as did Freud in arriving at his cognitive sequences, which are no longer so widely accepted.

Many basic psychoanalytic conceptions about drive, the number of drives, their allegiance to id or ego (or even such a notion as allegiance), and their developmental sequencing all need to be reconceptualized when confronted with the infant as observed.

Undifferentiation and Some of its Corollaries: "Normal Symbiosis," Transition Phenomena, Self/Objects

The idea of a period of undifferentiation that is subjectively experienced by the infant as a form of merger and dual-unity with mother is very problematic, as we have seen, but at the same time it has great appeal. By locating at a specific point in lived time those powerful human feelings of a background sense of well-being in union with another, it gratifies the wish for an actual psychobiological wellspring from which such feelings originate and to which one could possibly return. Weil (1970) accomplishes the same with her "basic core."

Ultimately, this kind of notion is a statement of belief about whether the essential state of human existence is one of aloneness or togetherness (Hamilton 1982). It chooses togetherness, and in doing so it sets up the most basic sense of connectedness, affiliation, attachment, and security as givens. No active process is needed for the infant to acquire or develop towards this basic sense. Nor is a basic attachment theory with purposeful moving parts and stages a necessity. Only a theory of separation and individuation is required to move the infant on developmentally, which Mahler goes on to provide.[3]

---

3. Once "normal symbiosis" has been developmentally positioned, so to speak, even as an act of belief, then the schedule for the next phases of development has already been implied. Separation/individuation or something very like it must necessarily follow to undo or, at least, counterbalance the symbiotic phase in the sense of dialectically moving its work forward.

Attachment theory does the opposite. It makes the achievement of a basic sense of human connectedness the end point, not the starting point, of a long, active developmental course involving the interplay of predesigned and acquired behaviors.

From the point of view of core-relatedness, one assumes that pervasive feelings of connectedness and interpersonal well-being do occur during this period from two to seven months. One also assumes that these feelings do serve as an emotional reservoir of human connectedness. The process is not seen as a passive one, however, nor as one that is given a priori. It results from the infant's active construction of representations of interactions with self-regulating others (RIGs). The RIGs and their activated form of evoked companions become the repository of the feelings that Mahler describes so well but ascribes to dual-unity. The self-regulating other is not a given, however; it is an active construct, and it forms alongside the forming sense of self and other. In our view, the developmental tasks of Mahler's phase of normal symbiosis, together with her first phase of separation/individuation, are going on simultaneously during the period of core-relatedness. For Mahler, connectedness is the result of a failure in differentiation; for us it is a success of psychic functioning.

In a vein somewhat similar to Mahler's, the British object relations school also postulates an early undifferentiated phase, but with emphasis on initial relatedness. They assume that the infant "starts life in a state of total emotional identification with his mother" and gradually experiences separateness without losing the experience of relatedness (Guntrip 1971, p. 117). In a similar vein, Winnicott (1958) assumes that in the beginning the infant has not yet separated out the specific object from the "me." "In object relating, the subject allows certain alterations in the self to take place, of a kind that has caused us to invent the term cathexis. The object has become meaningful" (p. 72).

The object relations theorists make the same mistake as the ego psychologists in assuming an important initial period of undifferentiation, which they reify and imbue with subjective feelings of security and belongingness much as Mahler has done for her phase of symbiosis. In a sense, they push a symbiotic-like phase to the earliest point in life, where Mahler has placed autism. Unlike Mahler, however, they do not see the primary state of relatedness as something one grows out of during a separation/individuation–like phase. They see separateness and relatedness as concomitant and equal developmental lines. They thus avoid oscillating sequential phases in which one or the other (relatedness or separateness) is in dominance.

The developmental view of internalized objects put forward by Self Psychology is quite different from that described by classical psychoanalysis or ego psychology. Nonetheless, self psychologists either overtly or covertly also suggest that there exists an important phase of self/other undifferentiation during the first six months of life. Because of this view, they assume that one can speak only of a self emerging from a "self–selfobject *matrix*" or from a "self–self other *unit*" (Tolpin 1980, p. 49) or of the "emergence of a cohesive infantile self existing (initially) *within* a self object matrix" (Wolf 1980, p. 122). How different is this descriptively from the picture of normal autism and normal symbiosis, both of which are problematic as constructs and not supported by the observational data?

It is not clear why the theory of Self Psychology needs to adhere to the central tenets or timetable of traditional psychoanalytic developmental theory up through the first six months of life. Their theory clearly diverges from traditional theory after that point. (In fact, the notions of a sense of a core self and the construction of normal self-regulating others appears to be more in line with and useful to the general outlines of a theory of Self Psychology.)

The Developmental Fate of Self-Regulating Others

A central point of contention between Self Psychology and traditional psychoanalytic theory lies in the view that there is a lifelong need for "self-objects." Kohut emphasized the clinical reality of one person using some aspect of another person as a functional part of the self to provide a stabilizing structure against the fragmenting potential of stimulation and affect. That is what a selfobject is (1977). It is a catchall term for a variety of ongoing functional relationships with others that are necessary to provide the regulating structures that maintain and/or enhance self-cohesion. Kohut and others, in the course of their work, began to realize that the use of and need for "self-objects" was not limited to borderline disorders and manifest only in certain transference reactions seen in therapy. The users of "self-objects" included everyone, and the need for them became viewed as legitimate, healthy, and expectable at every stage of the normal life span.

It is this notion that places Self Psychology in opposition to traditional psychoanalytic accounts of development, which make the goal of maturity (in part) the achievement of a certain level of independence and autonomy from objects, by way of the processes of separation/individuation and internalization. The development of the "self-object," according to Self Psychology, is not a phase-specific product of normal symbiosis, but a lifelong developmental line (see Goldberg 1980). Both theoretical systems agree on the need for some functions and regulating structures that originally rely on another to become autonomous self functions. (In Self Psychology, "transmuting internalizations" accomplish the task that is the aim of "internalization" [Tolpin 1980].) The construction of the superego viewed as the repository of the prohibitions and moral standards of another is the extreme example of "structuralization." The difference between the two theories is not simply one of emphasis, Self Psychology stressing the development of self-objects that endure and even grow, and separation/individuation stressing those that dissolve and become autonomous self functions and structures. The difference is more one of the perceived nature of the self, or of humankind.

The theory developed here in the light of recent research considers these phenomena in terms of the memory of experiences of being with others and the ways in which these memories are retrieved and used. In the beginning, others exist "within" us only in the form of memories or imaginings, conscious or unconscious, of the experience of self being with them (RIGs). What, then, is needed to recall their presence from memory? And how abstract or automatic can the recall cue become? During the infancy period, before adequate symbolizing functions are available, the recall cue cannot be too abstract and the experience of being-with cannot be automatic; it must involve at least some degree of reliving the experience, the evoked companion. We are therefore necessarily concerned more with the development of memories of self-regulating-others (or, in Self Psychological terms, "self-objects"). Internalization of the type that superego functions represent is not yet at stake.

Teleologically, nature must create a baby whose capacity for this memory and recall of being with others can in later life adapt to the needs of varying cultures. A member of one society, such as a hunting-gathering group, may never be expected to be out of sight or earshot of close members of the group for more than minutes or hours, and then only rarely. In another society, the isolated person on the frontier may be the ideal. Similarly, there is a cultural range in the degree to which various roles, functions, feeling states, and so on are explicitly stated by the society or left more to individual invention for their internal and external form. This degree will determine how overt or abstract the recall cue can be.

Along a different line of approach, a group's overall reproductive pattern may have a great deal to do with the experience of falling in love, or it may have practically nothing to do with it. The capacity to fall in love greatly exercises the memorial and imagining capacity for being with another. To engage in sustained romantic love requires that the individual be given the opportunity through many life experiences to develop the ability to become imbued with the presence of an absent person, an almost constantly evoked companion.

In many ways, then, the need for and use of recall cues to call someone else into one's presence varies greatly. The infant therefore needs a memory system of being with others that is highly flexible, allowing for adaptation to life experience. Processes, rather than psychic structures, are required. The notion of becoming maturely independent of others and the notion of continually building and rebuilding a more extensive working set of "self-others" as a maturational goal are just opposite ends of the same spectrum. The infant must be equipped with the memorial capacities to do both or either as experience dictates.

Affect State–Dependent Experience

Psychoanalytic theory has implicitly given the very intense emotional states a special organizing role. Affects are privileged as attributes of experience, and high intensity affects are awarded an especially privileged status. It is not surprising that this should have happened, since Freud's original theories gave traumatic states the primary etiological role. In trauma, it was assumed, the intensity of experience disrupts the ability to cope with and assimilate information. It is this (often hidden) assumption that has guided so many theoreticians. Melanie Klein's (1952) designation of the "good" and "bad" breast and Kernberg's (1975, 1976) splitting of self-experience into "good" and "bad" are direct consequences. So is Pine's (1981) suggestion about the role of "intense moments." In a similar vein, Kohut (1977) speculates that if the empathic failures of parents are too large, the sense of a cohesive self will be thrown too far off balance and the infant will not be able to perform the needed internalization to restore equilibrium (see also Tolpin [1980]). The assumption behind this line of psychoanalytic thinking is that the most clinically important experiences (and their memory and representation) are affect state–dependent; in other words, the affect state acts as the cardinal organizing element, and the very intense affect states are the ones in which the most clinically relevant experiences are precipitated out. Extreme bliss or extreme frustration, for example, are more potent organizing experiences than mild or moderate contentment or frustration.

Some recent findings in memory research can be interpreted as partially supportive of this prevalent view. G. Bower (1981) demonstrated that mood influences the encoding and retrieval of memory, that what is remembered or recalled is affect state–dependent. Manic patients were taught a list of items. Much later, they were tested for recall. At the time of testing for recall, some of the patients were still manic while others were now depressed. The same procedure was followed for patients who were initially depressed during the learning phase and when tested for recall were either still depressed or now manic. The results showed that material learned in the manic state was more readily recalled when the patient was in the same mood state. Similar results applied to the depressed patients. For both groups, memory was mood-dependent to a significant extent. In another phase of the experiment, Bower altered the affect state through hypnosis and found essentially the same thing—that memory was partially affect state–dependent.

It is important to note that these experiments do not tell how "intense" an experience must be before it can exert significant "state-

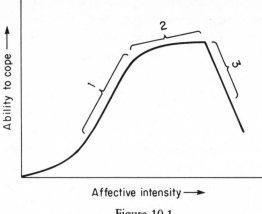

Figure 10.1

dependent" influences, nor do the psychoanalytic theories. Psycho-analytic theory usually makes the following distinctions: mild to moderate affect experience, intense affect experience, and traumatic affect experience. These could be schematized as in figure 10.1.

The mild to moderate intensity experiences (segment 1) are thought to play an insignificant role as organizers of memory. The intense experiences (segment 2) are thought to play an important role (compare Pine's "intense moment" [1981]). And the experiences that are so intense that the coping capacity to deal with them fails fall into the third segment of traumatic experiences. These may have particular potency as organizers of experience if they result in one-trial learning. (It is not always clear whether Klein and Kernberg see their formative experiences in segment 2 or segment 3.)

There are three main issues and problems with this conceptualization. The first is where to bound the segments. What constitute the boundary criteria for separate "states" that can produce *separate* state-dependent structures? Why could not this schematic be redrawn to show six, instead of three, separate and distinct segments? One then would end up with six separate state-dependent organizations of experience. On what basis can we divide the curve into discrete segments? There may be a natural break between segments 2 and 3, but even that is a supposition. Psychoanalytic theories more generally propose a discontinuity of experience between segments one and two. This issue is an empirical one. The separate states, however, may not be so discrete, and that leads to the second issue.

Can the different state-dependent experiences "speak to" one another? One of the classical notions of the traumatic state is that the traumatic experience is so state-dependent that it is entirely inaccessible under normal conditions and can only be re-experienced when the person is returned to the traumatic state, or close to it. Freud's original use of hypnosis was partially intended to permit patients to "revisit" experiences of trauma that were otherwise inaccessible.

Psychoanalytic theory has not been clear on the degree to which "intense moment"–dependent experiences are permeable. In other words, how available are such experiences to experiences in other states of affect intensity? Clearly, people do not create separate, impermeable states of experience that divide the intensity continuum into totally discontinuous, noncommunicating compartments like a string of pearls. Bower's experiment with mania and depression shows that these fairly intense mood states are not at all impermeable one to the other but are partially permeable; some information learned in one state can be recalled when in the other state. This issue, too, is an empirical one.

The third issue is that the more intense states are thought to have more state-dependent organizing power than the less intense states. This idea has intuitive appeal, but things may not be so simple as that. If intensity has reached the level of disorganizing adaptive capacities, the power to organize experience is dissipated. (Compare Sullivan's notion of the effect of extreme anxiety [1953].) The intense rather than the traumatic level might then be the most potent organizer. On the other hand, one can also argue that the capacity to take in the information to be organized would be best at a moderate rather than a high (let alone traumatic) level of intensity. In this case the moderate level of intensity would be the most potent organizer. This view is in accord with Demos's views:

> The bulk of psychic structure is created when both the "I" and the "we" experiences of the infant are going well. For example, the developmental literature is replete with descriptions of how the infant's behavior is enhanced in smooth interactions with a caregiver—interest is prolonged, variations on a theme and imitations of new behaviors occur, the infant's repertoire is expanded . . . At slightly later ages, Ainsworth has described how the securely attached infant will explore and play more freely in the presence of the attachment figure, and so on. Thus structure building is going on during good, empathic "we" experiences as well. What

happens then, during an empathic break? I am suggesting that the empathic break could be seen as presenting the infant with a challenge to her adaptive capacities, which, by and large, have developed in more optimal situations. (Demos 1980, p. 6)

In a similar vein, it has recently been seen in our laboratory that rather ordinary and very moderate affective experiences can be well remembered one week later (MacKain et al. 1985).

Sander (1983a) has speculated that infants learn a great deal about themselves when there are neither pressing physiological inner needs nor external social need—that is, when they are alone and in equilibrium. It is then that they can begin to discover aspects of self. Similarly, Sander (1983b) has maintained that normal interactions, at both low and high levels of affect, are the stuff of representations.

In therapy, however, things may look different. The therapeutic experience may favor the recollection of the higher intensity affective experiences (for many reasons beyond a bias in selection of material on the basis of theory). The privileged role of such experiences for the clinical infant therefore remains unchallenged, although for the observed infant, these questions are still open and undecided.[4]

Splitting: "Good" and "Bad" Experiences

Psychoanalytic theorists assume that the infant's view of the world during the intense moments of affective experience is the most important factor in the construction of object relations. When this view is combined with the assumption that experiences of pleasure and unpleasure in early life are the most relevant, as the pleasure principle predicts, the result is the notion that the first dichotomy of the world that an infant will make is between pleasurable ("good") and unpleasurable ("bad") experiences. This hedonically based split is thought to occur before the self/other dichotomy is achieved. Many psychoanalytic theorists, among them Kernberg (1968, 1975,

4. This general issue has also contributed to the greatly exaggerated notion that the observed infant is really a "cognitive" infant, while the clinical infant is an "affective" infant.

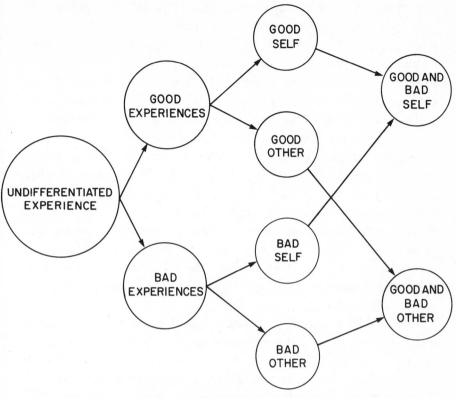

Figure 10.2

1976, 1982), would schematize the early developmental sequence as in figure 10.2.

The assumptions for this line of reasoning are as follows: (1) Hedonic experiences can and will override all other experiences and serve as the privileged organizing interpersonal event. (2) Infant experience is so hedonic tone–dependent that pleasurable and unpleasurable experiences cannot talk to each other, be cross-referenced, or integrated. Each is encapsulated from the other. (3) Accordingly, the infant is forced to do double bookkeeping with regard to experience and its memory. There is an interpersonal "world" that occurs or is re-evoked under the aegis of pleasurable feelings and another "world" under the aegis of unpleasurable feelings. There is also the cognitive interpersonal "world" that prevails under the conditions of neutral or less-than-peak states of hedonic tone. So the infant has to keep triple books, two affective and one cognitive. These three worlds cannot be mixed or integrated because of the

249

impermeability of state-dependent experiences. (4) This splitting into pleasurable and unpleasurable occurs prior to the formation of self/other differentiation as dated by the Mahlerian timetable. So when self and other do appear, they do so under the prevailing splitting influence of this already present good/bad dichotomy. (5) "Good" can be equated with pleasurable and "bad" with unpleasurable.

This account of subjective development is well tailored to the needs of the clinical infant glimpsed in certain adult patients. There is no question that one sees the phenomenon of splitting, usually associated with the internalization of the "good" and the externalization or projection of the "bad," as an important entity in adult patients with borderline disorders. The question is, how does this particular pathomorphic reconstruction of the development of a clinical infant square with knowledge of the observed infant? This particular case is important, because the Kleinian view (1952) and the version of it elaborated by Kernberg (1984) are very widely used conceptualizations.

The problems with this "split" clinical infant as an observable reality are several. The hedonic tone of an experience is certainly a potent attribute, but it is certainly not the only one and not demonstrably the more potent. Perhaps more important, it probably does not create relatively encapsulated hedonic tone–dependent experiences and memories. Hedonic tone–dependent experiences are simply not impermeable. (The majority of experiences a person encounters while manic are recallable when the person is non-manic or even depressed.)

Another problem is even more telling. If an infant had only two experiences with a breast, a pleasurable one and an unpleasurable one, then the Kernbergian position of hedonically split experience might be more tenable. But the infant has four to six or so a day, every day. And each one differs slightly with regard to pleasurableness. Under these conditions it should be less of a task to discover the invariants of what a breast or face looks or feels like, across the many shades of pleasure/unpleasure that fall upon them. Certainly the current hedonic tone of an experience (say, a pleasurable feeding) will imbue all the other attributes of the experience (what the breast looks like and feels like, how the mother's face looks, and so on) with certain feelings. An unpleasurable experience will imbue all those attributes with different feelings. That much is consistent with current notions. The problem lies in the dichotomization of experience into two types and the experiential isolation of the two types one from the other.[5]

Yet another problem with Kernberg's position lies in the timing of things. He has inherited the traditional timetable for self/other differentiation. This view is not able to take into account the likelihood that affective experiences are one of the major sources of *self-invariance*. That is, they will promote the discrimination of the self from the breast ("I have experienced this affect state in myself many times before in many circumstances. It's part of how I can be and can feel, and it is independent of the presence of the breast"). In other words, affective tone should induce the self/other dichotomy as readily as the good/bad dichotomy.

In the sequence according to Kernberg, the self and the other as separate entities cannot come together—cohere—until the cognitive infant can encompass the separate good and bad selves, in other words, until the neutral perceptual invariants are as strong as or stronger than the affective ones, at least at times. When that happens the infant can solidify the second great dichotomy, between self and other. Once that is done, there is a "place," so to speak—a self and an other—where the good and bad selves can "reside" in alternating ambivalence and later in simultaneous ambivalence.

Such a sequence raises all sorts of other questions. How can one postulate a "good self" and a "bad self" before there is a "self?"

---

5. Infants must learn about the world of affects as subjectivity both experienced in themselves and as seen in others. To do this they must come to appreciate that affects vary along the dimension of intensity (in terms of both hedonic value and activation). In order for infants to gain an integrated view of subjective and objective affect experience, they must have available to them a perceptual and experiential view of the spectrum of affect dimension as a continuous gradient (Stern et al. 1980; Lichtenberg 1983). In drawing arbitrary thresholds, the psychoanalytic theorists would fracture the infant's experience of the world of affect.

There is no question that state-dependent perception and memory do exist and may prove very helpful in considering the enormous influence of affect on perception and memory. Psychoanalysis assumed this to be the case long before the notion of state-dependence in its current form arrived on the scene. It is one of the great strengths of the psychoanalytic view. However, for the purposes of further understanding, psychoanalytic theorists must begin to frame this polemic in terms of state-dependence or some other current explanatory mode. And future research must address the issue of the extent of permeability between state-dependent phenomena. It seems very unlikely that the continuous gradient from weak to strong in pleasure and unpleasure should be perceived discontinuously. There is no clear survival or communicative advantage in that. The weaker end of the spectrum could never be used as a "signal" in the psychoanalytic sense, or as an intentional "signal" in the ethological sense, if continuity between weak and strong were interrupted.

What would "self" mean? What would mark the distinction between a "good experience" and a "good self"? Or, how do the "good" and "bad" selves interact through the medium of a nonaffective self, that is, a cognitive self that has enough self-coherence and continuity to encompass the "good" and "bad" selves?

In this view, then, the affective dichotomy (good/bad) precedes the self/other dichotomy. Findings from the observed infant permit no such assumption about sequence of dichotomies or privileged status of affect over cognition. Rather, both proceed simultaneously and remain permeable one to the other.

The final problem concerns the notion of "good" and "bad" psychic entities. It seems unavoidable that "bad" derives from "unpleasurable" and "good" from "pleasurable." The question is, when does the infant make the leap? "Good" and "bad" imply either standards, intentions, and/or morality. The infant can in no way make the connection between "pleasurable" and "good" or "unpleasurable" and "bad" at the level of core-relatedness, as suggested. It is only at the level of intersubjective relatedness that infants begin to conceive of the other as having intentions toward them, let alone malign intentions. Accordingly, it is a distortion of the infant's likely experience even to use the terms "good" and "bad" as freely substitutable with pleasurable and unpleasurable. The ontogenetic line from pleasurable to good is of extreme importance, but it is an issue of a later period of development than the one we are considering. Once again, the need to find in the infant events that are part of adult experience is misleading. Good and bad as encountered in the splitting of borderline patients requires a level of symbolization beyond the infant's capacity. A complex reindexing of memories and reorganization of experience is needed to *conceptualize* as well as to divide interpersonal experience affectively into the good and the bad. The same would be true for "safe" versus "frightening" (Sandler 1960). Splitting is, however, a fairly universal experience. It occurs not only in pathological forms in patients, as Kernberg and others point out, but probably in all of us in less intense forms. The point of this critique is not to suggest that splitting is not a pervasive human phenomena. It is, and it is ready-made for pathological elaboration, but it is the product of a post-infancy mind capable of many symbolic transformations and condensations on an hedonic theme. It is not a likely experience of infants as observed.

In spite of this critique, I do believe that infants will group interpersonal experiences into various pleasurable and unpleasurable categories, that is, into hedonic clusters. The forming of hedonic clusters of experiences, however, is different from dichotomizing or splitting all interpersonal experience along hedonic lines. For instance, if we consider an unpleasurable cluster of interactive experiences with mother as an entity analogous to a particular type of "working model of mother," then this cluster can also be conceived of as an assemblage of RIGs, all of which have a common theme that brings and ties them together as a working model. The common theme is an attribute of the experience, namely a certain degree and even quality of unpleasure. We can then speak of a negatively toned mother. The difference, for our purposes, between a negatively toned mother and an avoidantly attached working model of mother (for example) is the different attribute that acts as the common theme to tie together the various RIGs that form the two different constructs. The RIGs that are assembled to create the negatively toned mother share a hedonic tone and quality as the common attribute. The RIGs that are assembled to create an avoidantly attached working model of mother share contextual and attachment activating and deactivating attributes. Let us call them both working models, but of different kinds. The infant is bound to form many such working models. At a later date, after verbal relatedness is well established, the child or adult can, with the aid of symbols, re-index RIGs and various working models to form two superordinate categories that are imbued with the full meanings of "good" or "bad." In this way, an older child or adult can indeed "split" their interpersonal experience, but it is in fact not a splitting but rather an integration into a higher order categorization.

Fantasy versus Reality as the Central Issue in Ontogenic Theories

When Freud realized the extent to which his patients had been seduced or sexually approached by their parents in their fantasies, but not in actuality, he cast his lot and that of psychoanalysis with fantasy. Fantasy—experience as distorted by wishes and defenses—

firmly became the arena of inquiry. Reality—what actually happened, as determinable by a third party—was relegated to a background position, even considered clinically irrelevant by many. Since Freud's clinical concerns were with a patient's life as experienced subjectively, not as enacted objectively, his decision is easily understandable. Coupled with the postulate that the pleasure principle preceded or at least dominated the reality principle in development, this theoretical clinical position resulted in an ontogenetic theory of experience as fantasy, not of experience as reality. The units making up the steps or stages of developmental theory came to be such phenomena as wishes, distortions, delusions, and defensive resolutions.

It is in this tradition that Mahler and Klein have worked. A basic assumption of the notion of "normal symbiosis" is that even if infants could tell self from other, their defenses would prevent their doing so, in order to ward off anxiety or stress. Mahler postulates that from birth until two months the infant ego is protected by the stimulus barrier. After the barrier is gone, infants would be left with all the stresses and threats of being on their own, unless they replaced the reality of their separateness and aloneness with the "delusion" of a fused-with mother and thus a protected state. "The libidinal cathexis vested in the symbiotic orbit replaces the unborn instinctual stimulus barrier and protects the rudimentary ego from premature phase-unspecific strain, from stress traumatic [and in doing so creates a] *delusion* of a common boundary" (Mahler et al. 1975, p. 451). Normal symbiosis theory thus is based on a belief in infantile fantasy or distortion rather than a belief in reality perception. In a similar vein, Klein postulates the infant's basic subjective experiences as consisting of paranoid, schizoid, and depressive positions. These assumed infantile experiences operate outside of ongoing reality perceptions. Here, too, the units of a genetic theory are fantasy-based. (This notion may permit these theorists to ignore selected observational findings, but at considerable expense.)

The basic assumption that the appropriate units of a genetic theory are fantasies is open to serious question. One cannot disagree that subjective experience is the appropriate stuff for genetic theory, but how firm is the assumption that the most relevant subjective experiences of the infant are reality-distorting fantasies? And here we restrike a chord sounded before. If current findings from infancy studies fly against the notion that the pleasure principle developmentally precedes the reality principle, then why must wishes and defenses against reality be given a privileged and prior developmental position? Why must the sense of reality be seen as secondary in time and derivation, growing out of the loss of the need for fantasy and defense?

The position taken here is based on the opposite assumption—namely, that infants from the beginning mainly experience reality. Their subjective experiences suffer no distortion by virtue of wishes or defenses, but only those made inevitable by perceptual or cognitive immaturity or overgeneralization. Further, I assume here that the capacity for defensive—that is, psychodynamic—distortions of reality is a later-developing capacity, requiring more cognitive processes than are initially available.[6] The views presented here suggest that the usual genetic sequence should be reversed and that reality experience precedes fantasy distortions in development. This position leaves the infant unapproachable by psychodynamic considerations for an initial period, resulting in a non-psychodynamic beginning of life in the sense that the infant's experience is not the product of reality altering conflict resolution. This position is far closer to Kohut's and Bowlby's contention that pre-Oedipal pathology is due to deficits or reality-based events—rather than to conflicts, in the psychodynamic sense.

Deficit is the wrong concept, however, for these reality-based events. From a normative and prospective vantage, the infant experiences only interpersonal realities, not deficits (which cannot be experienced until much later in life) and not conflict-resolving distortions. It is the actual shape of interpersonal reality, specified by the interpersonal invariants that really exist, that helps determine the developmental course. Coping operations occur as reality-based adaptations. Defensive operations of the type that distort reality occur only after symbolic thinking is available. From this position, we can now take up again the all-important task addressed by A. Freud and ask what may be the nature, form, and developmental timetable of the earliest-appearing defensive operations, now that they have been repositioned as secondary reworkings of the infant's initially fairly accurate experience of interpersonal reality.

6. A reading of A. Freud's (1965) view of the ontogeny of defensive operations is compatible with this claim.

Chapter 11

Implications for the
Therapeutic Process
of Reconstructing
a Developmental Past

HOW MIGHT the developmental views presented here affect clinical practice? In particular, how might a therapist and a patient reconstruct a therapeutically effective narrative about the past? Two major features of this viewpoint have broad clinical implications. First, the traditional clinical-developmental issues such as orality, dependence, autonomy, and trust, have been disengaged from any one specific point or phase of origin in developmental time. These issues are seen here as developmental lines—that is, issues for life, not phases of life. They do not undergo a sensitive period, a presumed phase of ascendancy and predominance when relatively irreversible "fixations" could occur. It therefore can not be known in advance, on theoretical grounds, at what point in life a particular traditional clinical-developmental issue will receive its pathogenic origin.

Traditional theories assigned an age-specific sensitive phase of life for the initial impress of these issues. There was thus an actual moment in time toward which theory dictated we should direct our reconstructive inquiry. In fact, some understanding of the initial pathogenic events during the sensitive phase was not only practically desirable but theoretically essential for the fullest understanding of the pathology. From the point of view taken here, this situation no longer prevails. The actual point of origin for any of these traditional clinical-developmental issues could be anywhere along their continuous developmental line. No longer prescribed by theory, it poses a mystery and a challenge, and the therapist is freer to roam with the patient across the ages and through the domains of senses of the self, to discover where the reconstructive action will be most intense, unimpeded by too limiting theoretical prescriptions. This freedom permits the therapist to listen more evenly (much as Freud originally suggested) and to make the task of reconstruction more of a true adventure for both patient and therapist. There are fewer theoretical constraints on where they will arrive—in other words, fewer preconceptions about what the reconstructed clinical infant will look like.

The fact is that most experienced clinicians keep their developmental theories well in the background during active practice. They search with the patient through his or her remembered history to find the potent life-experience that provides the key therapeutic metaphor for understanding and changing the patient's life. This experience can be called the *narrative point of origin* of the pathology, regardless of when it occurred in actual developmental time. Once the metaphor has been found, the therapy proceeds forward and backward in time from that point of origin. And for the purposes of an effective therapeutic reconstruction, the therapy rarely if ever gets back to the preverbal ages, to an assumed *actual point of origin* of the pathology, even though there is theoretically supposed to be one. Most therapists would agree that one works with whatever reconstructive metaphor offers the most force and explanatory power about the patient's life, even though one can not get at the "original edition" of the metaphor. While the developmental theory is given lip service, the practice proceeds. There is widespread recognition that the developmental theories, when applied to a patient, do not

257

deliver any reliable actual point of origin for the traditional clinical-developmental issues. Such actual points of origin of pathology apply only to theoretical infants, who do not exist.

The second major point with broad clinical implications is that the period of emergence of each sense of self is most likely a sensitive period, for reasons given in chapter 9. It is the different domains of self-experience, rather than the traditional clinical-developmental issues, that are given a strong formative impress during a particular, and specifiable, developmental time slot. This implication sets up clinical predictions that are testable.

We will begin with some of the possible consequences of disengaging the traditional clinical-developmental issues from age-specific sensitive periods and then address some of the consequences of putting the domains of sense of self in their developmental place.

Implications of Viewing Traditional Clinical-Developmental Issues as Issues for Life

STRATEGIES FOR FINDING THE NARRATIVE ORIGIN OF A PROBLEM

The notion of a layering of different senses of the self as different forms of ongoing experience is potentially helpful in locating an organizing therapeutic metaphor. Take, for example, a patient whose major concern focuses on control and autonomy. In search of a key metaphor, one explores the clinical "feel" of the problem. A first question in identifying the feel is, what domain of relatedness is most prominent or active? The patient's current life and transference reactions provide the clues. Patients readily indicate which sense of the self is most at stake in the issue of control. Imagine three different kinds of mother-child relationships with regard to autonomy. The first mother operates under the assumption that it is necessary and desirable to control Johnny's body—that is, his physical acts—but not his words or feeling states. Those are his own business. A second mother may contest only Jenny's feeling states and intentions. And a third mother's vital personal sphere of control lies neither in what Jimmy does or feels, but only in what he says. That becomes her business. Each of these situations will result in a different clinical feel as to what the problem of autonomy is about, or which sense of self is at risk in the struggle.

The following case illustrates the issue of where to look for the narrative origin and key metaphor. A professional woman in her thirties complained of feeling unable to cope by herself, to initiate her own wishes and goals. She had taken a passive role in the conduct of her life, following what for her (given her family background and mental resources) was the path of least resistance and the path that someone else had urged or initiated. It was in this way that she had become a lawyer and gotten married. Her current and most acute source of suffering was her sense of paralysis in her law career. She felt that she had no control over her present situation or future course and that her life was in the hands of others. She felt helpless and furious. She frequently overreacted, and the over-reactions were placing her job in some jeopardy. When talking about her situation at work, she kept dwelling upon details that concerned her physical agency, especially the initiation and freedom of her *physical* acts: she wanted her office rearranged—flower pots, some books, a coffee table, all things she could move herself—and she had planned what was to be done, but somehow could not get herself to do it. She was furious with one of the senior partners for turning a common room into a special conference room, off-limits to all but senior partners. She seemed upset mainly at not being able to wander in there to see the view of the city, as she had before, not because it was any real inconvenience to her work or because she saw it as a demeaning statement about her lesser status. She most resented being deprived of her habitual walk and view.

Her concerns with her physical freedom to act made it feel as though the domain of core-relatedness and, in particular, the sense of agency were most involved. This impression was heightened by the fact that she felt no inability to initiate and control her life in the domains of intersubjective and verbal relatedness. She was very effective in addressing misunderstandings and empathic ruptures. With this in mind, we looked for any other times when her sense of a core self, and especially her physical agency, felt compromised. The life "moment" that made up the narrative point of origin for her therapy was found in a period of her life from age eight to ten, when she was largely bedridden with rheumatic fever and subacute bacterial endocarditis. This life period had been explored extensively earlier in treatment, when she had dwelled mainly on the depressive and depriving features of her illness. This time, however, we kept the therapeutic exploration closer to the feelings related to her sense of a core self. She then recalled that she had been ordered not to move about, even to walk to the window, and that even if she tried to do something or get somewhere, she was too physically fatigued. For anything physical to happen—to get upstairs or downstairs, to retrieve a book she wanted, to open the window—she had to wait for her mother or father to reappear and make it happen. She felt as though she had spent a lifelong season waiting for the "world to get activated and begin" at someone else's initiation.

This physically sick self, which had no agency and no capacity to initiate wished-for actions and which could not make "the world begin," became her narrative point of origin. It was this sense of self that she was now carrying about, and it became the pivotal metaphor for the "clinical infant" that was reconstructed. Once the metaphor was in place, she found it relatively easy to explore other manifestations of this historical event, and even some of its predispositions. Gradually, it helped her understand and deal with the acute distress she suffered at work. This metaphor acted as the fundamental referent for this aspect of her problems, and in her treatment she kept checking back to it, as to the North Star, to orient herself. This vignette makes several salient points for our purposes. First, the historical events ("traumatic" events) that served as the point of origin for the narrative occurred during the latency years. Regardless of her age, the major effect was in the domain of her sense of a core self. Because all senses of the self, once formed, remain active, growing, subjective processes throughout life, any one of them is vulnerable to deformations occurring at any life point. Similarly, since life issues such as autonomy or control are issues for the life span, they too are vulnerable at any life point.

The narrative point of origin can, and in this case probably does, correspond with the actual point of origin. The genesis of psychological problems may, but does not have to, have a developmental history that reaches back to infancy. Development of senses of the self is going on all the time, at all levels of "primitiveness." Development is not a succession of events left behind in history. It is a continuing process, constantly updated.

The second point to note is that the formative events that occurred during the patient's eighth to tenth years were the "first edition" of the problem. They were not necessarily a "re-edition" of earlier childhood events. We need not seek a theoretical actual origin point. One could then ask why she could not overcome the historical event, or trauma. Is it not necessary to look for earlier reasons that made her more susceptible to the trauma? Yes, it will be helpful to know about predispositions to susceptibility, but that is not the same as seeking an "original edition" in the earlier years.

Psychopathology when viewed from a developmental point of view is perhaps best seen on a continuum of pattern accumulation. At one extreme are actual neuroses, in which an isolated event (outside of the predictable and characteristic) impinges on the individual with pathogenic results. This kind of pathology has an actual point of origin that can occur at any point in development. And inevitably, the narrative point of origin and the actual point of origin are identical. There is no accumulation.

At the other extreme are the cumulative interactive patterns that can be observed very early, even at their initiation in infancy, and certainly during their continuation as development proceeds. These characteristic cumulative patterns result in character and personality types and, in the extreme, in personality disorders of the *DSM-III* Axis II types. These do not have an actual developmental point of origin in any meaningful sense. The insult (or pattern) is effectively present and acting at all developmental points. There is only accumulation. Naturally, the patterns start at only one point, the earliest point, but that does not assure that the contribution of this first point is more important quantitatively or even qualitatively than the contributions at later points.

Somewhere in the middle of the continuum is the situation in which characteristic cumulative developmental patterns are necessary but not sufficient to the pathogenic impact of an actual insult. In this case, the actual developmental point of origin is indeterminate and a matter for speculation.

This indeterminacy can be confusing for therapy. Most psychoanalysts would maintain that there is an earlier edition that either cannot be retrieved because of repression or cannot be recognized because of distortions or transformations between the primary and later editions. These postulations appear to be more theoretically than clinically based. It is certainly true that repression and distortions can hide an earlier edition; that is often the case in clinical work. It is not always the case, however, and even if it were, the unmasked earliest edition is rarely where theory predicts its origin point should be. To rescue this situation, theorists postulate an even earlier edition, hidden yet further in the past by repression and distortion. There is no end to the chase.[1]

When psychopathology is viewed from the clinical point of view, the primary task is to find the narrative point of origin—invariably, the key metaphor(s). Our theories about the actual point of origin tell us only how to conduct the therapeutic search for a narrative point of origin. Even in the case of character pathology, unless or until the therapy can come up with one narrative point of origin (even if it is actually no more important than a hundred other possible jump-in points), therapy will go more slowly. One of the major tasks of the therapist is to help the patient find a narrative point of origin, even as a working heuristic.

The third point of relevance to us is the way in which the domains of sense of self facilitate the identification of the narrative point of origin. The connection between the way the patient was feeling and acting in the present and the way she must have felt during her illness at age eight to ten seems so obvious that an astute clinician of almost any theoretical persuasion would soon enough have made the comparison: "Is the way you feel now at work at all like what it felt to be sick and limited in what you could do, when you were sick as a girl?" What then is the advantage of holding in mind a view of the development of senses of the self when listening to a patient? Speed and confidence in the therapeutic search process is one answer. With this patient, the connection made was not so obvious until after the fact, as is so often the case, because she had never been able to recover spontaneously the physical details of being sick and had dwelt in great detail on just the psychological features. Through the notion of domains of sense of self, it was easier and faster to find this narrative point of origin.

There is a final point to be noted in the vignette concerning the

1. The ultimate barrier to the "primary" editions of infancy may be the rendition into the verbal mode. This, however, is neither a repression nor a distortion in the dynamic sense.

lawyer. Sometimes the event that ought to constitute a narrative point of origin is clear to both therapist and patient, but the patient cannot get hold of it because the key experiences are not affectively available. The notion of different and coexisting levels of sense of self can inform the search for the affectively loaded experiences that, when recovered, can potentially serve as a narrative point of origin.

The affective component of the key experience usually resides primarily in one domain of relatedness (that is, in one sense of the self), and even in one feature of that domain—in the case of the lawyer, physical agency and freedom. The clinical question then becomes, what sense of the self carries the affect? And once the question is posed that way, a familiarity with the domains of self-experience can serve as a helpful guide. The procedure is no different from helping the patient to get or wander back "there"—into the experience—so that some part of the recalled event might trigger recall of the affective part, but it adds the particular sense of the self to the list of experienced components to use as a recall cue.

Another vignette will demonstrate how the process can work. A young man of nineteen had had a psychotic break three months earlier, precipitated by his girlfriend's leaving him. He acknowledged that this was the pivotal event. He could talk about his disappointment and sense of loss, but only rather intellectually. While he was clearly still mourning her loss, he had never cried or relived the pain or the pleasures of his relationship with her. He showed no feelings about the event. He even talked about the last night he saw her, before she finally wrote him a letter telling him it was over. They were necking in the back seat of a car, and she was sitting on his lap. Many questions were put to him to elicit his feelings towards her: "What happened the last night?" "Did you make out or just talk?" (general questions); "Did you sense a change in her?" "Was she behind her kiss?" (questions directed at the intersubjective domain); "What did it feel like to kiss her?" (a question directed at the domain of core-relatedness). None had unlocked his affect, but the next one was directed even deeper into his sense of a core self: "What was it like to have her full weight on your lap?" That question retrieved the affect and let him cry for the first time in three months. With a different patient, in whom, for instance, the shock and hurt were less in the loss and more in the sense of having been deceived, of being vulnerable, of not picking up the signals, and being angry about it, then a question such as "Was she behind her kiss?", which is addressed to a failure in intersubjectivity, might have unlocked the feeling of anger and humiliation.[2]

SEARCH STRATEGIES WHERE THE DIAGNOSIS IS ALREADY KNOWN

Different theories about a given diagnostic category have differing explanations of the central subjective experience of the illness and how it arises. For an example of widely differing views, let us look at what several authors have said about the state that Adler and Buie describe as an "experiential state of intensely painful aloneness" common to borderline patients (Adler and Buie 1979, p. 83). Each theory explains this feeling of loneliness differently.

Some authors have suggested that the experience of abandonment is the most critical to the borderline patient, that it engenders an aloneness that can only be alleviated by being held or fed or touched or "merged." Aloneness secondary to abandonment, then, is the primary experience that sets in motion various defenses (see Adler and Buie [1979]). In our view, this is the experience of aloneness at the level of core-relatedness.

Other authors (see Kohut [1971, 1977]) suggest that the fundamental determinant of aloneness in borderline patients is the absence

2. It may appear in the above description that uncovering the affect is more a problem of normal memory retrieval—did the therapist hit the right note (the effective retrieval cue) so that the patient resonated (recalled the lived episode with its attendant affect)?—rather than a problem of repression—a conflictually determined memory dysfunction. Two kinds of memory processes are involved, *involuntary memory* and *removing a repression*. Involuntary memory is perhaps best described by Proust in two well-known passages in *Swann's Way*: "And so it is with our own past. It is a labour in vain to attempt to recapture it: all the efforts of our intellect must prove futile. The past is hidden somewhere outside the realm, beyond the reach of intellect, in some material object (in the sensation which that material object will give us) which we do not suspect. And as for that object, it depends on chance whether we come upon it or not before we ourselves must die. . . . But when from a long-distant past nothing subsists, after the people are dead, after the things are broken and scattered, still, alone, more fragile, but with more vitality, more unsubstantial, more persistent, more faithful, the smell and taste of things remain poised a long time, like souls, ready to remind us, waiting and hoping for their moment, amid the ruins of all the rest; and bear unfaltering, in the tiny and almost impalpable drop of their essence, the vast structure of recollection" (Trans. C. K. Scott Moncrieff [New York: The Modern Library, 1928], pp. 61, 65).

Both processes of retrieval appear to be necessary, and complementary. It is the therapist's task to work on them simultaneously. For the "involuntary" component, this can best be done by leading the patient in the direction of that domain of self-experience where he or she is most likely to encounter the right "drop of . . . essence." For the repression, the usual therapeutic procedures are needed.

of empathic experience and/or the failure of a "sustaining object" that maintains psychological survival. Adler and Buie, in describing this kind of loneliness, refer to a patient who traced her "most unbearable loneliness" to her mother's empathic unavailability. In our view, this is the experience of aloneness at the level of intersubjective relatedness. (Adler and Buie focus on a failure of evocative memory as the underlying mechanism. This seems too limited.)

Still other authors have emphasized that it is the defenses against abandonment or against failures of gratification that provide the main explanation of the experience of aloneness. Meissner (1971) suggests that the desire to incorporate the object results in a fear of annihilating the object. A protective distance is set up to save the object from destruction, and it then becomes the secondary cause of the feeling of loneliness. Kernberg (1968, 1975, 1982, 1984) suggests that gratification failures lead to rage, which then forces the mechanism of splitting to occur to maintain both a "good" and a "bad" object. Splitting in turn results in a painful aloneness. In our view, these defense-based explanations of the loneliness experience belong at the level of verbal relatedness. Similarly, protecting the object from your own fury falls into the domain of a reorganized, verbally represented experience.

Probably all three views are correct, but none is all-inclusive. Each of these experiences of aloneness is the same feeling state experienced and elaborated in a different domain of self-experience. All are likely to happen, and three different qualities of feeling do not call for three different and mutually exclusive, dynamic etiologies. In order not to treat a patient with an inapplicable dynamic and in the wrong domain of relatedness, it is necessary to be alert to the clinical flavor of the feeling state, so that the patient, rather than an etiological theory, will guide the therapy to the sense of self that is most in pain.

All domains of relatedness will be involved in the illness, but usually one is experienced as more painful at any time. The therapist cannot know initially whether that domain is the most affected or whether it is the least affected and therefore the least defended. Some of the controversy over whether the empathic approach (as applied in Self Psychology) or the interpretive approach (as applied in traditional psychoanalysis) is more efficacious in the treatment of borderline patients is mitigated by the viewpoint taken here. An empathic approach will inevitably first encounter and address the failures in the domain of intersubjective relatedness. The patient usually experiences shock and then ultimately relief in discovering that someone is available who is capable and desirous of knowing what it feels like to be him or her. The relief and the opening up of interpersonal possibilities are enormous, almost irrespective of the particular content material that is discussed. (The literature is now replete with such examples other than Kohut's; for example, see Schwaber [1980b].) The content material, such as failure of gratification leading to rage, leading to splitting, resulting in loneliness, is in the domain of verbal relatedness and may be addressed only secondarily, as the background material through which the empathic understanding is achieved.

An interpretive approach, on the other hand, will inevitably first engage the content material as it exists in the domain of verbal relatedness. Any empathic understanding between patient and therapist falls to the background and is worked on almost secondarily in the course of interpretive work and usually later in the form of transference and countertransference.

In effect, the nature of the therapeutic approach determines which domain of experience will appear to be primarily distressed. Because one can expect problems in all the senses of self and in all domains of relatedness, the therapist will by virtue of the approach he or she chooses find the pathology predicted by the etiological theory that determined the choice of approach in the first place. The problem is that while all domains of relatedness will be affected, one is likely to be more severely compromised and will require not only more therapeutic attention but perhaps the initial attention that allows treatment to proceed. This fact requires the therapist to be flexible in approach. And most clinicians use neither approach exclusively; there is more flexibility in practice than their theoretical persuasion would suggest. All this suggests that instead of continuing to practice in apparent contradiction to the guiding theory, in order to treat patients more effectively, the guiding theories need to be more encompassing. The developmental lines presented here suggest one route.

SEARCH STRATEGIES WHERE THE AGE OF TRAUMA IS KNOWN

It is in the situation in which the age at which the trauma occurred has been identified that our developmental theories can be most helpful or harmful to therapy. To what extent are our clinical ears and minds pretuned by particular developmental theories to pick up only certain material and miss other material?

A case illustration serves best. A patient related that his mother was clinically depressed during the period of his life from twelve to thirty months and that his relatives said that at about that time he, an only child, had changed into a more somber and anxious child, needy but not always asking for assurance. His family recalled that he had occasional "silent tantrums" for which the triggering issue was his sudden, short-lived refusals to use words. These tantrums did not concern restrictions in his freedom of action. Speech development was normal. Mother stayed home with him during this time, occupied as a housewife. She was never hospitalized but was in treatment five days a week and quite "preoccupied with her problems." In spite of this, she was available enough that the boy appeared neither overly clingy nor resistant to her, and his exploratory behavior seemed normal as remembered by all. If anything, he appeared rather adventuresome.

At the age of thirty-four, when he first came to treatment, he was married with a two-year-old boy. He was functioning well enough at a junior level in a large corporation. His wife was a graduate student in the humanities and the more "intellectual" one. His presenting complaint was of a generalized depression, feelings of insecurity and not being understood, and episodes of enraged outbursts at his wife. The feelings of insecurity were experienced both at work and at home. For most of his life he had thought of himself as a risk-taker, but he was currently inhibited from taking a risk at work that involved an appropriate "betting on himself." He periodically yearned for a more stable job in which advancement would be less dependent on his initiations. Alternately, he wished that one of the more senior members would take him under his wing and serve as an unconditional patron. He had lost respect for himself for entertaining such wishes. He felt dependent on his wife and called her from work at least once a day, although she found the calls a nuisance. At times she complained that he would rather just hold her than make love with her.

It was mainly with his wife that he felt not understood. He felt that instead of just listening to him she always became defensive, so that he was confronted by an adversary rather than an ally. Even in issues that involved no criticism, when he simply wanted to explain how he felt about something, she would too quickly jump in with unasked-for suggestions about what to do or how to remedy a problem. When he wanted to be understood, he felt advised.

His explosions of temper arose most often in this context of not feeling understood. They took the form of a characteristic argument in which he would end up yelling something like, "You have words and labels and explanations for everything. And they are supposed to make sense, but they mean nothing to me. That's not what my life feels like to me." And while he raved, his wife would walk out of the room, shaken but saying coolly that he could not be talked to. He then would go after her in anger and fear, fear that he would strike her and that she would leave him. The fear was great enough that he backed off his position, retreating and apologizing to re-establish the previous level of contact with her. When this was accomplished, he felt less fearful and more secure, but sadder and more alone. At those moments, he burst out sobbing.

After one particularly explosive outburst on a Friday night, he came to my office Monday remarking that he had had a song in his head all weekend that he still could not get out. The song was "Reelin' in the Years," by Steely Dan, from the album "Can't Buy a Thrill." He remembered only some of the words:

> You wouldn't know a diamond
> If you held it in your hand
> The things you think are precious
> I can't understand ...
>
> Are you gathering up the tears
> Have you had enough of mine ...
>
> The things that pass for knowledge
> I can't understand

The therapeutic use of the known early history in such a case as this is determined by the features of the age period that seem most salient. And that is determined by what developmental theory is embraced.

268

Certain of this patient's problems—those in the area of security, fear of abandonment, wish for a patron, and inhibition of initiative— are readily accountable in the terminology of attachment theory or separation/individuation theory as patterns transformed across development. The comings and goings to and from mother during the twelve- to thirty-month age period make up a part of Mahler's practicing subphase of separation/individuation. They also exemplify the activation and deactivation of the attachment aim. For Mahler, the infant comes back to "refuel," or to get something that permits the infant to go back out and re-explore. What is the "something"? Mahler is not always clear, because the term "refueling" invites confusion with energic issues. But the metaphor implies a kind of ego infusion (via merging) that permits the infant to separate and explore again. For attachment theorists, these comings and goings help the infant to build up an internal working model of the mother that acts as a secure base to leave from and return to. In the terms used here, these are interactions with a self-regulating other that become generalized, represented, and activated. It is not difficult to imagine how a maternal depression could have an impact on these behavioral patterns and their representations. It remains to be traced how these early patterns survived the transformations of development, to present in the particular and not unrecognizable form that they assumed when this patient was thirty-four.

Mahler describes the appearance, around the middle of the second year, of a certain kind of seriousness, soberness, or deliberateness. A change in the infant's emotional and attitudinal aura occurs, away from the more carefree "world is my oyster" feeling previously given off. Mahler and her colleagues (Mahler, Pine, and Bergman 1975) have called this the "rapprochement crisis" that ushers in the "rapprochement subphase" of separation/individuation. They speculate that at this point infants have finally achieved enough separation/ individuation from mother to realize that they are not in fact all-powerful, that they are still dependent. This realization brings about the emotional-attitudinal change and a partial, temporary resetting of the attachment balance toward more attachment than exploration. Infants partially lose their omnipotence.

The impact of the mother's depression on the son's "rapprochement crisis" is not precisely predictable. On the one hand, one could imagine that his omnipotence lasted longer but on a less secure base.

On the other hand, one could postulate that he had less opportunity to develop an appropriate sense of omnipotence and had to give it up earlier. In any event, it is not clear how this early patterning was transformed over the next thirty-two years. Whatever the reason, his belief in his own powers at age thirty-four was slightly impaired.

So far, attachment or separation/individuation theory, or the notions of a self-regulating other and its representation provide plausible bridges between the early insult and current behavior. These occur mainly in the domain of the sense of a core self with a core other. However, they fall short of explaining the other two features of the current clinical picture, namely, the sense and pain of not being understood and the particular form of the patient's outbursts of rage. A consideration of the domain of intersubjective relatedness is needed.

At the same time that the practicing subphase of separation/individuation and attachment behaviors and the overt use of a self-regulating other are much in evidence, the sense of a subjective self and the domain of intersubjective relatedness also begin to form. These cast a different light on the comings and goings that occur during this first half of the second year. When the infant returns to mother, it is not only to be "refueled" or to deactivate the attachment system. It is a reaffirmation that the infant and mother (as separate entities) are sharing in what the infant experiences. For instance, an infant experiencing fear after wandering too far needs to know that his or her state of fear has been heard. It is more than a need to be held or soothed; it is also an intersubjective need to be understood. On a more positive note, the infant may look at mother while returning to her after playing with a box, as if to say, "Do you also experience, as I do, that this box is surprising and wonderful?" The mother somehow indicates "Yes, I do," usually through attunements, and off and away the infant goes. Or the infant's returns to mother may be in the service of confirming that the reality and/or fantasy of intersubjectivity is being actively maintained ("Touching this castle of blocks is still scary-wonderful, isn't it, Mom?"). The creation of intersubjective sharing permits the exploration and pursuit of curiosity. Even the level of the infant's fear or distress in the situation is partially negotiated by social referencing signals that occur in the domain of intersubjectivity, since they use the mother's feeling state as a tuner of the infant's. ("Is the block castle more scary than wonderful, or the other way around?")

What appears to happen in the early locomotor behavior of the toddler is this. When the infant has wandered much too far away, has been hurt, has been scared by something unexpected, or has become tired, the experience of returning to mother is almost solely at the level of core-relatedness. This is the attachment theory's description of what other analytic theories call regression or refueling. In less extreme conditions, we see a majority of returns to mother as having to do with subjective sharings—the re-establishment of the intersubjective state, which is not a given experience but which must be actively maintained. And much of the time, returnings to mother occur in both domains simultaneously. In fact, we often see infants who appear near the verge of fear make up or grab onto a handy experience for intersubjective testing and return to mother with a multiple agenda, a core agenda and an intersubjective one.

The returning of infants with multiple agendas is potentially of clinical importance, because some mothers find one agenda more acceptable than another. If a mother is less ready to soothe the fear, the infant will find a surprising number of intersubjective "excuses" to return. The use of intersubjective relatedness in the service of physical security is hardly unknown to us as clinicians and parents. The opposite also happens: some mothers are less available for intersubjective sharing but readily accept their physical capacity to calm fear. Once again the use of physical relatedness in the service of fantasied intersubjectivity is also well known to us as clinicians and parents.

To return to the question of how the mother's depressed behavior during these events might have had an impact later in life, it is not surprising that this man had a very keen sense of not being understood. He experienced a painful rupture in intersubjective relatedness when his wife would not or could not enter into and share his subjective experience, so far as that is possible. It is likely that a heightened sensitivity to this form of interpersonal disjunction was established during the period when he was one to two-and-one-half years old. It is very likely that because of her depressive "preoccupations" his mother was relatively less available for inter-subjective relatedness than for serving physically as a secure base of operations. The patient's painful feeling of not being understood seems to be most plausible and productively viewed in terms of intersubjective relatedness.

What then about the patient's particular form of enraged outbursts? During the period from eighteen to thirty months of age, the patient was in the formative phase of verbal relatedness. The advent of verbal relatedness permits the infant to begin to integrate experiences in the different domains of relatedness. For instance, the infant can now say the verbal equivalent of such core experiences as "I don't want to look at you," "I don't want you to look at me," and "I don't want to be near you." (Negativity begins around now.) The infant can also say the verbal equivalent of such intersubjective experiences as "Stay out of my excitement with this toy," and "I don't want to share my pleasure." The verbal equivalent may initially be something as impoverished as "NO!" or, some months later, "GO AWAY" or, even later, "I HATE YOU." The words are an attempt to tie together the infant's experiences in several domains. The verbal act of saying "NO!" is a statement of autonomy, separateness, and independence (Spitz 1957). At the same time it also refers to raw physical acts in the domain of core-relatedness, such as "I won't look at you," although the closest words the infant has to represent that personal knowledge residing in the core domain are "NO" or "GO AWAY."

This state of affairs both integrates and fractures experience and leads the infant into a crisis of self-comprehension. The self becomes a mystery. The infant is aware that there are levels and layers of self-experience that are to some extent estranged from the official experiences ratified by language. The previous harmony is broken.

I suggest that this crisis in self-comprehension is in large part responsible for the soberness seen at this period. This shift is a nonspecific consequence of a general crisis in self-comprehension and self-experience, brought about by the attempt (bound to partial failure) at the verbal representation of experience. It affects all life issues, with as many consequences for intimacy, trust, attachment, dependency, mastery, and so on as it has for separation or individuation.

This crisis in self-comprehension occurs because for the first time the infant experiences the self as divided, and rightly senses that no one else can rebind the division. The infant has not lost omnipotence but rather has lost experiential wholeness.

This version of what is going on is very different from Mahler's. It makes more comprehensible, however, the patient's outbursts at his wife when she insists on putting his subjective experiences into words. To him, his experiences somehow do not fit into her words. He is left confused, helpless, and infuriated. This is a current version of the crisis in infancy, when the need to verbalize preverbal experience results in fracturing. Parents are greatly needed for that buffering effect, and it is likely the patient's mother in her depression was not well disposed to help make this transition easier.

In sum, the greatest clinical value of the views put forth here lies in their suggesting search strategies to aid in the construction of therapeutically effective life narratives. The system presented urges a flexibility in theories about the developmental origin of pathology. It does so by offering some alternative explanations for well-known events, thus presenting a wider range of possibilities, and by emphasizing a developmental view that focuses on search strategies rather than answers about the timing of clinical origins.

Implications of Viewing the Different Senses of Self as the Subject Matter of Age-Specific Sensitive Periods

Each sense of the self has been allotted a formative phase when it first comes into existence—birth to two months for the sense of an emergent self, two to six months for the sense of a core self, seven to fifteen months for the sense of an intersubjective self, and eighteen to thirty months for the verbal sense of self. These formative phases can fruitfully be considered "sensitive periods" for the four senses of self, for reasons argued in chapter 9.

In the case of the lawyer cited earlier in this chapter, one would predict on theoretical grounds that there was, indeed, a predisposition for her problem, but that it occurred around the age of two to six months in the domain of a sense of a core self, especially agency, and not around age one to two-and-a-half years over the issues of autonomy and control. The battle is about the sense of core self-experience. The prize is self-agency; autonomy and control are only the local battlefields. The use of this clinical prediction is of limited value in a reconstruction, however, for the following reason. Even though the different domains of self-experience have replaced the traditional clinical-developmental issues as the subject matter for sensitive periods, they are less vulnerable to irreversible initial impresses, because all the domains of sense of self are viewed as active and still forming throughout life. They are not seen as the relics of past and finished developmental phases, as were the traditional clinical-developmental issues. The system stays more open to pathogenic insult, chronic or acute. Therefore, even in considering clinical problems in the different domains of self-experience, there are potentially many possible actual points of pathogenesis beyond the sensitive period. Again, the theory is less prescriptive with regard to actual points of pathological origin.

Nonetheless, this viewpoint does predict that environmental influences at formative periods of the different senses of self will result in relatively more pathology, or less easily reversible pathology, than later insults. In chapter 9 we discussed several of the more obvious predictions. In general, during the sensitive periods of formation answers to several questions about features of self-experience are being partially determined: What is the range of stimulations and events that will be subjectively perceived as self-experience? Which will be experienced as tolerable or disorganizing? What affective tones will be attached to all self-experiences in the different domains? How much actual interaction with self-regulating others is needed to maintain an undisturbed sense of self? Which self-experiences can be shared or communicated with ease and which with unease and foreboding? It is clear that a predictive working theory about these continuities would have considerable value in formulating the ontogeny of states of self pathology. It would also have much value within a traditional psychoanalytic approach, even if it were used only as a way of viewing and working with pre-Oedipal material and origins.

Epilogue

THE CENTRAL AIM of this book has been to describe the development of the infant's sense of self. I have tried to infer the infant's likely subjective experiences by considering the newly available experimental findings about infants in conjunction with clinical phenomena derived from practice. In this sense, it is a step towards a synthesis of the infant as observed and as clinically reconstructed, in the form of a working theory of the development of domains of self-experience.

The value of this working theory remains to be proved, and even its status as a hypothesis remains to be explored. Is it to be taken as a scientific hypothesis that can be evaluated by its confirming or invalidating current propositions, and by spawning studies that lead elsewhere? Or is it to be taken as a clinical metaphor to be used in practice, in which case the therapeutic efficacy of the metaphor can be determined?

It is my hope that it will prove to be both. As a hypothesis, this view calls attention to a variety of areas in which more experimentation is needed—in particular, studies on episodic memory and the role of affect in organizing experience, descriptive and theoretical efforts at providing a taxonomy of preverbal experience, and especially, renewed efforts to develop descriptive means to identify and trace interactive patterns across their developmental transformations. Also needed are prospective studies that test its hypothesis that age-specific insults will predict later pathology in specific domains of self-experience but will fail to predict pathology in specific traditional clinical-developmental issues. The scope of the field of inquiry that future experimentalists will find provocative, attractive, and challenging has, I hope, been expanded.

The view presented here is also intended to serve as a metaphor for clinical practice. It is likely that the clinical implications of this metaphor will come about slowly and indirectly. I suspect that the greatest force for change will happen through changing our view of who infants are, how they are related to others, what their subjective social experiences are likely to be, especially their sense of self, and how we search for past experience relevant for the creation of therapeutic narratives. Such a change filters its way through the thinking of therapists as they actively work with patients. As the picture of the reconstructed past of a patient's life becomes altered, the therapist finds it necessary to think and act differently. The constructs proposed in the last section of this book are intended to facilitate that process. Such a process of change takes many "generations" of patients. Exactly how this filtering and transforming process will translate into different techniques and theories of therapeutics is unpredictable. I have suggested some beginnings.

The second route for change is even more indirect and unpredictable, but perhaps the most potent. Besides being therapists or experimentalists, we are also parents, grandparents, and disseminators of information. The findings we relate and the theories we devise are ultimately information for new parents. Whether we intend it or not, the general educational nature of the work is inescapable. The process has already begun and is accelerating to alter the general view of the infant held by most people. Once parents see a different infant, that infant starts to become transformed by their new "sight" and ultimately becomes a different adult. Much of the book has described how such transformations between persons occur. Evolution as it is daily encountered in the guise of "human nature" acts as a conservative force in these matters, so that changing our general views of who infants are can change who they will become only to a certain degree. But it is exactly that degree of change that is at issue here. If seeing the infant as different begins to make the children, adolescents, and adults different enough a generation later, then we will be seeing different patients at that point—patients who will have experienced a somewhat different infancy and whose interpersonal worlds have developed slightly differently. The therapeutic encounter with this new patient will again require changes in clinical theory and search strategies.

Just as infants must develop, so must our theories about what they experience and who they are.

BIBLIOGRAPHY

Adler, G., and Buie, D. H. (1979). Aloneness and borderline psychopathology: The possible relevance of child developmental issues. *International Journal of Psychoanalysis, 60,* 83–96.

Ainsworth, M. D. S. (1969). Object relations, dependency and attachment: A theoretical review of the infant-mother relationship. *Child Development, 40,* 969–1026.

Ainsworth, M. D. S. (1979). Attachment as related to mother-infant interaction. In J. B. Rosenblatt, R. H. Hinde, C. Beer, and M. Bushell (Eds.), *Advances in the study of behavior* (pp. 1–51). New York: Academic Press.

Ainsworth, M. D. S., and Wittig, B. (1969). Attachment and exploratory behavior in one-year-olds in a stranger situation. In B. M. Foss (Ed.), *Determinants of infant behavior.* New York: Wiley.

Ainsworth, M. D. S., Blehar, M. C., Waters, E., and Wall, S. (1978). *Patterns of attachment.* Hillsdale, N.J.: Erlbaum.

Allen, T. W., Walker, K., Symonds, L., and Marcell, M. (1977). Intrasensory and intersensory perception of temporal sequences during infancy. *Developmental Psychology, 13,* 225–29.

Amsterdam, B. K. (1972). Mirror self-image reactions before age two. *Developmental Psychology, 5,* 297–305.

Arnold, M. G. (1970). *Feelings and emotions, the Loyola symposium.* New York: Academic Press.

Austin, J. (1962). *How to do things with words.* New York: Oxford University Press.

Baldwin, J. M. (1902). *Social and ethical interpretations in mental development.* New York: Macmillan.

Balint, M. (1937). Early developmental states of the ego primary object love. In M. Balint, *Primary love and psycho-analytic technique.* New York: Liveright.

Basch, M. F. (1983). Empathic understanding: A review of the concept and some theoretical considerations. *Journal of the American Psychoanalytic Association, 31*(1), 101–26.

Basch, M. F. (in press). The perception of reality and the disavowal of meaning. *Annals of Psychoanalysis, 11.*

Bates, E. (1976). *Language and context: The acquisition of pragmatics.* New York: Academic Press.

Bates, E. (1979). Intentions, conventions and symbols. In E. Bates (Ed.), *The emergence of symbols: Cognition and communication in infancy.* New York: Academic Press.

Bates, E., Benigni, L., Bretherton, I., Camaioni, L., and Volterra, V. (1979). Cognition and communication from nine to thirteen months: Correlational findings. In E. Bates (Ed.), *The emergence of symbols: Cognition and communication in infancy.* New York: Academic Press.

Bateson, G., Jackson, D., Haley, J., and Wakland, J. (1956). Toward a theory of schizophrenia. *Behavioral Science, 1,* 251–64.

Baudelaire, C. (1982). *Les fleurs du mal.* (R. Howard, Trans.). Boston: David R. Godine. (Original work published 1857)

Beebe, B. (1973). *Ontogeny of Positive Affect in the Third and Fourth Months of the Life of One Infant.* Doctoral dissertation, Columbia University, University Microfilms.

Beebe, B., and Gerstman, L. J. (1980). The "packaging" of maternal stimulation in relation to infant facial-visual engagement: A case study at four months. *Merrill-Palmer Quarterly, 26,* 321–39.

Beebe, B., and Kroner, J. (1985). Mother-infant facial mirroring. (In preparation)

Beebe, B., and Sloate, P. (1982). Assessment and treatment of difficulties in mother-infant attunement in the first three years of life: A case history. *Psychoanalytic Inquiry, 1*(4), 601–23.

Beebe, B., and Stern, D. N. (1977). Engagement-disengagement and early object experiences. In M. Freedman and S. Grand (Eds.), *Communicative structures and psychic structures.* New York: Plenum Press.

Bell, S. M. (1970). The development of the concept of object as related to infant-mother attachment. *Child Development, 41,* 291–313.

Benjamin, J. D. (1965). Developmental biology and psychoanalysis. In N. Greenfield and W. Lewis (Eds.), *Psychoanalysis and current biological thought.* Madison: University of Wisconsin Press.

Bennett, S. (1971). Infant-caretaker interactions. *Journal of the American Academy of Child Psychiatry, 10,* 321–35.

Berlyne, D. E. (1966). Curiosity and exploration. *Science, 153,* 25–33.

Bloom, L. (1973). *One word at a time: The use of single word utterances before syntax.* Hawthorne, N.Y.: Mouton.

Bloom, L. (1983). Of continuity and discontinuity, and the magic of language development. In R. Gollinkoff (Ed.), *The transition from pre-linguistic to linguistic communication.* Hillsdale, N.J.: Erlbaum.

Bower, G. (1981). Mood and memory. *American Psychologist, 36,* 129–48.

Bower, T. G. R. (1972). Object perception in the infant. *Perception, 1,* 15–30.

Bower, T. G. R. (1974). *Development in infancy.* San Francisco, Calif.: Freeman.

Bower, T. G. R. (1976). *The perceptual world of the child.* Cambridge, Mass.: Harvard University Press.

Bower, T. G. R. (1978). The infant's discovery of objects and mother. In E. Thoman (Ed.) *Origins of the infant's social responsiveness.* Hillsdale, N.J.: Erlbaum.

Bower, T. G. R., Broughton, J. M., and Moore, M. K. (1970). Demonstration of intention in the reaching behavior of neonate humans. *Nature, 228,* 679–80.

Bowlby, J. (1958). The nature of the child's tie to his mother. *International Journal of Psychoanalysis, 39,* 350–73.

Bowlby, J. (1960). Separation anxiety. *International Journal of Psychoanalysis, 41,* 89–113.

Bowlby, J. (1969). *Attachment and loss: Vol. 1. Attachment.* New York: Basic Books.

Bowlby, J. (1973). *Attachment and loss: Vol. 2. Separation: Anxiety and anger.* New York: Basic Books.

Bowlby, J. (1980). *Attachment and loss: Vol. 3. Loss: Sadness and depression.* New York: Basic Books.

Brazelton, T. B. (1980, May). *New knowledge about the infant from current research: Implications for psychoanalysis.* Paper presented at the American Psychoanalytic Association meeting, San Francisco, Calif.

Brazelton, T. B. (1982). Joint regulation of neonate-parent behavior. In E. Tronick (Ed.), *Social interchange in infancy.* Baltimore, Md.: University Park Press.

Brazelton, T. B., Koslowski, B., and Main, M. (1974). The origins of reciprocity: The early mother-infant interaction. In M. Lewis and L. A. Rosenblum (Eds.), *The effects of the infant on its caregiver.* New York: Wiley.

Brazelton, T. B., Yogman, M., Als, H., and Tronick, E. (1979). The infant as a focus for family reciprocity. In M. Lewis and L. A. Rosenblum (Eds.), *The child and its family.* New York: Plenum Press.

Bretherton, I. (in press). Attachment theory: Retrospect and prospect. In I. Bretherton and E. Waters (Eds.), *Monographs of the Society for Research in Child Development.*

Bretherton, I., and Bates, E. (1979). The emergence of intentional communication. In I. Uzgiris (Ed.), *New directions for child development, Vol. 4.* San Francisco, Calif.: Jossey-Bass.

Bretherton, I., McNew, S., and Beeghly-Smith, M. (1981). Early person knowledge as expressed in gestural and verbal communication: When do infants acquire a "theory of mind"? In M. E. Lamb and L. R. Sherrod (Eds.), *Infant social cognition.* Hillsdale, N.J.: Erlbaum.

Bretherton, I., and Waters, E. (in press). Growing points of attachment theory and research. *Monographs of the Society for Research in Child Development.*

Bronson, G. (1982). *Monographs on infancy: Vol. 2. The scanning patterns of human infants: implications for visual learning.* Norwood, N.J.: Ablex.

Brown, R. (1973). *A first language: The early stages.* Cambridge, Mass.: Harvard University Press.

Bruner, J. S. (1969). Modalities of memory. In G. Talland and N. Waugh (Eds.), *The pathology of memory.* New York: Academic Press.

Bruner, J. S. (1975). The ontogenesis of speech acts. *Journal of Child Language, 2,* 1–19.

Bruner, J. S. (1977). Early social interaction and language acquisition. In H. R. Schaffer (Ed.), *Studies in mother-infant interaction.* London: Academic Press.

Bruner, J. S. (1981). The social context of language acquisition. *Language and Communication, 1,* 155–78.

Bruner, J. S. (1983). *Child's talk: Learning to use language.* New York: Norton.

Burd, A. P., and Milewski, A. E. (1981, April). *Matching of facial gestures by young infants: Imitation or releasers?* Paper presented at the Meeting of the Society for Research in Child Development, Boston, Mass.

Butterworth, G., and Castello, M. (1976). Coordination of auditory and visual space in newborn human infants. *Perception, 5,* 155–60.

Call, J. D. (1980). Some prelinguistic aspects of language development. *Journal of American Psychoanalytic Association, 28,* 259–90.

Call, J. D., and Marschak, M. (1976). Styles and games in infancy. In E. Rexford, L. Sander, and A. Shapiro (Eds.), *Infant Psychiatry* (pp. 104–12). New Haven, Conn.: Yale University Press.

Call, J. D., Galenson, E., and Tyson, R. L. (Eds.). (1983). *Frontiers of infant psychiatry, Vol. 1.* New York: Basic Books.

Campos, J., and Stenberg, C. (1980). Perception of appraisal and emotion: The onset of social referencing. In M. E. Lamb and L. Sherrod (Eds.), *Infant social cognition.* Hillsdale, N.J.: Erlbaum.

Caron, A. J., and Caron, R. F. (1981). Processing of relational information as an index of infant risk. In S. L. Friedman and M. Sigman (Eds.), *Preterm birth and psychological development.* New York: Academic Press.

Cassirer, E. (1955). *The philosophy of symbolic forms of language, Vol. 1.* New Haven, Conn.: Yale University Press.

Cavell, M. (in press). *The self and separate minds.* New York: New York University Press.

Cicchetti, D., and Schneider-Rosen, K. (in press). An organizational approach to childhood depression. In M. Rutter, C. Izard, and P. Read (Eds.), *Depression in children: Developmental perspectives.* New York: Guilford.

Cicchetti, D., and Sroufe, L. A. (1978). An organizational view of affect: Illustration from the study of Down's syndrome infants. In M. Lewis and L. Rosenblum (Eds.), *The development of affect.* New York: Plenum Press.

Clarke-Stewart, K. A. (1973). Interactions between mothers and their young children: Characteristics and consequences. *Monographs of the Society of Research in Child Development, 37*(153).

Cohen, L. B., and Salapatek, P. (1975). *Infant perception: From sensation to cognition: Vol. 2. Perception of space, speech, and sound.* New York: Academic Press.

Collis, G. M., and Schaffer, H. R. (1975). Synchronization of visual attention in mother-infant pairs. *Journal of Child Psychiatry, 16,* 315–20.

Condon, W. S., and Ogston, W. D. (1967). A segmentation of behavior. *Journal of Psychiatric Research, 5,* 221–35.

Condon, W. S., and Sander, L. S. (1974). Neonate movement is synchronized with adult speech. *Science, 183,* 99–101.

Cooley, C. H. (1912). *Human nature and the social order.* New York: Scribner.

Cooper, A. M. (1980). *The place of self psychology in the history of depth psychology.* Paper presented at the Symposium on Reflections on Self Psychology, Boston Psychoanalytic Society and Institute, Boston, Mass.

Cramer, B. (1982a). Interaction réele, interaction fantasmatique: Réflections au sujet des thérapies et des observations de nourrissons. *Psychothérapies,* No. 1.

Cramer, B. (1982b). La psychiatrie du bébé. In R. Kreisler, M. Schappi, and M. Soule (Eds.). *La dynamique du nourrisson.* Paris: Editions E.S.F.

Cramer, B. (1984, September). *Modèles psychoanalytiques, modèles interactifs: Recoupment possible?* Paper presented at the International Symposium "Psychiatry-Psychoanalysis," Montreal, Canada.

Dahl, H., and Stengel, B. (1978). A classification of emotion words: A modification and partial test of De Rivera's decision theory of emotions. *Psychoanalysis and Contemporary Thought,* 1(2), 269–312.

Darwin, C. (1965). *The expression of the emotions in man and animals.* Chicago: University of Chicago Press. (Original work published 1872)

DeCasper, A. J. (1980, April). *Neonates perceive time just like adults.* Paper presented at the International Conference on Infancy Studies, New Haven, Conn.

DeCasper, A. J., and Fifer, W. P. (1980). Of human bonding: Newborns prefer their mothers' voices. *Science, 208,* 1174–76.

Defoe, D. (1964). *Moll Flanders.* New York: Signet Classics. (Original work published 1723)

Demany, L., McKenzie, B., and Vurpillot, E. (1977). Rhythm perception in early infancy. *Nature, 266,* 718–19.

Demos, V. (1980). Discussion of papers delivered by Drs. Sander and Stern. Presented at the Boston Symposium on the Psychology of the Self, Boston, Mass.

Demos, V. (1982a). Affect in early infancy: Physiology or psychology. *Psychoanalytic Inquiry,* 1, 533–74.

Demos, V. (1982b). The role of affect in early childhood. In E. Troneck (Ed.), *Social interchange in infancy.* Baltimore, Md.: University Park Press.

Demos, V. (1984). Empathy and affect: Reflections on infant experience. In J. Lichtenberg, M. Bernstein, and D. Silver (Eds.), *Empathy.* Hillsdale, N.J.: Erlbaum.

DeVore, I., and Konnor, M. J. (1974). Infancy in hunter-gatherer life: An ethological perspective. In N. White (Ed.), *Ethology and psychiatry.* Toronto: University of Toronto Press.

Dodd, B. (1979). Lip reading in infants: Attention to speech presented in- and out- of synchrony. *Cognitive Psychology, 11,* 478–84.

Donee, L. H. (1973, March). *Infants' development scanning patterns of face and non-face stimuli under various auditory conditions.* Paper presented at the Meeting of the Society for Research in Child Development, Philadelphia, Pa.

Dore, J. (1975). Holophrases, speech acts and language universals. *Journal of Child Language,* 2, 21–40.

Dore, J. (1979). Conversational acts and the acquisition of language. In E. Ochs and B. Schieffelin (Eds.), *Developmental pragmatics.* New York: Academic Press.

Dore, J. (1985). Holophases revisited, dialogically. In M. Barrett (Ed.), *Children's single word speech.* London: Wiley.

Dunn, J. (1982). Comment: Problems and promises in the study of affect and intention. In E. Tronick (Ed.), *Social interchange in infancy.* Baltimore, Md.: University Park Press.

Dunn, J., and Kendrick, C. (1979). Interaction between young siblings in the context of family relationships. In M. Lewis and L. Rosenblum (Eds.), *The child and its family: The genesis of behavior, Vol. 2.* New York: Plenum Press.

Dunn, J., and Kendrick, C. (1982). *Siblings: Love, envy and understanding.* Cambridge: Harvard University Press.

Easterbrook, M. A., and Lamb, M. E. (1979). The relationship between quality of infant-mother attachment and infant competence in initial encounters with peers. *Child Development,* 50, 380–87.

Eimas, P. D., Siqueland, E. R., Jusczyk, P., and Vigorito, J. (1971). Speech perception in infants, *Science, 171,* 303–306.

Eimas, P. D., Siqueland, E. R., Jusczyk, P., and Vigorito, J. (1978). Speech perception in infants. In L. Bloom (Ed.), *Readings in language development.* New York: Wiley.

Eisenstein, S. (1957). *Film form and the film sense.* (J. Leyda, Trans.). New York: Meridian Books.

Ekman, P. (1971). Universals and cultural differences in facial expressions of emotion. In J. K. Cole (Ed.), *Nebraska symposium on motivation, Vol. 19.* Lincoln: University of Nebraska Press.

Ekman, P., Levenson, R. W., Friesen, W. V. (1983). Autonomic nervous system activity distinguishes among emotions. *Science, 221,* 1208–10.

Emde, R. N. (1980a). Levels of meaning for infant emotions: A biosocial view. In W. A. Collins (Ed.), *Development of cognition, affect, and social relations.* Hillsdale, N.J.: Erlbaum.

Emde, R. N. (1980b). Toward a psychoanalytic theory of affect. In S. I. Greenspan and G. H. Pollock (Eds.), *Infancy and early childhood. The course of life: Psychoanalytic contributions towards understanding personality development, Vol. I.* Washington, D.C.: National Institute of Mental Health.

Emde, R. N. (1983, March). *The affective core.* Paper presented at the Second World Congress of Infant Psychiatry, Cannes, France.

Emde, R. N., Gaensbauer, T., and Harmon, R. (1976). Emotional expression in infancy: A biobehavioral study. *Psychological Issues Monograph Series, 10*(1), No. 37.

Emde, R. N., Klingman, D. H., Reich, J. H., and Wade, J. D. (1978). Emotional expression in infancy: I. Initial studies of social signaling and an emergent model. In M. Lewis and L. Rosenblum, (Eds.), *The development of affect.* New York: Plenum Press.

Emde, R. N., and Sorce, J. E. (1983). The rewards of infancy: Emotional availability and maternal referencing. In J. D. Call, E. Galenson, and R. Tyson (Eds.), *Frontiers of infant psychiatry, Vol. 2.* New York: Basic Books.

Erikson, E. H. (1950). *Childhood and society.* New York: Norton.

Escalona, S. K. (1953). Emotional development in the first year of life. In M. Senn (Ed.), *Problems of infancy and childhood.* Packawack Lake, N.J.: Foundation Press.

Escalona, S. K. (1968). *The roots of individuality.* Chicago: Aldine.

Esman, A. H. (1983). The "stimulus barrier": A review and reconsideration. In A. Solnit and R. Eissler (Eds.), *The psychoanalytic study of the child, Vol. 38* (pp. 193–207). New Haven, Conn.: Yale University Press.

Fagan, J. F. (1973). Infants' delayed recognition memory and forgetting. *Journal of Experimental Child Psychology, 16,* 424–50.

Fagan, J. F. (1976). Infants' recognition of invariant features of faces. *Child Development, 47,* 627–38.

Fagan, J. F. (1977). Infant's recognition of invariant features of faces. *Child Development, 48,* 68–78.

Fagan, J. F., and Singer, L. T. (1983). Infant recognition memory as a measure of intelligence. In L. P. Lipsitt and C. K. Rovee-Collier (Eds.), *Advances in infancy research, Vol. 2.* Norwood, N.J.: Ablex.

Fairbairn, W. R. D. (1954). *An object relations theory of the personality.* New York: Basic Books.

Fantz, R. (1963). Pattern vision in newborn infants. *Science, 140,* 296–97.

Ferguson, C. A. (1964). Baby talk in six languages. In J. Gumperz and D. Hymes (Eds.), *The Ethnography of Communication, 66,* 103–14.

Fernald, A. (1982). *Acoustic determinants of infant preferences for "motherese."* Unpublished doctoral dissertation, University of Oregon.

Fernald, A. (1984). The perceptual and affective salience of mother's speech to infants. In L. Fagans, C. Garvey, and R. Golinkoff (Eds.), *The origin and growth of communication.* Norwood, N.J.: Ablex.

Fernald, A., and Mazzie, C. (1983, April). *Pitch-marking of new and old information in mother's speech.* Paper presented at the Meeting of the Society for Research in Child Development, Detroit, Mich.

Field, T. M. (1977). Effects of early separation, interactive deficits and experimental manipulations on mother-infant face-to-face interaction. *Child Development, 48,* 763–71.

Field, T. M. (1978). The three R's of infant-adult interactions: Rhythms, repertoires and responsivity. *Journal of Pediatric Psychology, 3,* 131–36.

Field, T. M. (in press). Attachment as psychological attunement: Being on the same wavelength. In M. Reite and T. Field (Eds.), *The psychobiology of attachment.* New York: Academic Press.

Field, T. M., and Fox, N. (Eds.). (in press). *Social perception in infants.* Norwood, N.J.: Ablex.

Field, T. M., Woodson, R., Greenberg, R., and Cohen, D. (1982). Discrimination and imitation of facial expressions by neonates. *Science, 218,* 179–81.

Fogel, A. (1982). Affect dynamics in early infancy: Affective tolerance. In T. Field and A. Fogel (Eds.), *Emotions and interaction: Normal and high-risk infants.* Hillsdale, N.J.: Erlbaum.

Fogel, A. (1977). Temporal organization in mother-infant face-to-face interaction. In H. R. Schaffer (Ed.), *Studies in mother-infant interaction.* New York: Academic Press.

Fogel, A., Diamond, G. R., Langhorst, B. H., and Demas, V. (1981). Affective and cognitive aspects of the two-month-old's participation in face-to-face interaction with its mother. In E. Tronick (Ed.), *Joint regulation of behavior.* Cambridge, England: Cambridge University Press.

Fraiberg, S. H. (1969). Libidinal constancy and mental representation. In R. Eissler et al. (Eds.), *The psychoanalytic study of the child, Vol. 24* (pp. 9–47). New York: International Universities Press.

Fraiberg, S. H. (1971). Smiling and strange reactions in blind infants. In J. Hellmuth (Ed.), *Studies in abnormalities: Vol. 2. Exceptional infant* (pp. 110–27). New York: Brunner/Mazel.

Fraiberg, S. H. (1980). *Clinical studies in infant mental health: The first year of life.* New York: Basic Books.

Fraiberg, S. H., Adelson, E., and Shapiro, V. (1975). Ghosts in the nursery: A psychoanalytic approach to the problem of impaired infant-mother relationships. *Journal of American Academy of Child Psychiatry, 14,* 387–422.

Francis, P. L., Self, P. A., and Noble, C. A. (1981, March). *Imitation within the context of mother-newborn interaction.* Paper presented at the Annual Eastern Psychological Association, New York.

Freedman, D. (1964). Smiling in blind infants and the issue of innate vs. acquired. *Journal of Child Psychology and Psychiatry, 5,* 171–84.

Freud, A. (1966). *Writings of Anna Freud: Vol. 6. Normality and pathology in childhood: Assessments in development.* New York: International Universities Press.

Freud, S. (1955). *The interpretation of dreams,* (J. Strachey, Ed.). New York: Basic Books. (Original work published in 1900)

Freud, S. (1962). *Three essays on the theory of sexuality.* New York: Basic Books. (Original work published in 1905)

Freud, S. (1957). Repression. In *The standard edition of the complete psychological works of Sigmund Freud,* Vol. 14. (143–58). London: Hogarth Press. (Original work published in 1915)

Freud, S. (1959). Mourning and melancholia. In *Collected papers,* Vol. 4 (pp. 152–170). New York: Basic Books. (Original work published in 1917)

Freud, S. (1955). Beyond the pleasure principle. In *The standard edition of the complete psychological works of Sigmund Freud,* Vol. 18 (pp. 4–67). London: Hogarth Press. (Original work published in 1920)

Friedlander, B. Z. (1970). Receptive language development in infancy. *Merrill-Palmer Quarterly, 16,* 7–51.

Friedman, L. (1980). Barren prospect of a representational world. *Psychoanalytic Quarterly, 49,* 215–33.

Friedman, L. (1982). *The interplay of evocation.* Paper presented at the Postgraduate Center for Mental Health, New York.

Galenson, E., and Roiphe, H. (1974). The emergence of genital awareness during the second year of life. In R. Friedman, R. Richart, and R. Vandeivides (Eds.), *Sex differences in behavior* (pp. 223–31). New York: Wiley.

Garfinkel, H. (1967). *Studies in ethnomethodology.* Englewood Cliffs, N.J.: Prentice-Hall.

Garmenzy, N., and Rutter, M. (1983). *Stress, coping and development in children.* New York: McGraw Hill.

Gautier, Y. (1984, September). *De la psychoanalyse et la psychiatrie du nourrisson: Un long et difficile cheminement.* Paper presented at the International Symposium "Psychiatry-Psychoanalysis," Montreal, Canada.

Gediman, H. K. (1971). The concept of stimulus barrier. *International Journal of Psychoanalysis, 52,* 243–57.

Ghosh, R. K. (1979). *Aesthetic theory and art: A study in Susanne K. Langer* (p. 29). Delhi, India: Ajanta Publications.

Gibson, E. J. (1969). *Principles of perceptual learning and development.* New York: Appleton-Century-Crofts.

Gibson, E. J., Owsley, C., and Johnston, J. (1978). Perception of invariants by five-month-old infants: Differentiation of two types of motion. *Developmental Psychology, 14,* 407–15.

Gibson, J. J. (1950). *The perception of the visual world.* Boston: Houghton Mifflin.

Gibson, J. J. (1979). *The ecological approach to visual perception.* Boston: Houghton Mifflin.

Glick, J. (1983, March). *Piaget, Vygotsky and Werner.* Paper presented at the Meeting of the Society for Research in Child Development, Detroit, Mich.

Glover, E. (1945). Examination of the Klein system of child psychology. In R. Eissler et al. (Eds.), *The psychoanalytic study of the child, Vol. 1* (pp. 75–118). New York: International Universities Press.

Goldberg, A. (Ed.). (1980). *Advances in self psychology.* New York: International Universities Press.

Golinkoff, R. (Ed.). (1983). *The transition from pre-linguistic to linguistic communication.* Hillsdale, N.J.: Erlbaum.

Greenfield, P., and Smith, J. H. (1976). *Language beyond syntax: The development of semantic structure.* New York: Academic Press.

Greenspan, S. I. (1981). *Clinical infant reports: No. 1. Psychopathology and adaptation in infancy in early childhood.* New York: International Universities Press.

Greenspan, S. I., and Lourie, R. (1981). Developmental and structuralist approaches to the classification of adaptive and personality organizations: Infancy and early childhood. *American Journal of Psychiatry, 138,* 725–35.

Grossmann, K., and Grossmann, K. E. (in press). Maternal sensitivity and newborn orientation responses as related to quality of attachment in northern Germany. In I. Bretherton and E. Waterns (Eds.), *Monographs of the Society for Research in Child Development.*

Gunther, M. (1961). Infant behavior at the breast. In B. M. Foss (Ed.), *Determinants of infant behavior, Vol. 2.* London: Methuen.

Guntrip, J. S. (1971). *Psychoanalytic theory, therapy, and the self.* New York: Basic Books.

Habermas, T. (1972). *Knowledge and human interests.* London: Heinemann.

Hainline, L. (1978). Developmental changes in visual scanning of face and non-face patterns by infants. *Journal of Exceptional Child Psychology, 25,* 90–115.

Haith, M. M. (1966). Response of the human newborn to visual movement. *Journal of Experimental Child Psychology, 3,* 235–43.

Haith, M. M. (1980). *Rules that babies look by.* Hillsdale, N.J.: Erlbaum.

Haith, M. M., Bergman, T., and Moore, M. J. (1977). Eye contact and face scanning in early infancy. *Science, 198,* 853–55.

Halliday, M. A. (1975). *Learning how to mean: Exploration in the development of language.* London: Edward Arnold.

Hamilton, V. (1982). *Narcissus and Oedipus: The children of psychoanalysis.* London: Rutledge and Kegan Paul.

Hamlyn, D. W. (1974). Person-perception and our understanding of others. In T. Mischel (Ed.), *Understanding other persons.* Oxford: Blackwell.

Harding, C. G. (1982). Development of the intention to communicate. *Human Development, 25,* 140–51.

Harding, C. G., and Golinkoff, R. (1979). The origins of intentional vocalizations in prelinguistic infants. *Child Development, 50,* 33–40.

Harper, R. C., Kenigsberg, K., Sia, G., Horn, D., Stern, D. N., and Bongiovi, V. (1980). Ziphophagus conjoined twins: A 300 year review of the obstetric, morphopathologic neonatal and surgical parameters. *American Journal of Obstetrics and Gynecology, 137,* 617–29.

Hartmann, H. (1958). *Ego psychology and the problem of adaption* (D. Rapaport, Trans.). New York: International Universities Press.

Hartmann, H., Kris, E., and Lowenstein, R. M. (1946). Comments on the formation of psychic structure. In *Psychological issues monographs: No. 14. Papers on psychoanalytic psychology* (pp. 27–55). New York: International Universities Press.

Herzog, J. (1980). Sleep disturbances and father hunger in 18- to 20-month-old boys: The Erlkoenig Syndrome. In A. Solnit et al. (Eds.), *The Psychoanalytic Study of the Child, Vol. 35* (pp. 219–36). New Haven, Conn.: Yale University Press.

Hinde, R. A. (1979). *Towards understanding relationships.* London: Academic Press.

Hinde, R. A. (1982). Attachment: Some conceptual and biological issues. In C. M. Parks and J. Stevenson-Hinde (Eds.), *The place of attachment in human behavior.* New York: Basic Books.

Hinde, R. A., and Bateson, P. (1984). Discontinuities versus continuities in behavioral development and the neglect of process. *International Journal of Behavioral Development, 7,* 129–43.

Hofer, M. A. (1980). *The roots of human behavior.* San Francisco, Calif.: Freedman.

Hofer, M. A. (1983, March). Relationships as regulators: A psychobiological perspective on development. Presented (as the Presidential Address) to the American Psychosomatic Society, New York.

Hoffman, M. L. (1977). Empathy, its development and pre-social implications. *Nebraska Symposium on Motivation, 25,* 169–217.

Hoffman, M. L. (1978). Toward a theory of empathic arousal and development. In M. Lewis and L. A. Rosenblum (Eds.), *The development of affect.* New York: Plenum Press.

Holquist, M. (1982). The politics of representation. In S. J. Greenblatt (Ed.), *Allegory and representation.* Baltimore, Md.: John Hopkins University Press.

Humphrey, K., Tees, R. C., and Werker, J. (1979). Auditory-visual integration of temporal relations in infants. *Canadian Journal of Psychology, 33,* 347–52.

Hutt, C., and Ounsted, C. (1966). The biological significance of gaze aversion with particular reference to the syndrome of infantile autism. *Behavioral Science, 11,* 346–56.

Izard, C. E. (1971). *The face of emotion.* New York: Appleton-Century-Crofts.

Izard, C. E. (1977). *Human emotions.* New York: Plenum Press.

Izard, C. E. (1978). On the ontogenesis of emotions and emotion-cognition relationship in infancy. In M. Lewis and L. A. Rosenblum (Eds.), *The development of affect.* New York: Plenum Press.

Kagan, J. (1981). *The second year of life: The emergence of self awareness.* Cambridge, Mass.: Harvard University Press.

Kagan, J. (1984). *The nature of the child.* New York: Basic Books.

Kagan, J., Kearsley, R. B., and Zelazo, P. R. (1978). *Infancy: Its place in human development.* Cambridge, Mass.: Harvard University Press.

Karmel, B. Z., Hoffman, R., and Fegy, M. (1974). Processing of contour information by human infants evidenced by pattern dependent evoked potentials. *Child Development, 45,* 39–48.

Kaye, K. (1979). Thickening thin data: The maternal role in developing communication and language. In M. Bullowa (Ed.), *Before speech.* Cambridge: Cambridge University Press.

Kaye, K. (1982). *The mental and social life of babies.* Chicago: University of Chicago Press.

Kernberg, O. F. (1968). The treatment of patients with borderline personality organization. *International Journal of Psychoanalysis, 49,* 600–19.

Kernberg, O. F. (1975). *Borderline conditions and pathological narcissism.* New York: Aronson.

Kernberg, O. F. (1976). *Object relations theory and clinical psychoanalysis.* New York: Aronson.

Kernberg, O. F. (1980). *Internal world and external reality: Object relations theory applied.* New York: Aronson.

Kernberg, O. F. (1984). *Severe personality disorders: Psychotherapeutic strategies.* New Haven, Conn.: Yale University Press.

Kessen, W., Haith, M. M., and Salapatek, P. (1970). Human infancy: A bibliography and guide. In P. Mussen (Ed.), *Carmichael's manual of child psychology.* New York: Wiley.

Kestenberg, J. S., and Sossin, K. M. (1979). *Movement patterns in development, Vol. 2.* New York: Dance Notation Bureau Press.

Klaus, M., and Kennell, J. (1976). *Maternal-infant bonding.* St. Louis: Mosey.

Klein, D. F. (1982). Anxiety reconceptualized. In D. F. Klein and J. Robkin (Eds.), *Anxiety: New research and current concepts.* New York: Raven Press.

Klein, Melanie (1952). *Developments in psycho-analysis.* (J. Rivere, Ed.). London: Hogarth Press.

Klein, Milton (1980). On Mahler's autistic and symbiotic phases. An exposition and evolution. *Psychoanalysis and Contemporary Thought, 4*(1), 69–105.

Klinnert, M. D. (1978). *Facial expression and social referencing.* Unpublished doctoral dissertation prospectus. Psychology Department, University of Denver.

Klinnert, M. D., Campos, J. J., Sorce, J. F., Emde, R. N., and Svejda, M. (1983). Emotions as behavior regulators: Social referencing in infancy. In R. Plutchik and H. Kellerman (Eds.), *Emotion: Theory, research and experience, Vol. 2.* New York: Academic Press.

Kohut, H. (1971). *The analysis of the self.* New York: International Universities Press.

Kohut, H. (1977). *The restoration of the self.* New York: International Universities Press.

Kohut, H. (1983). Selected problems of self psychological theory. In J. Lichtenberg and S. Kaplan (Eds.), *Reflections on self psychology.* Hillsdale, N.J.: Analytic Press.

Kohut, H. (in press). Introspection, empathy, and the semi-circle of mental health. *International Journal of Psychoanalysis.*

Kreisler, L., and Cramer, B. (1981). Sur les bases cliniques de la psychiatrie du nourrisson. *La Psychiatrie de l'Enfant, 24,* 1–15.

Kreisler, L., Fair, M., and Soulé, M. (1974). *L'enfant et son corps.* Paris: Presse Universitaires de France.

Kuhl, P., and Meltzoff, A. (1982). The bimodal perception of speech in infancy. *Science, 218,* 1138–41.

Labov, W., and Fanshel, D. (1977). *Therapeutic discourse.* New York: Academic Press.

Lacan, J. (1977). *Ecrits* (pp. 1–7). New York: Norton.

Lamb, M. E., and Sherrod, L. R. (Eds.). (1981). *Infant social cognition.* Hillsdale, N.J.: Erlbaum.

Langer, S. K. (1967). *MIND: An essay on human feeling, Vol. 1.* Baltimore, Md.: Johns Hopkins Universities Press.

Lashley, K. S. (1951). The problem of serial order in behavior. In L. A. Jeffres (Ed.), *Cerebral mechanisms in behavior.* New York: Wiley.

Lawson, K. R. (1980). Spatial and temporal congruity and auditory-visual integration in infants. *Developmental Psychology, 16,* 185–192.

Lebovici, S. (1983). *Le nourrisson, La mère et le psychoanalyste: Les interactions precoces.* Paris: Editions du Centurion.

Lee, B., and Noam, G. G. (1983). *Developmental approaches to the self.* New York: Plenum Press.

Lewcowicz, D. J. (in press). Bisensory response to temporal frequency in four-month-old infants. *Developmental Psychology.*

Lewcowicz, D. J., and Turkewitz, G. (1980). Cross-modal equivalence in early infancy: Audio-visual intensity matching. *Developmental Psychology, 16,* 597–607.

Lewcowicz, D. J., and Turkewitz, G. (1981). Intersensory interaction in newborns: Modification of visual preference following exposure to sound. *Child Development, 52,* 327–32.

Lewis, M., and Brooks-Gunn, J. (1979). *Social cognition and the acquisition of self.* New York: Plenum Press.

Lewis, M., and Rosenblum, L. A. (Eds.). (1974). *The origins of fear.* New York: Wiley.

Lewis, M., and Rosenblum, L. A. (1978). *The development of affect.* New York: Plenum Press.

286

Lewis, M., Feiring, L., McGoffog, L., and Jaskin, J. (In press). Predicting psychopathology in six-year-olds from early social relations. *Child Development.*

Lichtenberg, J. D. (1981). Implications for psychoanalytic theory of research on the neonate. *International Review of Psychoanalysis, 8,* 35–52.

Lichtenberg, J. D. (1983). *Psychoanalysis and infant research.* Hillsdale, N.J.: Analytic Press.

Lichtenberg, J. D., and Kaplan, S. (Eds.). (1983). *Reflections on self psychology.* Hillsdale, N.J.: Analytic Press.

Lichtenstein, H. (1961). Identity and sexuality: A study of their interpersonal relationships in man. *Journal of American Psychoanalytic Association, 9,* 179–260.

Lieberman, A. F. (1977). Preschoolers' competence with a peer: Relations with attachment and peer experience. *Child Development, 48,* 1277–87.

Lipps, T. (1906). Das wissen von fremden ichen. *Psychologische Untersuchung, 1,* 694–722.

Lipsitt, L. P. (1976). Developmental psychobiology comes of age. In L. P. Lipsitt (Ed.), *Developmental psychobiology: The significance of infancy.* Hillsdale, N.J.: Erlbaum.

Lipsitt, L. P. (Ed.). (1983). *Advances in infancy research, Vol. 2.* Norwood, N.J.: Ablex.

Lutz, C. (1982). The domain of emotion words on Ifaluk. *American Ethnologist, 9,* 113–28.

Lyons-Ruth, K. (1977). Bimodal perception in infancy: Response to audio-visual incongruity. *Child Development, 48,* 820–27.

MacFarlane, J. (1975). Olfaction in the development of social preferences in the human neonate. In M. Hofer (Ed.), *Parent-infant interaction.* Amsterdam: Elsevier.

MacKain, K., Stern, D. N., Goldfield, A., and Moeller, B. (1985). *The identification of correspondence between an infant's internal affective state and the facial display of that affect by an other.* Unpublished manuscript.

MacKain, K., Studdert-Kennedy, M., Spieker, S., and Stern, D. N. (1982, March). *Infant perception of auditory-visual relations for speech.* Paper presented at the International Conference of Infancy Studies, Austin, Tex.

MacKain, K., Studdert-Kennedy, M., Spieker, S., and Stern, D. N. (1983). Infant intermodal speech perception is a left-hemisphere function. *Science, 219,* 1347–49.

MacMurray, J. (1961). *Persons in relation.* London: Faber and Faber.

McCall, R. B. (1979). Qualitative transitions in behavioral development in the first three years of life. In M. H. Bornstein and W. Kessen (Ed.), *Psychological development from infancy.* Hillsdale, N.J.: Erlbaum.

McCall, R. B., Eichhorn, D., and Hogarty, P. (1977). Transitions in early mental development. *Monographs of the Society for Research in Child Development, 42*(1177).

McDevitt, J. B. (1979). The role of internalization in the development of object relations during the separation-individuation phase. *Journal of American Psychoanalytic Association, 27,* 327–43.

McGurk, H., and MacDonald, J. (1976). Hearing lips and seeing voices. *Nature, 264*(5588), 746–48.

Mahler, M. S., and Furer, M. (1968). *On human symbiosis and the vicissitudes of individuation.* New York: International Universities Press.

Mahler, M. S., Pine, F., and Bergman, A. (1975). *The psychological birth of the human infant.* New York: Basic Books.

Main, M. (1977). Sicherheit und wissen. In K. E. Grossman (Ed.), *Entwicklung der Lernfahigkeit in der sozialen umwelt.* Munich: Kinder Verlag.

Main, M., and Kaplan, N. (in press). Security in infancy, childhood and adulthood: A move to the level of representation. In I. Bretherton and E. Waterns (Eds.), *Monographs of the Society for Research in Child Development.*

Main, M., and Weston, D. (1981). The quality of the toddler's relationships to mother and father: Related to conflict behavior and readiness to establish new relationships. *Child Development, 52,* 932–40.

Malatesta, C. Z., and Haviland, J. M. (1983). Learning display rules: The socialization of emotion in infancy. *Child Development, 53,* 991–1003.

Malatesta, C. Z., and Izard, C. E. (1982). The ontogenesis of human social signals: From biological imperative to symbol utilization. In N. Fox and R. J. Davidson (Eds.), *Affective development: A psychological perspective.* Hillsdale, N.J.: Erlbaum.

Mandler, G. (1975). *Mind and emotion.* New York: Wiley.

Maratos, O. (1973). *The origin and development of imitation in the first six months of life.* Unpublished doctoral dissertation, University of Geneva.

Marks, L. F. (1978). *The unity of the senses: Interrelations among the modalities.* New York: Academic Press.

Matas, L., Arend, R., and Sroufe, L. A. (1978). Continuity of adaptation in the second year: The relationship between quality of attachment and later competence. *Child Development, 49,* 547–56.

Mead, G. H. (1934). *Mind, self and society: From the standpoint of a social behaviorist.* Chicago: University of Chicago Press.

Meissner, W. W. (1971). Notes on identification: II. Clarification of related concepts. *Psychoanalytic Quarterly, 40,* 277–302.

Meltzoff, A. N. (1981). Imitation, intermodal co-ordination and representation in early infancy. In G. Butterworth (Ed.), *Infancy and epistemology.* London: Harvester Press.

Meltzoff, A. N., and Borton, W. (1979). Intermodal matching by human neonates. *Nature, 282,* 403–4.

Meltzoff, A. N., and Moore, M. K. (1977). Imitation of facial and manual gestures by human neonates. *Science, 198,* 75–78.

Meltzoff, A. N., and Moore, M. K. (1983). The origins of imitation in infancy: Paradigm, phenomena and theories. In L. P. Lipsitt (Ed.), *Advances in infancy research.* Norwood, N.J.: Ablex.

Mendelson, M. J., and Haith, M. M. (1976). The relation between audition and vision in the human newborn. *Monographs of the Society for Research in Child Development, 41*(167).

Messer, D. J., and Vietze, P. M. (in press). Timing and transitions in mother-infant gaze. *Child Development.*

Miller, C. L., and Byrne, J. M. (1984). The role of temporal cues in the development of language and communication. In L. Feagans, C. Garvey, and R. Golinkoff (Eds.), *The origin and growth of communication.* Norwood, N.J.: Ablex.

Miyake, K., Chen, S., and Campos, J. J. (in press). Infant temperament, mother's mode of interaction, and attachment. In I. Bretherton and E. Waterns (Eds.), *Monographs of the Society for Research in Child Development.*

Moes, E. J. (1980, April). *The nature of representation and the development of consciousness and language in infancy: A criticism of Moore and Meltzoff's "neo-Piagetian" approach.* Paper presented at the International Conference on Infant Studies, New Haven, Conn.

Moore, M. K., and Meltzoff, A. N. (1978). Object permanence, imitation and language development in infancy: Toward a neo-Piagetian perspective on communicative and cognitive development. In F. D. Minifie and L. L. Lloyd (Eds.), *Communicative and cognitive abilities: Early behavioral assessment.* Baltimore, Md.: University Park Press.

Morrongiello, B. A. (1984). Auditory temporal pattern perception in six- and twelve-month-old infants. *Developmental Psychology, 20,* 441–48.

Moss, H. A. (1967). Sex, age and state as determinant of mother-infant interaction. *Merrill-Palmer Quarterly, 13,* 19–36.

Murphy, C. M., and Messer, D. J. (1977). Mothers, infants and pointing: A study of a gesture. In H. R. Schaffer (Ed.), *Studies in mother-infant interaction.* London: Academic Press.

Nachman, P. (1982). Memory for stimuli reacted to with positive and neutral affect in seven-month-old infants. Unpublished doctoral dissertation, Columbia University.

Nachman, P., and Stern, D. N. (1983). *Recall memory for emotional experience in pre-linguistic infants.* Paper presented at the National Clinical Infancy Fellows Conference, Yale University, New Haven, Conn.

Nelson, K. (1973). Structure and strategy in learning to talk. *Monographs of the Society for Research in Child Development, 48*(149).

Nelson, K. (1978). How young children represent knowledge of their world in and out of language. In R. S. Siegler (Ed.), *Children's thinking: What develops?* Hillsdale, N.J.: Erlbaum.

Nelson, K., and Greundel, J. M. (1979). *From personal episode to social script.* Paper presented at the Biennial Meeting of the Society for Research in Child Development, San Francisco, Calif.

Nelson, K., and Greundel, J. M. (1981). Generalized event representations: Basic building blocks of cognitive development. In M. E. Lamb and A. L. Brown (Eds.), *Advances in developmental psychology, Vol. 1.* Hillsdale, N.J.: Erlbaum.

Nelson, K., and Ross, G. (1980). The generalities and specifics of long-term memory in infants and young children. *New Directions for Child Development, 10,* 87–101.

Newson, J. (1977). An intersubjective approach to the systematic description of mother-infant interaction. In H. R. Schaffer (Ed.), *Studies in mother-infant interaction.* New York: Academic Press.

Ninio, A., and Bruner, J. (1978). The achievement and antecedents of labelling. *Journal of Child Language, 5,* 1–15.

Olson, G. M., and Strauss, M. S. (1984). The development of infant memory. In M. Moscovitch (Ed.), *Infant memory.* New York: Plenum Press.

Ornstein, P. H. (1979). Remarks on the central position of empathy in psychoanalysis. *Bulletin of the Association of Psychoanalytic Medicine, 18,* 95–108.

Osofsky, J. D. (1985). *Attachment theory and research and the psychoanalytic process.* Unpublished manuscript.

Papoušek, H., and Papoušek, M. (1979). Early ontogeny of human social interaction: Its biological roots and social dimensions. In M. von Cranach, K. Foppa, W. Lepenies, and P. Ploog (Eds.), *Human ethology: Claims and limits of a new discipline.* Cambridge: Cambridge University Press.

Papoušek, M., and Papoušek, H. (1981). Musical elements in the infant's vocalization: Their significance for communication, cognition and creativity. In L. P. Lipsitt (Ed.), *Advances in Infancy Research.* Norwood, N.J.: Ablex.

Peterfreund, E. (1978). Some critical comments on psychoanalytic conceptualizations of infancy. *International Journal of Psychoanalysis, 59,* 427–41.

Piaget, J. (1952). *The origins of intelligence in children.* New York: International Universities Press.

Piaget, J. (1954). *The construction of reality in the child* (M. Cook, Trans.). New York: Basic Books. (Original work published 1937)

Pine, F. (1981). In the beginning: Contributions to a psychoanalytic developmental psychology. *International Review of Psychoanalysis, 8,* 15–33.

Pinol-Douriez, M. (1983, March). *Fantasy interactions or "proto representations"? The cognitive value of affect-sharing in early interactions.* Paper presented at the World Association of Infant Psychiatry, Cannes, France.

Plutchik, R. (1980). *The emotions: A psychoevolutionary synthesis.* New York: Harper & Row.

Reite, M., Short, R., Seiler, C., and Pauley, J. D. (1981). Attachment, loss and depression. *Journal of Child Psychology and Psychiatry, 22,* 141–69.

Ricoeur, P. (1977). The question of proof in Freud's psychoanalytic writings. *Journal of American Psychoanalytic Association, 25,* 835–71.

Rosch, E. (1978). Principle of categorization. In E. Rosch and B. B. Floyd (Eds.), *Cognition and categorization.* Hillsdale, N.J.: Erlbaum.

Rose, S. A. (1979). Cross-modal transfer in infants: Relationship to prematurity and socioeconomic background. *Developmental Psychology, 14,* 643–82.

Rose, S. A., Blank, M. S., and Bridger, W. H. (1972). Intermodal and intramodal retention of visual and tactual information in young children. *Developmental Psychology, 6,* 482–86.

Rovee-Collier, C. K., and Fagan, J. W. (1981). The retrieval of memory in early infancy. In L. P. Lipsitt (Ed.), *Advances in infancy research, Vol. 1.* Norwood, N.J.: Ablex.

Rovee-Collier, C. K., and Lipsitt, L. P. (1981). Learning, adaptation, and memory. In P. M. Stratton (Ed.), *Psychobiology of the human newborn.* New York: Wiley.

Rovee-Collier, C. K., Sullivan, M. W., Enright, M., Lucas, D., and Fagan, J. W. (1980). Reactivism of infant memory. *Science, 208,* 1159–61.

Ruff, H. A. (1980). The development of perception and recognition of objects. *Child Development, 51,* 981–92.

Sagi, A., and Hoffman, M. L. (1976). Empathic distress in the newborn. *Developmental Psychology, 12,* 175–76.

Salapatek, P. (1975). Pattern perception in early infancy. In I. Cohen and P. Salapatek (Eds.), *Infant perception: From sensation to cognition, Vol. 1.* New York: Academic Press.

Sameroff, A. J. (1983). Developmental systems: Context and evolution. In W. Kessen (Ed.), *Mussen's handbook of child psychology, Vol. 1.* New York: Wiley.

Sameroff, A. J. (1984, May). *Comparative perspectives on early motivation.* Paper presented at the Third Triennial Meeting of the Developmental Biology Research Group, Estes Park, Colo.

Sameroff, A. J., and Chandler, M. (1975). Reproductive risk and the continuum of caretaking casualty. In F. D. Horowitz (Ed.), *Review of child development research, Vol. 4.* Chicago: University of Chicago Press.

Sander, L. W. (1962). Issues in early mother-child interaction. *Journal of American Academy of Child Psychiatry, 1,* 141–66.

Sander, L. W. (1964). Adaptive relationships in early mother-child interaction. *Journal of the American Academy of Child Psychiatry, 3,* 231–64.

Sander, L. W. (1980). New knowledge about the infant from current research: Implications for psychoanalysis. *Journal of American Psychoanalytic Association, 28,* 181–98.

Sander, L. W. (1983a). Polarity, paradox, and the organizing process in development. In J. D. Call, E. Galenson, and R. L. Tyson (Eds.), *Frontiers of infant psychiatry,* Vol. 1. New York: Basic Books.

Sander, L. W. (1983b). To begin with—reflections on ontogeny. In J. Lichtenberg and S. Kaplan. *Reflection on self psychology.* Hillsdale, N.J.: Analytic Press.

Sandler, J. (1960). The background of safety. *International Journal of Psychoanalysis, 41,* 352–56.

Scaife, M., and Bruner, J. S. (1975). The capacity for joint visual attention in the infant. *Nature, 253,* 265–66.

Schafer, R. (1968). Generative empathy in the treatment situation. *Psychoanalytic Quarterly, 28,* 342–73.

Schafer, R. (1981). Narration in the psychoanalytic dialogue. In W. J. T. Mitchell (Ed.), *On narrative.* Chicago: University of Chicago Press.

Schaffer, H. R. (1977). *Studies in infancy.* London: Academic Press.

Schaffer, H. R., Collis, G. M., and Parsons, G. (1977). Vocal interchange and visual regard in verbal and pre-verbal children. In H. R. Schaffer (Ed.), *Studies in mother-infant interaction.* London: Academic Press.

Schaffer, H. R., Greenwood, A., and Parry, M. H. (1972). The onset of wariness. *Child Development, 43,* 65–75.

Scheflin, A. E. (1964). The significance of posture in communication systems. *Psychiatry, 27,* 4.

Scherer, K. (1979). Nonlinguistic vocal indicators of emotion and psychopathology. In C. E. Izard (Ed.), *Emotions in personality and psychopathology.* New York: Plenum Press.

Schneirla, T. C. (1959). An evolutionary and developmental theory of biphasic processes underlying approach and withdrawal. In M. R. Jones (Ed.), *Nebraska symposium on motivation.* Lincoln: University of Nebraska Press.

Schneirla, T. C. (1965). Aspects of stimulation and organization in approach/withdrawal processes underlying vertebrate behavioral development. In D. S. Lehrman, R. A. Hinde, and E. Shaw (Eds.), *Advances in the study of behavior, Vol. 1.* New York: Academic Press.

Schwaber, E. (1980a). Response to discussion of Paul Tolpin. In A. Goldberg (Ed.), *Advances in self psychology.* New York: International Universities Press.

Schwaber, E. (1980b). Self psychology and the concept of psychopathology: A case presentation.

In A. Goldberg (Ed.), *Advances in self psychology*. New York: International Universities Press.

Schwaber, E. (1981). Empathy: A mode of analytic listening. *Psychoanalytic Inquiry, 1*, 357–92.

Searle, J. R. (1969). *Speech acts: An essay in the philosophy of language*. New York: Cambridge University Press.

Shane, M., and Shane, E. (1980). Psychoanalytic developmental theories of the self: An integration. In A. Goldberg (Ed.), *Advances in self psychology*. New York: International Universities Press.

Shank, R. C. (1982). *Dynamic memory: A theory of reminding and learning in computers and people*. New York: Cambridge University Press.

Shank, R. C., and Abelson, R. (1975). *Scripts, plans and knowledge*. Proceedings of the Fourth International Joint Conference on Artificial Intelligence, Tbilis, U.S.S.R.

Shank, R. C., and Abelson, R. (1977). *Scripts, plans, goals, and understanding*. Hillsdale, N.J.: Erlbaum.

Sherrod, L. R. (1981). Issues in cognitive-perceptual development: The special case of social stimuli. In M. E. Lamb and L. R. Sherrod (Eds.), *Infant social cognition*. Hillsdale, N.J.: Erlbaum.

Shields, M. M. (1978). The child as psychologist: Contriving the social world. In A. Lock (Ed.), *Action, gesture and symbol*. New York: Academic Press.

Simner, M. (1971). Newborns' response to the cry of another infant. *Developmental Psychology, 5*, 136–50.

Siqueland, E. R., and Delucia, C. A. (1969). Visual reinforcement of non-nutritive sucking in human infants. *Science, 165*, 1144–46.

Snow, C. (1972). Mother's speech to children learning language. *Child Development, 43*, 549–65.

Sokolov, E. N. (1960). Neuronal models and the orienting reflex. In M. A. B. Brazier (Ed.), *The central nervous system and behavior*. New York: Josiah Macy, Jr. Foundation.

Spelke, E. S. (1976). Infants' intermodal perception of events. *Cognitive Psychology, 8*, 553–60.

Spelke, E. S. (1979). Perceiving bimodally specified events in infancy. *Developmental Psychology, 15*, 626–36.

Spelke, E. S. (1980). Innate constraints on intermodal perception. A discussion of E. J. Gibson, "The development of knowledge of intermodal unity: Two views," Paper presented to the Piaget Society.

Spelke, E. S. (1982). The development of intermodal perception. In L. B. Cohen and P. Salapatek (Eds.), *Handbook of infant perception*. New York: Academic Press.

Spelke, E. S. (1983). *The infant's perception of objects*. Paper presented at the New School for Social Research, New York.

Spelke, E. S., and Cortelyou, A. (1981). Perceptual aspects of social knowing: Looking and listening in infancy. In M. E. Lamb and L. R. Sherrod (Eds.), *Infant social cognition*. Hillsdale, N.J.: Erlbaum.

Spense, D. P. (1976). Clinical interpretation: Some comments on the nature of the evidence. *Psychoanalysis and Contemporary Science, 5*, 367–88.

Spieker, S. J. (1982). *Infant recognition of invariant categories of faces: Person, identity and facial expression*. Unpublished doctoral dissertation, Cornell University.

Spitz, R. A. (1950). Anxiety in infancy: A study of its manifestations in the first year of life. *International Journal of Psychoanalysis, 31*, 138–43.

Spitz, R. A. (1957). *No and yes: On the genesis of human communication*. New York: International Universities Press.

Spitz, R. A. (1959). *A genetic field theory of ego formation*. New York: International Universities Press.

Spitz, R. A. (1965). *The first year of life*. New York: International Universities Press.

Sroufe, L. A. (1979). The coherence of individual development: Early care, attachment and subsequent developmental issues. *American Psychologist, 34*, 834–41.

291

Sroufe, L. A. (1985). An organizational perspective on the self. Unpublished manuscript.

Sroufe, L. A. (in press). Attachment classification from the perspective of the infant-caregiver relationship and infant temperament. *Child Development.*

Sroufe, L. A., and Fleeson, J. (1984). Attachment and the construction of relationships. In W. W. Hartup and Z. Rubin, *Relationships and development.* New York: Cambridge University Press.

Sroufe, L. A., and Rutter, M. (1984). The Domain of developmental Psychopathology. *Child Development, 55*(1), 17–29.

Sroufe, L. A., and Waters, E. (1977). Attachment as an organizational construct. *Child Development, 48,* 1184–99.

Stechler, G., and Carpenter, G. (1967). A viewpoint on early affective development. In J. Hellmath (Ed.), *The exceptional infant, No. 1* (pp. 163–89). Seattle: Special Child Publications.

Stechler, G., and Kaplan, S. (1980). The development of the self: A psychoanalytic perspective. In A. Solnit et al. (Eds.), *The psychoanalytic study of the child, Vol. 35* (p. 35). New Haven: Yale University Press.

Stern, D. N. (1971). A micro-analysis of mother-infant interaction: Behaviors regulating social contact between a mother and her three-and-a-half-month-old twins. *Journal of American Academy of Child Psychiatry, 10,* 501–17.

Stern, D. N. (1974a). The goal and structure of mother-infant play. *Journal of American Academy of Child Psychiatry, 13,* 402–21.

Stern, D. N. (1974b). Mother and infant at play: The dyadic interaction involving facial, vocal and gaze behaviors. In M. Lewis and L. A. Rosenblum (Eds.), *The effect of the infant on its caregiver.* New York: Wiley.

Stern, D. N. (1977). *The first relationship: Infant and mother.* Cambridge, Mass.: Harvard University Press.

Stern, D. N. (1980). *The early development of schemas of self, of other, and of various experiences of "self with other."* Paper presented at the Symposium on Reflections on Self Psychology, Boston Psychoanalytic Society and Institute, Boston, Mass.

Stern, D. N. (1985). Affect attunement. In J. D. Call, E. Galenson, and R. L. Tyson (Eds.), *Frontiers of infant psychiatry, Vol. 2.* New York: Basic Books.

Stern, D. N., and Gibbon, J. (1978). Temporal expectancies of social behavior in mother-infant play. In E. B. Thoman (Ed.), *Origins of the infant's social responsiveness.* Hillsdale, N.J.: Erlbaum.

Stern, D. N., Barnett, R. K., and Spieker, S. (1983). Early transmission of affect: Some research issues. In J. D. Call, F. Galenson, and R. L. Tyson (Eds.), *Frontiers of infant psychiatry.* New York: Basic Books.

Stern, D. N., MacKain, K., and Spieker, S. (1982). Intonation contours as signals in maternal speech to prelinguistic infants. *Developmental Psychology, 18,* 727–35.

Stern, D. N., Beebe, B., Jaffe, J., and Bennett, S. L. (1977). The infant's stimulus world during social interaction: A study of caregiver behaviors with particular reference to repetition and timing. In H. R. Schaffer (Ed.), *Studies in mother-infant interaction.* London: Academic Press.

Stern, D. N., Hofer, L., Haft, W., and Dore, J. (in press). Affect attunement: The sharing of feeling states between mother and infant by means of inter-modal fluency. In T. Field and N. Fox (Eds.), *Social perception in infants.* Norwood, N.J.: Ablex.

Stern, D. N., Jaffe, J., Beebe, B., and Bennett, S. L. (1974). Vocalizing in unison and in alternation: Two modes of communication within the mother-infant dyad. *Annals of the New York Academy of Science, 263,* 89–100.

Stolerow, R. D., Brandhoft, B., and Atwood, G. E. (1983). Intersubjectivity in psychoanalytic treatment. *Bulletin of the Menninger Clinic, 47*(2), 117–28.

Strain, B., and Vietze, P. (1975, March). *Early dialogues: The structure of reciprocal infant-mother vocalizations.* Paper presented at the Meeting of the Society for Research in Child Development, Denver, Colo.

Strauss, M. S. (1979). Abstraction of proto typical information by adults and ten-month-old infants. *Journal of Experimental Psychology: Human Learning and Memory, 5,* 618–32.

292

BIBLIOGRAPHY

Sullivan, H. S. (1953). *The interpersonal theory of psychiatry.* New York: Norton.

Sullivan, J. W., and Horowitz, F. D. (1983). Infant intermodal perception and maternal multimodal stimulation: Implications for language development. In L. P. Lipsitt (Ed.), *Advances in infancy research, Vol. 2.* Norwood, N.J.: Ablex.

Thoman, E. B., and Acebo, C. (1983). The first affections of infancy. In R. W. Bell, J. W. Elias, R. L. Greene, and J. H. Harvey (Eds.), *Texas Tech interfaces in psychology: I. Developmental psychobiology and neuropsychology.* Lubbock, Tex.: Texas Tech University Press.

Thomas, A., Chess, S., and Birch, H. G. (1970). The origins of personality. *Scientific American, 223,* 102–4.

Tolpin, M. (1971). On the beginning of a cohesive self. In R. Eissler et al. (Eds.), *The Psychoanalytic Study of the Child, Vol. 26* (pp. 316–54). New York: International Universities Press.

Tolpin, M. (1980). Discussion of psychoanalytic developmental theories of the self: An integration by M. Shane and E. Shane. In A. Goldberg (Ed.), *Advances in self psychology.* New York: International Universities Press.

Tomkins, S. S. (1962). *Affect, imagery and consciousness: Vol. I. The positive affects.* New York: Springer.

Tompkins, S. S. (1963). *Affect, imagery, consciousness: Vol. II. The negative affects.* New York: Springer.

Tompkins, S. S. (1981). The quest for primary motives: Biography and autobiography of an idea. *Journal of Personal Social Psychology, 41,* 306–29.

Trevarthan, C. (1974). Psychobiology of speech development. In E. Lenneberg (Ed.), Language and Brain: Developmental Aspects. *Neurobiology Sciences Research Program Bulletin, 12,* 570–85.

Trevarthan, C. (1977). Descriptive analyses of infant communicative behavior. In H. R. Schaffer (Ed.), *Studies in mother-infant interaction.* New York: Academic Press.

Trevarthan, C. (1979). Communication and cooperation in early infancy: A description of primary intersubjectivity. In M. M. Bullowa (Ed.), *Before speech: The beginning of interpersonal communication.* New York: Cambridge University Press.

Trevarthan, C. (1980). The foundations of intersubjectivity: Development of interpersonal and cooperative understanding in infants. In D. R. Olson (Ed.), *The social foundation of language and thought: Essays in honor of Jerome Bruner.* New York: Norton.

Trevarthan, C., and Hubley, P. (1978). Secondary intersubjectivity: Confidence, confiders and acts of meaning in the first year. In A. Lock (Ed.), *Action, gesture and symbol.* New York: Academic Press.

Tronick, E., Als, H., and Adamson, L. (1979). Structure of early face-to-face communicative interactions. In M. Bullowa (Ed.), *Before speech: The beginning of interpersonal communication.* New York: Cambridge University Press.

Tronick, E., Als, H., and Brazelton, T. B. (1977). The infant's capacity to regulate mutuality in face-to-face interaction. *Journal of Communication, 27,* 74–80.

Tronick, E., Als, H., Adamson, L., Wise, S., and Brazelton, T. B. (1978). The infant's response to intrapment between contradictory messages in face-to-face interaction. *Journal of Child Psychiatry, 17,* 1–13.

Tulving, E. (1972). Episodic and semantic memory. In E. Tulving and W. Donaldson (Eds.), *Organization of memory.* New York: Academic Press.

Ungerer, J. A., Brody, L. R., and Zelazo, P. (1978). Long term memory for speech in two- to four-week-old infants. *Infant Behavior and Development, 1,* 177–186.

Uzgiris, I. C. (1974). Patterns of vocal and gestural imitation in infants. In L. J. Stone, H. T. Smith, and L. B. Murphy (Eds.), *The competent infant.* London: Tavistock.

Uzgiris, I. C. (1981). Two functions of imitation during infancy. *International Journal of Behavioral Development, 4,* 1–12.

Uzgiris, I. C. (1984). Imitation in infancy: Its interpersonal aspects. In M. Perlmutter (Ed.), *Parent-child interaction in child development. The Minnesota symposium on child psychology, Vol. 17.* Hillsdale, N.J.: Erlbaum.

Vischer, F. T. (1863). *Kritische gange, Vol. 2.* (p. 86). (No. 5, second ed.).

Vygotsky, L. S. (1962). *Thought and language* (E. Haufmann and G. Vakar, Eds. and Trans.). Cambridge, Mass.: M.I.T. Press.

Vygotsky, L. S. (1966). Development of the higher mental functions. In A. N. Leontier (Ed.), *Psychological research in the U.S.S.R.* Moscow: Progress Publishers.

Waddington, C. H. (1940). *Organizers and genes.* Cambridge: Cambridge University Press.

Wagner, S., and Sakowitz, L. (1983, March). *Intersensory and intrasensory recognition: A quantitative and developmental evaluation.* Paper presented at the Meeting of the Society for Research in Child Development, Detroit, Mich.

Walker, A. S., Bahrick, L. E., and Neisser, U. (1980). *Selective looking to multimodal events by infants.* Paper presented at the International Conference on Infancy Studies, New Haven, Conn.

Walker-Andrews, A. S., and Lennon, E. M. (1984). *Auditory-visual perception of changing distance.* Paper presented at the International Conference of Infancy Studies, New York.

Wallon, H. (1949). *Les origines du caractère chez l'enfant: Les préludes du sentiment de personnalité* (2nd ed.). Paris: Presses Universitaires de France.

Washburn, K. J. (1984). *Development of categorization of rhythmic patterns in infancy.* Paper presented at the International Conference of Infant Studies, New York.

Waters, E. (1978). The reliability and stability of individual differences in infant-mother attachment. *Child Development, 49,* 483–94.

Waters, E., Wippman, J., and Sroufe, L. A. (1980). Attachment, positive affect and competence in the peer group: Two studies of construct validation. *Child Development, 51,* 208–16.

Watson, J. S. (1979). Perception of contingency as a determinant of social responsiveness. In E. Thomas (Ed.), *The origins of social responsiveness.* Hillsdale, N.J.: Erlbaum.

Watson, J. S. (1980). *Bases of causal inference in infancy: Time, space, and sensory relations.* Paper presented at the International Conference on Infant Studies, New Haven, Conn.

Weil, A. M. (1970). The basic core. In R. Eissler et al. (Eds.), *The Psychoanalytic Study of the Child, Vol. 25* (pp. 442–60). New York: International Universities Press.

Werner, H. (1948). *The comparative psychology of mental development.* New York: International Universities Press.

Werner, H., and Kaplan, B. (1963). *Symbol formation: An organismic-developmental approach to language and expression of thought.* New York: Wiley.

Winnicott, D. W. (1958). *Collected papers.* London: Tavistock.

Winnicott, D. W. (1965). *The maturational processes and the facilitating environment.* New York: International Universities Press.

Winnicott, D. W. (1971). *Playing and reality.* New York: Basic Books.

Wolf, E. S. (1980). Developmental line of self-object relations. In A. Goldberg (Ed.), *Advances in self psychology.* New York: International Universities Press.

Wolff, P. H. (1966). The causes, controls and organization of behavior in the neonate. *Psychological Issues, 5,* 17.

Wolff, P. H. (1969). The natural history of crying and other vocalizations in infancy. In B. M. Foss (Ed.), *Determinants of infant behavior, Vol. 4.* London: Methuen.

Worthheimer, M. (1961). Psychomotor coordination of auditory visual space at birth. *Science, 134,* 1692.

Yogman, M. W. (1982). Development of the father-infant relationship. In H. Fitzgerald, B. M. Lester, and M. W. Yogman (Eds.), *Theory and research in behavioral peadiatric, Vol. 1.* New York: Plenum Press.

Zajonc, R. B. (1980). Feeling and thinking: Preferences need no inferences. *American Psychologist, 35*(2), 151–75.

Zahn-Waxler, C., and Radke-Yarrow, M. (1982). The development of altruism: Alternative research strategies. In N. Eisenberg-Berg (Ed.), *The development of prosocial behavior.* New York: Academic Press.

Zahn-Waxler, C., Radke-Yarrow, M., and King, R. (1979). Child rearing and children's prosocial initiations towards victims of distress. *Child Development, 50,* 319–30.

INDEX

Abelson, R., 95

Acebo, C., 66 *n*14, 132

Activation contours: amodal representation and, 59; vitality affects and, 57

Actual point of origin: of pathology, 257, 260, 262

Adler, G., 264, 265

Affect: in infant, 41–42; memory and, 245

Affect appraisal, 201–2

Affect attunement, 138–61; affect contagion and, 143; affect matching and, 143; alternative conceptualizations of, 142–45; art and, 158–61; authenticity in, 217–18; dance and, 158; definition of, 140–42; echoing and, 144; empathy and, 145; evidence for, 146–52; intensity of, 153; language and, 161; mirroring and, 144–45; music and, 158; painting and, 158–59; poetry and, 155; qualitative properties of, 153–54; sculpture and, 158; temporal qualities of, 153; underlying mechanisms for, 152–54; vitality affects and, 156–61. *See also* Misattunement; Non-attunement; Selective attunement; Tuning

Affect categories, 66

Affect contagion, affect attunement and, 143

Affect expression, 50–51

Affect intensity: as self-experience, 102

Affect matching: affect attunement and, 143

Affect memory. *See* Memory

Affect state-dependent experience, 244–48

Ainsworth, M. D. S., 25, 44, 186, 187, 247

Alert inactivity, 39–40, 42, 232–33, 236

Alexander Nevsky (Eisenstein), 155 *n*5

Alienating effect: of language, 174–82

Alienation, 136

Allen, T. W., 49

Aloneness, 136, 240

Amnesia, infantile, 98 *n*10

Amodal perception, 47–53

Amodal representation: activation contours and, 59

Amsterdam, B. K., 165

Anxiety disorders: tolerance for stimulation and, 189–91

Arend, R., 187 *n*2

Aristotle, 154

Arnold, M. G., 55 *n*7

Art: affective attunement and, 158–61; cross-sensory analogy and, 155, 158

Aspects of the True Self (Berghash), 159 *n*7

Attachment: evoked companion and, 114–19; as self-experience, 102–3; working model of, 114–19

Attachment patterns: psychopathology and, 187–88

Attachment research, 186–88

Attachment theory, 25, 137, 240–41

Attentional focus: sharing of, 129–30

Attunement, selective. *See* Selective attunement

Atwood, G. E., 219

Austin, J., 217

Authenticity: in affect attunement, 217–18; in parent's behavior, 214–17

Autism, 241

Autistic phase, normal. *See* Normal autistic phase

Autonomous ego functions. *See* Ego functions

Autonomy: mother-child relationship and, 258–59

Baby faces, 73
Baby talk, 72–73
Baker, Susan, 78
Baldwin, J. M., 8, 127
Balint, M., 44
Barnett, Roanne, 78
Basch, M. F., 145, 210, 220, 227
Bates, E., 124, 130, 133
Bateson, G., 23–24 *n*9, 180
Beebe, B., 21, 22, 84, 102, 139, 194, 195
Behavioral sciences: sense of self and, 6
Benjamin, J. D., 232
Bennett, S., 66
Berghash, Mark, 159 *n*7
Bergman, A., 44, 234, 269
Berlyne, D. E., 41
Bloom, L., 130, 168
Body-touching games, 73
Borderline disorders, 220; self-objects and, 243
Borton, W., 47, 153
Bower, G., 245, 247
Bower, T. G. R., 48, 51, 77, 130 *n*2, 152, 155, 175
Bowlby, J., 25, 44, 113, 118, 186, 202, 233 *n*1, 235, 255
Brandhoft, B., 219
Brazelton, T. B., 5, 37, 63, 75, 131 *n*3, 139, 190, 233
Bretherton, I., 25, 114, 124, 130, 171, 178
British object relations school, 44, 101, 241
Bronson, G., 37, 61, 88
Brooks-Gunn, J., 165
Brown, R., 130, 168
Bruner, J. S., 42, 91, 129, 130, 133, 168, 169, 173
Buie, D. H., 264, 265
Burd, A. P., 51
Butterworth, G., 82
Byrne, J. M., 49

Call, J. D., 5, 75, 164
Campos, J., 132, 187, 220

Caron, A. J., 189
Caron, R. F., 189
Carpenter, G., 66, 233
Cassirer, E., 29
Castello, M., 82
Categorical affects, 53; vitality affects and, 55
Causal inference: in infancy, 81
Cavell, M., 126
Chandler, M., 23–24 *n*9
Chen, S., 187
Chomsky, N., 168
Cicchetti, D., 23 *n*9, 66, 188, 201
Clarke-Stewart, K. A., 171
Clinical infant: clinical practice and, 14; observed infant and, 13–18, 231
Clinical issues: developmental process and, 10–12
Clinical practice: clinical infant and, 14
Clinical reality, 4
Cognition: infant, 41–42
Cognitive appraisal, 201
Cognitive development: Generalized Event Structures and, 97
Cohen, L. B., 41, 88
Coherence: of form, 87–89; of intensity structure, 86–87; of motion, 83; of temporal structure, 83–86
Collis, G. M., 129
Colored hearing, 154
Communication: intentional, 130–31
Communion: interpersonal, 148
Companion, evoked. *See* Evoked companion
Condon, W. S., 83, 84
Consciousness, states of: in the infant, 66
Constitutional capacities: psychopathology and, 191
Cooley, C. H., 8
Cooper, A. M., 8
Core-relatedness, 192–203; core self and, 27; intersubjective relatedness and, 125; overstimulation and, 194–97; psychopathology and, 202–3; understimulation and, 197–202
Core self, 11, 26–27, 69–123; core-relatedness and, 27; self-affectivity and,

71; self-agency and, 71; self-coherence and, 71; self-history and, 71; self-regulating other and, 105
Correspondences (Baudelaire), 155
Cortelyou, A., 85
Cosmic psychic isolation. *See* Isolation
Cramer, B., 15, 121 *n*7, 134, 224
Cross-modal fluency, 51
Cross-sensory analogy, art and, 155

Dahl, H., 55 *n*7
Dance: affect attunement and, 158; vitality affects and, 56–57
Darwin, C., 54–55, 56, 57 *n*8, 179
DeCasper, A. J., 49, 64, 92
Deferred imitation. *See* Imitation
DeLucia, C. A., 40
Demany, L., 49
Demos, V., 66 *n*14, 132, 145, 247, 248
Denial, 227
Developmental past: reconstruction of, 256–74
Developmental progression: clinical issues and, 10–12; and the developing senses of self, 25–26; and the developmentalist perspective, 24–25; and the psychoanalytic perspective, 18–23; quantum leaps in, 8–9; sense of self and, 26–34; subject matter of, 18–26
Developmental psychology perspective: on developmental progression, 24–25
DeVore, I., 237
Disavowal, 227–29; language and, 227
Disavowed self, 229
Disney, Walt, 155–56 *n*5
Dodd, B., 85, 107
Donee, L. H., 62, 63
Dore, J., 130, 131, 166 *n*1, 168, 171, 172, 173, 205, 215
Double-bind message, 180
DSM-III phenomenology, 192, 223; personality disorders in, 261
Dual-unity: with mother, 240
Dunn, J., 131
Dynamic memory. *See* Memory

Easterbrook, M. A., 187 *n*2
Echoing: affect attunement and, 144
Ego functions: autonomous, 135–36
Ego instincts: id instincts and, 238–40
Eichhorn, D., 8
Eimas, P. D., 107
Ekman, P., 55 *n*6, 90
Emdee, R. N., 8, 37, 65, 66, 72, 87 *n*4, 93, 131, 132, 220, 221
Emergent relatedness, 28, 30–31, 188–92; emergent self and, 28; feeding and, 236–37
Emergent self, 11, 37–68; emergent relatedness and, 28; other and, 47–64; process and product in, 45–47
Empathy, 125–26; affect attunement and, 145; intersubjectivity and, 219–20
Enthusiasm: in infant, 208; exthusiasm and, 209, 223
Episodic memory. *See* Memory
Erikson, E. H., 15, 19, 20, 232, 235, 236
Escalona, S. K., 45, 189
Esman, A. H., 232, 234
Ethology, 137
Evoked companion, 111–22, 193–95; RIG and, 114–19; working model of attachment and, 114–19
Exaggerated behaviors, 73
Excitation: handling of, 232–35; optimal level of, 74–75
Experience organization, the infant's, 65–68
Exthusiasm: enthusiasm and, 209, 223

Fagan, J. F., 62, 88, 91, 92, 189
Fair, M., 134
Fairbairn, W. R. D., 44, 128
Falling in love. *See* Love
False self, 209–10; true self and, 227–28
Fanshel, D., 180, 216
Fantasy: reality versus, 253–55
Fantasy distortions: reality experience and, 255
Fantz, R., 40

Feeding: emergent relatedness and, 236
Feeding problem, 225–26
Fegy, M., 61
Feldman, Carol, 173
Ferguson, C. A., 73
Fernald, A., 58 *n*9, 73, 122 *n*8
Field, T. M., 41, 50, 63, 75, 111 *n*4, 139
Fifer, W. P., 64, 92
Fischer, Canbell, 160
Fleeson, J., 25, 114
Fogel, A., 66 *n*14, 75
Form, coherence of. *See* Coherence
Form and Emotion in Photography (Metropolitan Museum of Art, New York), 159 *n*7
Fox, N., 41
Fraiberg, S. H., 55 *n*6, 91 *n*7, 121, 134
Francis, P. L., 139
Freedman, D., 55 *n*6
Freud, A., 34 *n*14, 255
Freud, S., 11, 15, 18, 19, 20, 44, 65, 100, 117 *n*6, 118, 210, 232, 233, 235, 238, 240, 245, 253, 257
Friedman, L., 43 *n*2, 113 *n*5

Gaensbauer, T., 8
Galenson, E., 5, 210
Garfinkel, H., 180
Garmenzy, N., 23–24 *n*9, 188
Gautier, Y., 15
Gediman, H. K., 232
Generalized Event Structures: cognitive development and, 97
Generalized memory. *See* Memory
Gerstman, L. J., 84
Ghosh, R. K., 158
Gibbon, J., 49
Gibson, E. J., 42, 45, 83, 88, 155
Gibson, J. J., 42, 45, 155
Glick, J., 169, 170
Glover, E., 239
Goldberg, A., 243
Golinkoff, R., 130, 164, 169
Gradient information. *See* Information

Greenfield, P., 168
Greenspan, S. I., 24, 37, 42, 191
Greundel, J. M., 91 *n*7, 95, 97, 98 *n*10
Grossman, K. E., 187
Gunther, M., 94, 96
Guntrip, J. S., 44, 241

Habermas, T., 126
Habituation/dishabituation paradigm, 40–41
Hadiks, R., 77–78
Haft, Wendy, 205
Hainline, L., 61, 62
Haith, M. M., 37, 49, 61, 62, 82
Halliday, M. A., 130
Hamilton, V., 240
Hamlyn, D. W., 126
Harding, C. G., 130
Harmon, R., 8
Harper, R. C., 78
Hartmann, H., 135, 239
Haviland, J. M., 139
Hedonic experiences, 249–53
Hedonic tone, 65–66
Herzog, J., 166, 167
Hinde, R. A., 23–24 *n*9, 25, 90, 126
Hofer, Lynn, 185, 205, 206
Hofer, M. A., 111 *n*4
Hoffman, M. L., 61, 143, 145, 166
Hogarty, P., 8
Holquist, Michael, 169
Homeostasis, 42–45. *See also* Physiological regulation
Hubley, P., 124, 128, 131 *n*3, 133, 134
Humphrey, K., 49
Hunger: satiation and, 237
Hutt, G., 191

"I'm gonna get you" game. *See* Suspense games
Id instincts: ego instincts and, 238–40

Imitation, 138–42; deferred, 143, 163–65

Inanimate things: self-regulating experiences with, 122–23

Infancy: perspectives and approaches to, 13–34; psychopathology and, 4

Infant development: relatedness domains and, 31–34

Infant observation. *See* Young infant observation

Infantile amnesia. *See* Amnesia

Information: gradient, 179–80; crossmodal transfer of, 48–50

Intense states, 247

Intensity structure: coherence of. *See* Coherence

Intentional communication. *See* Communication

Intentions: sharing of, 130–31

Interaffectivity, 132–33

Interattentionality, 130–31

Intermodal fluency, 152

Internal states: verbal account of, 178–79

Internalization, 173, 236

Interpersonal communion. *See* Communion

Interpretation: maternal, 134

Intersubjective relatedness, 128–37, 203–11; core-relatedness and, 125; evidence for, 128–33; leap to, 133–37; loneliness and, 265; non-attunement and, 204–97; psychopathology and, 223–26; selective attunement and, 207–11; subjective self and, 27

Intersubjective union, 209

Intersubjectivity: focus on, 127–28; empathy and, 219–20

Intonational signals, 180

Isolation: cosmic psychic, 136

Izard, C. E., 55 *n*6, 66, 89, 139, 143

Kagan, J., 8, 23–24 *n*9, 41, 42, 117 *n*6, 164, 165

Kaplan, S., 25, 26, 29, 46 *n*3, 108, 114, 174

Karmel, B. Z., 61

Kaye, K., 75, 139, 143, 165

Kearsley, R. B., 8, 23–24 *n*9

Kendrick, C., 131

Kennel, J., 233 *n*1, 237 *n*2

Kernberg, O. F., 245, 246, 248, 250, 251, 252, 265

Kessen, W., 41, 61, 233

Kestenberg, J. S., 159 *n*7

Klaus, M., 233 *n*1, 237 *n*2

Klein, D. F., 190

Klein, Melanie, 15, 26, 44, 245, 246, 250, 254

Klein, Milton, 19, 234

Kleinert, M. D., 131, 132, 220, 221

Kohut, H., 8, 15, 26, 144, 219, 229, 237, 242, 245, 255, 264, 266

Kreisler, L., 15, 134

Kris, E., 135

Kroner, J., 102

Kuhl, P., 50, 154

Labow, W., 180, 216

Lacan, J., 144

Lamb, M. E., 41, 187 *n*2

Langer, S. K., 54, 158, 160

Language, 162–63, 168–69; affect attunement and, 161; alienating effect of, 174–82; disavowal and, 227; memory and, 178; nonverbal global experience and, 175; reality distortion and, 182; repression and, 227; self-other relatedness and, 170–74; use of, 168–69; verbal relatedness and, 162–63; world knowledge and, 175–78

Language acquisition, 169, 170–74; narrative making and, 174; separation and, 172; as transitional phenomenon, 172–73; union and, 172

Lashley, K. S., 77

Lawson, K. R., 85

Learning disabilities: cross-modal transfer and, 188–89

Lebovici, S., 5, 15, 134, 205–6 *n*6

Lee, B., 26

Lennon, E. M., 88
Lewcowicz, D. J., 48, 49, 87
Lewis, M., 66 *n*14, 165, 187, 201
Libido theory, 238
Lichtenberg, J. D., 5, 15, 164, 166, 234, 251 *n*5
Lichtenstein, H., 207
Lieberman, A. F., 187 *n*2
Lipps, T., 143
Lipsitt, L. P., 41, 66, 91, 92
Locus unity: self-coherence and, 82–83
Loneliness: intersubjective relatedness and, 265
Lourie, R., 37
Love, falling in, 100, 244
Lowenstein, R. M., 135
Lutz, C., 55 *n*6
Lyons-Ruth, K., 85

McCall, R. B., 8, 23–24 *n*9, 117 *n*6
McDevitt, J. B., 94
MacFarlane, J., 39
McGurk, H., 50
MacKain, K., 50, 73, 132, 154, 248
MacMurray, J., 126, 128, 171
Maconald, J., 50
Mahler, M. S., 15, 18, 19, 20–21, 26, 44, 70, 101, 114, 144, 202, 234, 235, 240, 241, 254, 269, 273
Main, M., 25, 114, 119, 187 *n*2
Malatesta, C. Z., 139, 143
Mandler, G., 66
Maratos, O., 50
Marks, L. F., 154–55
Marschak, M., 75
Marwick, Helen, 215
Masturbation: in children, 210, 229–30
Matas, L., 187 *n*2
Maternal interpretation. *See* Interpretation
Maternal misattunement. *See* Misattunement
Mazzie, C., 122 *n*8
Mead, G. H., 8
Meissner, W. W., 265
Meltzoff, A. N., 47, 48, 50, 51, 153, 154

Memory: affect, 91–94, affect and, 245; dynamic, 98–99; episodic, 94–99; generalized episodes in, 95, 177; language and, 178; mood and, 245; motor, 90–94; perceptual, 90–94; recall, 91–94, 117; recognition, 91–94; specific episodes in, 95, 117. *See also* Self-history
Mendelson, M. J., 82
Merger: with mother, 240; primary, 104–5; secondary, 104–5
Messer, D. J., 21, 22 *n*5, 81, 129
Metaphor: organizing therapeutic, 258–60
Milewski, A. E., 51
Miller, C. L., 49
Mirroring, 220; affect attunement and, 144–45
Misattunement, 148–49; maternal, 211–14; tuning and, 211–26
Miyake, K., 187
Moes, E. J., 48
Moll Flanders (Defoe), 58
Mood: memory and, 245
Moore, M. K., 48, 50, 51
Morrongiello, B. A., 49
Moss, H. A., 139
Mother: dual-unity with, 240; merger with, 240
Mother-child relationships: autonomy and, 258–59
Motion: coherence of. *See* Coherence
Motor memory. *See* Memory
Motor plans, 77–78, 80. *See also* Sensorimotor schemas
Mourning process, 100
Mouth: as erotogenic zone, 235
Murphy, C. M., 129
Music: affect attunement and, 158; vitality affects and, 56

Nachman, P., 93
Narrated self, 174
Narrative making: language and, 174
Narrative point of origin: of pathology, 258–64

Nelson, K., 91 *n*7, 95, 97, 98 *n*10, 171, 172, 173
Newson, J., 134
Ninio, A., 130
Noam, G. G., 26
Nonattunement: intersubjective relatedness and, 204–7
Nonverbal global experience: language and, 175
Normal autism, 232–35
Normal symbiosis, 254; undifferentiation and, 240–42

Observational data, psychoanalysis and, 5
Observed infant: clinical infant and, 13–18, 231; seen with clinical eye, 185–230
Ogston, W. D., 83
Olson, G. M., 91
One-year phobias, 224
Orality, 235–37, 256
Origin. *See* Actual origin; Narrative origin
Ornstein, P. H., 145, 219
Osofsky, J. D., 25
Ounstead, C., 191
Overattunement: in parent's behavior, 218–19
Overstimulation, 194–96; core-relatedness and, 194–97

Painting: affect attunement and, 158–59
Papoušek, H., 80, 139
Papoušek, M., 80, 139
Parent's behavior: authenticity of, 214–17; overattunement in, 218–19; unauthentic attunement in, 217–18
Pavlov, I. P., 111 *n*4, 115
Peek-a-boo game. *See* Suspense games
Perception: infant, 41–42. *See also* Amodal perception; Physiognomic perception

Perceptual memory. *See* Memory
Perceptual unity, 51
Personality disorders: in *DSM-III* phenomenology, 261
Personification: of things, 122–23
Peterfreund, E., 19, 234
Phobias. *See* One-year phobias
Physiognomic perception, 53
Physiological regulation, 42–45. *See also* Homeostasis
Piaget, J., 29, 37, 45, 46, 48, 52, 64–65, 78, 91, 129, 131 *n*3, 133, 143, 155, 163, 164, 240
Pictures at an Exhibition (Mussorgsky), 155 *n*5
Pine, F., 23 *n*8, 44, 234, 245, 246, 269
Pinol-Douriez, M., 134
Pleasure principle, 65, 103, 233, 248; reality principle and, 238–39, 254
Plutchik, R., 55 *n*7
Pointing: infant's, 129; mother's, 129
Poetry: affect attunement and, 155
Preverbal infant: sense of self in, 6–8
Preverbal subjective life: psychoanalysis and, 7
Primary merger. *See* Merger
Private self: true self and, 229
Prohibition: act of, 215–17, 222
Prokofiev, S., 155 *n*5
Proprioception: modality of, 50–51
Psychodynamic formulation: of case, viii
Psychopathology, 261; attachment patterns and, 187–88; constitutional capacities and, 191; core-relatedness and, 202–03; infancy and, 4; intersubjective relatedness and, 223–26
Psychoanalysis: observational data and, 4–5; preverbal subjective life and, 7. *See also* Clinical infant; Clinical issues
Psychoanalytic perspective: on developmental progression, 18–23

Radke-Yarrow, M., 166
Rapprochement crisis, 269
Reality: fantasy versus, 253–55

Reality distortion: language and, 182

Reality experience: fantasy distortions and, 255

Reality principle: pleasure principle and, 238–39, 254

Recall memory. *See* Memory

Recognition memory. *See* Memory

Reelin' in the Years (Steely Dan), 268

Reite, M., 111 *n*4

Relatedness. *See* Emergent relatedness; Intersubjective relatedness

Repression: language and, 227

Ricoeur, P., 15, 16

RIGs, 97–99; evoked companion and, 114–19

Roiphe, H., 210

Rose, S. A., 48, 189

Rosenblum, L. A., 66 *n*14, 201

Ross, G., 95

Rovee-Collier, C. K., 91, 92

Rutter, M., 23–24 *n*9, 83, 88, 188

Sagi, A., 143

Sakowitz, L., 49

Salapatek, P., 41, 61, 62, 88

Sameroff, A. J., 23 *n*7, 23–24 *n*9, 46, 59

Sander, L. W., 5, 20, 24, 37, 42, 66, 84, 104, 248, 252

Satiation: hunger and, 237

Scaife, M., 129

Schafer, R., 15, 16 *n*1, 220

Schaffer, H. R., 75, 81, 107 *n*3, 117 *n*6, 129, 145

Scheflin, A. E., 107 *n*3

Scherer, K., 180

Schneider-Rosen, K., 23 *n*9, 188

Schneirla, T. C., 57 *n*8, 66, 201

Schwaber, E., 219, 266

Sculpture: affect attunement and, 158

Searle, J. R., 217

Secondary merger. *See* Merger

Selective attunement: intersubjective relatedness and, 207–11

Self: versus other, 69–99; with other, 100–123; word and, 172

Self-affectivity, 89–90; core self and, 71

Self-agency: core self and, 71

Self-coherence, 82–89; coherence of form and, 87–89; coherence of intensity structure and, 83–86; coherence of locus and, 82–83; coherence of motion and, 83; coherence of temporal structure and, 83–86; core self and, 71

Self-cohesion: maternal empathy and, 220

Self-events: invariant, 89–90

Self-experience: of affect intensity, 102; of attachment, 102–3

Self-history, 90–94; core self and, 71

Self-invariants: identification of, 72–94; integration of, 94–99

Self-objects, 242; borderline disorders and, 243

Self/other dichotomy, 248–53

Self/other fusion, 101. *See also* Self/other undifferentiation

Self/other relatedness: language and, 170–74

Self/other similarity, 107–8

Self/other undifferentiation, 101, 242. *See also* Self/other fusion

Self Psychology, 26, 108, 219, 220, 242, 243, 265

Self-regulating experiences: with inanimate things, 122–23

Self-regulating other, 102, 242–44; core self and, 105

Sense of other, 51

Senses: unity of. *See* Unity of senses

Senses of self: age-specific sensitive periods and, 273–74; behavioral sciences and, 6; developmental progression of, 26–34. *See also* Core self; Emergent self; Subjective self; Verbal self

Sensorimotor schemas, 78. *See also* Motor plans

Sensory correspondence, 154

Service de Guidance Infantile (Geneva), 224

Shane, E., 26

Shane, M., 26

Shank, R. C., 95, 96, 98 *n*10, 99

Sherrod, L. R., 40, 41, 61, 63, 64, 122

Shields, M. M., 130, 134
Simner, M., 143
Sincerity conditions, 217
Singer, L. T., 189
Siqueland, E. R., 40
Sleeping problems, 203
Sloate, P., 22, 195
Smith, J. H., 168
Snow, C., 73
Social experiences: relating of, 61–64
Social referencing, 132, 220–23
Sokolov, E. N., 41
Somatic state regulation, 103–4
Soothing technique, 58
Sorce, J. E., 132, 221
Sossin, M., 159 n7
Soulé, M., 134
Specific episodes: in memory. See Memory
Speech act theory, 217
Spelke, E. S., 48, 83, 85
Spence, D. P., 15
Spieker, S. J., 73, 88 n5
Spitz, R. A., 20, 37, 67, 72, 80, 131 n3, 272
Splitting, 248–53
Sroufe, L. A., 23 n9, 25, 66, 114, 187 n2, 188, 189, 201
Stechler, G., 26, 46 n3, 66, 108, 114, 233
Stenberg, C., 221
Stengel, B., 55 n7
Stern, D. N., 21, 22, 49, 72, 73, 75, 81, 84, 87, 93, 107, 121 n7, 134, 139, 146, 173, 179, 194, 195, 205, 233, 251 n5
Still-face procedure, 149
Stimulus barrier, 232–35
Stimulation: handling, 232–35; optimal range, 74–75. See also Tolerance for stimulation
Stolerow, R. D., 26, 219
Strain, B., 81
Strauss, M. S., 91, 97
Subjective experience: of infant, 64–68; sense of self and, 3–12
Subjective self, 11, 124–61; intersubjective relatedness and, 27

Subjective world: of infant and mother, 119–21
Sullivan, H. S., 44, 85, 128, 210, 229, 230, 247
Suspense games: "I'm gonna get you" game, 102, 106; peek-a-boo game, 101–2, 105, 106, 110, 116; tickle the tummy game, 106; walking fingers game, 106
Swan's Way (Proust), 264 n2
Symbiosis: normal. See Normal symbiosis
Symbiotic psychosis, 105 n2
Symbolic play, 163, 166; capacity for, 166–68
Synesthesia, 154

Temperamental differences: continuity of, 189
Temporal structure: coherence of. See Coherence
Therapeutic reconstructions, 231–55
Thoman, E. B., 66 n14, 132
Thomas, A., 189
Thumb-to-mouth sensorimotor schema, 59–60
Tickle the tummy game. See Suspense games
Togetherness, 240
Tolerance for stimulation: anxiety disorders and, 189–91
Tolpin, M., 26, 242, 243, 245
Tompkins, S. S., 57 n8, 66 n14
Total psychic transparency. See Transparency
Transition phenomena: undifferentiation and, 240–42
Transparency: total psychic, 136
Traumatic states, 245–47
Trevarthan, C., 50, 107, 124, 128, 130, 131 n3, 133, 134, 134–35 n4, 139, 144
Tronick, E., 75, 102, 132, 149
True self: false self and, 228; private self and, 229
Tulving, E., 94

Tuning: misattunement and, 211–26
Turkewitz, G., 48, 87
Tyson, R. L., 5

Unauthentic attunements: in parent's behavior, 217–18
Understimulation: core-relatedness and, 199–202
Undifferentiation: normal symbiosis and, 240–42; self/objects and, 240–42; transition phenomena and, 240–42
Unity of senses, 154–56
Uzgiris, I. C., 50, 139

Verbal account: of internal states, 178–79
Verbal relatedness, 226–30; language and, 162–63; verbal self and, 28
Verbal self, 11, 162–82; capacity for symbolic play and, 166–68; objective view of self and, 165–66; use of language and, 168–69; verbal relatedness and, 28
Vietze, P. M., 21, 22 *n*5, 81
Visual-haptic schema, 48
Vitality affects, 53–61; activation contours and, 57; affect attunement and, 156–61; categorical affects and, 55; communication of, 157–61; dance and, 56–57; music and, 56
Vocalization, 81
Vygotsky, L. S., 128, 130 *n*2, 134, 170, 171, 240

Waddington, C. H., 23–24 *n*9
Wagner, S., 49, 86
Walker-Andrews, A. S., 88
Walking fingers game. *See* Suspense games
Wallon, H., 127
Waters, E., 25, 187 *n*2
Watson, J. S., 81
Watson, Rita, 173
Weil, A. M., 240
Werner, H., 29, 53–54, 67, 174, 176
Weston, D., 187 *n*2
Winnicott, D. W., 90, 101, 122, 123, 172, 173, 199, 200, 202, 210, 229, 241
Wippman, J., 187 *n*2
Wittig, B., 25
Wolf, E. S., 66, 108, 109, 242
Wolff, P. H., 39, 143, 232
Word: self and, 172
World knowledge: language and, 175–78
Worthheimer, M., 82

Yogman, M. W., 189–90 *n*3
Young infant: clinical view of, 42–45; parental view of, 42–45
Young infant observation: research in, 38–42

Zahn-Waxler, C., 166
Zajonc, R. B., 66
Zelazo, P. R., 8, 23–24 *n*9

PORTRAITS FROM A SHOOTING GALLERY

PORTRAITS FROM
A SHOOTING GALLERY

Life Styles from the Drug Addict World

by SEYMOUR FIDDLE

RESEARCH SOCIOLOGIST, EXODUS HOUSE

HARPER AND ROW, PUBLISHERS

NEW YORK
EVANSTON
AND LONDON

1817

LIBRARY OF CONGRESS CATALOG CARD NUMBER: 67–13711

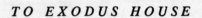

TO EXODUS HOUSE

Contents

Acknowledgments		ix
Foreword by Lynn L. Hageman		xi
Preface by Donald B. Louria		xiii
Author's Preface		xv

PART I. MYTHS AND SUBSTANCE OF ADDICTION

CHAPTER 1	Mysteries and Models	3
CHAPTER 2	Notes on the Heroin Addict and His Culture	21
CHAPTER 3	"The Life"	55

PART II. PORTRAITS AND CAMEOS

PORTRAIT OF	Billie	89
CAMEO 1	Howie—An Angry Loser	158
CAMEO 2	Lilly—Separate, Unequal, and Sad	162
CAMEO 3	Bert—Divided, He Retreats	165
CAMEO 4	Annie—The Prehensile Cat	168
PORTRAIT OF	Manny	171
CAMEO 5	Johnny—Sluggard and Victim	243

CAMEO 6   Joseph—Between Anger and Sadness   245

CAMEO 7   Artie—A Man Beside Himself   248

CAMEO 8   Ronnie—The Would-Be Master of His Fate   250

PORTRAIT OF   Justis   253

PART III. THE CHALLENGE OF ADDICTION

CHAPTER 1   The Unity and Diversity of Addiction   323

CHAPTER 2   Treatment   326

Glossary   345

Index   349

Acknowledgments

First, I would like to express my indebtedness to the hundreds of addicts and former addicts whose lives, over the years, have taught me to respect the diversity of addiction. In particular, I want to thank the three men who gave written permission to publish material from their taped interviews.

Next, let me express my general appreciation to the staff of Exodus House, all of whom have shared in my research, continuously offering me stimulation and wisdom. I should like particularly to acknowledge the manner in which the Rev. Lynn Hageman has debated, criticized, and amplified my views over the years. The Associate Director of Exodus House, the Rev. Stephen Chinlund, gave the first draft of this book a critical and constructive reading.

I would be remiss if I did not also mention the Rev. Norman C. Eddy, formerly the director of the East Harlem Protestant Parish Narcotics Committee, and Dr. Beatrice B. Berle, through whose grant by the Health Research Council of New York City, under the auspices of Cornell Medical College, I first became involved in the problem of addiction.

To Miss Evelyn Jaburek, Miss Caroline Cross, and to my wife, Adele, I wish to express my gratitude for not only typing and retyping the manuscript, but generally for making helpful suggestions. To my wife and my two children, Lorraine and Joan, who have endured my oscillating moods during the period of writing and rewriting, I owe a special thanks.

Finally, I would thank my editor, Norbert Slepyan, of Harper & Row, and Edward Ziegler, also of Harper & Row, who first suggested that I take time out to build a book around some of my tapes.

I have not included specific references to the philosophical and scientific literature from which I have drawn or derived the ideas underlying this book. They are too numerous to mention, especially those that pertain to the existential standpoint. Let me, however, point out that the concept of addict life style is a fusion of ideas drawn from the work of Alfred Adler and from Harry Stack Sullivan and his students. I have particularly found value in the work of Jane Pearce and Saul Newton, *The Conditions of Human Growth*. The lines from the *Purgatorio* are taken from the translation by John Ciardi, published by the New American Library.

SEYMOUR FIDDLE

New York City
November, 1966

Foreword

BY LYNN L. HAGEMAN
Director, Exodus House

Seymour Fiddle's *Portraits from a Shooting Gallery* is not an easy book despite its warmly humanistic concern. I say "not easy" because *Portraits from a Shooting Gallery* is profoundly ideological in an age that seems to have only contempt for ideas systematically pursued.

This is not to suggest that Mr. Fiddle has written *Portraits* as pure speculation. Quite the contrary, he has framed his ideology out of a personal confrontation with the culture of addiction as he has seen it during the past six years in his work with Exodus House. When he develops typology that appears "far out" to the academician, we may be sure that the "far-outness" is more an indication of the distance felt to exist between the ivory tower and the street than it is a judgment on the merits of the typology. No sophistication of questionnaire technique, no elaboration of statistical method, no cybernetic codifications, as yet, can substitute for the hundreds of days and nights spent in immediate personal confrontation with the addicts in prisons, hospitals, rehabilitation programs, and most important, the junkie on the street.

It must be made clear that the author of this volume has at no point pursued this quest for fact and truth in isolation. Rather, the entire staff and clientele of Exodus House has eagerly provided data and anecdotes as grist for the sociologist's mill, as well as providing the harshest of criticism that professionals and "grass rooters" can muster. In this day of vast research operations with the concomitant bane or blessing of the scholarly wheeler-dealer-operators, Exodus House has been fortunate in finding a committed researcher who has no qualms over the prospect of sixteen-hour days, grubby working conditions, and primitive resources. It is fair to assume that Mr. Fiddle has found compensations in terms of an unparalleled access to raw human research material in the midst of fellow workers who are similarly committed. The reader will find this indirectly reflected throughout *Portraits*.

Portraits is only an introduction to a complex world in which the reader is confronted with a new and strange culture that has its own hierarchies of value and authority, its own myths and heroes, its own economics and market systems, and its own matters of ultimate concern. And yet the reader will find that there is actually less of the strange and alien than there is of underlying identity between his own needs, fears, and commitments, and those of the members of the Addict Culture. Somehow, the apparent strangeness of that culture is only the strangeness of caricature which in distortion reveals the underlying motifs that shape all our lives.

Preface

BY DONALD B. LOURIA
Chairman, New York Council on Drug Addiction

Narcotic addiction is an enormous problem in many urban centers. Fifty percent of the nation's heroin abusers reside in New York City. In this city alone, in order to support their habit, they steal goods worth an estimated $500,000 to $1 million yearly. Over twenty percent of all crimes against property can be related to drug abuse. The addict sins not only against society but also against himself; his life becomes mired in the drug experience; he becomes a pariah, a thief, often a forger, and sometimes a venal pusher. Women turn to prostitution. Added to this life of degradation and depravity is the constant risk of heroin overdose or liver infection (hepatitis). It is startling to realize that one percent of the addict population die every year of heroin overdose.

The persistence and severity of the problem demands an understanding of the genesis of drug abuse and of the addict himself.

Seymour Fiddle has made a major contribution by providing a conceptual framework buttressed by detailed interviews with members of the addict subculture. He thus moves us substantially along the road to answering a basic enigma: Why should one person in a depressed neighborhood turn to drugs and another person from the same environment eschew drug abuse?

The book is valuable for an additional reason: It permits us to focus on the role of voluntary agencies in the antiaddiction fight. At present New York State has implemented a truly monumental program designed civilly to commit and effectively to rehabilitate addicts rather than jail them. New York State has been joined in this laudable effort by New York City and the federal government. No governmental program can succeed unless there is an active partnership between the public units and private, nonprofit, voluntary organizations. Among the latter, Exodus House deserves special recognition. Long active in the antiaddiction battle, first as part of the East Harlem Protestant Parish, under Reverend Norman Eddy, and now as Exodus House under the leadership of Reverend Lynn Hageman, it has contributed immeasurably to the community. Often the fight has been lonely and discouraging, without funds or support. Now the aid of governmental structures should make the task of voluntary organizations such as Exodus House easier and more effective.

But the antiaddiction forces must be a triumvirate made up of government, voluntary groups, and the public. Thus far the public is aroused but not fully committed to the battle. This articulate and eloquent book should help in obtaining that crucial commitment.

Author's Preface

Since the late spring of 1960 I have been gathering a diversity of materials on the lives of the addicted and the way in which they are formed—or, as some would say, deformed.

I have used a "pentagonal" approach. That is, material has been gathered in various ways. Sometimes it has been obtained as a *direct result of a service* done for the addict. It may be part of a screening process, as when a man seeking entrance into East Harlem's Exodus House is seen by the writer as part of the general stress testing which determines whether or not he can take the rigorous program of our organization. A good deal of the material is obtained in hospitals where men have sought individual counseling. These patients agreed, in effect, to exchange whatever wisdom I had for whatever insights they had. There were many sources, but rarely were formalized questionnaires addressed to the addicts. There was in my mind a general outline of questions, but hardly ever was the outline followed in any specific order.

There was a *protest* element in this research approach. I was protesting to the addicts, in effect, that they were not being reasonable in allowing themselves to be absorbed in a fruitless and endless battle with the law. Wouldn't it be better, I would say, if you found a more rational form of existence than addiction? On the other hand, I was protesting on behalf of the addicts, and in a number of papers I have attempted to give their point of view and their sense of what was happening to them. Some men would come expressly to protest and I have been a concerned though, I hope, neutral listener.

A third way in which I have been able to secure material has been through the writing of *stories, plays,* and *poems,* hopefully to be read by addicts as well as nonaddicts, but to be commented upon by the addicts as to the veracity of the insights. It was helpful from time to time to have an addict say that what I had said made sense. It was equally relevant if, for example, he felt no resonance in a story.

A fourth approach has been that of straight *observation*—walking and talking with addicts in diversified places, including prisons, hospitals, the streets, their homes, and other locales where they are found. Through this sort of direct confrontation I have sought to establish the addict within the context of his cultural habitat.

Finally, I have been trying to see the addicts in terms of a set of *basic concepts* that would apply not only to addiction to drugs but to addiction in general. As time has gone on I have sought to construct a series of conceptual schemes ranging from the purely poetical to the impersonally "scientific," hoping that this set of ideas would be of value not only to myself but to anyone who is interested in the problem of addiction.

In general, I have not paid people to talk to me. Service has been the payment for their trust, action, and advice. However, in at least one case I felt that, regarding publication, a man deserves money for giving the publisher the right to publish his life story. It should be said, however, that the question of money came *after* the taping.

The taped material has been selected to illustrate some of the processes and patterns described in the text, but because of obvious space limitations, many points do not find their taped echo. All three of the men whose portraits are presented have given their written consent to the publication of their tapes.

I should emphasize that the portraits and cameos have been chosen to represent various styles of addict life. Other portraits could have been selected to illustrate the unities and diversities of addict existence. I do not think that I can be accused of "loading the dice" in favor of any over-all theory of addiction although I must admit the tapes will show a certain predilection for one or another theory of psychodynamics. I hope that each reader will give the material the attention it deserves and will himself try to interpret the materials, understanding that what is needed is a dialogue and not a set of formulae which will answer all questions about drug addiction.

Finally, let me add that I do not rely exclusively upon these tapes for my understanding and interpretation of the individual life in question. Very often I know a good deal about a man before I see him in an interview. If a man comes to Exodus House for help, we will have seen each other often, particularly after he is screened by me in interviews. So, for example, the man I called Joseph, whose cameo appears in this book, was seen by me and, as a matter of fact, came to me on his own while he was in a pretherapy stage, to unload himself of terrible problems that had been besetting him. These counseling sessions merged neatly, imperceptibly into screening sessions and I have since seen him after these taping sessions when he has brought me individual dreams or problems for consultation. In short, the taping material was part of a research relationship which is, in turn, part of a larger relationship that the man and I have to the Exodus House Program. I receive insights and cues from other members of the staff so that my own personal biases are, at least in part, counteracted. If the reader will understand this, he will also understand that sometimes I cannot give the full basis for my interpretation of a particular point because the source material may have been given to me outside the tape situation and in confidence. Obviously, I cannot discuss in any detail the admission by a man of some homosexual act of which he is very ashamed unless he authorized me to do so. Acts which the man would not want to reveal in public obviously cannot be discussed, but they will necessarily affect me and my interpretation of the man's life. I do believe that I have been scrupulous in protecting such confidences and also in preserving accuracy.

PART I

MYTHS AND SUBSTANCE
OF ADDICTION

CHAPTER 1

Mysteries and Models

The Existential Drugs

Laymen who read about drug addiction are by now fairly familiar with the names of drugs which plague the police, upset public health officials, and produce the outlines of a social problem. Heroin, morphine, marijuana, cocaine, and now the barbiturates, amphetamines and hallucinogens such as LSD, these are some of the principal villains or heroes in this great drama, the designation of each depending upon the position of the observer.

Some of the characteristics which allegedly inhere in drugs are as familiar as these names. Yet we have to be especially careful in assessing and classifying drugs. The name that is given to a drug classification may in some subtle way even affect the behavior of the person who uses it. Take, for example, the common notion that alcohol is a "stimulant." Pharmacologically, as is known to some people, alcohol is a depressant, for it relaxes the central nervous system. However, the fact that it is called a stimulant and does at first *briefly* act as one influences people who look to alcohol for a "lift."

In the middle years of the 1960's a great deal of public attention has been focused on LSD-25, with the term "mind altering" or "mind expanding" being applied to the drug. It is no accident that in a *Life* magazine article photographs of intellectuals such as mathematicians were presented with captions of a line or two purporting to

3

describe the intellectual functions of the drug. One had to be careful to take into account the photographs, also included in the article, showing the utter terror generated by LSD and indicating the "mind-annihilating" possibilities contained within it.

From a sociological perspective, there is a shortcoming in classifying drugs merely according to their apparent psychophysical or physiological effects. These are relevant, but they do not encompass the whole "nature" of the drug. I want now to suggest an over-all category for psychochemical drugs such as those I have been talking about. Let us call them "existential."

I am suggesting here that the person who takes these drugs, be they narcotics, barbiturates, amphetamines, hallucinogens, or others, is making a decision, whether he knows it or not, which can significantly alter the course of his life. The unwanted life change may occur in part because of the drug's real or fancied pharmacological, physiological, or pyschological basis. But as important or perhaps even more important is its sociological status. Drugs which are illegal to possess or to sell involve the user, whether he likes it or not, in a potential or actual intrusion by the state into his own life. This is not an accidental feature. If a person smokes marijuana in New York City he is exposing himself to some, though slight, possibility for intervention by the police. The chances for intrusion will rise for drugs such as heroin, and, paradoxically, for LSD thanks to the publicity given to it. From a user's point of view, this illegality and the threats of punishment come to be attributes of the drug itself.

The existential drugs represent the *stretching of human limits* in an age in which wide-ranging scientific exploration has included penetration to the limits of "inner" space, that which is within man himself. The heroin addict, as I shall show, has massive social pressure on him. The LSD user experiences a recurrent unpredictable internal explosion. Existential drugs can be seen as personal expeditions to explore what man is really like and how far he can go and still remain human. These explorations, scientific and lay, come as no accident in an age in which concentration camps have been turned into laboratories for macabre experiments testing the human equation grotesquely and raising the question of what makes up human nature.

By virtue of their pharmacological, physiological, psychological, and sociological attributes, existential drugs perform in an almost routine way similar kinds of existential testing. Users and addicts experience private worlds in which they "stand out" by challenging some aspect of their nature. One day—some day—they wake up to discover they have passed the point of no return. Sometimes this is done almost consciously, if only as a matter of rationalization. The user may seek to find out about his inner nature by treating his body as a kind of test tube and acting as the observer of his own reactions. But he is doing more than that. Because these are existential drugs, he is also testing the impact of his conduct upon a given social system with its legal machinery and moral fiber. If he uses amphetamines in Greenwich Village he knows that he will find small groups of people who will welcome him—if he also has supplies or a "connection." He also knows that if he takes peak amounts of the drug he runs the danger of a quasi-psychotic response and looks, almost instinctively, to the group to help him weather the trauma caused by the chemical. What is more existential in character than a challenge to one's own sanity? This is the frequent effect of the amphetamines and LSD. But equally upsetting to the equilibrium of a person, and equally a challenge to the very structure of his existence, is a drug such as heroin, which exposes him to a whole culture tied to the underworld, the prison world, and the hospital world, in which a leading question is how to get rid of the habit. If the amphetamines directly assault the mind and, hence, the psychological basis of one's own existence, the opiates and particularly heroin call into question control over one's own existence. Existential drugs and reactions in effect take over the responsibilities of life itself. The observer has the feeling that, at a certain point, if the person becomes excessively involved in the drug, it is hard to know who is talking, the person or the drug. The very nature of freedom is continually re-examined by addicts in their behavior.

Drugs such as doriden hypnotize the mind of the user and particularly the addict (who pops them down like candy) to the point of amnesia and irrationality. What can the man say of his life if, after taking doses of this drug, he cannot recall what he has done for hours at a stretch and discovers, sometimes to his horror, from eyewitnesses that he acted in a way he would "ordinarily" not act?

Does this not suggest that this existential drug sets up a connection between the surface life a man lives and a life he might live, a subterranean existence, that waits below, a porter knocking for admission? In many cases, these existential drugs appear to be the force that volatilizes or energizes a whole sublife quite unknown to the conscious existence of a man and yet in some cases detectable in advance by professional psychiatrists. A point I again want to make is that existential drugs may expose the total or near total nature of the drugtaker, thereby expanding our awareness of his nature and raising the question of his "real identity."

For example, drugtakers insist that marijuana is "not a drug" but just a luxurious cigarette. Anyone who works with people who take existential drugs will have had the experience of being given an apparently logical demonstration that the law regulating the possession and sale of marijuana is irrational. The nub of the proof consists in demonstrating that there are people who use marijuana and never become addicted to other drugs. From this sort of reasoning, the "pro-reefers" argue that any law which is so horrendous as to arrest a man for the possession of a reefer has to be founded in injustice and irrationality. A second line is to point out that one form of marijuana is used as a medication in India, but the same person will not face the fact that marijuana, with the name and quality of hashish, has been blamed for producing several thousand psychotic patients in Morocco.

From my point of view, however, marijuana fits into the category of existential drugs. Not only does it affect the quality of a man's perception of reality, it does more:

Men speak of the giggling perspective it gives them or the frightening perspective occasionally experienced. It makes them more self-conscious—more aware of their being perceived by the outsider. I interpret its reaction as making a man's real identity secondary to his social image. Aside from this, again I would emphasize that its illegality and the chances for the law's intervention are a part of the enterprise of smoking "pot." It is true that in many areas such as East Harlem, where pot is smoked by potheads as well as potential addicts, the police rarely arrest a person for possession of a "reefer." (The exception is where someone openly flaunts the police by smoking a reefer right under their noses.) But the fact that the law is on the books means that when the police make a raid on an apartment they always may justify their intervention if they find reefers. What is a real fact is that when these items are reported to newspapers marijuana is included with narcotics. This kind of error is socially real and a part of the existential reality of being a pot smoker. An error is an error, but is it only an error to the person who is subject to punishment? The truth is he may serve a portion of his real life in prison because of it.

I think it no accident that programs such as Synanon, Daytop Village, and Exodus House, in which drug abstinence is a goal, actively discourage this "smoking." In the history of these programs —and this has happened at least once in each program—the arrest of a man off "hard" drugs for possession of a reefer and his imprisonment for six months has brought home to the members the manner in which "this harmless cigarette that can hurt no one" can bring a man part of the way from the progress he had been making. The law that puts a man in jail for six months for smoking a cigarette sounds horrendous, but it is a reality that each rehabilitation program must reckon with and each addict who has to learn to respect his own existence and values also must face it.

In such ways are these substances "existential." But they are so not only in these terms but in others even more closely related to the concepts of the existentialist philosophers, which we shall examine shortly.

Vogue and Mystery

Mr. G. is an addict. The first day after he came out of jail he took a shot of heroin, but then was able to keep away from "the stuff" for over a week. On the day in question he had visited with his parole officer, had had a good chat with him, and, it being a sunny day in May, he had then decided to walk uptown. Halfway to his destination he met, by "accident," an old flame of his who was on drugs. She complimented him on his appearance, said that she hoped he would keep on doing good, but wouldn't he like to visit her apartment? He said he would like to visit her apartment, and they went up together. According to him, he went there only to sleep with her, but before they got into bed she decided to inject herself with heroin and offered him some. He took a shot and then they went to bed. He spent the whole afternoon there with her, "taking off" several times.

While talking with me the following day he kept asking himself why he had done it. Why had he accepted her invitation, knowing what she really had in mind? Why would she, on the one hand, praise him and, on the other hand, try to entrap him? He felt more and more sure that her reason for doing it was that he was a good hustler, that he could make money for her, and that she could "lay back" and use him to get her heroin. Because he had thought that she liked him for himself, this left him bitter. But why, oh, why, was he letting himself go back into heroin that way?

G.'s story embodies a number of the elements of a modern mystery which a number of vogue words that have come into existence purport to explain. There are some who think in terms of "conditioning theory," while others find it more useful to think of bad habits generally. Still others find the enemy to be "modern society" and particularly "the misery of the downtrodden classes." None of these explanations really seems to help G. satisfactorily explain to himself why, feeling good, being brimful of good intentions, and enjoying a bright May day, he should let himself, against his better judgment, be lured down a poppied road to perdition. The event in its specific details remains a mystery to him.

I start from the penumbra of mystery to reinforce an important point: because of its complications, nobody is really an expert or authority in the field of addiction, and certainly no one can claim to be *the* authority. I say this also because there are repeated claimants to the title of expert and because there is in this field a coterie who are happy to classify and pigeonhole others, feeling that in doing so they have maintained contact with reality.

Recently I heard of a test being given to a number of alleged ex-addicts at a nationally known rehabilitation project. The men were asked to name ten "experts" in the field. The testees were apparently marked according to whether they believed that the number of articles published by a man, as well as his fame in certain cities, was a valid criterion for expertise. Where we have a vogue problem—and drug addiction is one—some of the worst aspects of our promotional civilization—its market mentality, its gross search for publicity, and its divorce from reality—come to the fore. I hope that in this discussion we can be forthright in our acceptance of our limitations in order that we may together explore where more knowledge and understanding are needed.

What does this mystery entail for social scientists?

First, we might ask whether social scientists may not look to the pharmacologists for specific help in understanding the cumulative effects of various drugs upon the user. I am unsatisfied by the reassurances that addicts give me, or those I hear from certain doctors and scientists, that heroin does not really affect the body as much as, let us say, alcohol. Nor am I impressed by the solemn argumentation of "potheads" that "you never heard of anyone getting lung cancer from marijuana, but you know how dangerous cigarettes are. Why can't we smoke our reefers?" For me, the model of pharmacological research is to be found in the painstaking, widespread studies made on cigarettes. There has been no comparable study for marijuana or heroin. When the pharmacologists will have been as well funded as the tobacco research men are, perhaps we will learn significant things about the electrochemical and physiological long-term effects of "existential drugs."

In a similar way, I think we may have been led down a false path by the speed with which the *barbiturates* produce damage to the brain. By comparison with barbiturates, heroin appears to be a relatively harmless drug. Certainly if heroin is regulated, common sense would suggest that so too should be the barbiturates. Meanwhile I am not persuaded by assertions that heroin is innocuous. We need long-range studies on different kinds of constitutions and personalities before accepting the use of existential drugs as merely a private pastime.

But this order of inquiry, while vital to general theory about addiction, does not, I repeat, come close to the kind of question that G. raises. Just why does a reasonable-sounding man act so unreasonably? Why does a man with a plan, real or alleged, permit it to be altered by the appearance of another person with her own plans?

Of course, in our psychologically oriented age, the easy temptation is to answer in terms of G.'s passivity or his frustrations or any of the other variables I alluded to above. I believe a good case could be made in psychological terms, but it would not get at the mystery of this recurrent phenomenon of a man permitting his life to be so contingent that a stray particle across its path diverts it. Even granting the relevance of the psychological variables, there is, I believe, a larger issue at stake that may well take us into the very heart of our civilization's darkness. It is a mystery of mysteries which G. is pointing to when he laments his own lack of will power. He is raising questions of a cosmic significance when he seems to act as though he was predestined to take another shot. Was all this determined some time before meeting the girl? Was perhaps even the decision to go for a walk in some latent way connected to something deeper lying within him and awaiting response? I think his lamentation applies to the nature of our democratic way of life and to the genuine rarity of nobility and excellence. For is he not saying that he wishes he were not somehow obliged to consider the feelings of the other? Does he not wish he were noble enough to feel that he did not have to obey? In a later section I shall return to this theme in discussing the myth of Don Quixote as it applies to the addicts.

In the meanwhile, what I am trying to say here is that we must retain an empirical but existential attitude. We must invoke the knowledge given to us by pharmacology, physiology, psychology, and sociology, but also be prepared to see in addiction a mystery that may go beyond merely empirical realms and have a long-run cosmic meaning.

The Place of Stereotypes in the Treatment of the Addict

There is a favorite game played by many social scientists, consisting in drawing up a list of stereotypes and then showing how superior social science is to the layman's knowledge. It is valuable and important for us to be aware of some of the more glaring misconceptions about the drug addict and his life. I became convinced of this when, invited to speak about sociological aspects of drug addiction, I had to suffer through a technicolor film full of misstatements and errors about addicts. The fact that it was apparently sponsored by the State Education Department only increased my awareness of the place of stereotypes in the treatment of the addict. What could one expect from less official sources if the producers of this film actually believed, as the film action suggested, that the man who pushes marijuana lures innocent virgins into the use of heroin by first inducing them to smoke pot and then tempting them with the virtues of heroin, all in rapid fashion?

It would be of some value if a reputable organization, assisted by people who work with addicts, could make a survey of leading groups in communities where addicts are and are not found, to get an idea of the true quality and quantity of the images of addiction. In the absence of such a study, let me set forth some of the stereotypes I have encountered as held by laymen, the police, addicts themselves, and professional people. Once more, I do not imply that I or anyone else has "the whole truth" about addiction or its images. I do suggest that there is a hierarchy of knowledge or, if you wish, of burnt fingers and stubbed toes, and that this kind of experience, ever more complicated and ever more intense, is what distinguishes those of us who work with addicts from those of us who just verbalize about them.

THE HOSTILE LAYMAN

The stereotypes of the hostile layman are perhaps projections of his own anxieties more than they are of the facts of the case. However, they do mirror a certain reality more appropriate to a past age than to the present.

The hostile layman visualizes the drug addict in aggressive terms. For example, he may characterize "the addict" as a sex fiend, this idea being an anachronism from a period when cocaine was the dominantly preferred drug. He may add to this sexual idea that of pure violence, and see the drug addict as an assaultive or murderous character. Sometimes the hostile layman is aware of the legendary interpersonal slickness of the drug addict, and in that case he depicts him in terms not of violence but of aggressive lies and schemes. At this point the image he draws comes close to that of some addicts themselves.

Excluded from the hostile layman's viewpoint of an addict as violent or nonviolent is any possibility that addicts, as human beings, will have a rather complicated set of defenses for their conduct and a complicated body of sentiment and sensitivity which can be harnessed for their rehabilitation. The notion that an addict might feel guilty about what he does is excluded from this kind of thinking.

THE FRIENDLY LAYMAN

Stated in broadest terms, the friendly layman has accepted the notion of the addict as a sick person. This leads him to visualize the addict as a man who belongs in a hospital under care. What the specific ailment is, he is likely not to know, or perhaps his theory will vary depending on his own psychological understanding and training. He may be thinking of other compulsions which he has observed. He sympathetically emphasizes withdrawal symptoms as a basis for his opinion of why a person remains "hooked."

Characteristically, the friendly type of layman sees the addict as essentially passive, but moved out of his nonviolence by forces outside his control, especially the pain of withdrawal. It is to the friendly layman that the stereotyped picture of the addict kicking his habit under impossible duress makes its basic appeal even though the contemporary addict rarely develops that kind of habit because of the depreciating quality of the drug on the market.

THE POLICE IMAGE

The experience of the police at once makes them better acquainted with the addict than are most professionals, and yet at the same time it may distort their perception of the information they get. This is understandable because their system of informers places in their hands an unrivaled body of personal information about the patterns and the ways of local addicts as well as about their participation or non-participation in crimes. On the other hand, the police see the addicts "at their worst." They see them under the spur of need or pseudo need. They see them living in basements and on roofs. They see them violating even their own negative codes. They see how addicts can be manipulated under temptation with drugs, or with the threat of forced withdrawal. The police rarely see the addict engaging in a purely voluntary humane act.

And the result is that, whatever they may publicly say, some policemen who work with addicts may treat them, if not as animals, then as subhumans. It is only in the light of these stereotypes that one can account for the repeated, independently presented reports about police brutality offered by numerous addicts coming in on their own to agencies such as Exodus House. Stories are legion of police compelling addicts to strip down in hallways and to submit to search even though other people are walking in and out.

The police theory concerning proper treatment of addicts follows from their denigrating stereotype. Stern discipline on the street, swift arrest, and enforced stay behind bars—this is policy. Whether the place of confinement should be called a hospital or a prison and whether or not the prisoner should have psychiatric help mark the difference in attitude between the moderate and the conservative policeman.

For the policeman, unlike the friendly layman, the "pushers" are not the main target. The friendly layman believes that the good kid is lured by the malevolent pusher, for whom he would advocate long-term sentences. The police are not deceived by this distinction, and point out that addicts actually induce other addicts by example if not by actual persuasion. However, police spokesmen are willing to accept extended imprisonment for pushers because so many addicts, in fact, do push.

As I suggested, there are moderate policemen who believe that some kind of compulsory hospitalization for an extended period would be more satisfactory than other methods. They believe that only through such strong measures will the evil and deficient character of the weak addict be transformed and matured.

Such a view of the addict is a result of the peculiar combination of detailed information and the policeman's own aggressive stance toward what he feels to be a menace to society.

THE MEDICAL STEREOTYPES

I suppose that the opinions of doctors vary with the quality and frequency of their interaction with addicts. Leaving aside these differences, which, of course, are important, I have the impression that psychiatrists who work with addicts sometimes relate to them also in terms of their own general approach to the emotionally disturbed. Freudians and neo-Freudians appear to have different styles and approaches to addicts, although they tend to converge in their practices. However, where a medical practitioner does tend to be biased, the word most frequently used by those who have contact with the addict is "immature." The adjective presupposes a perspective, that of the conventional social class system to which the professional belongs, and in which "maturity" seems too often to mean taking on the emotional tone of the new professional classes.

Doctors particularly resent the addict's patterns of self-medication and self-classification. Listening to group therapy and "bull sessions," I am continually amazed that doctors do not understand the place of addict knowledge and expertise in the preservation of the addict's own personal identity. When addicts insist that they are not immature they are not thinking along the same lines as professionals. An addict feels he is responsible when he is meeting the needs of his habit. The doctor who calls him "irresponsible" is thinking in terms of his duties to his family or to himself. When the addict emphasizes his cleverness, intelligence, and reasoning powers he is thinking of his ability to maintain a habit. The doctor who emphasizes his lack of judgment is thinking of the high cost the addict is paying for his way of life. A synthesis of both points of view would obviate this stereotyping process.

In listening to doctors, I also find that they share with the friendly layman a tendency to assume that addicts are nonviolent people. Sometimes they are rudely shocked when a specific addict "acts up" because he is deprived of his methadone or other medication. But the doctors tend to say this is the exception to the rule. In a similar way, these doctors are prone to put stress on the voluntary nature of treatment and only with some experience do a number of them come to favor a more flexible treatment system.

THE EX-ADDICTS' STEREOTYPES

In places such as Synanon and Exodus House ex-addicts are an integral part of the treatment process. How do they view their former associates? No generalizations are possible since different ex-addicts in different programs seem to act differently and to think differently. There is one thing, however, I believe they have in common: the ex-addict finds it essential to distinguish himself from his former associates, intellectually and emotionally. He finds it convenient, if not essential, to think that to be an addict is to be stupid.

He may or may not accept the psychiatric or psychological vocabulary or concepts, since these might vary with his own education and background. But some ex-addicts tend to be more favorable to or to find more utility in their own experience than in contact with professional doctors. More than one ex-addict has told me that he thinks he learned a lot as an addict, and he would never have learned about human nature had he "not gone to school in the street as a junkie." Implied in this dualism—that of a stupid addict with "educative addiction experience"—is the notion that through suffering a person taps levels of experience which cannot be gotten any other way. Whether nonaddicts suffer the same way, whether in fact they do not learn by their own suffering, is a question not often articulated by these ex-addicts.

What is also striking about some ex-addicts is their willingness to "buy" one-word clichés about their associates. Thus, the epithet "stupid" used so often by Synanon may have its rehabilitation impact, but is scarcely suitable in describing tens of thousands of men and women of the most diversified kinds. Or when an ex-addict who has gone to the Psychiatric Hospital at Rio Piedras for rehabilitation comes home, refers to ex-addicts as "psychopaths," and emphasizes exclusively his own skill as an addict in manipulating, he is again overemphasizing one dimension of the problem. As the portraits and cameos presented in this book indicate, there is a rich diversity of addict life styles.

THE ADDICTS THEMSELVES

Finally, I must point out that in talking with addicts over the years I, as well as others in the field, have been impressed with the mixture of truth and error in their self-descriptions. I am not speaking here merely of their facile attempts to justify what they do on the basis of survival needs, which certainly suggest a "psychopathic" concern with physiological needs. I am thinking rather of their attempts to depict themselves as essentially innocent people who are normal, or as normal as "anybody else," if they have their drug. The picture is of a group of men and women who, like diabetics, "function" when they have their particular form of insulin, which in this case is the drug. The onus is at once transferred, of course, from the individual to society or to society's agents, such as the police. Thus, the addict's stereotype presupposes a ritual drama in which he is the immediate victim and the police the immediate villain. Beyond that, there is the ultimate victim which, of course, is not only the addict, but society, which, by generating brutalizing pressures upon the addict, causes him to make depredations on a large scale and to waste his labor power and talent.

There are addicts who stress the high percentage of talented members among them. For many years, from many addicts, I have heard talk of artistic, musical, literary, and other talent. I must confess, however, that, while there is a considerable body of folk literature called "Toasts"* among them, and while I have seen some good paintings done by addicts, read an occasional good poem by an addict, and have enjoyed many jam sessions by addict musicians, it is my opinion that they appreciate or believe they appreciate more than they create. Here, too, the argument seems to be implied that were they given their heroin they would produce much more for the national cultural capital. They imply, too, that there is something about heroin itself which would enable them to do this. (Other addicts, who are more careful, are inclined to scout the myth of addict talent and to deny that heroin encourages the development of such talent.)

* Definitions of addict jargon are given in a Glossary on page 345.

Like the friendly critic, the addict sees himself as an essentially passive or nonviolent person and argues that only the exceptional addict resorts to violence. When it is pointed out to him that there are increasing numbers of men who "take off" addicts, as well as nonaddicts, he is forced to admit that the facts are correct but that these people are operating under extreme psychological conditions or are atypical. The image is of an aggressive society and an unaggressive addict.

Addicts are also somewhat ambivalent on the question of their own stealing patterns. On the one hand, they will usually deny that they like to steal. They will say that their habit forces them to steal. On the other hand, close interviewing will bring out that, even before many of them became drug users, some types of addicts were actively engaged in antisocial activities which occasionally, if not frequently, involved the taking of property. The fact that among these were some men who did not reach the eyes of the law is helpful in preserving the stereotype.

In general, the addict's mechanism for preserving his stereotype is to deny the validity or relevance of evidence which suggests a wide range of patterns beyond that described in the addict's own stereotype.

A particularly curious illustration of these tendencies appears in interviewing men who have pushed drugs for any length of time. Aware of the general popular indignation against "pushers," the man who is pushing or who has pushed will say he didn't make a profit out of his activities. All he did was to cover his need for drugs, his rent, and some money for clothing, and so on. This is true even of the "successful" pusher. By showing himself and, presumably, his auditor that he makes no profit, he gives himself the image of a nonprofit businessman, an altruistic person. Generally this is followed by a request that the police turn their attention to the upper echelon of the hierarchy and away from the small fry. The pusher does not properly calculate and evaluate how much money he is making because his frame of reference is that of the Profit System. By importing an ideal from the square culture, the pushing addict is able to escape what he feels is the popular scorn for the pusher and the profiteer.

Although stereotypes are rigid constructs, I have the impression that some of the groups who hold them about the addict are not immutably devoted to them. First, there are many groups who, in point of fact, are indifferent to addicts and do not harbor strong ideas about the subject. If they have stereotypes, and it is likely that they do, these ideas are changeable. This is true even of those who are hostile laymen living in a neighborhood which may be a market area or be near a market area. This is all the more true, I believe, of hostile laymen who have little to do directly with the addicts, but who pick up attitudes through newspaper reports and hearsay.

I think that newspapers, particularly the yellow press, do a disservice both to the public and to the addicts by their repeated sensationalizing of information, even information which seems to be concerned with helping the addict. I would extend this comment even to reports on nonaddictive drugs such as LSD. While I would not attribute the increase in usage of LSD to newspaper and magazine articles, there is little doubt in my mind that giving notoriety to drug use, and particularly showing fairly intelligent and/or creative people making use of the drug for "mind expanding needs," gives a hallmark of sanction to more unstable adolescents and early adults who are looking for "kicks" or "instant communion," and who want to find a rationalization for indulging in LSD. (Similarly the "epidemic" of heroin use in the 1950's was sparked by its notorious use by prominent jazz musicians.)

Veteran addicts in the 1960's have told me repeatedly about their own feelings that the press in the early 1950's was actually calling the attention of youngsters who had no knowledge of drugs to the "kicks" that could be gotten from them. Television programs have shown drug addicts at work with the whole apparatus being visible. I find it amazing that these programs did not call forth protests from parents of youngsters of an impressionable age. These programs may have been designed to alert the public and to break old stereotypes, but they also create new ones.

Some critics will argue that I have constructed new stereotypes, that in point of fact the categories or opinions set forth above are not faithful representations which would result from an exact sampling of respective populations. For example, would all doctors or laymen or ex-addicts share the tendencies described?

I have not been able to determine through my qualitative research all shades of opinion about addiction and their relative frequencies. What I hope the reader will gather from my sketchy presentation is, first, a recognition of the incompleteness of current opinion about drug addiction; second, an idea of the unfairness of much of that opinion; third, and perhaps most important, a sense of the pariahhood of addiction. It is essentially the evidence of the alienated condition, of the anguish of the addicts, as I shall call it, which shows up time and again when nonaddicts speak "in confident ignorance" of this much-misunderstood minority group. Anyone who has seen an ex-addict vehemently calling an addict stupid comes to realize that such an ex-addict is now as concerned with keeping himself from the temptations of addiction as in treating the addict. The so-called friendly layman may turn out to be someone who is really using the addict or the addict's thefts for his own gain, and hence views the addict not as a person but as an object.

I do not say that there are not those among us who can relate to the addict as a person, but I would suggest that honest examination will show that, thanks to such conditions as the consequences of the laws governing the addict, as well as the power of the popular morality concerning drug use, some degree of separation between the addict and one who is trying to work with him is inevitable.

In this regard, we may compare the alcoholic with the drug addict. Medical textbooks used to describe the addict and the alcoholic in similar terms, stressing their common unreliability and attraction to their respective drugs. But until recently an alcoholic was never referred to as an addict. I believe that part of this linguistic distinction comes from the fact that there have always been many more alcoholics than drug users, but part of the explanation also lies in the associations of drug use. One of these associations is with the laboratory, and it has always seemed to the popular mind, as shown in mass media, movies, and stories, that anyone who makes his body a laboratory is a man apart. A Frankenstein monster walking among us would be the implied image. Secondly, I believe that there is in this attitude to the drug a residue of hostility toward contributions from the Orient. The image of the mysterious, inscrutable Oriental may well linger in the attitude toward the opiate and the opiate user. At any rate, the joint effect of these two associations added to the historical treatment of the addict and his response to those laws have given us a picture of a man apart. The various categories of opinion I have described above reflect this picture in various ways.

CHAPTER 2

Notes on the Heroin Addict and His Culture

Some Types of Addict Life Style

Earlier I pointed out some of the leading contenders for *the* addict stereotype, and I suggested that it would be good to realize how diversified are the addicts. Let me now point out that in a truly scientific description of addiction, or even of one addict, we should have knowledge on four levels of reality: the pharmacological, the physiological, the psychological, and the sociological. At the present stage of drug addiction study, it is not possible to set up equations or models describing the interaction of these variables. On the other hand, to say that we need basic research on all these levels is almost superfluous. This pressing need explains why no one is in a position to be satisfied about the way he classifies addicts and addiction.

From time to time we do find writers purporting to give shorthand summaries of what they take to be the essence of the addict. I pointed out some of the phrases earlier. Let me add that the word "irresponsible" or the phrases "escaping from reality" and, more recently, "character disorders" are used to summarize the nature of their problem.

I have the impression that sometimes this sort of oversimplification is partly a result of too little contact with addicts and partly, where there is contact, a result of the nature of the addicts themselves. That there are few inspiring and exuberant figures among the addicted discourages some nonaddicts from enjoying being with them. Or if they do exuberate under the influence of heroin, a little knowledge and insight reveals that the man or woman is playing Pagliacci to the crowd. So, for example, a man I know has a fund of bittersweet shafting humor, and his appearance in a street crowd is a moment for big smiles and guffaws. He presents this picture to his friends, but to a psychiatrist whom he trusts he describes his depression at being unable to reconcile himself to an identity crisis of being caught between Jewish and Negro parents. Or another man whose humor is much more bizarre and whose conversation is more difficult to follow is the butt and source of humor. But, again, the addicts who enjoy his talk do not sense the multiple conflicts he has about his identity. I suspect that not many professionals enjoy working with so dolorous a problem. Hence there is a tendency to paint the addict in somber, monotonous colors.

Let me now suggest that it is useful to think of a number of characteristic life styles that overlap. We have to consider men who range from mildly to severely disturbed, as tending to live out fairly pathological lives, often in the absence of the drug itself.

Let me, in a preliminary way, warn the reader that what follows is a tentative exploration, and that I, myself, have more than one way of classifying the lives of the drug addicts. Classifications, after all, depend upon the purposes of the classifier at the time as well as the state of his own orientation to the problem. Moreover, it is likely that some other person who has worked with addicts may come up with quite a different classification. *What counts is that the reader feel the resemblances and differences between the people he knows as nonaddicts and those who take drugs.*

I would also like to emphasize the fact that, to a degree, these are imperfect ideal types. I do not wish to caricature Max Weber's concept of ideal types, and, to repeat, I do not want to risk the accusation that I have constructed stereotypes in their place. As the reader will soon see, I have chosen my types according to the way in which an addict's behavior will reflect some special emphasis or basic feeling about his world. These types of existence are *tendencies* and may well overlap in concrete reality. What I have done is to take the gamble that these tendencies may be isolated for the purpose of illuminating the lives of drug addicts.

First, let me give an over-all view of these types, always remembering that there are many more available and that I have selected those that I regard as theoretically significant.

The drugtaker, especially the illegal drugtaker, has to concern himself almost entirely with getting money and acquiring the drugs on which he depends. To do so, he has to manipulate reality, himself and others, behind a pretense whose style and content will vary with the individual. I suggest that one form of the drugtaking "life" puts its main stress and gets its predominant form from the "phoniness" flowing from this "economic sphere." I classify this form of existence as the *life of pseudo self* or the *pseudo life*.

A second form seems to survive by sheer apathy and passivity. The user "rents out his works," and in other ways exemplifies the *passive life*.

A third form of existence is shaped by the manner in which a man will keep on using drugs even though the original meanings of drugtaking have disappeared. This kind of *obsessional life* streams from the frequent cycle or movement detectable in many drug addicts; from enchantment to disenchantment, from "charisma" to routine, from enthusiasm to ritual. The content of this life seems less important than its frames of reference.

A fourth form of life among drugtakers is an expression of antagonism to the society which frames laws making the life of the addict a burden and to the "responsible citizens" who look down upon the drug addict as a mere animal being. This expression of hostility or resentment I take to be a part of the *paranoid life*.

Next, I wish to call attention to the *depressed life* as the abiding and predominant tone of the man or woman who keeps on resorting to drugs and who experiences only negative gratification and a corresponding psychological change within him.

Finally, there is the man who uses the drug to express the dividedness and alienation he sees in and around him. This is the *retreatist life pattern*.

THE PSEUDO LIFE

The pseudo life is lived out most dramatically by the con man. It is organized around a set of "false signals" beamed to observers by the drug user to set up impressions about his own intentions, attributes, and history. This life pattern feels like real life, but is counterfeit. It is predatory in nature, in that the con man receives rewards of profit and kicks for implanting ideas which his victim misinterprets. Essential to the pseudo life is the establishment of pseudo identities, masquerades, and false self-images which the drugtaker may even join his victim in believing. The irony of such an existence is that at length the person can experience vitality only from the mistakes he causes others to make. Furthermore, his success is usually based on his exploitation of phoniness in his victim, which means, in turn, that the addict becomes increasingly certain that the world outside of him is totally fraudulent.

At bottom the pseudo life is a parasitical one, in which one person, by distorted communication, uses others' strengths and weaknesses upon which to batten. Given the nature of the premises and conclusions that govern such a life, it is almost to be expected that a person existing by it would in the course of things need to believe his own distortions.

A person who lives the pseudo life may or may not experience guilt feelings concerning these tendentious messages. In the typical case, guilt is at a minimum. This has to do with the fact that the pseudo life arises because a person may have been warped or so threatened that his physical survival at one time or another in his life appeared to be a matter of chance. For a person who feels continuously threatened with extinction, the vital lie, like the Platonic myth, carries its own justification. Naturally, if a person comes to believe that the pseudo life is real, he has no need to experience guilt. The existential cave in which he lives, with its distorted shadows, becomes existence itself.

The pseudo life is lived in the ambit of a series of markets, and the person experiences himself competing with other " personalities" to make the best impression. Consciously or not, he distrusts others who are going through the same sort of pseudo life, and he is easily tempted to put down others whom he doesn't trust anyway.

Though most men in conventional and unconventional society engage in some self-misrepresentation, the drugtaker of the type I have in mind is dependent upon such false images for his very existence. He would destroy anyone—in theory—who destroys these images which he worships as the source and strength of his existence. Without his "front" he is nothing.

It follows from these attributes that the person who lives the pseudo life is living on thin ice and must continually be anxious. One use of the drug for such a man is precisely for control of his anxiety so that he can carry out his masquerade with aplomb and success. Another consequence of the pseudo life and its anxiety is the underlying and terrible *sense of rage* at having continually to bring truth and error into consistency. The fact of the strain of continually acting out a myth that can be questioned at any point almost suggests that the person who lives the pseudo life wants to be punished, wants to be caught by some terrible agency which will administer punishment that in some way he may deserve. He wants to be damaged, even destroyed, even as he wishes to damage and destroy the manipulated other, especially the naïve observer, the square, who will be taken in by the con game which turns out to be one element in the conning of the pseudo life.

In fact, the one who lives a pseudo life may come to depend on a drug such as heroin in order to permit him to carry out the "acting" that is its indispensable element. Moreover, by becoming dependent on the drug he gets a sense of reality, a relentless and real drive to get money to get his drug. Hence imperatives generated by the compulsion to take more drugs give a reality core to a fake life.

THE PARANOID LIFE

If in the pseudo life drugs provide a substance of reality which gives a flow to a life of fiction, the paranoid life has no such problems. The man who lives such a life is overly conscious of the impact of what he feels to be a hostile reality. He does not "act" or "pretend" that his messages are real. He "knows" that his reality is hostile and that it calls for appropriate reactions. In the pseudo life reality is a kind of thin ice. The paranoid life is reality composed of steamy stalactites all aimed at the person himself. Such a man needs drugs to quell the anxieties and the rages that engulf him when he considers his misfortune in being born out of joint or at a time which is manifestly inhuman.

If life is so dangerous, then the person who lives it must be eternally vigilant, for this is the price of his survival as well as his liberty. The vigilance that is eternal is full of stress and strain, and this is costly to him physically, psychologically, and socially. These costs must be paid, and it is to the interest of the person who lives the paranoid life that he gets the society that hates him to pay for it. The drugtaker's paranoid life contains its own justifications for making depredations upon the society that bars him from his drug or from alleviating the strain of enduring life within a hostile world.

The paranoid life is lonely because it is based on the premise of the need for suspicion of other people. Its spirit is that the only person you can trust is yourself, and this is itself problematical given the way in which the paranoid life induces a man to dangerously impulsive acts of violence without rhyme or reason. Even on drugs of the narcotic type, people who live the paranoid life may not be fully appeased and may go around looking as though they want to destroy anyone or anything in sight. One mechanism by which the paranoid tends to reduce his own fears and rage is through derogation of others. After all, if you can feel honestly that some people, if not all people, are inferior to you in strength or in cunning or reputation, to that extent you have reduced the effectiveness of the hostile world's attempts to destroy you. You are not at home in the world, but at the same time you have reduced its jungle aspect by just so much.

The paranoid mode of life also has as an element something of a search for paradise. Paradoxically, the person who is enraged with the world around him may often be trying in some way to restore some lost period of innocence, of joy now denied him. The memory of this period may be one of the themes in his life. Hence we would expect that some people who live this life may react to a drug such as heroin as though they were children suckling at the breasts of their mothers.

THE PASSIVE LIFE

This is the label most commonly used in articles and books about addicts. As in a play such as *The Connection,* the theater and the films, when describing the addict, have sought to dramatize this form of existence. Actually one can distinguish at least three variants of the passive life: the indifferent, the dependent, and the aggressive.

The indifferent form has as its theme "I can't do much about life, but then it really isn't worthwhile anyway." This kind of feeling, I suppose, is found among all addicts, but in this indifferent life the feeling of worthlessness of living comes to the surface in an emphatic way. The man who is a "greasy junkie" just doesn't think it worth the effort to do anything except get his fix. Off drugs, he says he has no "drive," and looks around to depend on welfare or chance opportunities. For him there is little of the blasé attitude found among the "cool" youngsters. His indifference stems from weariness or apathy, a sense of defeat which may be there even though he has not really fought and lost. In a sense he depends on not being open so as not to have to fight.

The second form is that of the dependent man. He may care somewhat for his situation or his life, but faced with the complexity and, as he sees it, the cruelty of reality he decides that it is better to look around for some strong figure to make life a little easier, maybe a strong woman or a strong program or a strong father. In any case, he will essentially transfer the responsibilities of growing up and fulfilling his social obligations to some other person. The formula is, "If I have no strength, I'll borrow it." On drugs, he is likely to be the sort of person who acts as a flunky or who, if he is lured into burglarizing, will be the lookout. He will not initiate forays but may well carry suggestions to others about possible "scores" by which they can make money.

Thirdly, there is the passive person who at times surprises everyone by striking out in an aggressive way. This passive man cares even more about himself than the dependent one and really deplores his own impotence and passivity. For one reason or another, and often through anxiety, he is simply unable to get a measure of self-control. His despair mounts and, with the despair, irritation, embarrassment, and anger generated by people upon whom he might be depending, and he will then, unwittingly or wittingly, hurt somebody verbally or physically. Sometimes his aggression is turned inward. He acts as though shooting up his drug were a form of punishment.

Often in the addict culture he has a bad reputation. He is unreliable, moody. Often he takes the drug wholly unconsciously to offset these periodical outbursts. His formula seems to be, "If I can't create, at least I'll destroy." Whatever the variation, such passive lives find a pharmacological resonance in the nature of heroin. The depressant that relaxes them is an echo of their own desire not to move the world *but to be moved along with it*.

THE DEPRESSED EXISTENCE

The "depressed life" really makes an extended system of puns out of the word "depressant," going beyond pharmacological discussions of the effect of the drug upon the central nervous system.

As regards the future, the depressed life is a movement downward. The person feels as though his chances for failure, no matter how defined, are greater than his chances for success. As regards the present, he experiences the time as oppressive, boring, empty, in short, a bale of hours that keeps him from moving. Finally, the inertia of the present and the pessimistic sense of the future are extended back in time to the past, although they may be intermingled with some gay colors of good fortune that is no longer retrievable.

Since all experiences within time tend to be against the individual, understandably he seeks some kind of resolution in an existence out of time. Hence the depressed life is accompanied by frequent ideas of, and even attempts at, suicide. Death appears to be more of a friendly stranger than it would be to other people. The upshot of this and the other attributes of the depressed life is a distinctive gray coloration placed upon one's existence. There are no highs, or almost no highs, and no lows, or almost no lows, except through the direct intervention of the drug. One of the functions of the drug for the depressed life is to reintroduce ebb and flow on a regular and apparently spontaneous basis. It seems to call for some kind of exciting break. Depending on a number of factors, the depressed life may invoke the use of amphetamines, hallucinogens, cocaine and marijuana, among others. These would be a sort of salt and pepper to life's meal. On the other hand, others of the depressed life may invoke barbiturates, heroin, and hypnotics and experience them as "stimulants." This may be contrary to the expectations of the pharmacologists, but has been observed by more than one of us in the case of addicts.

From the point of view I have been espousing, it is understandable that the depressed life begs for existential drugs. One of the effects of drugs of any kind is to introduce a mood element which varies the emotional tone of the person through introducing contrasts in the height and depth of the emotions. The depressed person then gets the simulacrum of real life with its joys and sorrows—something he has missed in his attempt to curb some deep fear he has about the expression of rage or other strong emotion.

THE OBSESSIONAL LIFE

The obsessional life is oriented around ritual and codes with a compulsive obedience to both. Though the codes may tend to be those of the underworld, the man or woman who adheres to them justifies such adherence in lofty, noble terms. The obsessional life attains a measure of strength and clarity, as well as of consistency, because it follows certain professions even to the point of self-destruction. How often do some veteran addicts speak with nostalgia of the old days when addicts were addicts, and were looked up to by everybody? The obsessional person may achieve his clarity through contrast with the youngsters, who have no such codes and who apparently live only by impulse and greed.

The obsessional life is a life apparently under the control of the intellect. Here are planning, memory, and reasoning, although all three are under the control of a form of thinking that may have been appropriate to an earlier period in the person's life.

It is characteristic of the obsessional life that it scouts the emotions and suppresses spontaneous displays toward others. The obsessional life seeks in drugs the way of extinguishing the need for tender emotions. It is possible that a Freudian might find in some of these older drug addicts, and especially in the case of men who started using drugs in their thirties or late twenties, a marked Oedipal relationship. In other cases I have the impression that this form of existence is given a certain color and concretion by the use of drugs. The person who can't relax and enjoy himself may be able to do so on drugs. But then, in turn, the drugs themselves and the way of life become incorporated within an obsessional way of thinking so that the addict may appear to be strong but really depends on such a frame of reference as the underworld to allow him a kind of clarity. There is in this sort of life, therefore, a dialectic between spontaneous emotions and set frames of reference.

THE RETREATIST LIFE

Finally, there are those who have a life relatively withdrawn from those around them. Full of anxiety about their neighbors, friends, and family, they prefer to constrict their lives, to set up various façades so as to appear to be normal and to look about vigilantly lest they be forced to expose themselves to some dread danger. Characteristically, they evoke sympathy on the part of their family, for example, the mother or grandmother, but in response they try to pull their rescuer down to the same level of anxiety. The great fear is that of falling apart and for this fear they will use drugs to give a sense of illusory integration. Drugs also give a support to the party wall that separates one's life from that of others.

Such a person is continually involved in a vicious circle where he misperceives the intentions of those around him because he is so anxious. In order to correct the injuries and damages that result from these misperceptions, and to calm himself, he uses drugs. He thereby "elevates" himself all the more, psychologically and socially, and intensifies the chances for misperception. In turn, the damages that produce a sense of disorganization compel him to withdraw all the more, constricting his life all the more, and therefore increasing the chances for misperception. This continuing system of ever-narrowing ripples brings this life closer to something approaching schizophrenia. It is this form of life which has caught the attention of those experts who label all drug addicts as retreatists. In my opinion, it is only one of the types of drug life forms.

This series of life styles, in theory, could be found in the same men before drugs and after their addiction. So far as I know, no long-range research on the impact of addiction on prior life patterns has as yet been carried out.

Until then we will not know whether, and how, a man's addict life style is affected by his preaddiction pattern. Even the effect of the age at which a man began his addiction is not certain, though there appears to be a tendency for some of these late developing addicts to have suffered from a severe obsessional pattern, such as is illustrated by the case of "Manny," reproduced later in the text.

We also need research on what might be called the Jekyll-Hyde complex. A significant number of men report puzzlement and disturbance because, while using drugs, they act quite differently when they do and do not have their drugs. Is this sense of "personality cycling" related to some deeper life style? If existential drugs alter lives radically, then answers to these specific questions are needed.

Finally, I would call the reader's attention to a persistent regressive tendency, a tendency to be infantile, that in varying degrees places a strain upon the addict's basic life style. The infantile desire of the hooked man to have all that he wants when he wants it is a tug in a backward direction. As a result, each of the six life patterns is crisscrossed by "oral tendencies" and "dependency." One can imagine the inner conflicts besetting a man who has been raised in a strict Catholic family when he finds himself violating binding norms because of a need to feed himself like a baby on chemicals that are frowned upon, first, by society and then by himself after he is hooked. Apparently this regressive pattern is most conspicuous in those who even before they were on drugs emphatically showed these demanding traits.

The Curse of the Necessary Extra Dimension

From the point of view of masses of addicted men trying to understand themselves in their moments of intoxicated despair and despondency, there is at least one curse upon them to which they feel they have an answer. I would call it the curse of the necessary added dimension. In an offbeat way the addicted man comes to feel that through his encounter with heroin, and to some extent with the other existential drugs, his life has been altered against his will so as to make him feel that without the drug "something is missing." Without his drug he feels as naked as a scholar without a frame of reference.

The drug experience, repeated not merely for days but for months and years, leaves behind a residue which it is useful to think of as a synthetic instinct. One addicted to an existential drug acts as though he had been changed fundamentally, in that there dwells within him a force requiring its own autonomous satisfactions. It seems to have a memory, will, and style of its own though no addict on the drugs acts identically with another. There are at least minute differences in preferences and sometimes behavioral differences as when, for example, one man may nod continuously and another manage to avoid nodding at least in public.

This synthetic instinct is a convenient name to summarize a series of internalized expectations which create in the addict himself, a feeling of being qualitatively different from anyone else who does not use existential drugs and part of a potential chemical brotherhood with those who do. If the addict does not feel genuinely like a blood brother to his fellow addicts, the reason lies in the manner in which the constant pressure of the contemporary market divides addict from addict as each seeks to minimize his dissatisfactions and all too often interferes with the satisfactions of others.

It is in the nature of existential drugs that after a while the cumulative residue of the experience of daily and continual ingestions makes him feel that he is only normal if he has the extra dimension of chemicalization within himself. I cannot stress too much my feeling that the year 1898, in which heroin was discovered, was a great watershed in human history, for this was the year of the discovery of a process by which man can actually transform the terms of his existence by chemical reaction. Morphine is powerful, but heroin is more so. Man's self-transformation in the direction of simplification, in the direction of adding one single dimension that, in turn, would become more important than all the others, was the crucial meaning of 1898. Whereas in his theory of relativity Einstein gave us an added fourth dimension that *fitted into* three others, heroin became an added dimension that took over the rest of life.

Thus when a heroin addict says that he is missing something and identifies the missing component with the drug itself, I think it would be wrong to assume that he is completely correct in his identification. It is part of the curse of the added dimension for its victim to see merely the surface of his needs. The addict may well crave drugs, but in turn this craving submerges or smothers other needs, other things that he is missing, so that he is feeding the chemical alien within him.

In order that I not be accused of being melodramatic and of falling victim to the hysteria of the popular attitudes, let me explain further that I am not thinking here merely of the chemical by itself, but of the whole complex about which heroin and existential drugs tend to become centered. The man on drugs often has a relentlessly powerful drive that, as is well known, takes energy away from all other spheres of life. He feels a diminished and sometimes extinguished interest in love and sex, although some perverted kind of gratification is obtained from the fact that heroin increases the capacity to prolong the erection. Food is generally less appetizing and less interesting to the man on drugs. He walks and runs, but generally in service to the need to get money and the drug. Thinking and imagining tend to be more and more focused around the needs of the synthetic instinct and not of the natural processes of life.

And yet this total involvement becomes, itself, identified as an added dimension to life. When a man says he is missing *something,* he does not say overtly what is really the case—that he is missing *everything.* A kind of misperception occurs—the whole is identified with one part—but this misperception itself is evidence of the tremendous power that grips the addict.

The idea of an imperious added dimension leads me to make another distinction that may be helpful in understanding the rehabilitation process. The term "detoxification" is used to describe that early stage of any rehabilitation process in which a man's current physical need for heroin is removed as well as any current supply within him. As is generally expressed by workers in the field, getting rid of man's physical dependence is nowadays a simple matter and the real problem of rehabilitation is "working upon his mental dependence or psychological dependence."

From the point of view I am expressing, there is an ambiguity here. I think we must distinguish detoxification from another process I would call "dechemicalization," which is at once chemical, physiological, psychological, and social. Dechemicalization is the process whereby a man is weaned away from the need for the added dimension of drug commitment. The synthetic instinct and the synthetic personality which it generates over time are obstacles to his rehabilitation. Getting rid of this pattern of remembering the experience of having one's body yearn for and be gratified by the added dimension is, however, more than "mental." Some have called it brainwashing, a period of deconditioning or reconditioning, a period of meeting and resolving anxieties that were the trigger for a man's reaching for a chemical; it is a process of reactivating a man's expectations so that he could enjoy life in a new way and without the curse of looking for the added dimension in a chemical that would control him. In any rehabilitation process dechemicalization merges imperceptibly with the reconstitution of the human being himself.

Earlier in this section I suggested what the reader might think is a forced parallel between the discovery of heroin in 1898 and the advancement of the theory of relativity in 1905. I now want to show a deeper parallelism by noting how the very idea of an added dimension of chemicalization in the drug addict connects to the notion of time. Specifically, at least in relation to addicts, I am told that some of heroin's power lies in the drug's *apparent* capacity to bring about rapidly what occurs either more slowly or not at all. I would extend this comment to the other existential drugs, addictive or not. LSD, for example, seems to serve the needs some adolescents in college have for "instant genius." Heroin gives a number of apparent instant gratifications of a seemingly magical kind. Some pills, such as doridens, give instant courage. In short, whatever you value, there seems to be some drug that will give it to you, or at least the appearance of it, in foreshortened time. Time, as a dimension, is thus annihilated magically and replaced by the processes of a drug.

That the experience of time itself is affected by the taking of drugs is well known. How often have amphetamine addicts told us of how they will stare for hours between two steps of working with a tape recorder or stare for hours at a spot that they want to clean before moving to it. Or people who smoke pot will talk about how time seems to be slowed. In short, the added dimension of chemicalization gives the relativity of time a new twist. I would believe, as a matter of fact, that the more we explore the world of the drug addict the more we will see that there are subdimensions within the added dimension, and that one of these is a version of time. Within this subuniverse of addiction basic research may well uncover replicas of the world outside, but replicas turned inside out or in directions we cannot yet fully appreciate.

Jean Paul Sartre says of man, "We are anguish," maintaining that suffering is essentially a part of the human state. If the addict life is a caricature of existence in the "square" world, then one would expect that anguish would be part and parcel of addiction. Yet it is sometimes said that addicts are not anguished, that they feel nothing. Indeed, it is the contention of many addicts and ex-addicts that they do not suffer, that they are pleasure-loving and happy-go-lucky as long as things go right. They point particularly to the "nod" as evidence of this. These forceful assertions notwithstanding, anguish is very much at the heart of addiction, and to what extent this is so can be seen through examining first the nod and then other specimens of addict conduct.

THE AMBIGUITIES OF "THE NOD"

The nod, or "high," is a stereotyped form of addict conduct that results from the ingestion of good heroin. Its quality and depth vary in part with "the system" or tolerance of the addict as well as the quality of the heroin ingested. It is, first of all, useful to see that there are three levels of the nod corresponding to the unconscious, preconscious, and conscious levels in the Freudian topography of the mind. In the very deep nod there is true oblivion; then, moving up, there is the less intense nod in which a man is vaguely aware of the life both inside and outside himself; finally, there is the superficial nod in which he is fitfully awake and asleep, and often falsely conscious of what is happening around him. In the deep nod the man loses touch with the reality outside, and in the superficial nod he is easily irritated into angry awareness.

There is no doubt that the nod is valued as such by addicts. They prefer to nod rather than to sleep. Sleeping, they say, keeps a man from enjoying the nod.

The nod is therefore the culmination of the shot and represents the narcotization and apparent stimulation which the addict craves. It represents the end of striving, the cessation in varying degrees of all troubled reflection as well as the abandonment of all other projects except that of the quest for apparent euphoria and homeostasis.

The nod produces anguish because its standards are ever escalating beyond the capacity of the addict to be satisfied. In the nod, at any of its levels, the addict experiences an expectation of a certain stimulus, and it is in the nature of heroin addiction that as time goes on the nod becomes harder and harder to achieve. This is a Sisyphian task, doomed to failure and anguish, this attempt to meet the internalized expectations of the nod.

Furthermore, an observer watching a man nodding with his head between his knees in a womblike position finds it hard to resist interpreting the image of the addict as a man striving to become newly reborn and detached from some warm inner life at present. This, too, constitutes an unintentional but apparently very real source of frustration to the addict. The nod is a temporary experience; it promises much and in the long run yields only a taste of ashes.

Let us not forget, finally, that the "nod" corresponds with "le néant," or nothingness, which Sartre has found to be the central challenge of human existence. It is part of the cosmic irony of drug addiction that the users of drugs at first see this nothingness as an explosion and are surprised when it does not take place. Then they drink soda pop because their mouth is dry and, lo, they vomit. This period of heaving serves as a contact point of revulsion and nausea to the immediately following experience of euphoria. It is the frame of reference one suspects for euphoria.

As an addict becomes a veteran, his chances for vomiting decrease provided he sticks to heroin. But because of the deteriorating quality of the drug and hence the user's recourse to pills of all kinds and to liquor, vomiting and the presence of its smell continue to plague him. Moreover, the addict who is run down and not eating well may develop indigestion, and may vomit. For some men vomiting becomes a kind of punishment, a means by which the body hurts itself for continuing to be involved in drug addiction. Vomiting, therefore, may in some cases become the overt expression of the anguish of existing as an addict—a psychosomatic moral purgative.

A LIFE OF CONTINGENCY: A DISPENSABLE BEING

But there are other features of the life of the addict by which one can detect its existential anguish. As Sartre has more than once emphasized, it is when a person becomes aware of contingency, that is, the fact that he is dispensable, as is everything around him, that he experiences anguish. It is hard to think of any group that is as aware of its contingency as the addicts. An addict soon learns that he is almost nothing socially, and that the market is everything. Not only must he treat himself as an object, but as a trivial one to boot. If he is arrested, he knows that there will be someone to take his place. Even if he is a pusher, he knows that his arrest today will only mean that tomorrow some other addict will be more than eager to assume the same risks. When he enters jail he knows that he is taking the place of someone who has just been released, that he will be given a number which, from his point of view, is purely accidental, that he will casually be assigned a cell with another person, and that his stay will leave no great impression upon the prison or the population.

He knows, too, that only a few people may think about him, maybe only his mother, and that the world will little note his absence. If he has been a good connection, there will be some men eager to see him again, but only to use him. He knows, therefore, that his presence or absence is of importance only to people like himself, and only in a limited and transient way. This latent anguish bedevils the addict and produces, at bottom, a cynical attitude toward his life. To become completely interchangeable and replaceable, like peat in a bog, and really to have no personal justification that will stand up to inquiry even by himself, in the long run means he must fall short when judged by what might be called existential standards, the standards of the good and valid life. The way seems open only to hopeless nihilism or else to a resolute decision to be responsible to oneself.

It is one of the ironies of drug addiction that a man is compelled, even against his will, to feed his habit, and then to rationalize this as a form of responsibility. But even this feeling of pride in maintaining one's habit yields to a deeper feeling of being indispensable only in a limited way, of being a creature to oneself or at least to a fraction of oneself. In sum, the addict experiences the anguish of being incomplete.

THE THROWBACK TO THE HUNTING ECONOMY

There is even more. There is the feeling that as an addict one is performing acts which fearfully resemble those of a primitive society based on a hunting economy. One is atavistic, a throwback to the time when the ground one ran on led to sites from which one would throw long spears at running targets. In today's urban metropolis the streets and the houses are protected, and the addict hunts, knowing he is hunted by the police and the watchmen and the other squares. The addicts themselves report only the anguish of the overt state of being hunted, but I believe that the larger meanings of their lives, the hunted being hunter and the hunter being hunted, are particular examples of the larger problem that besets them. They live an anachronistic kind of life without many parallels in a life that they were presumably prepared for in their childhood. Even addicts who as children roamed the streets instead of attending school are not likely to have experienced in anticipation the extreme violations and rigid structure of rules and regulations that the adolescent and adult addicts encounter. Alone, and without legal name, the addicted maraud the streets hoping to be invisible, seized by the desire to make some use of any special situation and recover something from the dread they experience.

MARKET CONDUCT AS SOURCE AND SIGN OF ANGUISH

Like surrealists, they withdraw ordinary meanings from the environment around them. "Everything is Everything," for instance, means nothing wrong is happening. A slang synonym would be

"Every*body*'s cool" where Everything equals everybody. They withdraw words from the vocabulary of market interaction. In their stead, a grunt, a sign, or a monosyllable is assured, and an entire transaction rooted in cliché and a pattern is performed. Words in some contexts give the addict the feeling that he is being "phony." (There are some men who are unable to give their autobiographies without being prompted and feel the need for a shot in order to relax and talk.) In the market they may experience the anguish of having withdrawn from the whole sphere of language. Of course, there are others who reverse this process, who experience the anguish of overtalking, who are unable to keep from "running off at the mouth," and typically reveal more than they intend.

But the most exquisite source of anguish lies in the misperception by the addict that what he does is purely his business and not instinct with the public interest. The addicts profess to follow in this regard a doctrine of laissez-faire individualism. Each man ought to be allowed to pursue his habit as long as he doesn't hurt anybody else. Like people who are addicted to food, sex, money, or any other object, they will brook no interference with the pursuit of their "pleasure" even if it counterworks toward pain. A perennial source of anguish for the addicts is that society considers their drugs to be involved with the public interest, and that therefore the users of those drugs may not be heard to complain that their lives are altered by the drug and in ways which cause them anguish.

When an addict says out loud that he could cut off the hand that plunges the needle into the arm that contains so many thousands of dollars he is doing more than engaging in hyperbole. He is experiencing his own hand as something alien to himself, as a creature that rests on forces independent of its owner, alive, androgynous, and existing on its own. His hand becomes as detached from him as the rest of the world. Symbolically speaking, the heroin addict in his anguish appears to be experiencing the world somewhat as does an LSD patient who, under the drug, painted herself as a series of detached organs. I believe that in one way or another the existential drugs produce in their habitual users an anguish such as they are rarely able to express except by the arts, and then only if they have sufficient talent.

SYSTEMS OF IMPOTENCE AND ANGUISH

Finally, let us not forget the humble day-by-day facts of the addict's life which cause him a profound anguish. The addict inherits a body of norms, laws, and customs, which are his burden and which bind him in a system of impotence. There is a tragicomic predicament here that I believe has gone unnoticed both by addicts and by commentators on addiction. On the one hand, the addict, as does Don Quixote, fancies himself a bit of a knight, a curious manipulator of persons and things, and able to control his fate. He is of the opinion that he is a fantastical power person. On the other hand, the realities are that the addict, as a pariah, has a minimum of social power. He is not at all in charge of his fate, but has to respond within grave limits.

Another way of looking at this matter of power and impotence is to ask just what kind of technical or general knowledge an addict needs to fulfill his role as an addict. He actually is an unspecialized person whose mind is afloat with as many bits of data as is the mind of the ordinary nonaddict, but who, unlike the ordinary man, does not really have the obligation to know something in specialized detail beyond that required by the womanly task of buying for his own "needs," in a market which in his case happens to be an illegal one.

There is a special predicament inherent in the situation of the man who can never really know if he knows enough about the world to function in it. He has no defined set of skills, but if he is a good hustler he has to be prepared to act spontaneously, to improvise, to assume airs and bluff his way through situations. The fate of having to rely upon pseudo knowledge or unwanted criminal technique is one more undercurrent generating the anguish about which I have been speaking.

The addict's anguish is intensified at a conscious level when he reads or hears about programs being contemplated for his situation, and then compares those allocations with the funding of problems such as alcoholism and mental disease, and then beyond that when he compares the pitifully small amount of money for the treatment of drug addicts with, say, the space and war programs. This is not merely a repetition of the comparison between public and private realms to which I have alluded. It is also a reinforcement of the addict's private experience, which he shares with other people, that he does not count. Of course, the fact that he generally does not vote and usually cannot vote because of his record furthers his sense of impotence and gives him the feeling of being as weak as a cigarette paper tiger cub, a being who can wheel and deal on the private level but has to remain silent on the public level. Moreover, the anguish of being an addict is not diminished by allocations to agencies; according to the addicts, it is only when their problem has publicly hit the middle classes that the street addicts are benefited. More than one addict has bitterly told me that it is only because newspapers, radio, and television have learned that there are nice middle-class white drug users in Yonkers, Long Island, Poughkeepsie, and elsewhere that the governor and the mayor of New York are concerning themselves with giving large amounts of money for the rehabilitation of addicts. What counts here is not the degree of the addicts' misperception of reality but their resentment at a policy apparently meant for them and their betterment, but generated only when a different class of the population becomes incorporated into the addict life pattern.

When the addicts, like other minority groups, observe the slowness of legislation and the added slow-footedness of society in putting this legislation into practice, they express their anguish in the form of cynicism about politicians and the hypocrisy of the square society. They become aware that the rapid action that seems to accompany the passing of legislation is an illusion, and they experience the slow realization that, chanceless and placeless, they will still be faced with the same dry gray world.

INTRINSIC ANGUISH

Let me reiterate that anguish lies at the very heart of the idea of addiction. Addicts are not merely anguished; they are *anguish*. The honeymoon of exquisite pleasure from the drug, I have observed, is the very antithesis of anguish, but it is in the nature of this process that the addict needs more and more of the same drug to get approximately his initial pleasurable experience. Anguish results when he discovers more and more that not only does he have to take more and more of the drug, with its attendant social and economic consequences, but that these progressive increases do not take him much closer to his goal. After a while, all he can do is to get the imitation of normality, and normality is no longer the pre-drug state of his body-mind. His becomes an endless task of expending all his time and committing his body only to satisfy the needs of some new, synthetic man that he never intended to make. The ultimate anguish is the frustration of being compelled to serve an ingrown alien master and to have no political recourse, no fourteenth amendment to invoke to emancipate himself.

Still there are limits to the negative side of anguish, and it is only fair to point out before concluding this section that addicts are past masters at the art of exploiting this intrinsic suffering. Elsewhere I allude to the fact that addicts objectively are exploited though they may not experience it subjectively. One of the reasons for this discrepancy is that they themselves exploit their own condition. They particularly play upon the guilt—real or fancied—of significant members of their circle, especially their relatives and friends, as long as that guilt still directs the person who feels it to offer some kind of compensation for the addict in his woe. Drug addicts, like alcoholics, seem to radiate this kind of suffering. Those who are accustomed to associating with them develop a kind of extrasensory perception that permits them, even imposes upon them, the knowledge that the addict is suffering and that the square can alleviate that suffering by crossing the addict's palm with silver. However, in my mind this sort of petty con game is scarcely a reward commensurate with the enormous suffering I have already described.

In such key ways is it true that at the heart of the addict's life is anguish and not pleasure, as used to be popularly supposed? Far from being a purely hedonistic creature, the addict lives a life of complex pain-and-pleasure blends.

The Drug Addict as an Existentialist Creature

Over the years in working with the addicted, my colleagues at Exodus House and I—and, I am sure, other people in other places—have noted striking resemblances between the problems of the addicted and the problems of modern man as described by prominent existentialist thinkers.* Of course, no one would deny that men as complex as Heidegger, Kierkegaard, Sartre, Marcel, and Nietzsche, to take only a few of the leading names, differ radically in their emphases and even in their points of view on some questions. Still, as commentators have pointed out, they have jointly outlined a series of related problems about the moral and personal crises of our time. Theirs is the image of a world in dissolution. The terms of their description thus properly apply, if only by coincidence, to a specific kind of man, *homo addictus,* who lives under the extreme strain of the law and order of twentieth-century America. We have already seen some of this applicability in the anguish suffered by the addict, a condition examined with more general relevance by Sartre.

It will, I believe, help to keep the context clear if I set forth some of those leading problems, based on a kind of intuitive consensus to be found among these existentialist thinkers. For the addict mirrors more or less the existentialist's idea of the essence of each of these modern issues.

UNCERTAINTY, AMBIGUITY, AND ANXIETY

Each thinker has in his own way discussed the modern loss of absolute and universally verifiable frames of reference common to all mankind, frames which had once afforded men a sense of place and direction. With these reference points a man could know without effort where he stood, where he had come from, and where he was going. Instead, man has continually to create, in a world that is always in a state of becoming. Man creates a place for himself, but that place is always potential. In this universe a man feels that he is a small burdened creature, that he has lost that golden support that helped earlier generations.

How does the addict fit into this image? As I have suggested in the case of G. and his unintended return to drugs, there is a pro-

---

* Note that I am talking mainly about their *description* of how man is, not their *prescription* of what he ought to be. But, if only negatively, the latter is involved in this analysis.

found uncertainty that grays the life of the addict. As I said earlier, the addict becomes mystified after a while by the forces within him that make him act the way he does. He is also continually uncertain, and tragically so, as to whether in fact he or society is right about using drugs. (I do not speak here of surface verbalizations, but about what a man will say in a long probing interview, where he has a chance to feel that honesty would not be held against him.) This uncertainty is hooked into anxiety, which is one of the forces that keep a man using drugs. Furthermore, the loss of a sense of the sacred means that many men, who in early childhood were exposed to some kind of religious involvement or who even may have had an intense affiliation to it, keep looking for the sacred in a chemical equivalent, such as heroin. In a gray, desacralized world, the collective temptation will always be to replace the holy with a synthetic equivalent.

ALIENATION

It is now almost a platitude to say with the existentialists that modern man is alienated from the world around him. The world of massive developments in technology, culture, and society leaves the individual with the feeling that his is a world not only that he never made but a world he could never have conceived of. Those who have talent complain of the leveling of civilization that prevents any sort of authentic selfhood and existence. Those without talent seek to justify their existence through synthetic experiences. Neither group is satisfied; each remains alienated from the life it projects into the future. The world is seen as a hostile and sometimes confusing scene in which the individual really is not at home.

The addict—especially if he lives the paranoid life, feeling himself to be something of a monad in a group of monads—experiences bitter loneliness. Unlike the lonely alcoholic, the addict is labeled as a pariah by law and morality, and is squeezed down and out of the society if his social identity is revealed. He did not make the laws, such as the Harrison Act, that govern his *de facto* status nor any of the subsequent statutes and bureaucratic interpretations which set the rules of the game he plays. The basic attitudes about him preceded his existence on earth. Thus he experiences himself as a stranger amid strangers, and even acts in an ambiguous way toward fellow addicts, depending upon the state of the market for drugs and his position within that market. Who is more alienated from his fellows and the world than the man with a market mentality in a mass society which keeps his market illegal?

NAUSEA

I would propose the term "existential attitude" to account for the feeling of disgust about oneself that Sartre earlier wrote about. It assumes that the person orients himself to his life as a whole and to the effect of one part on another. "Nausea" is the disgust a person feels in the middle of the night, sleepless and restless and thinking about the life he did lead, the life he is about to lead, and the life he could have led had he made different choices. It is the disgust a man experiences when he compares how he should have lived his life and the form he actually had given to it, and the life he actually is about to lead. If the gap is enormous, the terror that results is proportionate and the sense of disgust or nausea parallels it. The failure to live up to these existential norms is one of the attributes of the moral crisis that the existentialists have signaled to us.

Do addicts experience a parallel nausea about themselves, a specter which calls for them in a unique way?

Class-conscious commentators might feel that this idea does not really apply to addicts, that it really is an attribute of a middle-class citizen in an affluent society. His hunger and biological needs satisfied, he has the time and the surplus to lie back and ask about the meaning of life and his place in the world. Experiences with users suggest to me that these existential attitudes also affect the addicted. Even men who are "strung out" so that their whole lives are focused around the drug will say that when they get high they start to think about themselves. Often a man gets to the point where the shot yields a kind of good feeling immediately interfused by his guilt, anger, and resentment at having yielded to temptation. Each such shot, I submit, is a deflection from a life path that the addict would like to take but cannot, and which leaves him filled with a disgust that may interfere with the feeling that he is getting "straight" from the drug. Living as they do in an extreme situation such as those described by the existentialists, the addicts are continually aware of how life is contingent for them so that every day brings the possibilities not only of death but of maiming, imprisonment, and disease. In short, each day brings the possibility of a radical alteration in the course of their lives, but in a way they do not really plan. This condition of impermanence and provisionality generates a continual sense of nausea in veteran addicts whom one meets. It gives a lie to those who cynically believe that addicts do not "really" want to kick their habit. They do and do not, of course, and the complicated ambiguities of their situation confuse their self-feeling and generate the disgust they have for themselves and their fellows. The existence of this nausea also runs counter to the superficial statement, given freely by the addicts to hit-and-run journalists and researchers, that they have no feeling. On the contrary, addicts have many feelings, depending on the state of their being, and one of them is precisely disgust.

ABSURDITY

Existentialist thinkers have discovered that human conduct, when alienated and under extreme pressure, will become reduced to an absurdity, a living equivalent to the logical process of *reductio ad absurdum*. The contradictions in man's being are multiple and exposed in glaring fashion under pressure of circumstances.

Addicts live a life of absurdity, a life full of pathos and irony. Under the stress of their need, and circumscribed by law and morality, they act the role of a fool more often than they realize. When G., on his way to becoming an ex-addict, veers course under the surface subtlety of a charming female, he is acting absurdly. To act absurdly in this case is to act against one's interests, short term or long term, and all the while to pretend not to notice it or to engage in semantic thought play by which to be weak is to be strong, to be inferior is to be superior, to be stupid is to be intelligent; in short, to be negative is to be positive. The contradictions of one's life are not transcended except in words. This is the case of the addict who has to keep on doing something that he really is unable to control. He may accept help on one level, but he continually sets up situations that may prevent his ever being helped or helping himself.

A special form of absurdity that bedevils addicts and those who wish to further their rehabilitation goes under the name of self-sabotage. How many times have we heard that So-and-so, who was "doing fine" and staying off drugs, has decided in the flush of prosperity that he is going to marry a certain girl and settle down and have a family? This means also that he will buy a car when, in fact, the money he is making is just enough to support him and his minor habits and permit him to feel that he is on his way. How many addicts have committed the absurdity of premature commitment? How many have misjudged themselves badly? The number is absurdly large, and in all such cases those of us with a darker temperament would suggest that perhaps this kind of self-damage is rooted in the character of the man and in his need for self-punishment. The fact of the matter is that even as the nations of the world set up situations that can only produce mass destruction, so the addicts in their small way set up the silly traps in which they are going to fall under the pressure of the hunt for money and drugs.

THE NECESSITY OF CHOICE AND RESPONSIBILITY

Existentialist thinkers never weary of telling us that we have no option of whether or not to choose, and that even the lack of choosing is itself a decision and a choice made. The men who were fighting the Nazis in the Resistance, of course, made a very clear choice that involved their whole lives. It is in extreme situations, where a man is "between the sword and the wall," that he reveals not only his nature but the ultimate value he holds. Forced choices used in certain psychological tests (e.g., Allport-Vernon, *Study of Values*) are taken to be barometers of the course of a person's life. To choose is an integral part of life, and in so saying the existentialist tends to identify himself with the active life as opposed to the contemplative one. But choices are also made by philosophers.

What about the addicts? Are we not told time and again that they are "irresponsible" and "passive" and let themselves be moved or float into situations that they have not made? Are they not too immature and too incompetent to adhere to the rugged individualism that appears to be the American equivalent to this existentialist tenet? If one talks long enough to addicts, one discovers that they do have an individualism of their own. As I will show in presenting their social types, they put down the man who is a beggar, who does not dare forage for his own heroin. But they also will put down the man who is unable to choose between his loyalty to his fellows and his loyalty to the police. Many men drop more scorn upon "ratting" or informing than upon being a "creep." They recognize that under the pressure of police threat certain men, such as the man who faces a long prison term or the youngster who is easily intimidated or cajoled, will betray their fellows. Recognizing these weaklings, as they are called, does not mean that they are condoned. The addict values the man who is responsible to his fellows in this context and says nothing to the police.

Secondly, an addict will argue that he is "responsible" for keeping up his habit. That is to say, he will go out and steal, and so on, and do all the things a good hustler would do in order to get the money he needs to support himself. When one argues with an addict that he is not supporting his real self, he will shrug his shoulders and say this is a matter of point of view. Moreover, addicts under pressure agree in principle with the existentialists that they must choose, but their choice is socially wrong. They differ from the middle-class rehabilitation worker in that they attribute responsibility to themselves in areas which sound irresponsible to the "square."

Another example of this existentialist-at-work appears when addicts who have pushed will insist that they never or almost never "turned on"—that is, gave a shot to—a nonaddict. One cannot believe them in every case, because certainly somebody gave the new user his first shot. The repeated protestations by some men that they did not share in this process sound like masked guilt or shame at having chosen to give a man or a woman a fix with an idea of hooking them so as to make them vulnerable for future exploitation. Recruitment involves at least some planning and choice and a taking on of responsibilities for oneself through choosing to involve others in one's fate.

A similar question of irresponsible "pulling down" takes place when a man who has previously been addicted comes out of jail.

There are always some pushers around who will sell to him, choosing as a rationalization the "fact" that if they don't sell to him someone else will. The man chooses to buy, and knows the consequences, and the addict pushers choose to sell him, and they know the consequences. Both would agree that this is an act taken in full awareness, and that each can be punished for it; but the admission stems from a sense of responsibility that does not go very far. Even here the addict seems to caricature the Sartrean individualist who glories in his capacities and powers, and who seeks to advance his own destiny and boundaries even at the expense of others. It is no accident that both in Sartre's heroes and among the addicts the constant threat of failure to fulfill the norms of this extreme form of individualism generates anxiety, anguish, despair, and the nausea of not living up to one's own highest norms: to choose by existential norms.

"THE PRIMACY OF PERSONAL EXPERIENCE OVER ABSTRACTIONS"

I borrow this phrase from the philosopher William Barrett in his study of existential philosophy, *Irrational Man*. Barrett has rightly observed that the existentialists seek to be in touch with the modern temper and modern experience. For them, man is the center of the world or at least is put into a world of "contingencies, discontinuity in which the center's experience [is] irreducibly plural and personal." Each of the existentialists, from Nietzsche on, has been concerned about stripping some aspect of traditional beliefs away to uncover what core of reality, if any, still remains and, going beyond that, has sought to inspect the future through his philosophy. All of them have in short been prophets as well as philosophers. The characteristic existentialist orientation and philosophy has been toward the "immediate and qualitative, the existent and the actual—towards 'concreteness and adequacy.' "

How does the addict exemplify this aspect of existentialism?

First of all, the addicts repeatedly deny that a nonaddict can really know what it is like to be an addict in its good or bad, favorable or unfavorable aspects. "You can't tell what a shot feels like unless you try it yourself." Or again, "You can't know what it is to be hunted by the police unless it happens to you." In these and other "sentences," the addict is stating the incommensurability of his life against the square's and attributing the unbridgeable gap between the two to the uniqueness of the addict's experience. This experience, like so much of the experience recounted by the existentialists, is dark and unfathomable, and somehow embraces the conscious, pre-conscious, and unconscious. In contrast, the addict may scorn many professional efforts to understand him and mock psychiatric or sociological jargon which he, of course, will use on other occasions for its prestige effect.

Secondly, any representative survey of a group of street addicts is likely to show a higher percentage of men claiming to be artistically gifted than profess mathematical or scientific endowment. Part of the explanation lies in education, but only part. A man who day after day "cooks up" a chemical so that even the very smell of the match may induce sickness in him,* carefully draws heroin up a needle, then injects it into his veins and waits for a response, is primed for an experience. He centers his whole life around that experience, and hence it is understandable that he becomes in some degree accustomed to evaluating life in experiential terms. He becomes more concrete minded in that sense. Understandably, even the more intelligent and well read among the addicted tend to see the world as a complicated sensory affair rather than as a set of axioms from which other theorems are to be deduced. I am not implying that addicts lack capacity to make abstractions. However, there is a tendency on their part to prefer the traditional artistic medium. It seems to me to be a fruitful line of research to ask whether there is any accident in the fact that many avant-garde poets have dabbled in the drugs, starting from Baudelaire. In the modern addict culture, of course, there are many intimate connections between the sphere of jazz and that of drugs.

THE IMPERATIVE TO UNMASK

I have said before that one of the tenets of existentialism is that a man is homeless. A particular expression of this homelessness is

* In the cooking-up process some addicts develop an association between phosphorus, the symptoms of sickness, and the magical effect of heroin in removing those symptoms. After a while the smell of the burnt match, itself, can induce the symptoms—an interesting example of conditioning effect.

modern man's long-run propensity to strip away from himself all rationalizations and all alibis, and to dispense with or to attack the use of idols which he himself may have depended upon. The existentialists, such as Sartre, identify the idolatrous with the conventional, but in so doing Sartre identifies the modern temper with the attack on humbug. The man who cannot rely upon traditional forms, even humbug, feels stripped, naked, and faceless. The unmasking process, however, is a separate one, for it involves as its highest values the idea that, while truth is relative, the relative is real.

The unmasking process goes on at all times among the addicted, and its particular target is conventional society. How often have we been told by an addict that those who oppose his use of drugs really would themselves like a shot but dare not ask for one? In contrast, an addict will point out that alcoholics get d.t.'s, that cigarette smokers get lung cancer, and that middle-class people use pills of all kinds without anybody making any fuss about it. He will unmask the pretenses of police going through their ritual drama of arresting a certain quota of addicts in order to satisfy the public's demand that the taxpayer's money be used effectively. The addicts continually are unmasking social workers and psychiatrists. It is very likely that there is no agency that has not been threatened with "exposure" by paranoidal addicts. He who lives an alienated life cannot stand the existence of others who outwardly at least seem to be at home in our society.

On the other hand, it should be clear that many addicts who are as immature as nonaddicts tend to rationalize their own positions by using a welter of projections and alibis. They resist the unmasking process when it is applied to themselves. In that sense, a part of the rehabilitation of the addict consists in assisting him to direct his unmasking powers to himself. Rehabilitation—I shall elaborate this theme—has existentialist elements in it.

THE OMNIPRESENCE OF TIME AS A PROBLEM FOR MAN

The existential thinkers are poignantly aware that man, concrete living man as opposed to abstract man, belongs in a historical habitat, and that to understand his present he has to understand the time that was and the time that is to be. Whether we are reading Heidegger or Sartre, we become aware more and more of the burden of time and the responsibility that man has to make use of that time. The existentialist's critique of "civilization" and his resentment at the leveling of man by mass culture gets its most stunning effect in the apparently remote discussions about the omnipresence of time. He raises questions about the time-and-life-consuming impact of television, radio, mass sports, and yellow journalism.

Faced with the secularization of world views and a growing awareness, or at least a growing belief, that the only time that counts is the time on earth, modern man can only look to death as the boundary that makes him sorrowful but conscious of his finitude. It is here that Sartre, for example, as a novelist has shown the banality of existence and Hannah Arendt has taught us about the banality of evil. The existentialists have cuttingly and incisively characterized modern man as a creature who is obliged to handle time and create his own life while frequently being aware of the fact that he is assuming a godly role beyond his capacities.

And what of the addicts and their position with regard to time? Elsewhere I treat elements of this problem, but let me here tackle it from another vantage point: that of time as a historical burden. Addicts are continually complaining that they have nothing to do. They are often like little children whose TV set is cut off, and who face a long rainy day. Time is a dreadful foe. Even waiting around for hours for a pusher to appear does not really meet the need of filling the space between now and then. Every day is a burden of history, a burden of watching or feeling some second move by a leaden giant. The burden is so intense and the lack of timepieces is so manifest that some addicts even become proficient in keeping time through cigarettes. Since, due to economic reasons, they generally smoke nonfilter king-sized cigarettes, they have a standard unit of time, the length it takes for the cigarette to become a butt. They keep track of the number of cigarettes smoked and get a rough calculation of the passing of time, if they are too lazy to go to a center or an agency where there is a clock. If they go to an agency they are continually aware of the time and, of course, will interrupt the most diversified kinds of conversation at the witching hour, the time for the pusher to appear.

In some hospitals, no matter how many activities the recreational director gives them, there will always be some men who will say that there is nothing to do. Just as Heidegger said that man is the creature who is shot through with time from head to foot, so too do we who work with the addict notice that this man who apparently takes himself out of time through the use of a shot feels that he is dominated by the slow passing of time. Addicts compare the conditions of life as they were in the past with those of the present, and always adversely. The addict feels a *resentment* toward present time because he cannot handle it. His future is one more dimension that he feels is imposed upon him and, as I have shown elsewhere, he seems to try to control it through heroin, but discovers to his dismay that the history of addiction, including the history of its control, unmasks his pretenses to escape the toils of time.

THE NEED TO CREATE AN AUTHENTIC SELF

So far I have outlined the portrayal of man's life as depicted by a consensus of existentialist thinkers. It is a life which is insignificant, alienated in a hostile world, and strange. These existentialist iconoclasts would also break the images of convention. In their novels, plays, and essays they have sought to free insignificant man from stale, received images of himself that, in their view, prevent the natural development of his potentialities to transcend himself. To put this in a formula, not only is God dead but so, too, is man, and it is the quest of the existentialists to renew man by stripping from him the false burdens he carries. Their negative stance and their delving into nothingness are intended to help man become more authentic. This is the meaning of their iconoclasm.

Among the addicted there are two divergent tendencies, one looking toward a kind of authentic existence and the other toward a synthetic personality and synthetic life. On the one hand, there is a continual plunging into suffering and danger, a daily guerrilla warfare against a society which would alienate them. In this continual encounter with Nothingness there emerges the feeling of being "for real." The man who is in constant danger of death, knowing it at first hand, is an approximation of the existentialist position that in an extreme crisis, against the wall of fate and in front of the needle of temptation, a man sees his true self emerging. Contrariwise, there is the continual resort to drugs which makes a man feel not his real self but himself as narcotized or overstimulated. Drugs may bring out tendencies that differ in kind and emphasis from the undrugged self.

In talking to the addicted and letting them "run off at the mouth" about life itself, I have been moved from time to time by this real uncertainty about their own relationship to their selves. If I may speak of the existential attitude that directs a person to search for and create his authentic life, then I would repeat that many of the addicted feel frustrated and disgusted at themselves for not being more honest and successful in achieving this form of authenticity. I suspect, too, that this yearning to be "for real," when given an opportunity to function positively, may be a strong force pulling a man off drugs and promoting his rehabilitation. But before that happens, men will go through stages when they will not know which of their selves is normal, the self on drugs or the self off drugs, and only the passage of time and development will clarify in a man's mind just who he is and who he is not. If we remember also that there has been a tendency for addicts of all kinds to mix up their drugs and to switch from drug to drug, from depressant to stimulant, and more recently even to sample the hallucinogens, then we know that the use of drugs to discover one's real self, so often recommended by literary and artistic figures, runs the danger that the search may derange or damage the self in the process, even as the inspection of certain precious objects may unintentionally destroy them.

CHAPTER 3

"The Life"

A Pressure-Cooker Universe

If we had to characterize in one sentence the life of the typical addicts (whatever their form of existence) in the United States under contemporary legal conditions, that sentence would run something like this: They live a life of continuous pressure interspersed by moments of relaxation and gratification, which inevitably lead to more continuous pressure. This is, of course, a general statement, and I shall try to show in what cases it holds and in what cases it is only partly true.

Let me start by describing briefly four principal kinds of addicts as seen from the point of view of addicts themselves, and expressed in their own language. Upon examination it turns out that this "typology" is based on two criteria. First, does the addict in question take risks? Second, does he profit from the risks?

The first type of addict is called variously the good hustler, the boss hustler, the ace hustler, the five-star hustler, and so on. He is the ideal of many addicts and his characteristics are that he takes considerable risks, but profits from them. By this I mean that he is always "out there" trying to make money or at least trying to get heroin in ways which fit within the mores of the addict culture of which he is a part, if not of the conventional society upon which he may be preying directly or indirectly. The risks will vary in quality and quantity from time to time and from person to person. So, too, will the rewards. A man who may be a good hustler in one neighborhood may be deemed to be rather "a creep" elsewhere. In fact, veteran addicts insist that there are fewer and fewer good hustlers, particularly in the new generation. This, however, is in part a reflection of the permanent split, ever-changing in nature, between youth and age in the addict world. Among the kinds of activities that fit into the category of good hustler and good hustling would stand the man who was a good burglar, confidence man, forger, pickpocket, or shoplifter. Among the females it would include the prostitute ("the hustling broad") and the shoplifter ("booster"). It need only be added that the very nature of the term "hustler" indicates the kind of continuous pressure under which this type of addict lives.*

Second is the category of persons ambiguously referred to as being "into" something. The essence of this type is that he takes a minimum risk and yet gets an appreciable reward. If we examine this structural situation we can see that this man really has cornered a market on something or someone. He has inserted himself into a strategic position in which his knowledge, attitude, body, mind, or whatever is vital to the ongoing concern of someone or some group. He is heroin to someone else's needs. His services or even his silence being essential, he is assured of money or the drug or both.

Among the situations where this happens may be named the blackmailer, as in the case of the young man who gets a homosexual "up tight" and is able to extort money from his family; the female addict who entrances an established pusher and exchanges her charms for his heroin; and the working addict who is able "to make himself a partner in the firm" because he is a trusted employee and is able continuously to extract items from the store or company and sell them on the black market for money. The person who is "into" something is under pressure to keep his connection and corner alive, but the pressure is not nearly of the same order and intensity as that of a good hustler. It should be added that few addicts are able to maintain themselves in this position for a long time, at least among those

---

* There are some good hustlers, such as payroll robbers, who do not go out every day to steal and in that sense do not have the same distribution of pressures as other good hustlers. They "lay up" after every big haul. However, they qualitatively experience greater risks because of the tension from the threat of long terms in jail if and when they are apprehended.

whom one meets in the streets, prison, hospitals, or treatment agencies.

Third would be the person who is variously called "the fool" or "flunky" and whose structural essence lies in the fact that he takes larger risks but regularly gets very little from them. He exposes himself to maximum pressure and yet scarcely survives as an addict. Why he does this seems to vary from person to person, but two extreme types come to mind.

On the one hand, there is the young man or woman who has no skills and has just begun to get a big habit. Desperately eager to be part of the great big blooming addict culture, this chemical cub voluntarily does something which cannot produce much money but can lead to great danger. Such would be the person who carries the pusher's supplies around with him from the connection to the place where he is going to sell or at least stash drugs. The other extreme would be a veteran addict who is afraid to steal because he is known to the police as a burglar or a man who has had successful connections with pushing but no longer has the money or is no longer trusted by the connection. He, too, may do menial jobs such as steering people to pushers or buying drugs for them if they have no connections themselves and getting for his pains a "taste" of the drug. Since he transmits the drug to the third party, under the law he is technically committing a sale. He, too, is exposed to pressure of arrest and a sense of being desperate on a continuous basis. Quite often he looks like a "greasy junkie," and this very appearance is what permits him to function. If a good hustler goes to "cop" and wants to know who is a junkie, this sort of poverty is a living ad, notifying him that he can ask this person hopefully to do him the favor of buying his drugs for him.

Finally, there is the "creep," a term loosely used but having among its meanings reference to the man who takes no risks that count and who gets no big rewards. This is a man who apparently has withdrawn from the downdraft of competition, who is afraid of the police, afraid of addicts, afraid of middle- and lower-class society, and yet clings to his habit. He lives by begging fixes or money from anyone, does petty errands of all kinds for all sorts of people, and is generally looked down upon. Sometimes, in fact, he may get only small rewards at a time, but because of the way his day runs he may actually get a total amount of heroin, for example, that is larger than that of even a good hustler. The man who goes around with a needle in his pocket or in his mouth and offers it to others who have no needle, in exchange for a taste, may do that ten or fifteen times in the course of the day and thereby acquire a big habit. If that happens, it is not likely that he will stay in this category; he will be compelled to go out and get more money for himself because there will be days when only a few people will come around to give him a free fix. In that case it is likely that this man will be arrested since he does not have much competence or confidence as a hustler. Hence this man is under a peculiar kind of pressure which mounts when he is more lucky than his skills would permit him to be.

With these four social types of addicts before us and with some idea of the respective pressures upon them, let me now sketch out a typical day of a man who is a good hustler. Since he is an ideal type he will give us, I believe, a good picture of just what life in a pressure-cooker universe feels like.

If he is a good hustler, as I said, he will tend to have a rather "big habit." This means that on any day he may be using an average of $15 worth of heroin. But there will be periods when his habit will treble, depending on his hustling luck. (Note that I have not placed all pushers in one category. Pushers are found in all categories depending on the circumstances and type of pushing.) The day will begin in a way which depends upon the hustler's self-control. If he is able to save one bag from the night before, then he has his indispensable "morning shot." In that situation his pressure will begin a little later than if he has not been able to resist the temptation to shoot up all the drugs that he got the day before or the night before. Assume for a moment that he has not had this control, an assumption which is often a reality. He has to go out in the street somewhat "sick" because during the nighttime his habit "came down," that is to say, he developed symptoms. If he is sick he has to get his drug right away. The magical drug will make him straight again. He knows this, and "to cop" becomes an imperative drive. If he is too sick to hustle in any meaningful way he will go out and even beg his fix. This does not make him a creep in his own eyes because he will pay back the person from whom he borrows or he will justify it as being a temporary aberration due to his pressure. Or he may go to borrow money from his family, although this is not very likely for most men who have full-blown habits. The family has "cut them loose," that is, it has ejected them from the home for some time.

However, it may be that despite all his relentless and angry maneuverings he has not been able to get any money from those who ordinarily have money or would give it to him if they had. Now his habit is making him more and more desperate, and he will have to turn to more obviously illegal measures. What he will do will depend on circumstance. If at that juncture someone tells him that there is a "sting" that he knows about, he will immediately go with him if he believes the man can help to get money at once. Otherwise he will take some brief chance that opportunity presents. It may be that he passes a car in which he sees a tape recorder. It may be that he sees, through a hallway, an open door where a housewife has gone out to a neighbor. The opportunities are as diversified as life itself, and under the pressure of the urge to get straight the hustler's senses will appear to him to be more acute than ever before. His sensorium will transform reality into a treasure house of possibilities. At least this is how many hustlers describe what happens under the spur of need. The addict makes his foray, goes to a fence, which may be formal or informal—a neighbor, storekeeper, or pusher—and gets his money, and then his drug. What counts in these situations is speed, and so it may well be that he will bring whatever item he has directly to the pusher, who will then drive a mean bargain, knowing by observation that his customer feels himself to be without real options. Under these circumstances, from what I have learned, men will sell tape recorders that would legally yield upward of $50 to $100 for a few bags of drugs, which would ordinarily cost $3 to $4 each.

Once he has "taken off," that is, injected the heroin, the hustler feels the diminution of pressure. At least this is the case if the bags he has bought have any small measure of heroin in them. What happens increasingly, however, is that he may be sold defective heroin. It may be cut excessively,* or it may be diluted with barbiturates so

---

* The amount of heroin in the bags sold in any market on any day is variable. Different men also have different tolerance levels. As a result, they tend to be vague about what would be a minimum permissible amount of

that he gets an illusory kind of high. If the hustler we are following is frustrated at this point, it can be predicted that the so-called passive addict will become a violent man, and his target will be the pusher who sold him "the garbage." However, the addict has to find him first, and under the circumstances described it is unlikely that he will. If that is true, then he has to go out looking for another pusher, but before he can do that he has to get more money. His sickness becoming steadily worse, the pressure understandably mounts. The degree of desperation may lead him to violate his norms of conduct. A man who ordinarily would not attack another human being for money will, under such need, snatch a woman's pocketbook, but if that is not possible because the police are around, he may wait in a hallway, stop a person, beg him for money, and if refused, take it at knife point. In short, the pressure is converted into everbolder exploits even against his own wishes, anxieties, and philosophy of life. At any rate, this too can lead to his getting money, and we may assume that he gets "straight."

The day now lies before him under the premises of the situation I have been outlining. With somewhat more optimism, our hero or antihero can now put to use his resources and habitual point of view. Of course, if he is concerned about being arrested for anything he has done while desperate, then it is likely that he will immediately decamp from the neighborhood where he is too well known and for the next few days will treat his old haunts as "hot." This does not mean that he will change his economic or maintenance pattern. It simply means that he will go to buy in another neighborhood where he has connections. It is characteristic of a good hustler that he does not confine his purchasing of drugs to one area. He will be known or have connections in several neighborhoods so that precisely under the conditions here described he can be more flexible about his habits. He is also flexible about the areas in which he does his depredations. If he is a booster he will recognize the fact that he can "burn out" a certain department store. He will therefore respect the store detec-

---

heroin in a bag. But where a man's symptoms are not removed by his shot, he is sure that the bag has been cut excessively. He knows that the pusher has put too much milk sugar or "manida" (baby food) into the bag to stretch the heroin.

tives and move from place to place as the days pass. The good hustler will also not stick to one particular form of activity. He may intersperse a burglary within a series of boostings. He may even decide that he is too tired of the hassle. If he makes a particularly large amount of money through a windfall, as, for example, when he stumbles upon a cache of dollar bills in a house he is burglarizing, he may buy a large amount of heroin and go into business as a pusher.

For most addicts becoming a pusher means a drop in pressure. This may seem paradoxical to a layman who has been told truthfully that there is continuous police effort to arrest pushers. But the fact of the matter is that the pusher addict in the 1960's has often been more concerned with the danger from other addicts than from the police. The so-called "take-off artist" is omnipresent in market areas, and if he is not going to be paid off, this means even more of a threat of having his supply of drugs or his money forcibly taken. The police, even when they are accused of having "rats," of shaking down pushers, or of being unfair to them in any way, do not really constitute that much pressure upon many pushers. At least from what I understand in talking to them, they do not experience the police as being that much on their backs. There are far more addicts around at any time than narcotics squad people or plainclothesmen.

But to go back to our hustler, his day will depend upon his fortune and upon the capital he has available. If the premise is that he has no capital, then one can be assured that he is going to have to settle for even petty acquisitions. He has to get his fix and that means he has to have money. As a result, the man who is a proletarian without any capital to back him will have to compromise with his own norms and become something less than a good hustler.

On the other hand, if he has been lucky recently and has not wasted his money, he may well have a supply of drugs stashed away without even the thought of selling it. Such a man will have a minimum of pressure upon him to go out and steal in any one day, and can either "lay up" and use his drugs or, as sometimes happens, he can just use his drugs casually and plan for a new coup. This situation is most uncommon among most of the known addicts one meets. The amount of control required seems to be too much for them. I know of one case where a man with two comrades was able to get some $17,000 from a great jewelry theft. He shot up this amount of money in cocaine, a highly volatile and expensive drug, in a very short time—a matter of a week or ten days. As the addicts themselves say easy come easy go and fast money just disappears down the rabbit hole.

Under the premise of a small amount of cash available at any time or a lack of drugs, the hustling addict's day begins in the morning and only ends late at night when he goes to sleep. In fact, as one of them put it to me, an addict has to have a 25-hour day. Where his luck is bad and he has to work through the night, an addict who is a good hustler may be forced to buy "bombitas," an amphetamine derivative that keeps him awake. Some men do not sleep for days or apparently do not. They spend their time looking for stings. Nor do they feel exploited under this burden; they feel they are their own master and their own slave.

Out of this continuous pressure comes what can be called a physical stereotype of a man who is hustling. He may be keeping his clothing somewhat clean, but he loses weight; he looks tired and sounds tired; from time to time there is a rather desperate, lonely look about him; he has little time or no time at all for sex except in so far as through sex he may be able to get money from dependent women; he becomes the very model of alienation from society.

The fact that this is the life of an idealized type of person introduces one of the ironies within the addict society. Here we have people who are supposed to be passive, narcotized by the drug, and yet they are continuously on the go. In a sense, pharmacology points one way and cultural pressure the other. The drug, a depressant, is supposed to relax them and it does. It is supposed to narcotize conflicts and it does. It is supposed to produce a nod that extracts them from reality and it does ideally. And yet, because of the economic setup of which they are a part, because of the money that has to be got and the angles that have to be played, the man who would be happy merely contemplating the world, seeing life pass before him, and experiencing it in a depressed way, a paranoid way, a pseudo-vital way, and so on, is forced to go out and spend his days, his weeks, and his months in continuous activity and hyperactivity.

I have spoken here of the life of the heroin addict. Similar comments may be made for the amphetamine addict, but they would be of a different order. Here the hyperactivity is not as yet linked to economic pressures, but to the effect of the drug itself as well as to the expectations within the groups of people who use the drug. Barbiturate addicts, who are fewer in number, as well as doriden addicts, live a differently confused kind of life full of chaos, accident, and aggression, but they too follow the paradox of a pharmacology leading in one way toward passivity and of a cultural pressure leading in other ways toward violent activity.

The Magic Market as a Supporting Structure

Of course, a reasonable man would ask just what makes a person submit to such horrendous pressure. Surely anyone with half a brain or any degree of morality if given the chance to stop would stop. But, as every layman knows, many addicts just don't stop even if they have the chance. Society gives them opportunity to go into hospitals to detoxify. What happens is that they may or may not stay for the regular time but, as is well known, even if they do they are likely to take up their old life again. Skeptics even say that they go to the hospital just to cut down on their habits so that upon leaving they can enjoy the drug once more. How can one explain such "irrational" conduct? In fact, if one talks to more astute addicts, one learns that they are painfully aware of the contradiction between reason and their conduct. They themselves know how in their lives they had been perfectly aware of the high costs they pay for staying "in the life." They know that they are simply heading for prison or disease or death if they keep up their habit. They appreciate, to a point, their own "stupidity" and freely admit that the life makes no sense. And yet there they are, day in and day out, going through the same kind of "changes."

The concept of a magic market will help clear up some of the mystery.* This general term is useful in embracing the life of the

---

* In my own thinking I distinguish "White Magic Markets" from "Black Magic Markets," but the distinction would take us too far from the line of our argument. I am speaking here of the "White Magic Pattern."

addict in so far as it has a magical luster and imports this luster to the addict and the things he does. He feels that he is the object or subject of remarkable forces whose essence exists in the disproportionate effect of small efforts. Things happen that cannot be explained by natural laws, but which affect the addict. In short, the magic market serves as a system of control and power to meet or correct the life of continuous pressure being placed upon the addict.

The principal element in the magic market is heroin. (Similar comments might, of course, be made about the other drugs, but for purposes of clarity and immediacy I am going to speak exclusively of heroin.) The pharmacology textbooks list a number of the effects of this drug upon the person who ingests it. It is safe to say that no text enumerates the functions attributed to the drug by the addicts and by those who observe them, which would include their families, psychiatrists, social workers, and the police. The belief in its potency and the magic is tied in with the grip heroin has over its user. Briefly, it seems to meet every apparent need that the addict can experience. From another point of view, it meets pseudo needs which he deems to be real.

The addict acts as though heroin helps him meet his needs for interaction, for moving away from, toward, or against other people. A man who feels that he lacks confidence in the presence of others and wants to get close to them may need to take a drug in order to overcome his diffidence. A man who wants to blot out reality and escape from others can use a drug for that purpose. Or a man who wants to be aggressive, who, for example, fears stealing but has to steal to get his heroin, will take a shot to go out to steal, get his money, and then buy heroin, and so on and on.

Besides the incapacity to interact, a man may feel simply incompetent. He may feel sexually incompetent. In that case, as I have mentioned, a shot of heroin will delay his orgasm long enough so that he can give gratification to more than one woman if need be. Certainly it makes him feel like a giant. Or a man who says that he needs a shot to work will take heroin and work for some time. Such, at least, are claims being made for the white magic.

Also, there is the man who wants prestige among his fellows. Taking a shot will give him the satisfaction of knowing that he is part of a secret fraternity sharing the arcana of chemistry that only the elite can experience.

Furthermore, heroin gives a sense of rhythm, rule, norm to life. The morning shot, afternoon shot, and evening shot, for example, are mecca points in the course of the day. For the man who is not working, is afraid to work, or cannot work, these consumption points are in part the equivalent of the workingman's daily schedule. Conversely, by giving a "kick" the drug interrupts "boring" routines.

Heroin and its magic market gratify the thirst for new experience. Intrigue and uncertainty in the market correspond to the wish for "action" and "mystery" within. The compulsion to get and use a dubious "bag" makes for adventure and satisfies the need for excitement.

Heroin gives symbolical significance, a meaning to life. Events, persons, objects, places—all can be characterized in the light of the need for heroin. What people say about things is transmuted in a one-dimensional manner, and simplified significance is placed upon things which ordinarily would have a more complex meaning. It follows that dependence upon heroin means dependence upon a highly simplified but paradoxical medium. If all of reality is perceived through the eyes and frame of drug use, then, as in a play or novel by Gênet, life is refracted in a strange way. A word that sounds harmless to squares may become charged with meaning to a drug addict. Or an object that is perceived casually by a respectable person takes on a more philosophical or pragmatic value for an addict. So, if a woman in a crowded bus opens her purse and pills drop out, this is a matter for concern and solicitude on the part of those hanging from the straps. But an addict looking on will later comment that it's amazing how squares can be hooked and nobody pays any mind to it, but if an addict were to have those pills—"Man!" he says, "he won't hear the end of it."

A teen-ager to whom schools are boring, meaningless places, feels a special thirst for significance in his life that he may not recognize as such. For him, drugs kill a void. Through them he finds a way of imputing meanings to things that otherwise would be meaningless.

In addition, an addict can achieve a sense of integration through drugs. At least, he may claim that he feels more at home with himself, that his anxieties about not being whole are resolved. Becoming "straight" is a kind of chemical normalization at best and yields a feeling of putting the parts of himself in order. The addict expects the drug to do what he has not done or will not do: put a point to his life and impart a sense of congruence to the various parts of his person. Unable to abide the kind of conflicts generated within and without him, he nullifies them in an act of chemical poetry. Some "authorities" would phrase these functions in terms of getting identity, and it is evident that some men who don't have clear boundaries on themselves claim to get these from confrontation with the drug as well as with the entire addict life.

Finally, but not the least important for the addict is the magical way in which a man who has been getting sick because he hasn't received his dosage of heroin can alter his conduct and characteristic appearance instantaneously when he takes a shot. In fact, some "authorities" are inclined to believe that the main reason a drug addict keeps on using is that he fears the agonies of withdrawal. The theory is that drug addicts become drug addicts when they become aware of the connection between the heroin and the removal of pain. Once they learn that they can check the withdrawal symptoms by the administration of the dose they are hooked.

However, this is not the whole story, since men will use a drug immediately upon coming out of jail when they no longer have any dread of withdrawal. They will use it when they are anxious about their capacities and their relationship to the universe around them. Furthermore, though the heroin has become weaker and weaker over the years and withdrawal pain has become weaker and weaker, the men have not ceased getting hooked nor has it been easier for a man to kick the mental habit he has developed. Still, this is one of the magical functions imputed to the drug and should not be minimized.

If we examine this impressive set of claims, it surely cannot be doubted that if they are even only half consummated they represent heroin to be genuinely magical. We are in the realm of myth, with heroin as a divine or heroic substance. But there is more to being a drug addict than just using heroin, and we find other areas of magic that keep him involved in this life.

The heroin addict's language and his communication patterns generally appear to have for him a magical potency. One who listens long enough to addicts, especially those who live the pseudo life, learns that they are extremely proud of being able to hustle money by "sweet-talking broads," by language, gesture, and communication generally. Or it may be a case of selling a building to a "chump," the building, of course, not being owned by himself. Again, one persuades a nurse to give more medication than the doctor prescribed. The language of the addict is a complex one, depending upon the addict, and tends to bridge several strata of society when it is maximally developed. So the addict is proud of being able to talk like a square, if he can, and also to "rap" like someone who was "in the life.* A significant number of addicts develop keen powers of persuasion, and they treat this as something of a magical process.

Actually, communication in this form of life is tied in with a process known as "psyching," which is, roughly speaking, the application of common sense and intuition in detecting the strengths and flaws of a person one wishes to victimize. Addicts are sometimes thought to have poor judgment about their own lives, and this is true. Yet, paradoxically, a person who may be a poor judge of his own decisions may be able to detect weaknesses in people who apparently are more mature in their judgment. In fact, he seems to feel a kind of symbiosis or partnership-in-dependency in people who may be strong along certain lines and weak along others. By appealing to their strength and showing his weakness, by using language which embodies this conscious and unconscious awareness, he gets the money for his drug.

But if I have observed correctly in my work with the addicted, there is an even more intimate connection between language and the person of the addict. When talking to some addicts, at least, I get the feeling that they have found a reality, an identity in language itself. They talk freely of being actors, good or bad. I think that some of them find a pseudo identity in the language process, as-

---

* The reader will notice how very little addict jargon intrudes into the taped materials. These men wanted to show that they knew more than "street language." During rehabilitation words such as "square," responsibility, orientation, therapy, etc., undergo changes in meaning.

suming a stance in life that is more verbal than realistic. They do *speechify,* but *are* not. This kind of magical process, whereby *to be* is merely a verb, seems to be important for giving a sense of integrity to some of these men. (The person who lives what I call the pseudo life especially seems to rely on this magical process.)

The addict finds still a third kind of magic in the ambiguities of existence, particularly those of a disordered existence. The term "overlay" gives us an opening wedge into understanding the phenomenon. An overlay is a verbal assertion of a motive, intention, attitude, or conduct that is respectable and given out to all those who have to be influenced. It actually, however, conceals beneath its surface one or more other intentions, attitudes, motives, or what have you. So, for example, if an addict wants to protect himself when he goes to cop drugs he may get his mother to give him an errand to do in the same area. This would give him an explanation. This sort of conduct is not, of course, confined to addicts, but the point is that because of the continuous pressure upon them, they are forced into full-time invention of these overlays to the point of becoming craftsmen of the overlay. The person who practices the pseudo life, of course, really has one continuous overlay or ambiguity in his life so that he may blur distinction between what is real and what is not. What is magical here is the use of ambiguities beyond those he, the person himself, manufactures. That is to say, the addict becomes able to detect ambiguities in situations where people not so trained or interested would see only a smooth surface.

Consider, for example, the matter of a urine test for the detection of heroin. Both addicts and ex-addicts are astonishingly able to raise questions in the mind of anyone who administers these tests as to their efficiency and effectiveness. A man's urine test will come back labeled "questionable," which would indicate that the laboratory felt there was some technical doubt about the amount of heroin used. Or quinine might appear, which would suggest that their man had taken a shot or that the shot was a "dummy"—that is, without any drug. In both cases which do produce a certain amount of doubt for the agency administering the test it will be amazing to see how the addict and "ex-addict" will adopt a strategy to confound even the trained worker. They sense the ambiguities in the lab reports even without knowing that they are called questionable. One ploy will be that of asking in a kind of plaintive way just what reason the agency has to play games with a man they know is off drugs. Or, in a paranoical mode, they might ask, in effect, who their enemy is or whether the agency simply wants to get rid of them. Yet it is certain that the tests are valid. The addict is competing with the lab, using word magic to play upon professional uncertainties due to certain ambiguities in the results. The presence of quinine might be accounted for sometimes by quinine water, but where the man denies drinking quinine water the results are pretty clear. The ambiguity he plays upon is the ambiguity of the conscience of the professional, which he knows or senses. From a few gestures he expands the ambiguity into a tactical position in his favor.

There is also the magic of perception under the impact of need. I have alluded before to the manner in which, under the pressure of being sick, a man will see opportunities that apparently do not exist. There is, I believe, a magical element in this process. Consider, after all, what happens when the addict is walking along the street and peers into a typewriter store. He sees the owner moving toward the back, there are no customers in the store. Looking around for a policeman, he sees none. Timing the matter correctly, he darts into the store quietly, lifts up a typewriter, moves out, and has it under his coat, keeps on peering into the store so that the typewriter is touching the window, but covered by his coat. The owner comes back curious. He asks the man if he wants anything. The man says no, moves away into a hallway next door and then out into the back yard adjoining the house, over a roof, and then out to another street, where he finds a shopping bag, and delivers the typewriter to a fence. As experienced by the addict, this is a magical process of transforming an item in the store into heroin in his pocket.

This is what we may call rational magic compared to a man under barbiturates who will engage in irrational magic. Though an officer is ten feet away from him, he will try to open the door of a car that contains something he wants. The officer may come around, tap him on the shoulder, and the drug user may try to push him away. More than one barbiturate addict has had to be beaten over the head by an officer as he tried to ransack a car in the very presence of the officer. However, common to both rational and irrational magic is the idea that by playing roles that hide risks one can transform property belonging to another into heroin and subsequently into one's person. The man on the spur of heroin is more conscious of his chances and provides a "cooler" overlay—the barbiturate addict simply ignores reality in order to get at what he wants.

Finally, there are addicts whose appearance has a magical quality of making them invisible. The greasy junkie who is always down on his luck, who has shoes with toes that turn outward and falling socks, often can pass as an alcoholic bum in many areas. He may be the last person that some officers would stop because he so easily shuffles along hiding his identity behind his poverty. Or, again, some of them stand in the shadows of hallways, merging with the darkness as they nod, trying to hold themselves erect and never really being noticed by those hurrying by. There is in this capacity to hide a safety mechanism that is hard to appreciate if one is not himself continually under pressure from the police. In short, this is a phenomenological mystique that fits into a magical system. Since there are varying attractions among the different techniques used, as well as competition among the users, we speak of the system as a magic market which cumulatively grips and draws men and women back into addiction—even against their will.

Realities—Hidden and Otherwise

Things magical, then, do not exhaust the universe of addiction. Rather, they give it a romantic aura, furnishing a semblance of plausibility to an addict's persistent system of denial. To a man who denies that he is addicted or that, if he is addicted, he can't stop when he wants to, or that there is any point in stopping, in short, for one who participates in any of the other intricate network of denials which refresh him, the implicit belief in magic is helpful support. But surrounding the magical realm is social reality itself, the outer shell of the addict's anguish. I want now to turn to this reality and penetrate its structure. The reader will bear in mind, as I have suggested in the beginning, that this reality is still full of mystery, secrecy, and darkness. The thousands upon thousands of addicts generate a culture of their own. I want to examine its structure vertically and horizontally, indicating where magical beliefs and practices play a part.

ERSATZ TOTALITARIANISM: THE SUBSTITUTE CULTURE

How are these thousands of addicts ruled? I put this question in a Pickwickian way in order to bring out certain features of their lives. Anyone who works long enough with the addicted hears ugly rumors about gangsterism and racketeers. The name Mafia inevitably crops up. It should be immediately said for most of the addicted men and women that these names refer to fairly invisible personages, with the exception that certain of the lower echelons of the racketeering hierarchy have earlier in their lives perhaps known men who became addicted. But here, too, there is a tendency toward a sharp cleavage between the distribution hierarchy and the bottom layers of the addict world. Though there is such alienation, it is important to understand how it feels to be one of the thousands of men and women who support the pyramidal structure.

The top levels of the distribution hierarchy correspond to an illegal upper class. This class, which I will dub Invisible Illegal Personages, or I.I.P.'s, for short, has two branches. There are, first, respectable or so-called respectable people who allegedly contribute large sums of capital to in-between connections. They ask no questions, and at some later time, they receive their original investment plus a profit, again without raising questions as to how the money was used and whence the profit sprang. About these people one only hears vague rumors even from those who claim to be knowledgeable.

The second branch of this illegal upper class is a specifically criminal group associated directly with the underworld though not necessarily in the good graces of the lords of the underworld. They are called renegades, according to some of the addicted men who profess to know about these things. It is freely said that at the Mafia's Apalachin Meeting in 1957, there was a real breach between generations, and that the renegades are those who rebelled against orders to pull out of the narcotics trade. Apparently they were lured by the prospect of continuing high profits and also high dangers in this traffic. It may be speculated that this group has retained its international connections, receives the money from the more respectable groups, and transmits it to the appropriate quarters.

Much about this criminal upper class's motivations and behavior is unclear. It is far too easy to say that these people just want profit or even that they just want power. We simply do not know enough about them; their motives and psychology remain a real mystery to social science.

However, it is no mystery that these people try to hide their movements and their motives. Even if their identity is suspected by the Federal Bureau of Narcotics, which may have them on a list of wanted men, what goes on remains obscure even to police specializing in this work.

The secret of their structure was described to a man, who, though using drugs, was sufficiently respected by certain of his hierarchy friends in that he could entertain the idea of getting large amounts of drugs from them. He was speculating out loud to one friend who has Mafia connections that if he wanted to organize a drug traffic ring he would start with four trusted people who didn't know each other, and they, in turn, would separately entrust their money or heroin to four others, and so on. The Mafia man looked up and said that this is precisely the way it was done. Every man knows only a certain man above him or a certain few men above or below him so that the higher one goes toward the upper class, fewer and fewer of the people have any direct connections with them, and the more remote is the connection between the drug and the man occupying a high position.

As one goes down the hierarchy one passes through wider and wider strata, from wholesalers who deal in kilos to considerable pushers who deal in smaller weights, ounces ("pieces"), and then to the street level. At the street level one encounters a blend of non-using and using pushers, with the nonusers being a slender minority in the 1960's. With the exception of these nonusers, there is very little profit being made at the lower level. A certain amount of profit comes to some exceptional pushers who are addicted. A certain amount of money comes to young people who are beginning in the business but whose lot is generally to become an addict through contact with the drug. And most important of all, because of the widespread resort to informers, the average life expectancy of a pusher as a pusher is quite limited. Estimates vary, but it is a safe guess that the police know that a certain person is pushing within a few weeks of his beginning, and then it is only a matter of time and the police's own plans as to when, despite his bravado, he is going to be arrested and sent to jail. The police have their own unenviable task of Sisyphus because no sooner do they arrest a pusher than another addict has taken his place. This pattern is due to the fact that pushing is considered by some men to be easier, and that some men are unable to "hustle" by stealing or doing other illegal acts.

At the bottom of this socioeconomic pyramid are the addicted men numbering, as I have said, in the tens of thousands in the United States. Within the perspective of addict society, the addicted man is in the most technical sense of the term a proletarian. His "property" basically consists of his own labor power and the strength, intelligence, and daring he can bring to the use of his life. He has no one employer (except himself) and in effect is actually working for the benefit or profit of the invisible hierarchy above him. From a nominal point of view, he seems to be self-employed or engaged in joint ventures, but this is merely a façade. That is to say, when he goes out in the street in the morning and looks around for a sting, or illegal enterprise, and joins up with three others because there is more likelihood of four making money than one, he seems to be an independent entrepreneur. In fact, there are some men who seem to have been bitten by the bug of enterprise, for they speak of themselves as though they were independent misadventure capitalists.

However, once they get their money they inevitably spend almost all of it on drugs, the money going to the pusher and then in varying ways up the ladder to the weight dealers and then the I.I.P.'s. In short, they seem to be hiring themselves out in the long run, not for their own profit but for the profit of the hierarchy which is their invisible employer. I am suggesting as an image that we have a hierarchy that employs a vast proletarian mass that hires itself out and that this hiring-out process is disguised by apparent freedom. The entrepreneurial role serves only to give to the proletarian the feeling that he is his own boss. I am suggesting that this illusion, this romantic laissez-faireism and individualism of many addicts is the kind of myth that narcotizes the addict as much as does his own heroin.

In what sense may we call this system totalitarian?

In the first place, the locus of power obviously lies in the mists of the illegal upper class. Addicts are somewhat ambivalent and variable about how they feel toward this upper class; some report being quite unconcerned about it. Others who envy the money coming to these people may do so because they also envy their control over heroin. They are split as to whether they would like the police to arrest the "big shots." If this happens, they, the addicts, are without drugs. Hence a man's current interest in rehabilitation is a factor in his opinion about the drug hierarchy. In so far as the man is hooked and involved in the culture he depends upon the whims and caprices of those upper-class people—remember that the illegal upper class may not be "upper" in the conventional society—for subsidizing his heroin. In effect, he works as a proletarian in order to give the incentive to these classes of people to keep the international trade in heroin going.

But is this totalitarian? It is if we recognize the fact that the addicted man is like the ordinary citizen of a totalitarian state who is forced to do things according to an imposed rigid scheme benefiting the ruling classes. The addict who complains bitterly that he does not feel like stealing or undergoing all the risks of arrest and so on is like the "little man" who has to labor long hours, accept rationing, and undergo humiliation from state-paid bureaucrats, uniformed officers, and storm troopers. The proletarian character of the addict, his legal defenselessness, and his general weakness make him not only dependent on heroin but absolutely subservient to the I.I.P.'s.

It is totalitarian also in the sense that a Kafkaesque society is totalitarian, in that fluctuations in the addict's life and in the market which governs that life come to him not as options but as social imperatives. He may defer orders or change orders that affect him, but he does not see them and he experiences them only as adversity or good fortune. His fate seems to be in the hands of people at different levels of the hierarchy. He does not see these people; he does not know them nor would he recognize them if he met them. These nameless personages can inspire in him a kind of quaking analogous to that generated by the storm trooper or Gestapo in Nazi Germany. The difference is that this totalitarianism is invisible, and not a known impersonal elite, and its power over addicts is not fear of tortures such as those of a star chamber or Gestapo headquarters, but rather that generated by anxiety that one's supply of heroin will be cut off. This terror seems to be strong even when the quality of the heroin is severely cut, as it has been in the 1960's.

It follows that between the illegal upper or capitalist class and the illegal proletarian class there is not conflict, but a moving class accommodation. This moving equilibrium is profitable to the first and borne by the second. The addicts find themselves "hooked" to a system they fall into and only suspect in outline form. The illegal upper class is able to divert from and to the conventional class system funds of money that appear not to be traceable by the usual accounting methods. A worldwide trade concentrated on the American continent, but especially on the big cities of the United States and more particularly on New York City, serves to energize a deviant class system which is an axis for the underworld. I have been told by more than one addict that every time an enterprising housewife puts five cents on a number in East Harlem she is contributing, whether she knows it or not, to a narcotics ring. I think that this is somewhat exaggerated because today the distribution of narcotics is less centralized than it was in the 1950's, and, as I have indicated, it seems to be fractured among a number of renegade groups as well as some independents with particularly good connections on ships coming from overseas.

Still, if there is accommodation, I believe that not much gratification comes to the proletarian class from any leadership in the illegal capitalist class. The proper contrast, I think, is between this situation and that of the peasants in feudal society. Whatever exploitations and depredations took place on the peasants and their families, they seem to have had some sense that the class or elite that controlled them in some way was a model, the embodiment of certain ideals they respected. From time to time the lord of the manor would be visible. This is not the situation, as I have said, of the illegal capitalist class, which remains largely invisible to the proletarians, which performs no honorific or exemplary function for them, and which seems to be utterly indifferent to their fate. But its invisibility gives it a magical quality in some circles.

It is because the addicts are involved in a market or series of markets that they are exposed to the winds of circumstance and the whim of their invisible leadership. They have no legal "talent," no court of appeals, and no unions to protect them from the giant trafficker. The result is that this mass of addicts resembles an aggregate of monads, each claiming a certain identity from his status as an addict but each using his own resources to fend for himself. Each is compelled or prepared to exploit his fellow addicts as well as himself to keep up his habit, obliged thereby also to subsidize the illegal capitalist class. He cannot look to this elite for emotional solidarity or any formulas to give meaning to his addiction. The top is not only invisible but inaudible. It does not protect the mass of addicts from the incursions of state power but is prepared blithely and freely to throw them in large fractions to the police to give the police a record and divert them from themselves. In this strange totalitarian society the masses of men learn that they and fractions of their lives are expendable.

In the beginning of this section I indicated that the addict culture is a substitute culture. In what sense is this true? Briefly, I think that the life of the addict is not only a parody of the life of the nonaddict but comes to serve as a substitute for the man or woman who is unable or unwilling to share in the life around him. I think the word "escape" is used too loosely in this connection because a person who escapes has a rather specific sphere from which he is fleeing and a specific sphere into which he goes. The act of escaping may also be rather affirmative, even aggressive, whereas the addicts who try to find this substitute for the square existence seem to float into addiction casually rather than through any design. Later on, as I have indicated, after repeated encounters with the drug and with addiction, a man may half-consciously fall back on the drug to cope with his problems.

There is an "ersatz" quality to addiction even when it is most real. In speaking to addicts who are still using and still subject to the immediate trauma of the problem I have the feeling that I am talking to men who are living an "as if" existence. They are living as though they did not have to eat good food and sleep well. They are living as if the bulk of life were unnecessary, that, for example, the major industries of the United States could be dispensed with. They act as though there were no wars, no problems of politics, no raging theological or social controversies going on all over the world.

This air of unreal abstraction is most conspicuously symbolized by the "nod" but is shown in their conversation when addicts are high on drugs. Whether it be in a hospital or a prison, in an agency or on the street, if they are left to themselves these men will talk unavoidably about who has the "stuff," who has the better "stuff," how "stuff" was in the past, the pressure of the police, events having to do with the comings and goings of men in jails, hospitals, and elsewhere, and, finally, deaths due to various causes, and speculations on those causes. The world of reality is narrowed to a spotlight for the theater of the absurd and in that spotlight a dancing nod occurs. The limited number of permutations and combinations is verbalized within a small area expressing vitality and that vitality is synthetic in that it flows from a preoccupation with a chemical.

In short, these thousands of people have tethered themselves to a substitute world, a narrow, self-limited and self-comforting world. If, from this narrow perspective, they look out at the penumbra that surrounds them, it is ironical that they claim to be "hip" and find the rest of the world inferior. Surely never was prejudice so designed to blind a man from his diseases in the present and his stuntedness in the future.

Money-and-heroin relationships exemplify this crazy minor reality. In a general way, I would feel it is correct to say that heroin is the money standard of addict culture. This does not mean that money is irrelevant but that rather there exists a kind of bimetallic standard comparable to the old gold-silver problem in nonaddict life. Addicts have a problem in relating money to heroin. Money comes from outside and retains some of its validity as a standard; heroin is a standard that is autonomous and autochthonous within the boundaries of addict life.

We first agree with most addicts that a user will turn everything or anything into money if he can. Under the pressure of desire to buy heroin an addict will perceive the possibilities for exploitation all around him and will act. Heroin is the Great Transformer. In this case it is money that is doing the transforming under the impact of the need for heroin.

Money is also a way of assessing the people who are potential victims. The con man, the mugger, the pickpocket—all these have to make quick assessments of the money worth of their victim at the point of the crime. Hence many addicts develop a capacity to ascribe a correct money status to a man or woman by virtue of his clothing and residence. Money is the standard of evaluation. The addict assesses his own fellows in part in terms of "hustling" ability where "hustling" means the capacity to get at least the money one needs.

Nonetheless, money is not the exclusive criterion for assessing people, events, or objects. Heroin is a competitor, and in the case of most people hooked on it it is perhaps the crucial criterion. One asks an addict, "What would you do if you had the following choice: you had ten dollars offered to you, on the one hand, and two bags of heroin, on the other?" He will tend to say that in most situations, he would take the two bags; since the man is hooked he needs heroin like an island, by definition, needs water, and by having the heroin on his person or available in his control he makes sure that he will not go sick.

Then, one asks the man, "Suppose there were a hundred dollars, and you had two bags offered to you also—which would you take?" Some will say that they would take the hundred dollars because the odds are they can get more than two bags. Then, if one adds that a "panic" period is on, where drugs are rare and hard to obtain even illegally, they will tend to say they would take the two bags. It is clear that where they prefer to take the money they feel they can use it to buy more heroin. They prefer the money in these cases as a means of improving their chances of getting more heroin.

The heroin is important in judging the worth of addicts and pushers. More exactly, the quantity and quality of a man's connection to heroin also distinguish him from his fellows. Agency workers who visit prisons are always being asked on the street when certain men are coming out. It is remarkable how rapidly information about prison comings and goings of their fellows is spread by street addicts, particularly about men who are "into something," and who can, in their turn, be exploited or at least be partners in exploitation involving money and heroin. This is often one of the reasons for a man's reinvolvement.

As the case of G. illustrates, a man who is a good hustler is someone that men and women in the addict culture do not want to lose. He brings capital and, hence, that much more impetus to the circulation of heroin into and down the addict society. From the point of view of the addict the man with good connections has a kind of magic which makes it worthwhile to cultivate his acquaintance. But if it is magic it is tinged with a good deal of realistic thinking. It leads the addicts to prefer not to make anyone an enemy for one cannot tell who will be on top tomorrow. As the slogan has it, "The Chances Go Around." However, it is especially those men who can bring capital or who have good connections with heroin who are respected, and of the two, the good hustler and the man with good connections, I believe it is the latter who would be preferred. Often, as a matter of fact, the man who is "into something" as regards drugs is confused with the good hustler and is called such by people who do not choose their words accurately (as many addicts do not). But the confusion, I think, shows how important are heroin connections. A man who does nothing more than sit around and occasionally go to a specific big connection is felt to be as vital a moving force as a man who makes stings, commits daring robberies, or forges or embezzles or cons, although he may not be as admired.

In short, there is a hierarchy of money-getting and a hierarchy of heroin-getting, and while the first is important and indeed vital to the circulation and distribution of heroin, from the point of view of the person who uses, access to heroin is the crucial element. You can always get money, in theory, but there are panics about heroin. There are no money panics in the eyes of the addicts.

We can see the effects of this dual standard of evaluation when a man decides that he wants to "straighten up" and become rehabilitated or, more exactly, wants to rehabilitate himself. The man who, on drugs, felt that he could always make money and did so is a little at a loss to know how to function and gauge his progress when he is "off." He discovers that he is "missing something," and does not know for sure what it is. It is significant that his first impulse is to feel that what he is missing is the drug, and then, secondarily, the excitement of the life. He observes with dismay that when he was on stuff (if he was a good hustler) he often had money anyway to use for his little expenses, to give away to his wife or girl friend or child or anyone else. On drugs he had the sense of gaining surplus value, which is to say, life was invested with a surplus element despite the enormous, relentless, and grinding pressure upon him. In contrast, off drugs, this is the common complaint, a man tends to have neither money nor heroin. The man who is trying to be rehabilitated is posed with the dilemma: if I sell drugs, I can get money, but if I have drugs, I'll get hooked.

A good part of this dilemma comes from the pre-eminent role of heroin in the evaluation process. The addict on drugs has incorporated within his psyche this dual standard, and in becoming or trying to become an ex-addict square he has to readjust his sights. He has now to put money in a new perspective. Particularly in the early period of transition, this does not mean that he has to give it the same value as it is given by middle-class people, but he has to learn how to handle his money as though it were crucial ("sacred"?). He cannot go around buying things indiscriminately because he does not have the money that can permit him this luxury. He has to budget his time as well as his money. He discovers, as a matter of fact, that money and time are now two of his principal standards of evaluating himself, with time now taking the place of heroin as a rival to money. He has to spend time without spending money and evaluate his week in the light of how profitably time has been spent just as on drugs he evaluated himself in terms of how much heroin he had got. The swift transformation of perspectives demanded of the addict is hampered, as I say, by repeated misperception of the place of money in his changing life.

Don Quixote Meets Señora Heroina

Frequently it is said that the addicted person under the influence of his particular existential drug is highly unrealistic and lacking in good judgment. This may not be true for specific individuals, especially those who have used heroin. Unless he is under the terrible pressure of immediate necessity for drugs, a heroin addict can use some degree of judgment to survive. However, in many areas of their lives men and women addicted to the existential drugs appear to follow in the footsteps of the famous Man from La Mancha, Don Quixote. In fact, talking to them, I have often had the impression that they are living out a particular version of the myth which I would call "Don Quixote Meets Señora Heroina," where heroin plays the role of Dulcinea. Let me explain the sort of conduct and statement which supports my feeling.

First of all, many of them—whatever their real class origins—act as though they were or had been part of an elite culture—the addict culture—membership in which, at one time or another, has been for a privileged few. I do not think it is an accident that the addicted refer to themselves as being hip, and scornfully refer to the outsiders as squares. Leaving aside any allusion to the origin of the word "hip" from opium society which itself was, of course, deemed an elite group, the heroin addicts also claim a special historical position in the underworld sun. They all refer to some golden age in which things were better than they are today, and that particular period will, of course, vary with the number of years the man has been using. If an addicted person began using in 1940, then *ipso facto* that becomes the golden year. If he began in 1950, that year is the starting point for the Fall, and so on. But in any case, by an astonishing magical trick, every man and woman who used the drugs can claim to have shared in paradise.

I say this is no accident because I feel that this idea of belonging to an elite culture is a protective device that permits the proletarianized addict to feel that he is part of a happy few who can understand the experience, the cosmic encounter. Especially the squares with their confident ignorance do not share this encounter. I say it protects them because, were they not so sheltered behind the cultural façade, many of them would likely never have become deeply involved in the drug. They are like alcoholics who need the protection of the estimated eighty million social drinkers in the United States in order to conceal their existence as a minority of some five or six million. The addicts cannot rely upon such extensive numbers, but they do exaggerate their place in the United States, giving anyone who listens estimates that go as wildly as one million heroin addicts. Whereas the alcoholic masquerades under a broad base of legitimate users of his drink, the addict feels he is protected by the exaggeratedly large numbers of illegal fellow sufferers.

Now, what is the rational basis for this elite status style? There is the claim to be "cool." This links the addict to the aristocratic appearance of being above pettiness and always being in control of his fate. The "cool" man with his "front" is like a mailed knight riding on his charger, indifferent to any of the petty obstacles and interferences around him.

The addicted also claim the special gift of intelligence which marks them off from the plebeians around them. There is an interesting kind of argument that they offer to demonstrate their higher IQ. "Could a square survive," they ask, "in the kind of jungle we live in? It takes brains, man, to keep up a habit that costs $35 to $40 a day—every day in the year. You don't get that kind of money if you're stupid or dull." Such is the reasoning. In Puerto Rico, a certain semblance of reality is lent to this element of the myth by the fact that the hospital at Rio Piedras has published reports of IQ studies, showing that the average of the users was higher than that of the nonusers. This study, however, was not controlled to compare people of comparable education, and, I think, only showed that addicts in Puerto Rico may have more education than nonaddicts.* (A number of the samples came from New York City.) Furthermore, a whole series of legends about "short con" and "long con" games helps to solidify the addicts' self-image as being particularly bright.

But this element of pseudo-aristocratic belief and myth breaks down after a man tries to move into or survive in any segment of relatively conventional society. It is then that he begins to feel inadequate and even stupid for what he has done and for what he is not able to do in the present. In fact, one of the elements of rehabilitation programs seems to be the frank reappraisal of a man's skills and attitudes and his introduction to himself under a new life.

Going on with the elements of a Don Quixote image, a man on drugs tends also to feel that he is hypersensitive, with the word

* Even where limited samples of addicted men show an average IQ somewhat higher than the norm, the difference is much less than that which they claim.

"sensitive" being used at various times to mean sentimental, overly responsive, aesthetic, and easily frustrated. Under any of these meanings, however, he seeks to put himself above the common cut of man or woman in order to ally himself with the artistic or aesthetic side of life's problems. As I have said earlier, I find it no accident, in the light of this myth, that so many men at one time or another claim to be artistically inclined and that in rehabilitation programs in the past so many of them "homed" into pottery, painting, and other artistic programs. The love of drama and the emphasis on style sometimes also appear to be accounted for by a certain homosexual strain in a number of these men. But in any case to be sensitive is to be a cut above other people.

But I have not yet reached the point at which a man begins to play the sorrowful knight. This is when he acts as though he were in heroic pursuit of an ideal which at one time was an ideal—namely, the qualities of heroin—and which is now only a faded tapestry. The myth seems to apply to the manner in which the addict will still cling to the hope that the next shot will not only make him "straight," will not only remove the symptoms of his sickness, but will give him a "buzz," or even an ecstatic "high." I think it is important to recognize the ambiguities in the addict's position. Knowing full well that the "stuff" is "garbage," he will tell himself and anyone who hears him that he has no hopes of anything better from the market than just getting "straight." But if one listens long enough one can detect the wistful hope that the erstwhile ideal is still operative and that, in fact, it is an ideal if only *something* will happen! And at one level of his consciousness he keeps hoping that it will happen. It is at this level that he retains his affiliation back to Don Quixote, insisting that Dulcinea is not a prostitute but is, in fact, his fair dream of ideal beauty.

The picture of the mad knight, symbolical of a feudalism out of joint and out of date, helps us also to feel the incongruities in the alienated position of today's addict as he experiences or refuses to experience the world that is oppressing him. Consider, for example, the almost monotonous way in which addicts will deny aspects of their lives to themselves and to those around them. For example, a young user will deny categorically that he is using; or if he is hooked, he will deny that he is hooked; or if he is hooked and admits that he is hooked, he will deny that he is a greasy junkie. What is is not, to the extent that it reduces him to a common run of humanity and deflates his grandiose fantasies. If we will not accept his fantasies or, like Sancho Panza, humor him he will disappear from us and find company among his fellows who may in some way share with him the impulse to restore a warm chemical feudalism—if only in fantasy. Is it any accident that these men sometimes call heroin "horse"? The man who rides the horse, which is also Mrs. Heroin, is bound to be an anguished metaphor, not sure if he is Don Quixote or a bagged Centaur.

Or, again, when he is either denying or affirming, we notice how impressed he is with the power of rhetoric and, as he goes through "his act" with utter "sincerity," explains to us why at this point he cannot go to a hospital, or why he has to break off an interview in order "to see his landlord who is waiting for him," when really what is involved is getting a shot that he has a sudden, imperious need to get. We recognize that here is a man who needs to feel that his very presence is influential and that we, who are the target of that influence, will feed his grandiosity.

Take, again, the manner in which heroin distorts the sexual life. Many men feel like sexual giants under the influence of heroin, but on the other side of the picture is diminished interest in sex. Still, men who are reared in the tradition of the ideal of "the big dick," the extended, rigid penis, derive a special nobility in their own minds from their capacity to outlast any woman or even several women in the course of a long night's work. I take this to be another component, however Paul Bunyanesque, in this whole peculiar myth.

Again let me emphasize the feeling of many men that they are heroes or at least negative heroes—that is, martyrs. When they speak about the police—and they are continually talking about them—there is always an unspoken undertone, at the very least, that it takes a person of heroic dimensions to endure the humiliations of the police, to escape their traps, to leap over roofs like Superman, then down fire escapes and into and around and under intricate nested basements. A man talking months later about such an exploit will glow with a certain enthusiasm—if he has been successful—about how he outwitted the police. Surely, says this undertone, anyone who does this is a hero and a genuine claimant for aristocratic recognition. The fact that at another level these men feel that they are petty offenders and are treated as such by the police does not fully deflate this element of their unconscious myth.

Addicted men are also proud if they can show off their good clothes and general taste. In fact, an addict shows he is a "good doer" (i.e., is successful) if he can maintain his role as a fashion plate. (Of course, it is only the exceptional addict who can afford a car, of whatever vintage. Watches, too, are a sign that a man is doing well or else is a skillful burglar.) Like his aristocratic equivalents, our chemical knight would like to be a model for style and, more generally, a sumptuary virtuoso.

Finally, let me point out the recurrent statement that anyone who interviews addicts will sooner or later hear from them that *they* are exceptions, that *they* are different from other addicts. After one has heard this statement over a hundred times, one is prepared to ask the one hundred and first if he hasn't noticed that there is something rather paradoxical about a group in which every one feels so different from the others. He will agree that this is true, but then say that he *really* is different, which leaves you, of course, precisely where you were before. The sense of belonging to an elite group turns out to refer to people who are not really elite except for you and me, and I don't know about you. This is the ultimate caricature and paradox within this unconscious quixotic myth. Their belief, never too clearly stated, that they are an elite group, turns out really to mean, at one level, that the speaker is himself an elite man if only society would recognize his great talents.

Together these elements make up a picture of a group that at one phase of its existence, one stage of its drug use, and one period of its development would make inordinate demands upon society. We see them demonstrating some of these demands in hospitals and squelching them in other places like prisons. It becomes one of the problems of rehabilitation for staff members to cope with this belief that is acted out in different ways by different men and with different degrees of insistence. Perhaps rehabilitation programs are saved by the fact that if they screen their candidates well it is likely that only those survive or mostly those survive who have either abandoned or successfully repressed their unconscious allegiance to this myth.

Let us turn now to some portraits and cameos which are intended to show the diversity of addicts. The portraits are tapes or sections of tapes with commentary and the cameos are brief analytical summaries of cases.

PART II

PORTRAITS AND CAMEOS

Portrait of Billie

Billie had been known to Exodus House in the years when it was called the East Harlem Protestant Parish Narcotics Committee. He had been sent to the United States Public Health Hospital in Lexington, Kentucky, and to other hospitals through the Narcotics Committee's referral services. Other members of the staff and I would meet him in New York City's Metropolitan Hospital or in the street so that there was a long-term but superficial relationship to him. One day during a period of his hospitalization I asked him if he would tape-record for me some of his memories.

In one of the taped sessions, not here included, I pointed out to Billie, who was twenty-five at the time, that his voice had an unusually sad tone, and this surprised him. He said that he was depressed almost all of the time but had never noticed that there was a sadness in his voice. There is always a sadness in his face whether off or on drugs. He is rarely off. There is good reason for a sense of hopelessness about himself—for something is always happening to him that gives him, if not dismay or irritation, at least embarrassment. After his last signing out from the hospital he was soon involved with other men in a roundup in which, as far as he could see, he was an innocent bystander. This led to his imprisonment for a short while before his acquittal and eventual release.

Billie is one of those many addicts who, through action or inaction, may unwittingly expose themselves to risks that do not add to their growth, but may imperil their very existence. The material that follows illustrates this point and shows its place in his life style, which ironically tends to favor a conservative outlook.

The two interviews I am including were held in a cubicle that one of the nurses kindly offered us in the interest of privacy. Outside from time to time one could hear the fire engines which so frequently scream through East Harlem that they almost become part of the routine of life. Billie sat there all eagerness and chain-smoking, wanting to be part of a book. From time to time patients would peer through a window and once there was an interruption to bring Billie his commissary. I had the impression that Billie was trying his best to give his all, hoping in his own way to enlighten the layman who would read his story about the real nature of the addict's life. Unlike the other histories recorded in this book, Billie's was oriented specifically around research. Like the others, however, each interview lasted about an hour and a half. During the first interview he was still under the influence of the methadone he was receiving as part of a detoxification program. During the second interview he was off drugs completely.

SEYMOUR FIDDLE. *Please see if you could give me the story of your life as you see it.*
BILLIE. The story of my life? Well, uh, my plans were when I was in high school that I started making plans for my future was to go to the university, if possible. Then I got involved with a group of fellas that were using drugs. You can't actually call them drug addicts because they weren't, you know, hooked or strung out, but they were joy popping like they call it, and I got involved with them, and they didn't uh ask me or force me to use drugs but I was curious and that's how I started using dope, through these fellas and uh . . . I thought I could give it up, y'know. I thought my will power is strong. I could give it up, but I enjoyed the kick and I continued till I got to this stage, and now, like seems . . . the outlook I got on life now is this that uh I don't feel right unless I've got some kind of buzz, you know. Like I don't feel normal or I got some kind of buzz in my head, and while I'm clean, even when I'm not hooked, I feel depressed all the time, and when I take off . . . even if there's not a nod, y'know, just the idea that I took off and I got a slight buzz that will make me

feel normal, happy, give me a complete different outlook on life and
. . . uh . . . this is the way I've been existing for the last nine years
or so since 1957.

[Billie's assuming not only that it isn't good to feel depressed but
also that it is necessary and right to take immediate action in the
form of self-medication to change the state. He also identifies
chemical state with mental outlook and arrives at the conclusion
that an injection produces a radically different outlook on life. This
superficial view of what an outlook is gives further apparent rational character to the whole business of drug use. This opening
statement also establishes his self-image as a depressed person.]

S.F. *How would you compare the way you act off drugs and on
drugs? On drugs, what differences are there?*
B. Well, off drugs, I'm very quiet . . . I uh . . . don't speak
practically at all. They have to force the words out of me . . . and I
. . . I get a feeling that I don't get along with people and that
it is very difficult for me to get along with people. But on drugs
I feel that everybody likes me, that I could speak better, that I know
everything is going down and I'm doing everything right whether I'm
not. I don't know whether I am or whether I'm not, but that's the
feeling that I get that I'm doing everything right. Now I don't know
if people have that feeling you know . . . when I'm drugged. I believe at times when I'm sober, when I'm not using drugs, I think well
maybe I made a fool out of myself, but I'm not sure, you know?
'Cause it is something like a split personality—with me.
S.F. *Really? You feel like a Jekyll and Hyde?*
B. Yeh . . . well, I get that feeling 'cause I change completely.
. . . I'm very quiet when I'm not high on anything, y'know . . . or
when I'm not on drugs . . . I'm very quiet, and when I am on drugs,
I speak a lot and I'm very bold, I'm very forward. I lose that complex.
. . . I don't know if it is a complex actually 'cause when I'm not on
drugs I don't feel like I have a complex. When I'm off drugs I don't
feel like that I have a complex. 'Cause if I had to speak to a person,
I would speak to a person. If I had to go to an interview, I would go
to an interview, y'know? That's not being on drugs so . . . but I'm

more bold when I'm . . . when I have the drug in me . . . so I don't know whether it is. . . .

S.F. *When you were not using anything years ago, before you ever began drugs, what kind of person were you like then?*

B. Well, I was young . . . I was seventeen. . . . Those years were to me, they were happy years. As a matter I recall back . . . they seem like the happiest years of my life.

S.F. *Why were they happy? Tell me how.*

B. Gawna school . . . I enjoyed school very much. I didn't cut classes, I didn't play hooky, and to me it was a ball to go to school, and every day was a new experience to me, y'know? 'Cause I was lookin' forward to doin' somethin' different . . . get together with my friends. We had a gang, get together plannin' dances, outings, goin' to the beach on Sundays, picnics, goin' to the movies on Sundays with your girl. Y'know, every day was like a new experience, but now the drugs took the place of all them things.

[Billie's effort to establish a period of adolescent paradise is not entirely convincing and certainly does open up more questions than he has asked himself. If he describes every day as "a new experience," then something was driving him to look for these new experiences and it was not a basic contentment with himself.]

S.F. *Everything?*

B. Everything. Now I don't do anything at all . . . except it's just . . . just think of the fix and even while you're taking, even while I'm taking off, I'm thinking how I'm gonna get the next fix. So everything, you know, evolves around drugs, everything . . . my whole life.

S.F. *Exactly how did you get involved for the first time, and when did it take place?*

B. Well, it was in school and I saw . . . I knew that a couple of my friends was doing something, and I was curious. I wasn't sure what they were doing at first. I thought they were drinking, and I was curious. I asked one of them, and he explained to me what he was doing. . . . They were skin-popping and I says I like to try, and he says no, I don't think you should try it. I says well, don't tell me what to do

. . . I got money. . . . I like to . . . Well, naturally when I told him I had money, y'know, they went for it, and they let me try it, and that's how I got involved. I skin-popped once, and after that I just kept on mainlining . . . 'cause I found out that through a mainline, it's a much quicker high, and you feel it faster and you enjoy it more.

S.F. *Had you heard about heroin before?*

B. No.

S.F. *Why were you so willing to take that, eager to take that shot?*

B. I was eager because of the way I saw my friends high. You know they—to me, they were having such a ball. You know like everything was . . . they were laughin' and carryin' on and they were having a ball like they were the "in" crowd and I was "out," you know. Well, I wasn't the only one that probably got involved in, you know, caught in that whirlpool, you know? There were two or three other guys got caught there too. Well, like uh . . . that's the way it seemed to me at the time. Like . . . uh . . . they were, you know, into something, and like I wasn't into anything.

S.F. *Isn't it very funny? You said that those were the happiest years of your life. Before you used drugs.*

B. Hmm. Hmm. That's the way it seems to me now.

S.F. *If you were so happy, why were you so curious about why they were happy? It doesn't make any sense, does it? If you are a happy person, why should you want to be jealous of and want to be in with the people who are enjoying themselves if you are enjoying yourself too?*

B. Yes, I was happy in the sense that we were doin' a lotta things.

S.F. *Such as?*

B. Like I said, outings, dances, going to movies on . . . well, like uh just . . . it could be like . . . just that certain day, you know, when this happened . . . maybe like they were happy and I was unhappy. It doesn't mean like when I say that those were the happiest days of my life that I was happy every minute, you know, can you understand what I mean?

S.F. *Does that mean that you want to be happy every minute?*

B. Probably so . . . but what I'm sayin' is that day when I seen them, jumpin' up and down and havin' a ball . . . I was already curious because I had dug them before.

S.F. *Oh, you had?*

B. Yeah—but I never approached them.

S.F. *Oh, I see.*

B. But this particular day I did. Y'understand? That's what happened. But like I said, I think those were the happiest days of my life 'cause after I got involved with drugs . . . I don't remember . . . I don't remember enjoying myself with a guy. I tried. I tried doin' everything that I did when I wasn't using drugs, but it wasn't the same. It wasn't the same at all, you know, I couldn't. Something . . . like something went out of me. Completely . . . I don't know. . . . I couldn't do, you know, or have the same fun that I had when I wasn't using drugs.

[Billie here is indicating the existential character of heroin. It not only "changes his outlook," it seems to have taken something out of him. This kind of observation, in varying words, is made by a great many addicts. There is a radical turning in a man's life when he becomes hooked on heroin.]

S.F. *Did this puzzle you? Make you worry at all?*

B. It puzzles me—I think about it, you know. There was a point when I was younger that I really worried about it, and I always had a solution for it . . . like uh . . . I say, well, the solution to this is to stop using narcotics and everything will go back to normal, to like it was, but it wasn't that easy, you know? When I would take off everything would be clear like I'll stop using drugs and that's it, but once I was sick, you know, the problem was there like, you know, I had to take off and then it would be the same thing. I would have a solution for it. But like there wasn't.

S.F. *In other words, when you took off you had the illusion that you had the solution?*

B. Right and the solution was clear—to stop using dope, but I couldn't, you know?

S.F. *Where were you born?*

B. In Puerto Rico.

S.F. *And how old were you when you came here to New York?*

B. Four years old.

S.F.   *Do you have any memories of Puerto Rico at all?*
B.   Very very little.
S.F.   *What do you remember?*
B.   I could recall the house we lived in. And . . . the little that I remember is very depressing. We had holes in the floor—I recall that. I recall when it rained how the rain used to come through the ceiling, through the roof, and I recall the muddy streets, you know. Things like that. But life itself, I don't recall—I just remember very little things.
S.F.   *Remember people?*
B.   Do I recall people? No. I recall falling through a window but they are very low. The houses in Puerto Rico are very low. I recall falling through a window with my cousin one time—we were playin' —things like that—little things that to me don't make no sense. I don't even know why I remember . . . why those things stand out, you know?

[But the fact that Billie's memories of Puerto Rico are mostly sad is itself no accident. It fits into his conception of himself as living a depressed life.]

S.F.   *Do you remember your father and mother being in Puerto Rico?*
B.   Oh, I remember my father. He was a . . . he was a chauffeur and when he used to come from work, he used to blow his horn, and he used to give me change, you know. It musta been pennies or somepin' every night when he used to come home. That I recall.
S.F.   *What did you do with the pennies?*
B.   I don't recall what I did with them. But I recall he used to blow his horn and I used to run out to meet him.

[This memory of the father blowing his horn would be a happy one were it not that it contrasts so much, as we shall see, with his very strained relationships with his father in New York.]

S.F.   *What kind of work did he do?*
B.   He was a chauffeur in Puerto Rico.

S.F. *Was he a chauffeur in a truck or a car?*

B. I can't recall if he was a chauffeur with a truck or a taxi or what. I know he was a chauffeur of some kind.

S.F. *How about your mother? What did she do?*

B. My mother . . . uh, I know she didn't work, but this I know 'cause I was told . . . but I know she didn't work.

S.F. *Who else was there in your family besides yourself and your mother and father?*

B. You mean when I was over there?

S.F. *Yes. Over there.*

B. My cousins. Four cousins and my aunt.

S.F. *You lived in the same house?*

B. We lived in the same house. I can't remember, you know, ever playing with them or anything like that.

S.F. *Do you remember coming over here on board a ship or plane?*

B. I remember . . . I remember a train station. That's all I remember when we were coming over. My mother left me alone with the luggage. That's all I remember.

S.F. *Do you remember, were you afraid?*

B. I don't remember. She told me later that I started wandering around the station crying, but that's because she told me. But I remember being left alone with the luggage, yes, I remember that.

S.F. *Then you came to New York.*

B. At that time—this was in 1944—there wasn't like flights from Puerto Rico to New York direct. They would have to stop over in Florida, and then to New York . . . that's what happened. . . . So we took the train from Florida to New York.

S.F. *Did you ever find out why they moved that year?*

B. Why we came over here? I was told that my father found a better position. Much better money in New York and he sent for us.

S.F. *Oh, at that time he was living in New York already?*

B. Yeah . . . he came ahead of us.

S.F. *And you came with your mother?*

B. Yes.

S.F. *Then when you arrived in New York, where did you live?*

B. We lived on 116th Street between Lexington and Park in Manhattan—the same place—I'm still living in the same place. That's uh

. . . twenty . . . twenty-one years now, twenty-one or twenty-two years. Twenty-two years, yeah.

[Billie's situation may seem exceptional to those who view the slum dweller as an uprooted person moving from ghetto place to ghetto place. It is ironical that whereas Billie might have considered living in the same home for twenty-one years or so with pride, this fact taken in conjunction with the comments that follow suggests how hemmed in and constricted he felt living at home.]

S.F.　*In the same house?*
B.　Same house.
S.F.　*In other words, your family never moved.*
B.　And I recall at one time—I must have been about ten years old —I used to detest it. I used to detest the neighborhood.
S.F.　*Why?*
B.　The house, everything. Just—I used to hate it. It got to a point where I didn't want to come home. You know, like we used to go to the movies, and at the movies, you see, you see different . . . I would see different environments . . . how people lived, you know, in the picture. . . . This was all . . . but then I . . . and then to come home and have to face, you know, a room crowded with people . . . I hated it.
S.F.　*Did you have any of your own books or any of your own toys?*
B.　I never had toys. They used to buy us clothes at Christmas. If we got any presents at all, it was clothes.
S.F.　*Well, what happened to your father's job?*
B.　He got the job all along. He kept the job. He was the one that was supporting the family. He had the job. He kept the job. He was a merchant seaman. I never got to see my father.

[A special study might be made of the relationship between merchant seamen fathers and delinquent or potentially delinquent children. Billy here is emphasizing one facet of this problem, the irregularity and infrequency of father-son contacts, especially where the father is working full time as a seaman.]

S.F. *Oh, he became a merchant seaman. That was the job. I see.*

B. Yeah. That was the job. He was a merchant seaman. And like . . . he was home something like maybe a month or a month and a half out of the year, and the rest of the time he was out. I never got to see him. Actually, when he came home, I was afraid to approach him like . . . you see kids, you know, "daddy!" And they run up to their father and throw their arms around him. Well, I was afraid to do like that 'cause he's very stern and very strict, you know. Had that look about him. Like I have a lot of respect for him. Or I had. Not no more. You know I lost him. I don't respect him no more.

S.F. *Why did you lose your respect?*

B. 'Cause uh . . . maybe it's my fault, but he left just last year. He got fed up and left.

S.F. *You mean he left the house?*

B. He left the house. 'Cause I was stealin' too much from him. You know? One time I took a hundred dollars from him.

S.F. *How much—a hundred?*

B. A hundred dollars. He had just come home from a trip. . . . He had his wallet, and he works hard for that money he makes, and I took a hundred dollars from his wallet.

S.F. *How much was there in the wallet?*

B. There was over three hundred dollars. But I didn't mean to . . . I didn't want to take a hundred dollars, you know? But it was like I needed sixty dollars, and they were in fifty-dollar bills, you know, and so I took two fifty-dollar bills. If there would have been smaller bills, I wouldn't have taken the hundred dollars. Anyway that's one of the big things to me, in my mind, is one of the things that really hurt him or got him aggravated to the point where he left.

[Observe how Billie, in effect, puts part of the blame for his taking the one hundred dollars on his father, the victim shares guilt with the thief. He is also projecting blame on the chance situation, the kinds of bills the father had in his wallet.]

S.F. *What position has your mother had about you? What has she done?*

B. What has she done? She doesn't approve. But like she'll—she'll tell me like "as long as I'm alive, you'll have a roof over your head." And she'll try to help me the best way she can. She doesn't approve of what I'm doin'. She doesn't like what I'm doin', you know? But she gave up too, she can't . . . she can't uh . . . she—she feels like there's no hope for me.

S.F.   *How do you feel?*

B.   I feel there's gotta be . . . there's gotta be some kind of hope 'cause I'm always looking . . . always looking for an outlet, for a way or means to get away from this. You know, I've spoken to my psychiatrist, and I told him, you know, that I want to get away from this, but I—I—it just seems like there's times when either I've left jail or the hospital and I really got my mind set on not using narcotics, you know? But I don't know what happens. I go back into the neighborhood, you know, same environment, and go right back into it. A day or two, a week . . . I'm right back where I started, but I really, I really go out at times, I'm not saying all the time, at times with my mind really made up not to use drugs, and I just slip back into the pit.

S.F.   *When were you first arrested?*

B.   About 1960.

S.F.   *What was the charge?*

B.   Acting in concert.

S.F.   *What does that mean there?*

B.   What does that mean?

S.F.   *In your case, what does it mean?*

B.   I was walking with a fella that had narcotics on him. I know he had narcotics 'cause we were gettin' down—we were gettin' together to get this half load in.

S.F.   *Was he a pusher?*

B.   No. He was another drug addict and uh . . . they caught him and they caught me. I thought they were gonna let me go 'cause they find the stuff on him, but no, they wrote us both up. They got him for possession, and they got me for acting in concert. I don't know if they observed me giving him money or what—I know they got me for acting in concert.

S.F.   *How much time did you spend?*

B.   I got a suspended sentence acting in concert, but I recall at that time my people still hadn't known I was using drugs. I started using drugs in 1957, and they didn't come to find out until I got arrested.

S.F. *How come you were able to hide it for three years?*

B. They weren't wise to, you know, what was happening. They didn't know what was a drug addict or the symptoms or how . . . their reactions, you know, or anything like that. You know? They weren't wise. You know, plus my father wasn't home. . . . Even when he was home he wasn't like to find out anything. It was very easy to fool my mother. So I got away with it.

S.F. *You have a brother, don't you—a younger brother?*

B. Yeah. On my father's side.

S.F. *Do you live with him too?*

B. He didn't live with us. He lived with my grandmother. She died just last year.

S.F. *How come he didn't live with your mother?*

B. I don't know. They didn't get along. For some reason or other. 'Cause his mother—my father married my mother while his mother was still alive, and I think that my father wasn't married to my brother's mother, y'understand? So it's . . . got a conflict there . . . that they . . . I know my brother didn't get along with my mother.

S.F. *So have you really been an only child in a way all along?*

B. That's right. True.

S.F. *You and your mother living in a house. Your father coming in and staying awhile, and then back to work.*

B. That's right.

S.F. *Would you say you were a spoiled child?*

B. Yes.

S.F. *How were you spoiled?*

B. In the sense that uh . . . not when I was younger 'cause when I was younger, we weren't doing so good when I came from Puerto Rico, but I say like from the age of like eight years old on, you know, like I got everything I wanted. You know, money, clothes, and I did anything like I wanted to do—stay up late—stay out in the street, and I got away with murder. You know?

[Those who lead depressed lives may be conveniently divided into two main categories. On the one hand, there are those who report a substantial period in their childhood when things were going well, and they knew and were given considerable—apparently excessive —freedom to enjoy material things. Often this was accompanied by much freedom in the streets. On the other hand, there are those who report receiving a minimum of material satisfactions from their parents, and who were forced to turn to the streets for what they wanted. The importance of relative deprivation and relative satisfaction in relation to the development of subsequent addict life needs to be explored.]

S.F. *Your mother wasn't after you to . . . ?*

B. No. No, she uh . . . she would tell me, you know, don't do this, don't do that, but like deep inside I know like she would say it, and mean it, but I could do it, and she wasn't gonna do anything about it, you know?

S.F. *You didn't believe she was going to punish you?*

B. Right. And she didn't. She never punished me.

S.F. *You said that you didn't play hooky.*

B. No.

S.F. *Did you get good marks?*

B. Average marks. English was my best subject. Math I was—I was very bad in math.

S.F. *Were you spending much time in the street during this period? After school?*

B. Yeah. I spent all the time in the street.

S.F. *You liked the street and you liked school too, both?*

B. Right, both.

S.F. *But you didn't like the house.*

B. Right. I spent very little time in the house. I would go in and grab a sandwich or something and run back out. The only time I was there in the house for two or three hours was if I had friends up there with me. You know?

S.F. *Didn't you ever talk much with your mother at all?*

B. No.

S.F. *What sort of person is she?*

B. She is an educated person. She understands English and she went up to, I believe, it was the second or first year high school, you know, which at that time was somethin,' somethin' at least in Puerto

Rico, you know? Because at that time in Puerto Rico you had to buy your books and what not, the way she tells me, so she knows enough. . . . She could have a better job than she has now and she doesn't. She does—what is it they call it? She packs. She does packing. In some firm.

S.F. *Does she work because she has to?*

B. Yes. She has to. I'm sorry to say, she has to.

S.F. *Because your father doesn't send her enough money?*

B. My father doesn't support us at all. You see he left. He left, and in a way she was glad he left because uh . . . my father has always been this type of person, he's had different women all his life, you know? And like she was fed up with that, you know? She was fed up with that. She would find lipstick on his collars and letters from other women, and what not, you know. Naturally, I imagine she felt bad that . . . you know? And she don't want that no more and so she figured if uh . . . if he leaves and still sends me money, he's gonna feel that I'm obligated to him in some kind of a way, you know? So I'd rather not have him send me anything, and you know, just forget it altogether.

[Notice how easily Billie slips into his mother's role and speaks as though *she* were talking. Although he may be exaggerating when he says she doesn't talk to him, what he really means is that between mother and child there is the kind of tie that permits them to rely on nonverbal communication. His own self-boundaries are not sharply defined.]

S.F. *How did these affairs look to you when you were younger? And how do you look at it now? Did it disturb you in any way that your father was that way?*

B. Well, when I was younger I didn't know my father was that way.

S.F. *No? Well, when did you first find out about it?*

B. I hated it. I thought it was disgusting.

S.F. *When did you find out about it for the first time?*

B. I believe when I was in junior high school. I must have been fourteen or fifteen.

S.F. *How did you find out about it?*

B. I saw my mother crying one time, and she explained it to me. She half explained it to me, you know. Not thoroughly, not completely, but I more or less could make out the rest for myself, and I hated it, and I thought it was disgusting. And I never felt any love for my father at all, and I thought that . . . I just couldn't stand him— I couldn't stand him. I still can't. I had respect for him. . . . I told you I had respect for him. It was like you would respect the cop in the street. That's how I respected him, you know? Because I was afraid he would hit me, you know. But not respect because he was my father. I just respected him because I was afraid of him. . . . He never laid a hand on me though.

S.F. *No; isn't that funny?*

B. But that's the way I felt about him. I didn't like him. I detested him for the way he treated my mother.

S.F. *Did you ever show this to him?*

B. He never sat down to speak with me or anything like . . . we never were that close, you know? I don't know if he noticed it, but like uh but we never were that close . . . like . . . I think he knew my feelings . . . or . . . I had the idea that I knew his feelings. I thought that he acted that way because he wanted respect, you know, like he wanted the whole household to respect him like he was the master, you understand? That's the way I felt. I don't know if I'm wrong. But he always had this stern look. And like uh . . . lunch would have to be ready at a certain time . . . had to be warm, you know. Had to be something that he liked and all of this, you know, and he liked that and he liked the way he acted and when he would come in very serious, he would never sit down and give you no kind of advice. . . . Even when he found out I was using drugs, he never pulled me over to talk to me. . . . The only time that he would ever talk to me was when he would get drunk and he would get drunk quite often, you know. That's the only time he would decide to give me advice. . . . I used to feel like chokin' him.

S.F. *What sort of advice did he give you?*

B. He gave the advice—if you can call this advice, you know. By sayin', I'm not workin', I'm not working like a horse so you could become a bum, and this is what, you know, I'm slaving for, you know, and things like that, you know? Things that are not really advice. . . .

It's more like threats they seem to me, you know. Like he says uh
. . . he would tell me, he always made me feel like I was responsible
for my mother, you know. In other words, since he wasn't home, I
had to be the man of the house. I had to take care of my mother, you
know. . . . He would tell me, like never mind, don't worry about
me. I don't want you to worry about me. I want you to worry about
your mother. She's the one that counts, you know . . . 'cause I'm a
man. I can take care of myself. I can sleep on a park bench if I have
to, but your mother, she's the one that counts. You have to take care
of her. That's what he would always tell me. He always would come
up with the same subject . . . like putting the weight on me like I
was married to her, you know. I wouldn't answer him. I wouldn't tell
him boo! 'Cause I was afraid of him like I tell you. But this, he
wouldn't say in a sober condition. This, he would only say when he
was drunk, and I detested it. I hated it, you know?

[Billie's statement that his father made him feel responsible for his
mother finds an echo in many situations and many cases. The
larger concepts of *apparent precocity* and *existential strain* are
worth exploring. Sexual precocity would be a familiar illustration.
Since it is very likely that the young man cannot fulfill adult requirements, this is a source of frustration, and hence, in Billie's
case, anger and depression.]

S.F.   *Did he ever take you out with his other women?*
B.   No. I would see the way he would act around other women, you
know? Like, let's say he was with a group of friends and there'd be a
couple of other women there. He was all smiles and very gay, then
he'd come home, and he'd have a long face, you know, like if the
world caved in on him.
S.F.   *Did he insult your mother or what?*
B.   No. He would be very serious and very stern . . . like depressed, you know? And a couple of times, he struck my mother, you
know? I'm ashamed to say this but he did.
S.F.   *When did he do that?*
B.   I never got to see it, you know? 'Cause like they had their room
their private room, but I would see my mother crying, and I put two

and two together, you know? And I knew that he struck my mother.

S.F. *How did you feel then when you made that inference?*

B. Well, what do you mean? When I would find this out? Well, I felt like beating on him, but like he's a much bigger man than me. I'm as small as my mother.

S.F. *How tall is he?*

B. He's about 5 feet 6 inches . . . something like that. I'm 5 feet 4 inches plus he's a merchant seaman with hands twice my size. He's very . . . built.

S.F. *Well-built.*

B. Yeah.

S.F. *Strong?*

B. Strong.

S.F. *So you could do nothing—you just watched him.*

B. I couldn't do nothing. And there was another thing about him. He's very cheap with his money, you know?

S.F. *What do you mean by that?*

B. I'm not ashamed to speak about these things because those are facts. . . . He's very cheap with his money . . . like he will send my mother a certain amount every fifteen days, and like outta that he expected her to pay the bills an-a-plus have money left over for, you know, to put in a bank, and like if she didn't prove to him where the money went like . . . it was a big stink over that, you know. He never bought me anything, not that I could recall . . . not in my later years. And I recall one time my brother—that's his son—the way I see it—that's his son, and he's got a right to support him or at least help him out whatever he needs, and one time my brother came over and he needed a pair of shoes, you know. So "Look, pop. Look how the shoes I'm walkin' around with. Can you give me money for a pair of shoes?" And he tol' him, "I haven't got no money for no shoes," you know? I recall it was for the holiday and things like that. That prove to me that he was cheap.

S.F. *Did you ever have any happy moments with your father?*

B. Yeah . . . I think, I think I did.

S.F. *Such as . . . you remember what the occasions were at all?*

B. We all went out on an outing at one time to Pelham Bay Park and we all had a very good time. He was happy, and we played ball, catch, you know, and we ate ice cream. He put his arms around me, you know. He treated me like I was a son. That's the only time I could recall.

S.F. *How come he was so different then?*

B. I don't know why that particular time he acted that way, but that's the way it was unless something good happened to him, you know? Extra good. That made him feel that way. I don't know if he needed . . . I don't know if he needs psychiatric help, but a few times in these drunken stupors, he used to get into, he try to jump out the window, you know?

[In associating his own condition and his problems with his father's drunkenness, Billie not only reminds us how often alcoholism in the father is associated with some addiction in the child, but also suggests that depressive life patterns may be handed down unconsciously.]

S.F. *Really?*

B. See . . . don't get me wrong. My father is not the type that gets drunk like every day, you know, all that. He loves . . . he likes to drink, but like he's the type that'll get drunk like when he comes home from a trip. Maybe he's been gone for two months. He comes home from a trip . . . he'll drink. He'll get drunk . . . he'll get drunk outta his head and uh . . . he also . . . he loves to drink at parties. Well, I know that he likes to drink when he's home, when he's not working, but while he's working he won't drink. That's the type of man he is.

S.F. *Did you ever have any feeling about why he was so accustomed to drinking so much? You never figured out why? You never thought why?*

B. No. I thought he did it to enjoy it. To me, he's a very nasty man. You know? At one time, at one time I was . . . I was high on goofballs, and goofballs make you get very nasty. . . . I don't know if you ever seen a person high on goofballs. They become very nasty and very . . . you know, you think you could lick the world, you know? And I tol' him, you know, uh . . . well, I don't want to say the language I tol' him . . .

S.F. *Say it . . . say it. What are you afraid of?*

B. I tol' him, "I'm gonna bus' your ass," you know? And uh . . . he almos' kill me, you know? If my mother wouldna been there, he woulda kill me . . . I don't know. . . . And there was a table in the middle of the living room . . . he kicked with his . . . he kicked it and he broke the legs. He went like this . . . four legs. . . . They went four ways, you know, four different ways when he kicked it. [Laughs] I said "Oh, my God!" You know, my mother got in the way and she tol' me "Get out! Get out! Leave! Leave!" And I got out. That's the only time I ever stood up to my father. And it wasn't because I was brave or anything. . . . I'm not gonna tell you that I was being brave or anything. It's just that under the influence of goof-balls . . .

S.F. *How did you feel after that about it?*

B. I was ashamed I did it and . . . and I was ascared to face him when he got home. Or to meet up with him again. That's the only time I ever faced up to him. I think it was a very stupid thing to do. I musta showed him right there the way I felt about him, you know. 'Cause uh . . . ya see, this is the way it happened. . . . I was standing in the living room tryin' to eat a plate of rice and beans, you know? And I was goofed up, and my face was like this, you know. In the plate of rice and beans. And he came in, and he says uh . . . "Looka ya son, looka ya son. He looks like a pig, ya know?" And I said, "Who are you to call me a pig? I'm gonna mess your ass, your cock's out." And you know, that's when it happen. He says "WHAT!" And then my mother jumped in . . . and I recall I didn't eat. I ran out of the house. But if she wouldna jumped in, he woulda killed me . . . he woulda killed me. One time . . . one time, at a dance, at a cement wall. It musta been cheap cement—that plaster of Paris—he put his fist through that wall, you know? He was drunk and this is the way he gets when he's drunk. And he was arguing with one of the relatives, you know, and for some reason or other he put his fist, and it went in so far that you could see to the—the—the wire that they have behind the plaster. You could see it. He's like a brute. At least to me, he looks that way . . . like a brute. . . . I tell ya . . . one of his hands would cover my face twice over. You could imagine his pulling on ropes.

S.F.   *Did you ever dream of him?*

B.   No.

S.F.   *Did you have nightmares about him?*

B.   No.

S.F.   *Any monster after you?*

B.   No. I've had dreams of—of—of monsters, you know.

S.F.   *What kind of monsters do you see?*

B.   There's one particular dream that stands out in my mind when I was younger in Puerto Rico, and I don't know why I remember this. Either I was four years old or less, but like I was sleeping with two of my cousins, and this bear-shaped figure . . . our bedroom was next to the kitchen, and in Puerto Rico, they had the custom of sleeping with their doors open. And the bear-shaped figure standing there like this in the doorway was white, you know? And I recall like I sat up in bed like this, and I looked at it, and he just stood there looking at me. And I recall running from my room and jumping into my aunt's—she was sleeping with her husband—I jumped into her bed, and got under the sheets. I recall that . . . that's all I recall.

S.F.   *What do you think it meant?*

B.   I don't know what it meant. I've also had dreams of little dolls— little dolls chasing me, you know? At times, in the dream, they're toy dolls, and then they're real dolls, you know, they're little human dolls chasing me, and I try to run but I can't get away from them, you know? I don't know what they mean.

S.F.   *What do you think of when you think of dolls? Think of anything in particular?*

B.   No. I don't know. I don't think of nothing in particular and these dolls are chasing me, and I try to get away from them, and they were around my legs, tryin' to pull me down, you know? Things like that. I hear that everybody dreams of being on ledges and falling off and jump off. . . . I have dreams like that quite often. Falling off a ledge or a cliff.

S.F.   *Never reaching the ground?*

B.   Never reaching the ground.

S.F.   *You wake up before then?*

B.   Right. And of taking off . . . yeah, sticking a spike into my arm, but never gettin' high, but doin' it, but I dreamt that also. Especially when like when I'm kicking . . . that happens to me when I'm kicking a lot in the Tombs. Or . . . when I'm kicking I always have a dream of taking off. . . . It must be because I'm thinking so much about it, you know, about, you know, taking off on drugs. I can't have it . . . I need it, you know?

S.F. *During these years when you were using, what was your main way of maintaining yourself? Getting your money for drugs?*

B. My mother. She always supported my habit.

S.F. *She wasn't able to support the whole habit, was she?*

B. No, not the whole habit completely. Part of it, and then I would go out and angle and steal whatever I could, you know, and that way . . . that's the way I always supported it.

S.F. *Was your mother working even when your father was still living with her?*

B. For periods of time, she worked. But not all of the time.

S.F. *So there were times when she couldn't support you.*

B. Oh, yes, she did because my father would . . . he sent like one hundred dollars every fifteen days.

S.F. *How big a habit did you have?*

B. I was just beginning to use drugs then in 1957. And I always used to . . . I think . . . this is what I think. . . . I think she knew I was using drugs . . . so I was doing something that wasn't right. . . . She had to because I would come home, I was throwin' up, I wouldn't eat, you know? I was losing weight. She had to know that there was somethin' wrong, but, you know, they say that mothers never want to admit to themselves that their angel is doin' somethin' wrong. That their son is a good boy. He wouldn't do nothing wrong, you know? Well, I think she knew . . . deep inside she knew, and she would give me money, you know?

S.F. *How much would she give you?*

B. She would give me ten, fifteen, twenty dollars. Not every day . . . like when this money would come in, and then like during the week every day . . . like, you know, a couple of dollars here, there . . . like that.

S.F. *But she really couldn't do that forever without your father starting to suspect. Maybe that's why they fought. Maybe they were quarreling about the money she gave you.*

B.   It's possible, but there was money in the bank. There was enough money in the bank at the time. You know? And the money that I was supposed to get for clothing, you know, and my allowance . . . it would all go to dope, you know? Everything would go to dope. Like I would exaggerate everything . . . like my high school pictures. I think they cost uh—uh . . . the whole thing cost about fourteen dollars and some change, and I said it cost twenty-five dollars. Everything . . . everything I would exaggerate . . . like if I had clothes in the cleaners to take out, and it was two dollars' worth of clothing, I'd say it was five dollars' worth of clothing, you know? Like that . . . and this I would do every day. Every day I had some new scheme. You know, a drug addict mind is something that's thinking all the time . . . he's always thinking of how to do this and how to do that. You probably know this already, right?

S.F.   *Hmm. But still, aside from your mother, there must have been some other regular way of making the money.*

B.   Yeah. I had . . . I always . . . I had a girl up, friends, you know? And there was a period when I worked, you know? When I graduated from high school, I worked for a little while.

S.F.   *Doing what?*

B.   Recreation work for the Park Department. It was only seasonal work, you know? I could've took the Civil Service exam and probably passed it if I woulda studied up on it, but I didn't bother. . . . I was already hooked and I didn't bother.

S.F.   *Were you able to get to work on time? Every day?*

B.   No. I was practically . . . either late or if I came in early, I was looking for some excuse to leave, you know, before lunch . . . and there was always something. I don't know how I kept that park job so long. You know, for the whole season . . . it didn't last eight months exactly . . . I think it lasted six and a half months. But I don't know how I kept it.

S.F.   *Were you living at home then with your mother?*

B.   Yes. I always did.

S.F.   *Never moved out?*

B.   Never. I tried. I was trying. And my mother's alone. She . . . my cousins, after they got a little older, they moved out of the apartment. . . . It was a good apartment . . . seven-room apartment

. . . you know? But there was quite a few of us though, you know? We were sleeping like two in a room, three in a room. After they got older, they moved out, you know? They got married . . . none of them use drugs, and so now it's just my mother and myself alone, and I feel bad. I feel bad about leaving her alone. I couldn't bring, you know, myself to that point where I . . .

S.F. *She's alone now. You're in the hospital. She's alone now, isn't she?*

B. Yeah, but she understands. You know, she knows I'm going back. You know, I'm going back home.

S.F. *You had these girl friends. Were you living with them or you lived with your mother?*

B. Living with my mother.

S.F. *Well, what was the arrangement between you and the girl? How did you . . .*

B. Well, uh . . . usually when I had a girl, it wouldn't be a drug addict. It would be a decent girl. Either they worked or go to school, but I can't see myself going out with a junkie broad. 'Cause I don't like the way they carry on what they have to do. I don't want to . . . I don't want to have nothin' to do with a junkie broad.

S.F. *Ever take off with one?*

B. Yes.

S.F. *Did you have any problems? Anything special take place?*

B. You mean like in having relations? Yeah.

S.F. *After you took off?*

B. Yeah, we had.

S.F. *Was it her idea or your . . .*

B. Her idea. It usually is the broad. Yeah. I don't know why stuff would—would—would uh upset a drug addict broad more than it would do to a man, you know? They usually start playing around, foolin' around or kissing you or tryin' to get you started. This is not all of them; some of them don't care.

S.F. *What's the effect of the drug on you? On your sex drive?*

B. None.

S.F. *None at all?*

B. I mean, if I have to . . . you know, do any . . . if I have to have any relations . . . I could do it. I could work out, but it doesn't stimulate me, like I don't get horny or anything like that.

S.F. *It doesn't decrease your interest in sex?*

B. Decrease? I don't even think about sex.

S.F. *That's what I mean. You have no interest in it.*

B. No, I don't. Not after I take off anyway. I have more interest in sex when I'm kicking. I think about it more. You know, when I'm going through withdrawal symptoms.

S.F. *Is that what happened here too? So far?*

B. Not so far 'cause I'm still on methadone. But it happens . . . yeah, it happens I think more about sex.

S.F. *You dream about sex?*

B. Yeah, you do. . . . I dream about sex.

S.F. *Any particular woman that you dream of?*

B. Yeah, there's one in particular, but not all the time. This childhood girl of mine that I went out with. . . . I think a lot about her, and dream with her a bit, quite a bit and uh . . .

S.F. *Have you seen her since? Outside of dreams I mean.*

B. Yeah, as a matter of fact, just about three weeks ago, like we got together. She has never married, and she is older than I am. She is twenty-seven years old. She has never married. She's got a little girl. It's not mine, you know? And uh every now and then, I don't know, for some reason or other, we get together. You know, she comes to see me, and she comes to see me at my house, and we have relations. She says that she's always, you know, felt the same way about me . . . that I've always been the one that, you know, she's loved. . . . I don't believe her really, you know. No, I don't believe her.

S.F. *Why not?*

B. 'Cause I don't. I think . . . I think that uh she's pushin'. I think she either wants to satisfy herself, you know, and I'm her tool. I'm the one she's gonna use to satisfy herself, you know? So that's what she comes for rather than spoil her reputation in the street with just anybody, you know? She knows with me, it's safe, you know. I'm not gonna go blabbing about it, so that's it. But I don't think she is really interested in me as far as really loving me or marrying me.

[He does not get enough personal gratification from satisfying this woman sexually. Any gratification he gets is circumscribed by his feeling of being a tool. Billie feels that he is dark compared to his girl friend. It may be that this color feeling contributes to his depressed life style.]

S.F. *Is she interested in somebody in particular? Is there another man?*

B. No. That's what I just finished telling you. She is twenty-seven years old, no, she doesn't have an older man. I guess when she, you know, when she gets horny, you know, when she gets in that mood, she comes to see me, you know, and satisfies herself, and that's it maybe till a week or two weeks from then. You know, again, the same thing.

S.F. *Does your mother know about her?*

B. Yes.

S.F. *What does she say about her?*

B. My mother, you know, likes her very much 'cause she's a nice girl. You know . . . very quiet.

S.F. *Do you ever intend to marry her?*

B. I wanted to at one time . . . but her people are very prejudiced, you know?

S.F. *Why?*

B. She's a Puerto Rican, but she's this type Puerto Rican. She's got light brownish hair with green eyes, light complexion like yours. She's a, she's a good-looking girl, you know, and her people always had high expectations for a man, you know? At one time, at one time while we were in high school, we even took our blood tests. We got the marriage certificate, you know. We went through all the thing, and all that she was doin' the age at that time . . . uh . . . let me see, yeah, she was under age.

S.F. *So were you.*

B. So was I . . . yeah. And uh . . . her people went and they sent her to Puerto Rico. They got her away fast when they saw like we were going too far. And, as a matter of fact, I used to go up to her house, and they barred me from going in the house. They got her to tell them everything we did together, you know.

S.F. *Were you sleeping with her then?*

B.   I busted her cherry and all that . . . you know, they got her to tell them all that and still an' all, they wouldn't accept me like to marry her.

S.F.   *She wasn't pregnant?*

B.   No. She was supposed to have got it apparently that one time. Some friend tol' her to take some quinine pills for bringing on the period, you know? And that's how . . . that's—that's what I could remember. That's the only time. I don't know whether she was really pregnant or not.

S.F.   *Now, at present, do you think you'll marry her?*

B.   If I do marry anybody, it'll be her, yeah.

S.F.   *I wonder what holds you back.*

B.   What would hold me back? The only thing that's holding me back is the condition I'm in. You know, I can't get outta this rut. That's what holds me back from doin' anything I want to do really.

S.F.   *Are you in love with her?*

B.   I believe I am. She's the only one I think of like I say. And there's been other girls after her. But they don't get my interest as much as this particular girl. But still and all, like I told you, I don't think she loves me.

S.F.   *You feel you love her, but she doesn't love you?*

B.   That's the way I feel. I don't think she really—she really cares. You know? She cares enough for me to satisfy her. But—but as far as makin' a home with me, I don't think she—she's really that interested. I might be mistaken, but then again, she shows an interest in a way, but it's not like . . . it's not . . . I feel . . . you know like . . . I feel she's not really . . . all mine. She's just—she . . . like I said, she's just using me as a tool.

S.F.   *You used this phrase again—twice now. Is there anybody else you think uses you like a tool when you're on drugs?*

B.   I can't think of any.

S.F.   *Do you ever feel that when you're an addict that somebody's making use of you? Exploiting you?*

B.   I can't think of anybody else.

S.F.   *Like people making money out of you.*

B.   No, nobody makes money outta me. No.

S.F. *Even the big pushers? Big connections?*

B. Well, I work for people, yeah. But it's been, you know, I made money for other people but it's been for my interest too, you know? For my benefit. I mean they've made more money than I have.

S.F. *You mean pushing.*

B. Yeah. But I had to—it was a must. You know? I didn't care whether they made twice as much as I was making. As long as I got what I wanted.

S.F. *As long as you got your fix.*

B. Right. But I never felt then that they were using me.

S.F. *Because you got what you wanted. You were not jealous of their money?*

B. No. It never bothered me. I thought about it. You know, I would think about it . . . it wouldn't bother me, you know. I wouldn't want it. You know, like I say, I want to be in his position. You know, I wouldn't think like that. I would think about it. Wow! He's cleaning up, but that's as far as it would go.

S.F. *In other words, when you're on drugs, which is more important to you, heroin or money?*

B. [Laughs] That's a difficult question. 'Cause the more money you have the more heroin you can buy, you know?

S.F. *But if you had—that famous question they ask you all the time —if you're hooked, right? Sitting in front of a desk, a man puts in front of you two bags of heroin from the street—*

B. There's stuff in the street . . .

S.F. *Right. Now, two bags with that kind of stuff, and say six dollars, right? Or maybe ten dollars, now which would you take? The two bags?*

B. Two bags.

S.F. *Of course. In that situation there's no question about it.*

B. Yeah. When it's that much amount of money.

S.F. *All right. Let's take two bags and one hundred dollars.*

B. You'd take one hundred dollars because you could buy five times as much.

S.F. *Now, suppose there's a panic: two bags and one hundred dollars.*

B.   You'd take the two bags. Yeah, of course.

S.F.   *So it depends on how things are outside.*

B.   That's right. Correct.

S.F.   *Interesting point.*

B.   Are you asking that I would feel like anybody—like they were using, I mean? Uh . . . I forgot to mention it. At times I have felt like I have been used . . . like a person would tell me—c'mon, you go cop, you know. I'm gonna give you a fix, you know? You gotta carry it. You gotta walk. Anything happens. It's yours. I felt they'd been using me, you know? Yeah, I forgot to mention that to you. And uh . . . other situations. A guy comes, you know . . . uses my works and uh . . . oh give me fifty cents or a dollar, you know? For using my works. At times I thought he's just using me 'cause I got something he wants, you know?

S.F.   *Did you ever feel that your mother was using you? Or you using your mother?*

B.   Yeah, I feel like I'm using my mother all the time . . . but then I—I feel that I can't—I can't help myself from using my mother 'cause I can't leave her . . . I can't leave the house. I feel like I'm obligated to stay with her because she's by herself.

S.F.   *Did she say so?*

B.   She never said so. She's never said this to me, but like I felt that she's content even though I'm using drugs to have me use drugs and be in the house. Like I feel . . . this is the way I feel at times. She tells me different. Like she would tell me that she doesn't want me to use drugs, but I feel that like she would rather have me use drugs and stay by her side the rest of my life, you know, rather than not use drugs and leave her. You understand what I mean? That's the way I feel. I might be wrong. She's never come out and said this, but this is the way I feel.

[Here is another example of "symbiosis," which by restricting the addict's growth serves further to accentuate the melancholy in his life. Note also how, in the next two paragraphs, what he thinks is a hypochondriacal pattern. One may be sure that he too has in the past faked or induced symptoms in order to get money from his mother.]

S.F.   *Has she been looking around for another man?*

B.   No. And she's fifty years old, but she's well preserved . . . you know, I mean, she can—she can get another man if she wanted, but she's not a bad-looking woman.

S.F.   *Why wouldn't she want to?*

B.   I have no idea. She says she's sick, you know. Like recently, the doctor found she had asthma, and that's another thing. At times I feel that she exaggerates this sickness more than what it is, you understand, like to keep me home. Keep me from going to the street . . . and all that. I think a lot about these things and I say to myself, no . . . I'm—I'm wrong, maybe I'm wrong, maybe that's not the way it is. But these are the thoughts that enter my mind. You know, like she fakes more than what it really is, like when she had a headache, she'll tie a handkerchief around her head and exaggerate . . . ohhh . . . ohhh! You know, and all that, you know? To have me stay home and feel sorry for her. 'Cause she knows I will stay home if I see she's ill.

S.F.   *She works now? You say, she had two jobs?*

B.   No, my father left, but she worked. She's working now. She's the one that's holding up the household.

S.F.   *Well, she can't, at this point, be making much money.*

B.   Uhh . . . forty-eight—forty-nine dollars a week.

S.F.   *She can't be supporting you too much.*

B.   No, not much. My grandfather helps her out.

S.F.   *Oh, he's still alive?*

B.   Yeah.

S.F.   *Her father?*

B.   Her father.

S.F.   *What does he do?*

B.   He doesn't do anything. He's on welfare.

S.F.   *Well, what did he do when he worked?*

B.   What did he do when he worked? Well, the way . . . the story I got when he worked in Puerto Rico, he owned a little stand, a little fruit stand, but I've never known him to work while he was over here in New York, you know? He helps out. He sells fruits out in the street, you know? He goes out for a few hours. 'Cause now the stuff out there in the street, it's so bad, you know, that I'm not that anxious to shoot that much dope in any more 'cause I know I'm not gonna get high, you know? So like I'll take off two or three times a day, and that's it, you know. I'll let it go at that 'cause I know no matter how much I shoot I'm never gonna get high unless I'm gonna shoot up a barrel. I know I'm not gonna get high. The thought of gettin' high is gone . . . I forgot about it.

S.F.   *The stuff doesn't make you high?*

B.   It doesn't get me high. You know. You might sit down . . . you might get off and sit down for a few minutes, smoke a couple of cigarettes, you know . . . close your eyes and talk with your boy, but I don't consider that being high. High is to be like they say, the good old days . . . when you would take off, you wasn't able to talk . . . you know? That was high. Not no more. You don't even see guys taking O.D.'s any more.

S.F.   *Did you ever have an O.D.?*

B.   Yes, I had two or three of 'em.

S.F.   *When?*

B.   When I started. But the dope was very good then. Like two guys would get high on a three-dollar bag, you know? I caught a few of these.

S.F.   *Were you rescued by somebody else or did you come out by yourself?*

B.   My friends. I was lucky that I was always with a friend. That would, you know, save me.

S.F.   *Do you ordinarily take off with somebody?*

B.   No. Most of the time I take off by myself.

S.F.   *You're not afraid of an O.D.?*

B.   No. [Laughs] Not now anyway. You know? And if I thought I would get one, I would—I would—I would be cautious against . . . you know, I would take steps so as not to try and get one. Like I say, I had a three-dollar bag, and this is supposed to be extra good, you know. I would put half of it in there, you know, and take a very little bit, you know, if I thought I was gonna get an O.D.

[This kind of caution about an overdose is cited sometimes by addicts as evidence that they are not "suicidal" when they take drugs. To my mind, it proves nothing either way. The fact of the matter is that in taking drugs an addict is relying upon chance and probabilities to guide him.]

S.F.   *You were in jail. No, the first time you had a suspended sentence. What was the second time you got in trouble called?*
B.   Uh . . . 1751.
S.F.   *What year was that?*
B.   In uh . . . 1961.
S.F.   *How long did you stay in jail?*
B.   Well, uh, my people got me out on bail, and then I uh did go back to court like for hearings, then to plead, and then for sentencing. I got six months, and I did the six months for that. It was broken down from a felony to a misdemeanor. 'Cause the 1751 is a felony. It was broken down from a felony to a misdemeanor. It was broken down to a 3305.
S.F.   *As soon as you got out, did you use right away?*
B.   The same day.
S.F.   *Why?*
B.   I was [Laughs] dying to get off. I can't explain to you why. . . . I recall in jail I would be tied up like this . . .
S.F.   *Tight? With a belt around . . . ?*
B.   Yeah. For practicing, you know?
S.F.   *An imaginary belt around your arm?*
B.   Just imagining what I was gonna do out in the street, you know? And the same day we got out . . . there was four of us together . . . I had uh sixty some odd dollars saved from the money I was gettin' from home, you know, and we all got high.
S.F.   *You bought a bundle?*
B.   No, we didn't. We bought loose bags. We came right over here to 103rd Street.
S.F.   *How is it you didn't think of buying a half load or a load? Couldn't get it?*
B.   The same day? Because we didn't . . . we didn't need that much to be high. You know? What would we do with the rest? Like everybody would shoot like three quarters of a bag or less 'cause everybody was clean. Could you imagine after four months . . . everybody's clean . . . so what—what . . .

S.F. *You weren't thinking of making any money out of it?*

B. No, I wasn't. After we did that we went downtown shopping. I recall I bought a pair of shoes and then . . . I didn't even go home. That's the only time I was in jail too. I didn't even go home.

S.F. *Why not?*

B. I don't know. I didn't even go home. I didn't even call up. As a matter of fact, when I did, I called up this girl I was talkin' to you about . . . that's the only one . . . the only person I called up.

S.F. *To tell her you were home.*

B. To tell her I was out. She tol' me . . . she tol' me—she tol' me I didn't write to you 'cause I was afraid that you, you know, are mad at me for finding out where you are. I thought you didn't want me to know where you are. But I'm glad to hear that you're home. I say, well, I'm home . . . I'll probably see you tonight.

S.F. *Did you?*

B. Yeah. I seen her that night. And uh it's a funny thing, I don't know why I didn't go home. I went to the movies.

S.F. *After you got high?*

B. Yeah, after I got high. And there was . . . my cousins were there . . . my mother, my aunt . . . like the whole family was waiting for me to come home. Like, in other words, a little reception —welcome home committee, you know? And I didn't go home. I showed about eight o'clock . . . and I had got outta there, it musta been a little after ten in the morning. And I showed up at eight o'clock at night. They thought that something had happened to me. They called up Riker's Island, and they said, well, he left this morning, you know. We don't know his whereabouts. And they were all worried about me. My mother was crying . . . you know. I felt bad about it. I felt shitty that I did a thing like that. It was such a good feeling to be free again, you know, [Laughs] you know? There was a couple of . . . there was a couple of guys waiting for us . . . you know, when the ferry docks on the other side? Well, there were a couple of junkies waiting for their friends, you know. They just happen to be there, and so they came along with us, and they showed us everything that was happening. . . . That's how we got high like that. I could remember it just like if it happened . . . yesterday.

[Billie is describing himself as though he were a man who had been freed from one prison and was trying to avoid going voluntarily into another. Getting high is as much a reward for the pains in Riker's Island as for the impending suffering in living with his mother.]

S.F.   *But in dreaming of that, it took several months, of course.*

B.   It was . . . it was so good to kick. Oh, what a terrific feeling to kick. . . . As a matter of fact, my knees were shaking, you know, on that ferry, and I was only four months . . . and I acted like I did twenty years. It was such a good feeling to know that I was cut loose, and I didn't have to worry about I'm a coward . . . and whistles and all that. Maybe that's why I didn't go home. . . . Maybe that's why I wanted a party that day. Actually, it wasn't no party. We got high, and I slept all through the picture. I nodded all through the picture, you know? I called it fun 'cause I had fun anyway even though I nodded all through the picture. I thought it was fun. I don't even re- member the name of the picture. Every now and then I would open my eyes and look at a scene, and then try to see it, and then nod like out. . . . That's what happened all through the movie.

S.F.   *You mention that you used goofballs. Have you ever been hooked on goofballs?*

B.   Yeah.

S.F.   *When was that?*

B.   Oh, '64 . . . '63 . . .

S.F.   *How much were you taking?*

B.   I used nembutals—nembutals. I used to use something like uh . . . ten at a clip, you know? And uh seconals, tuinols and cibas, but—but I never used them all together. Always, you know, separate. As a matter of fact, I was brought in here three times with an over- dose. The third time they wanted to send me to Bellevue, and if I tell you what I did, you won't believe me. I ran out this hospital in my pajamas.

S.F.   *Why?*

B.   I didn't want to go to Bellevue.

S.F.   *Were you afraid of being put away?*

B.   I was hooked on goofballs. I was hooked on stuff, and I didn't want to go to Bellevue. They tell me a week of observation, you know? Tears came out of my eyes. When that woman . . . it musta been a woman psychiatrist, when she told me, I would have to go for a week of observation, tears came out of my eyes.

S.F. *What had you been doing that made her do that?*

B. I had caught an overdose of barbiturates.

S.F. *That's no reason.*

B. But that was the third time. They thought I was trying to kill myself. That's what it was. They keep a record of them things, and it was the third time for me. Everybody said this guy is trying to kill himself, you know? So they wanted to send me to Bellevue, and I told her, I swear to you, I'm not trying to kill myself—it's just an accident.

S.F. *Three accidents? All three were accidents?*

B. All three were accidents. I don't think I was trying to kill myself. I was just a pig. I made a pig outta myself. I wasn't satisfied.

[Once more the ominous implication of the overdose for the depressed life. By focusing upon his greed and making a moral judgment about himself about which he feels bad, he escapes the implications of a possible suicidal pattern for himself.]

S.F. *You had been taking too much barbiturate?*

B. Yeah. I made a pig outta myself. I took too much. I was high, but I wanted to be higher.

S.F. *Did you ever sell barbiturates?*

B. Did I ever sell barbiturates? I probably did at times when I needed money to . . . to cop or something . . . you know. I needed more money, but most of the time I didn't because they were very difficult for me to get.

S.F. *How is it that some people have easy connections for getting pills and others don't have the connections? What's the reason?*

B. Well, I don't know. When I was using barbiturates I had this guy that drove a truck for a pharmaceutical firm . . . you know. I knew him. That's how I . . . I used to get like for a dollar I'd get fifty, sixty while the guys on the street get two pills.

S.F. *So you must've sold some of these.*

B. No, very rarely. If I did, I can't even recall if I did because most of the time, like I said, they were difficult to get and I was hooked on 'em, y'know? I was using stuff for the second time too, and if I did I really can't tell you that I did, but if I did, it was to cop because I was short or somethin' like that. But I really—I really can't recall makin' any sales of barbiturates. And then a lot of people don't like barbiturates.

S.F. *What effects do the barbiturates have upon you?*

B. Ohh man! I used to do way-out things. I used to . . . I used to do, you know, I didn't care who was lookin' at me. Like at the newsstand, if there was a magazine there, and I wanted it, I would take it. I didn't care who was there. There could be a cop standing right there. I would take it, you know? Things like that. Like I would go to kick a door in. You know, like you don't care. And like I told you before with my father, you know? Things like that.

S.F. *The pills didn't relax you apparently.*

B. No. They got me high. Then they drove me insane.

S.F. *Did you ever use the bombitas?*

B. Yeah, I have.

S.F. *Get hooked on them? Large amounts?*

B. Well, I never knew you could get hooked on bombitas.

S.F. *Perhaps psychologically you can.*

B. What! Mentally?

S.F. *Yes. No physical symptoms, but mainly the psychological.*

B. You could get physical symptoms?

S.F. *Some people when they take large amounts.*

B. Oh, well, I never take large amounts. I've used bombitas. I don't know . . . they don't thrill me. They call that a cheap coke high, you know? To me, it has no coke high . . . it peps you up a little bit, you know? It gives you a little energy, and you jump around for a little while, and boom! It's gone, and that's it. You know, I don't think it lasts more than forty-five minutes. . . . You're lucky, at least that's the way my system works.

S.F. *That's why you don't go for them in a big way.*

B. Yeah. . . . I think that's why I don't go for them.

[At this point the first interview ended. The second proceeds:]

S.F. *I wonder if you would tell me some of the adventures you have had, some of the times you were in great danger, as you saw it?*

B.   Well, for instance, just a couple of months ago, I had a half a load, meaning fifteen three-dollar bags, and a certain group of friends of mine knew that I had this half a load, and they followed me while I was on my way home after I copped. They followed me into my hallway. One of them grabbed me from behind. There was four of them . . . and one of them grabbed me from behind, and one of them put a knife at my throat. I couldn't move, but I didn't want to give up the stuff either 'cause that's how badly I needed it. I was sick and uh when I refused to give it up, one of them sliced the jacket I had on me. Actually, there was only three of them working on me. The one that held me by my neck, and the other was searching my pockets, but I had the half a load in my hand, you know, and I refused to give it up, so like I thought . . . I said to them "You're gonna have to kill me, cut me, but I'm not gonna give it up." You know. That's how much I wanted to take off . . . that's how sick I was, you know. We argued for about ten minutes there without them doing nothing, and without me doing nothing. Now it came that like they were getting like frustrated putting up with me, you know, without me giving this thing to them. They told me "Awright, give us half of it, and you keep the other half." But I could see, you know, I thought right away. I put two and two together. A half of this half a load is not enough for four guys. If I open my hand and start counting out bags, they gonna try to take it all because half is not enough for four guys, you know. So I told 'em, "Let me go, you know. Let me go in my house, and I'll give you—I'll throw the half of the load to you out the window." And they said, "No, 'cause we know you're not gonna open up the window." You know? We argued against this . . . it seemed like we were arguing for about fifteen minutes. Then one of them—he's supposed to be a good friend of mine too—he was drinking out of a soda, and he hit me across the head with the soda bottle, right here across my forehead, and I got about an inch scar here. They took five stitches, and uh when he hit me I blacked out . . . my head hit the wall and I blacked out. When I came to, there was blood running over my eyes, and I couldn't see too well because of the blood in my eyes, and the half a load was gone. That's one of the—

S.F.   *Were you buying those loads for yourself or also to sell?*

B. For myself, for my own use.

S.F. *At that time, you weren't selling?*

B. No.

S.F. *Now, these friends, how long had you known them?*

B. I grew up with them. You know, we used to take off together. The reason why I wouldn't sell dope is there's too many rats in the street. And like uh . . . you never know when a guy—a friend of yours—is coming to you as undercover agent, and cop offa you. Maybe once, twice, three times, they might even cop offa you six times. Next thing you know you're busted. They'll come up to you with a paper telling you you made two sales on January 16, you know? At twelve o'clock in the afternoon, something like that. You don't even remember, and here they are reading out of a paper what you did, and what you didn't do two months ago. So that's why I wouldn't bother selling dope. I did at one time, but that was many years ago. And I didn't sell dope, actually, I used to help somebody that sold dope.

S.F. *Now, after you blacked out and went to the hospital, what happened?*

B. I didn't go to the hospital right away. I found myself when I woke up. It musta been just a few seconds or maybe a minute, you know, a terrific . . . I saw stars in front of my eyes and I didn't know the cut was so deep. The bottle broke on my forehead, you know. A little lower and I would have lost an eye, and I saw stars. That's how hard this guy hit me with this bottle. When I woke up I took my handkerchief, I didn't even use a handkerchief. I didn't have my handkerchief. What I did, I got a chance to get my knife out of my pocket, which they didn't take, and I cut the inside of all my pockets out, and I used that as a handkerchief. And I put that over my forehead, you know, and I was walking around the street with a pipe and a knife in one hand, looking for these guys, and I didn't find one of them. But then like I couldna looked too long because I was sick. I recall I was sick. I musta just looked till about five or ten minutes, you know, and I gave up right away, and I ran upstairs, and I conned my mother outta some money. She gave me six dollars that day and I went out and bought two bags before I went to the hospital.

S.F. *What did she say when she saw you?*

B. She—she piled in. She said, "What—what happened to you?" There was blood all over my shirt, all over my pants, my shoes were bloody, you know, and I wouldn't stop bleeding, and this—this wasn't important to me even though it ached and it pained, and you know. I looked in the mirror and I saw it was a deep gash, you know, a deep groove, and I didn't care. It wasn't important to me. What came first was my sickness. Like I wanted to take care of that before anything else. So she gave me my money 'cause I—I wouldn't have gotten it so easy if I woulda just gone up there, you know. I woulda had to really bullshit in order to get it, you know? But she saw what had happened, and she knew that I had money on me before I left the house, and she knew I wasn't bullshit, and she knew I was telling her the truth. So she went and she gave me six dollars. I went out and copped, got straight, then I went to the hospital. I went to the Hospital for Joint Disease. . . . I sat there for half an hour. . . . They didn't take care of me . . . they say the doctor is busy now, what can you afford to pay—asking me all kinds of stupid questions, you know? I said, "Look, I'm gonna pay him, you know? Just help me. See what's gotta be done about this." They said, "Well, you have to sit down and wait." And she took my name—the receptionist. It says like "emergency," you know, and you expect a hospital where it says emergency you go in and you find doctors and nurses runnin' around. It was a room about as big as this room, you know, with a little desk at the end for the receptionist, and nobody there, with a door over here and a door over there. I say, "Wow!" I sat there for about half an hour thinking the doctor might come 'cause I didn't want to make this long trip to the hospital. So when the doctor didn't show, I jumped on the bus and came to the hospital—Metropolitan.

S.F. *What happened there?*

B. Here, they took care of me right away. The receptionist took my name . . . told me to go in through the door. I went in through the door, sat down. . . . The doctor didn't ask me how it happened or anything, you know. They said a laceration of the forehead, somethin' like that, and they lay me out one of them stretchers they got there, and they took the stitches. They gave me a couple of shots to freeze the area and they took five stitches. I asked the doctor "How many stitches you had to take?" He says only five and said I was lucky 'cause I was. I thought that my forehead would get puffed up, you know? Would be real swollen? And it didn't get swollen at all. You know? It got a little . . . it was a little lumpy here, you know? But not like I expected it. . . . I expected even my eyes to get dark, you know, black, but it was nothin' like that.

S.F. *After you recovered, did you see the same fellows again?*

B. I didn't do nothin'.

S.F. *But you saw them?*

B. It's a group of fellas and they stick together, and I knew I didn't stand a chance against four of them. So I didn't bother with them, but I did put out the wire that if I caught one of them alone I was gonna crack open their heads, you know? If I would catch one of 'em alone which is pretty impossible. These guys seem to go to bed together, get up together, you know. And that's why they do these things because they stick together . . . you know . . . it's like that old strain "United we stand, divided we fall," you know. If one of them was to walk up the street alone, they would get sliced up.

S.F. *Is this their main stick?*

B. I believe so. But I was surprised at their doing that to me because I knew them and that was the last thing I expected, and they gave me a chance, I copped, they saw me copping . . . they gave me a chance to walk out the block. They didn't do anything while I was in the street. They waited until I got into the hallway, you know, and when I got into the hallway, the door slammed—pam! Behind me— right? Now, I heard the door open up again, you know, but it didn't slam this time. They let it go easy like, you know, twht! They let it close easy and I looked now, and I say water, you know, and I saw one of them, you know, the one that was comin' up ahead, but like since I knew him I didn't spec anything like, you know? And the next thing, these guys are grabbing me to my neck.

S.F. *How had you got that money? Had you stolen some stuff to get that kind of money?*

B. I hate to say this, but I had beaten some people like.

S.F. *Yourself?*

B. Myself.

S.F. *How would you beat them?*

B.   It was some white boy, you know, some Italian kids from way up in the Bronx. I came home in the car . . . I had beat him in the afternoon, and I had to hide from them.

S.F.   *What do you mean by beating in that case?*

B.   I took their money. They sent me out to cop and, you know, I didn't show up again. I told them to wait for me in a certain place, and I didn't show up again. You know, I scrambled their money and I had to hide from them from about three o'clock in the afternoon till about eight because that's how long they stood around, you know. And I didn't come out till they left. I don't know whether they thought I got busted or what, you know? I know I didn't see them again. To this very day, I haven't seen them again.

S.F.   *So in that case you had exploited the Italians, and now you were exploited by your own friends.*

B.   Right. That's right. That's exactly how it happened.

S.F.   *In the end, your friends got the benefit of that.*

B.   And it really hurt me . . . it's guys that I knew, you know. Like if they woulda asked me for a fix, I woulda gave it to them because there was enough, you know. But they wanted it all, man, and like leave me with nothin', and they saw I was sick. Oh, as a matter of fact, I had cramps in my stomach. You know? I wasn't putting up no kind of resistance when they grabbed me. That's how sick I was, that's how weak I felt, you know, and when you're in that condition you . . . you can't put up no resistance—not even if there was one guy who felt better than you . . . you couldn't fight him probably. He would have the advantage over you. You understand what I mean? That's how it is. That's how sick I was that day.

S.F.   *Were any of them sick?*

B.   I think one of them was sick . . . the other three guys didn't look sick to me. The one that hit me with the bottle was sick. He got desperate . . . the other guys didn't wanna like really hurt me 'cause they knew me. Even though I know this guy—the guy that hit me with the bottle—I knew him for like . . . it's like when you know a person, an acquaintance, you know, you're not too tight with him, you know? Hey, what's happenin' and like that, you know? Like he wasn't that tight with me maybe that's why he built up his courage to hit me with that bottle. But the other guys, I could tell they didn't

want to hurt me. And maybe that's why I got enough courage to refuse 'cause I knew there wasn't . . . you know, these guys wasn't
gonna hurt me. I didn't expect this other guy to hit me with that bottle, but he did, as a matter of fact, he hadn't even finished the soda
before he hit me. . . . Like a third, a third of the soda was in the
bottle, and he hit me just like that—good thing it was a thin bottle—
that's one of the things that happened to me.

[Is it any wonder that when asked to describe an adventure involving great *danger* to himself, Billie tells a tale of *woe?* While there
is a danger, the real emphasis in his story is on his pain and suffering and injury and the betrayal by friends. Embodied in it also
is his realization that he got what was coming to him. Having exploited "the white boys," he is himself exploited by his long-time
associates. Far from this being an adventure with the thrill of
danger, it is another litany of suffering.]

B.   Another time I was high on goofballs, I recall it was a . . . this
happened about two years ago. We had that big blizzard snowstorm
in New York. This was 1965 or the beginning of '65, around there.
. . . I was high on goofballs, I recall I took the goofballs on 116th
Street and Madison Avenue, and I was with a friend of mine. . . .
Now my friend went down to a basement to take off, you know, and
I say "I'll sit out here in the hallway where it's warm and wait for
you." It was just beginning to snow, you know, but heavy like. And
I say to him, "I'll sit out here in the hallway and wait for you," you
know? That's all I recall. That's the last thing I recall, sitting in the
hallway . . . the next thing I knew, I was in a dark place, you
know, like it was freezing cold, and all I could say was "God help
me!" I kept repeating over and over, you know? And I would like
black out and like come to, you know, and getting conscious a little
bit, and saying "God help me, God help me," and black out again.
And this went on all night 'cause when I went out I was . . . I woke up
at 116th Street between Seventh and Lenox. Now imagine, from Madison Avenue all the way to Seventh and Lenox. Those are long blocks.
I don't know if you ever walked those blocks, but they're very long.
I woke up over there, and . . . the only reason I found my way

outta that—that alley—it was an alley—I had two dollars in my pocket, I recall. My pockets were turned inside out, my hat was gone. Somebody had taken the gloves I had, you know, and I didn't know I was in an alley. I didn't know where I was. All I remembered was cold, dark, and everywhere I touched it was snow, and I kept calling for this guy that was with me. I recall I kept calling his name, Carlos, you know. I kept saying "Carlo! Carlo!" You know? No answer, and I remember the wind . . . who-o-o! It was really cold. I recall when the light started breaking through, I saw where I was—in an alley, but I still didn't know I was between Seventh and Lenox now. I thought I was on Madison Avenue . . . in some yard or somepin', you know. As a matter of fact I thought I was in the same hallway in the same building, but in the yard. I didn't know the two dollars were missing, and I was in a stupor like . . . half frozen. I realized later on that the high from the barbiturate was gone. It was like I was half frozen, you know. And when a person is frozen, they get into a stupor like . . . they act like they drunk. You know? And I try to get up on my feet and I would fall on my chest. You know, actually my whole weight of my body. I couldn't stand up, so what I did was crawl to where the light was breaking through. The light was breaking through like . . . you know these old tenements? Where they got staircases leading to the yards and alleys and what not? That's the way I saw the light coming through, and the stairs were completely covered with snow . . . I couldn't, everything, I couldn't hold the banister because I kept slipping off so, with my hands, I started going like this all the ways till I got to the street, and when I got to the street I didn't see a car, no buses, it was like a nightmare. I'm telling you . . . you know, I was—I was scared. I thought I was—I thought, . . . as a matter of fact, . . . people that you would . . . I would see a person pass by to me, it seemed like every two hours, a person would come by, you know, like goin' to work. It was somethin' like six o'clock or six-thirty in the morning. Going to work, they'd be all wrapped up, and you wouldn't see no buses, no cars, no nothing, and I still didn't realize that the two dollars were gone. You know, that's how much of a stupor I was in. Now, I got out to the street. I tried to get up on my feet, and I would stumble again. I would stumble backwards, sideways, you know? And I don't know for how long this went on . . . how long I was trying to, you know, like stand on my feet to walk straight. I don't know for how long. . . . I recall that . . . this was like in the middle of the block, and I managed to crawl—you could say I actually crawled 'cause every time I tried to stand up I would fall. I managed to crawl to the corner of Lenox Avenue and 116th Street, and there—there was a few people, and like under an awning, you know, like waiting for a bus or a car. I don't know what they were waiting for, and I told 'em "Help me please!" They were Negroes. You know, I said "Help me please!" Now, could you imagine how I looked? I'll give you an idea how I looked. My hair was all white, you know, like icicles had formed on my hair, you know, ice and snow all over my eyebrows, on my eyelashes. My clothes was completely covered with snow, you know, so I musta looked like a bum to them. Everybody thought I was some kinda bum, and then they saw that I was in a stupor condition, and they ignored me, you know. And I was beggin' people to help me, and they ignored me. I'm tellin' you, it was like a nightmare. I never want to go through something like that again. And uh it got to a point where I gave up, I gave up askin' people. . . . I just leaned against the wall and then I sort of, you know, down like that and sat there like this . . . I don't know how long I . . .

S.F.   *With your head against the wall?*

B.   Yeah, with my head against the wall.

S.F.   *Eyes closed?*

B.   No. My eyes were open. And I recall a guy that I knew that lived in that neighborhood was on his way to work 'cause that morning they had called for volunteers to shovel snow, and this guy, you know, his name is Satch, he's a drug addict also, he was one of the volunteers, you know. I tol' him "Satch." I was able to recognize people, you know? Even though I couldn't stand up. . . . I was like in a stupor condition, you know, my mind wasn't completely gone—I was able to recognize people. I saw Satch. I called Satch, he walked over to me. I says "Satch, I'm in trouble—I can't get home, you know." He says "Wait for the bus," and he kept going, you know. He saw me in that condition, and he probably said, "Oh, this guy fucked over or somethin'." He kept goin'. He ignored me, and I just laid there. I gave up, you know? I just laid there against that wall . . . snow fallin' on me, and everythin', man. I don't know, it was going real heavy, and I don't know, this Puerto Rican fellow . . . he just, I don't know where he showed up . . . or what made him, what made him, you know, like notice me. You know, but he— or maybe he saw people half frozen before, and knew what the condition was. You know, he could see something in me that made him, you know, feel sorry for me, made him, you know, I needed help. Something attracted his attention toward me, a Puerto Rican. Now, every Negro person I asked refused to help me, you know, except for this Puerto Rican. He walked over to me, and in Spanish, he asked me, "What's the matter? You know you need help there?" And I don't know the guy from Adam. I never saw the guy in my life. I said "Please, I can't get home." He says, "Where do you live?" I says, "Between Lexington and Park." He says, "What are you doin' all the way out here? I gotta look at you." . . . I never saw the fellow before. . . . I thought he was sent from heaven, you know. I said, "I got two dollars in my pocket. Take it. Call a taxi." He looked down my pocket and said, "Your pockets are turned inside out, you don't have no money, you know." I said, "Oh-h-h." That was another shock, you know. I said, "How we gonna—how we gonna—we can't get a cab." He said, "That's not important because there are no buses running because the snow is so heavy." You could see for yourself, there's no cars, you know, nothing. He said, "Look, if I see a taxi coming or a bus, we'll jump on it. Don't worry, I'll pay." But we didn't see a bus or a cab coming, so he took my arm and put it around his back, and he actually had to drag me all the way to my house, and I recall, when I got home, my mother was still worried about me. And she was wonderin' where I was, you know, in that snow 'cause she knows I don't stay in nobody's house, you know. And like uh when she . . . knocked on the door—I knocked on the door. I lost my keys, and this guy was holding me up. My mother —"Oh, what happened to you?" You know? I saw tears in her eyes. She really felt bad to see me in that condition, and uh . . . this guy knew somepin', you know. He said, "Don't put his hands in hot water, wrap 'em up in a blanket or somepin', you know, but don't use hot water. Give him somepin' warm to drink, you know." He knew his business . . . like he knew what he was talkin' about, and my mother followed his instructions, you know, because he thought that my hands were frostbitten. They were already beginning to get all lumpy and the next day when I woke up I looked at my face, every exposed area like where I didn't have no clothing was all frostbitten, even my ears, my hands—wow! And painful too. I think if I woulda laid out there like a few more hours I coulda croaked, you know? I woulda died. . . . I woulda actually frozen, and I don't know how I wound up from Madison Avenue. I never did find out how I wound up from Madison Avenue all the way between Seventh and Lenox. . . . I never did find out.

S.F. *Did you ever think about how you lost that money?*

B. I never did. I always thought that a couple of guys came by the hallway, saw me, you know, picked me up, started walking with me, you know. I probably was in a—like they call—temporary amnesia. . . . I don't remember anything like what happened after I sat down in this long hallway . . . to wait for my boy. I don't recall anything. Maybe a couple of guys picked me up, and walked with me all the way down there, took my money and left me in some alley, you know. Or—or took me down an alley . . . took me down that yard, searched me where nobody could see them. After they got through searching me, they took the two dollars, took the hat, the gloves, and put me there. I'm—I'm—I thank God to this day, they didn't take my coat. The coat wasn't worthwhile takin' anyway 'cause, you know, . . . but if one of them had been up tight for a coat . . . I mean, he woulda taken it, man, you understand? And I really woulda been in trouble then.

S.F. *What barbiturates were you using?*

B. Tuinols. The big red and blue.

S.F. *How many had you had before?*

B. I had taken two previously, and then I had taken a shot of dope, and then when I sat in this hallway to wait for my boy, I had taken two just before I went into the hallway, but I recall I usually drank some hot coffee behind the goofballs. I didn't do that that day. I just took the two goofballs and went in the hallway.

S.F. *That's all you remember after that?*

B. That's all I remember. I remember sitting down and telling him, "I'll wait for you over here." And he says, "Okay. I'll be up in a few

minutes, you know?" And that was it. That's one of the worst experiences that I could recall. I mean to me, it's really terrible. You
know what it is to find yourself in agony and turn to people and they
all turn their backs on you? Like you're not even there, like you're
some kind of animal, you know? To me, it's a terrible experience. I
don't ever wanna go through something like that and I recall I
stopped using goofballs.

S.F.   *You did?*

B.   I did.

S.F.   *You haven't used any since?*

B.   No. I have taken goofballs, but not as excessively as I did at
that time. You know? 'Cause I used to take goofballs as if they were
M & M's. You know? I used to be popping them into my mouth like
crazy. I didn't care . . . until this happened to me, and there were
times when I used to get home, I mean I used to get home in a condition like all goofed up in a stupor, and I would wake up in the
morning, and start yelling at my mother, "Where's the bag I had in
my pocket?" Where's this . . . where's that, you know? I would
get beat for money . . . and uh . . . a whole lot of things. I was
taking goofballs, and I still won't give them up.

S.F.   *You mean the guys take advantage of you when you are on*
goofballs?

B.   I wouldn't know how I would lose my money. I would wanna
cop money, oh, man! Lose everything and sometimes I would get
home, and I wouldn't even recall how I got home, you know. And
when my mother knew that I was using goofballs, she used to keep
an eye out for me, and she would be looking out the window, and
she told me one time that—it was around three o'clock in the morning, you know—and like uh . . . I hadn't gotten home, you know?
And, you know, like at that time, everything is very quiet. This was
summertime, everything was very quiet, and uh, she heard some snoring in the hallway, you know? And she says, "I wonder if that's
Billie." And she opened the doorway quietly, you know, and she
went all the way down to the third floor, and she found me on the
third floor with my knees against one of the steps. You know, like
let's say this is one of the steps . . . my knees were against the
steps like this. I was with my head on another step, and the spike

hangin' out of my arm, you know? And there was two bags here, there were three goofballs layin' over there, the cooker over here, and I was like in that position.

S.F. *Bent over?*

B. Yeah, snoring, you know? And uh . . . she says she picked me up, you know? And that when she picked me up, I started goin' "Ugh—ugh." You know, I had been layin' there in that position for a long time so that step had dug into my knee in such a way that when I had to get up it was very painful, and I said "Awgh! Awgh!" But I don't recall this. . . . I don't recall this and next day I had to learn to ask her for the goofballs that she found. She gave me the stuff back. But the goofballs, she didn't want no part of that—she flushed 'em.

S.F. *How did you get involved with goofballs in the beginning?*

B. I just heard about it, and I wanted to try 'em out.

[Just as he has told us a story in which he was the victim of fate and goofballs, and not really an active agent, so too he interprets his own involvement as something of an accident in which a friend tells him about the goofballs, and he "wanted to try 'em out." The underlying burden of the bulk of this story and of his interpretation is that Billie is not responsible for hurting himself—it just happened that way. It seems to be the special function of passivity and irresponsibility for the depressed life that both attitudes serve to cut down on threatening and, hence, depressing facts. If he were to feel that he was actively responsible for taking the drugs, would he not feel that he ought to have done something and would not this make him feel more depressed? The risks of existence are to be minimized.]

S.F. *Who told you about them?*

B. A friend of mine he told me . . . like uh started off with cibas and doridens. I didn't dig too tough because they would dry my mouth too much and my lips, and it would make me very thirsty. So I gave doridens up for nembutal . . . I had to take too many of them to get high. I gave up nembutals for tuinols, but actually I tried all kinds of goofballs and uh . . . to me, at the beginning, since I didn't take too many, I would take one or two, then take off. I would really nod, and enjoy it, you know. . . . I would be very high—even if it was a weak bag. I'd feel it more and that's how I got involved with goofballs. You know, because I had the impression that if I had a couple of goofballs in me, and I would take a bag no matter how weak it was, I would get high, and then I didn't have to use as much stuff as I would have to use if I wasn't takin' goofballs. That's how I got involved actually. . . . After a while I got to a point where I was takin' so many goofballs, and I think my body was so saturated with goofballs that I would buy a bag or two and I would actually go back and tell the guy that he beat me 'cause I didn't feel the stuff. . . . That's how I got it. It got to a point where I think the goofball was overpowering the stuff, you know, and I would fight, and I was acting like a maniac, and walkin' around the streets like a bum, you know. I wouldn't shave, sometimes my pants were torn off, I was dirty, I didn't care where I sat. . . . Sometimes I would be all goofed up and lay down in the rain, you know, and even though I went through all these experiences, I wouldn't stop takin' 'em. . . . I wouldn't stop, you know? The girl I had told you about, she found me. She found me one morning. She was going to work in the corner on Lexington Avenue on 116th Street, in a stupor like, you know, and uh she helped me. That's one good thing about her, . . . she doesn't care like if people saw her. She just cared about my welfare, you know, took me and took me home. . . . She found me in that condition one time, and still and all, you see these . . . I'm telling you 'cause they were told back to me. But actually half of these things I don't even remember them. You know, like these stupors I used to get in. My mother would tell me, "Aren't you ashamed? Look at you with your pants torn and dirty, on the corner like a bum." You know. "She brought you home and look at how clean she is," you know. "She's goin' to work. You know that's embarrassing; that's embarrassing for her to have to do that, you know, but she did it because she had to. It embarrasses her, you know that? . . . You know it does." And I would say, "Yeah, ma, I know you're right," but I would continue on doing it, you know?

S.F. *How long were you really strung out on goofballs?*

B. For about a year . . . a good year and then the other year, it was like off and on, you know, off and on.

S.F. *Which was your favorite goofball? The one you liked best?*

B. Well, like I said, I liked all of 'em.

S.F. *Which one did you like best?*

B. At the end I stopped with the tuinol.

S.F. *Why?*

B. 'Cause it was the strongest.

S.F. *What do you mean by strongest?*

B. The one I would feel better than any other one. I would feel it better than the doridens, the cibas. I would feel it better than the nembutals, better than the seconals, better than any other barbiturate. It's a two-colored pill, two-tone, blue and red.

S.F. *Where would you feel it? You said you would feel good. Where?*

B. Where would I feel it? I would feel it in my head. I would go into these nods. That's how I would feel it. These—these like stupor nods like—like I told you before, I was very . . . like I didn't care if I was bowlegged. A friend of mine would come to me and say, "C'mon we gotta. There's a television in such and such a house, and let's go get it." I would . . . like I didn't care, you know? I mean things that I wouldn't ordinarily do.

[Here, again, an addict is making himself believe that he is not responsible for the crimes he commits and that he is really the victim of the drugs. Much of the antagonism to goofballs found among addicts is due to their being a source of weird conduct, but that antagonism is also a way of discharging the guilt about depredations upon the "pills" and presumably the pharmaceutical houses which make them.]

S.F. *Would you . . . suppose your friend came to you and said, "Look, there's a television set in that house." Would you then take the pills?*

B. No. I would have to be in this condition. I'm saying like . . . that's the condition I got into . . . like I didn't care. I would . . .

I would be so goofed up that I would do anything. A cop could be standing right there, and if there was a newsstand there, and I wanted to take a paper, I would take it. I wouldn't care if that cop was standing there, you know? That's the condition I got into. But this is when I was under the effect of these barbiturates. Never, never—like, in other words, I didn't have no heart, you know, I didn't have no heart unless I had these pills in me, and I caught about three overdoses on goofballs. I told you that.

S.F. *You said you had no heart unless you had goofballs. Did you have no heart when you had heroin?*

B. No, heroin would make me meek.

S.F. *Meek?*

B. Yeah. I would just wanna lay around and enjoy it. Goofballs is supposed to be like a sedative that's supposed to put you to sleep, but it doesn't. . . . It would make me like a wild man, you know? Run around, doing all kind of stupid things . . . begging people for money, things that ordinarily I would be ashamed to do. Begging people for money and all that. And even if I caught overdoses on barbiturates, I never gave them up, you know. I had to have all these experiences—that's why I have faith in God. You know?

S.F. *Why?*

B. Because of the experience I had. I coulda died in that alley. And all I could recall was yelling out to God. You know . . . and uh . . . this fella that came by. I don't know where he came from . . . when he helped me.

S.F. *Have you seen him since?*

B. No. I never saw him in my life. My mother gave him a cup of coffee.

S.F. *How did she act when you came in?*

B. Oh . . . oh . . . she . . . surprised and happy at the same time to see me 'cause she knew I was taking barbiturates, and she knew the kind of trouble I would get into, you know?

S.F. *Were there other times before when you had similar dangerous situations that you recall?*

B. No . . . uh . . . it's just that when I would be under the influence of these goofballs I would have money to cop, you know? And the money I got by begging people in the streets or if not by taking something from somewhere, you know, I was stealing my mother blind. You know? And uh . . . a lot of times I would lose my money. I would go out to cop and like the guys would just take the money out of my hand, you know? I'd be like this . . . in a stupor like, you know? So a lot of people would take advantage of me, you understand?

S.F. *Your friends?*

B. Friends. Most of the time I wouldn't even remember who would take the money. I would just like try to, you know, snap my brain out of the stupor for a minute to see the connection and all, you know, to see how it was. But this didn't happen very often. It happened a few times, you know. People took advantage of me this way, you know? And then, a lot of times, I would take off and come back screaming to the connection that it was a dummy what he sold me, you know, and it actually wasn't, you know? I'd come back and say, "Give me the bag." And he'd say, "What are you talkin' about? You took the bag already." You know? I would lose it, a whole lot of things like that under the effect of goofballs, you know. I didn't function right, I didn't think right. You know, like I would take the bag, you know, and I might think it was uh . . . a piece of paper, so I would probably throw it away. And then I would walk and maybe an hour later I would remember that I had copped a bag. . . . What did I do with it or I wouldn't remember that I shot it up, and then I would come back screaming to the connection. A lot of times they felt sorry for me or they just wanted to get me out of their hair. 'Cause I was like a pest.

S.F. *Really?*

B. Really. I'm tellin' you, like a pest. These goofballs would get me in a condition that, oh man! . . . Like, you know, I would do things that were awful, like I would bother—like waking up people four o'clock in the morning to ask them for money. You know, people that I knew, friends of mine, not—they didn't use drugs. I mean, like this lady that I know that owns a beauty parlor, and one night . . . like she likes me a little bit, you know. I recall one time knocking on the door at four o'clock in the morning to ask her for five dollars. . . . I was doing all kinds of—

S.F. *What did she say?*

B. She didn't give it to me. She slammed the door in my face. But the following day, I recall again, in her beauty parlor, I asked her for money, and she gave me a few dollars. But like I completely lost all sense of pride. I had no pride whatsoever, you understand? And I recall, I would fall. I had lumps all over my head, you know, scratches. My hands were always dirty. These pills, they actually get you like a bum. You don't take care of yourself . . . that's how I was and uh . . . one time I recall I was so high on goofballs I was like by the curb, and I started to keel over, you know—fall over? And this guy grabbed me just in time. My head woulda hit the side of the curb, and I think I woulda died right there and then. 'Cause when I would fall I wouldn't—when you're in these stupors, man, like you would fall and like uh . . . you don't try to protect yourself or, you know, try to break the fall or anything like that. You just like let yourself go. Your body's natural, like you're not expecting to fall, you know. That's how it used to be with me, and in 1963 I got hit by a car behind goofballs.

S.F. *What happened?*

B. I was gonna cop with a friend of mine, and we were crossing the street, Madison Avenue and 117th Street. We were gonna cross the street . . . there was a bus over here like this . . . we had the light, though, you know. I was high on goofballs, but not in one of these stupors, but I was high on goofballs, I recall. We had the light and there was a bus here, and we crossed in front of the bus. Now, after we crossed in front of the bus, the light changed while we were in the middle of the street. It wasn't one of these modern lights that gives you a warning—the yellow—with the yellow. It was one of these old-fashioned lights . . . the green would go off, you know, and there's just a few seconds before the red comes on—one of those. And I recall, we went in the middle of the street, and from behind the bus, shoots this car—an Oldsmobile. It shot, you know. My friend, he wasn't high on goofballs, you know? He sized up the car and ran over to the other side. But the car—bam!—hit me. It couldna been goin' too far, you know. It hit me, and it threw me and I landed like . . . the bus at the same time when the car hit me already started to move, you know. And—and when the car hit me it kept goin' a little bit, and I got like block between the bus and the car, you know. And my boy thought that the bus had run over me. He said—he screamed, "Billie!" And then he ran over across the street, and that aheh! When he ran over across the street that I was like laying out like this, and I got up and "What the fuck is happening, man!" And I got up and walked over to the sidewalk and I collapsed, you know. I collapsed again, and uh . . . they called the ambulance. . . . This— this, I remember, this cop that used to be on this beat. He came over and he says, "Ah, man, this guy's all right. He's not feeling no pain, man." You know, and I was. I was telling the people, "Get the fuck away from me, man. What are you looking at?" You know, "Get outta HERE!" You know, and the guy that was with me, "Get these people outta here, you know. What are you lookin' at?" They never seen somebody get hit by a car, you know? Because there was a crowd around me, you know? It's like a show there. And the ambulance came, and they took me to the uh . . . uh Harlem Hospital, and they laid me out on a stretcher. This leg, my left leg was puffed up like this, it puffed up. As a matter of fact, it swolled up so much that you could [Laughs] see it bulging through the pants, you know. And the shoe, I had to take the shoe off, you know, and everything, you know? I was laying there, they took me and took X rays of my leg. This whole side of my body, you know, where I got hit by the car. Oh, they probably took X rays of my whole body, but I know in particular, they were paying attention to this side of my body, you know. So, after they took the X rays, I had to wait for the results of the X rays to see if there were fractures or what before they could, you know, like cast and all that. And to me, it seemed like an eternity that I was laying in that stretcher there waiting, you know? So I gave my boy a dime, you know, my boy went into the ambulance with me. I gave him a dime. I said, "Call up my mother and tell her to come and get me outta this damn hospital. I'm not stayin' here another minute." And—and the nurse over there said, "But, mister, you can't leave, you can't leave! If you leave, we're not responsible for whatever happens to you," you know. I said, "I'm leaving, man, 'cause I'm tired of laying out on this stretcher," and I would see every now and then they would bring in like colored guys, cut up, this guy bleeding through his head. You know probably from five to one, you know. It was on a Saturday night, man, so you could imagine how that Emergency Ward looked in that Harlem Hospital. And uh . . . my mother came in a cab with my cousin and she took me right away to Mt. Sinai Hospital, you know? There they took X rays, you know. And they came back right away 'cause the Emergency Ward at Mt. Sinai Hospital says they take care of people right away. It's never like full actually, you know? And uh . . . they came right back right away. . . . They didn't see no fractures, but they say to come back the next day for more X rays, which I did, and uh . . . I recall, they gave me two pain killers. My leg was in pain . . . they said the only thing that's wrong with your leg is that your blood vessel's busted, you know? And that's what got your leg swollen, the blood vessel that broke from the impact so . . . uh, I was lucky there. . . . I didn't get, you know, no fractures or anything, and I recall, I left my mother right over there—right by the Mt. Sinai Hospital, and I cut out with my friend. We had about twenty dollars between us, you know. [Laughs] And I was just thinkin' of copping.

S.F.   *How long did it take before you recovered fully?*

B.   Oh, it took a good month before my leg went back to normal. I was walkin' around with a cane as a matter of fact.

S.F.   *But you still went on copping?*

B.   Yeah, I still went on copping.

S.F.   *Cane and all?*

B.   Cane and all. It [Laughs] didn't affect me . . . and I was walking with a limp. It was very difficult for me to get down the stairs, and we got four flights of stairs in my building, you know? But it didn't stop me from goin' out, man. I would go out after I bagged.

S.F.   *How were you making money then?*

B.   Oh, like my mother was supporting me . . . like I told you before. Most of the time like it was ma who was taking care of me, you know? And like she would be so worried about me getting into trouble and . . . and I stopped using goofballs there for a period again . . . after that accident 'cause I got like a little scared, you know? But once it was all over, I sued. . . . It was uh . . . what's the name of these people? Allstate. I never went to court, you know. 'Cause like the lawyer sent me some papers. I signed them with a public—a notary public and uh . . . the day I was supposed to go to court I was sick. I was so sick that I tol' him over the phone "I'm not going, man. Do whatever you want, get whatever you want from them." And I coulda got a couple thousand dollars, you know, but I dint—I blew it.

S.F. *How much did you get?*

B. Eight hundred and some odd dollars.

S.F. *That was your share?*

B. That was the whole thing. He took half of that. You know? I wound up with three hundred dollars and something because uh . . . almost one hundred dollars went to a private doctor . . . that he . . . it was his idea of me goin' to a private doctor, you know, to make it look good, you know? So that was it, and that money—three hundred and some odd dollars—I don't think it lasted a month. Then I really was shootin' dope and takin' goofballs like there was no tomorrow. . . . I really went beserk. . . . I gave my mother a hundred dollars but, you know, I think back, and I find myself a pretty miserable character because the way she looked out for me, the least I could have done was given her half of it, you know? But I didn't. She wanted me to put it in the bank. Some of it in the bank in case of an emergency . . . but I didn't.

["Handicapital" is a term that ought to be part of the vocabulary of social science. At least as it applies to the addicts, it would refer to the exploitation of one's disadvantages and sufferings in order to get money from them. I have been surprised at the involvement of addicts in lawsuits, particularly around negligence when they have been able, apparently, to claim no contributory negligence by not revealing the fact of their involvement in drugs at the time. At least no evidence about barbiturates, as in this case, came to light.]

S.F. *Did your father know about this business?*

B. He was overseas at the time. Yeah, he found out about it. Either my mother wrote to him, and told him about it, you know. But she wouldn't tell him the things that I was goin' through and the things that I would do. She'd tell him that I got into an accident.

. . . I got hit by a car, but not the condition I was under, you know, all goofed up and things like that. I believe it probably made very little difference to him, you know?

S.F. *Why do you say that?*

B. 'Cause like I said, you know . . . I told you before . . . he never showed any affection for me, you know. That's why I believe it didn't matter to him one way or another. Like, for instance, when his mother died just a year and a half ago, you know, my grand-mother, he was overseas at the time, and like you will figure if your mother dies that you would take a plane or try to, you know, as soon as possible. Maybe I'm wrong in thinking this, maybe he was at sea when this happened and, you know, there was no way of him gettin' back to the United States, but like uh . . . I always thought he coulda made it back here when his mother died, and you know, at-tend the funeral at least, but he didn't. Like he just sent flowers to New York. . . . A flower telegram, you know. He sent a big, big bouquet of roses, red roses, and that's all he did.

S.F. *Did you ever talk to him about it?*

B. About what? About when his mother died? No. We never spoke much like I said. Like the only time he would give me anything was when he was either drunk or feeling good or somethin'. He was very nasty with me.

S.F. *Did you feel crushed by him in some way?*

B. What do you mean "crushed"?

S.F. *Did you feel that somehow he was too much for you to take?*

B. Yeah, like I said, he scared me. I was scared of him. I had re-spect for him like I would respect a cop on the corner, you know. When he would walk into the house, if there was laughter and gaiety in the house, it would die out . . . he was like a plague, man, you know. That's how I always interpreted it. If we were having fun in the house, if he would walk in, everybody would keep quiet, you know, and lookin' at television. Nobody would dare say hey—ay, you know, or laugh, you know, and everybody would like know that he . . . his presence in the room . . . you know, he would let it be known, man. . . . That's just the way he acted . . . you know, and I hated it.

S.F. *Now, once you started to use drugs, then you didn't travel very much?*

B.   I didn't go nowhere. All the money was goin' in my veins. That's right.

S.F. *Did you stick to one area, like to East Harlem?*

B.   Hmm. I useta travel a little. There were times when I hung around 100th Street, and times when I was on Madison Avenue and 112th Street. There was a time when I hung around 110th Street and Lexington; there was a time when I hung around on . . . on Madison between Madison and Fifth and Lenox, you know? Over there towards the West Side.

S.F. *What was the reason you chose one area at one time, and then moved?*

B.   Because there used to be good dope in this section, then that's the section I used to go and hang out. You know, I used to follow the dope.

S.F. *Really. How did you find out about it?*

B.   You would hear it from people. That they got a good bag at such and such a place, you know? I would go and find out. Till that place got burnt out or whatever happened, you know? And they got a good bag over there, and I would go over there. But these last few years, like, I don't know, I don't know if it's that I'm more mature, got more sense than to go into neighborhoods that I'm not sure or that I don't know or to get involved with people that I don't know, but these last few years I been hanging around my own neighborhood, around people that I know—

S.F. *Why?*

[For the man living the depressed life, "maturation," far from expanding his horizons and increasing the number of places to which he could go, has tended to mean that as time went on, more and more, he restricted himself to those areas and those areas alone where he felt perfectly safe. The depressed life becomes exceedingly conservative.]

[In the next few minutes of the interview, which have been deleted here, Billie described how he had had a fairly active role in a juvenile gang as a kind of adviser. It is possible that his depressed life style serves to moderate group aggression.]

B.   I mean, I knew what a drug addict was, you know, like they would take drugs . . . inject somethin' into their vein—that's, that's all I knew, you know?

S.F.   *You saw them?*

B.   No, I never did see them, you know. But it wasn't like . . . I wasn't like curious then, you know. It didn't bug me like . . . I knew of them . . . I didn't know what drugs were or what kind of high it gave you or anything like that, but I knew that drugs existed, you know. And like I knew people took drugs. I mean, I couldn't tell a drug addict apart from another person . . . I wasn't that experienced, you know? But I knew drugs existed, that much I knew, you know? I wasn't tempted then. Maybe it was because I had more things to do then . . . hanging out with this group . . . dances, girls, parties, you know.

S.F.   *Skin-pop?*

B.   Once. Skin-popped once. I skin-popped because it was the first time, and if I would mainline I would catch an O.D. I saw him mainline, and I saw the way he got right away. He started nodding and I felt very curious, you know, like . . . it tempted me like I wanted to know . . . ha . . . you know, how it felt to feel that quick rush. He told me, you know, you feel a quick rush and boss high and all this and that. So after I skin-popped, that was it. . . . I kept on mainlining.

S.F.   *How old were you?*

B.   Seventeen—almost eighteen.

S.F.   *Right. Almost a year or two had passed and something had changed in your life. What was new about your life that . . .*

B.   What was new? From not being curious about heroin to being curious about it?

S.F.   *Right. What had changed in your life? Anything?*

B.   I don't know. I have no idea. To me, everything seemed the same.

S.F.   *Really.*

B. Yeah . . . I had no idea what—what made me, you know, feel this way, that changed my attitude towards drugs in any way like . . . like I told you before, like I was just curious about it. You know, the guys in high school had taken it—that I knew. I always see them jumpin' aroun', being so gay, you know, having a ball, smoking, talking. Like this bugged me, and I got to such a point that I had to try it, man. But I don't think nothing had changed. Like I was still having a good time when I started using drugs.

S.F. *In the opening months or the opening year, you had a good time too, didn't you? On drugs?*

B. Yeah . . . yeah. The first year at least or the first two years . . . it was a ball, actually a ball.

S.F. *Tell me why it was a ball and how it was a ball.*

B. I wasn't hooked on heroin and like I would do it maybe once a week or twice a week, you know? Sometimes, I would do it three days in a row . . . it didn't bother me, you know? I felt more effect from it, you know. I recall I first used drugs . . . like I used to throw my guts up. I was vomiting and sick . . . I would turn cold, you know, chill sweat, cold sweat comin' out of my body and everythin', but like this would be all gone after half an hour or so, and then came that good feeling that lasted hours, you know? That's what I cared about. And even though it made me sick, you know, and like I knew I was gonna get sick when I took the drug, it didn't stop me from takin' it, you know. I continued to take it, you know, 'cause I knew what was comin' behind it, you know. And I would like the first few years, like uh . . . my people didn't know I was using drugs . . . like my character didn't change much . . . at least I don't think so. My mother, if she did know, she never let me know about it that she knew or she didn't want to admit to herself that I was using drugs, you know. But I would come home vomiting, you know, and would lay stretch out in bed and sweat and vomit. . . . I couldn't keep nothin' down and she would see me like goin' into these deep nods and all that, and she would ask me, "What's the matter with you?" I'd say, "I'm sleepy, tired," and that—hah. And she would let it go at that. She wouldn't ask me any more questions.

[In the earlier years or, better, the earlier months of drug use, the depressed individual experiences what he takes to be joy. This synthetic equivalent is something that reminds him of what he thinks people who are happy feel like. The heroin also, of course, serves to alleviate the anger. This is embodied in a depression, and hence to that extent is experienced as a relief.]

S.F. *Was she giving you money then too?*

B. Yeah . . . I was getting an allowance and I had money. I had a little money in the bank . . . not much. . . . I think I had about close to a hundred dollars. I had a little bank book, you know?

S.F. *During these years, were you also working?*

B. No. I worked . . . I recall I had a job in a grocery store when I was uh . . . but I hadn't started to use drugs then. But I recall, this job I had in a grocery store, I used to save my money, buy clothing with it . . . things like that.

S.F. *That's before you used drugs.*

B. Right.

S.F. *Now, once you started to use drugs, you were seventeen. What happened to the job?*

B. I didn't have the job.

S.F. *You didn't have any job at all?*

B. No. I didn't have a job.

S.F. *How did you spend your time during this period?*

B. While I was using drugs?

S.F. *Yes. During the first year or two.*

B. I'd be getting high, and sometimes like uh . . . I was scared to go home in that condition, you know, like in a stupor condition, you know. And I would lay around on rooftops or go into a park and nod and wait till it wears off a little bit before I went home. That's how I spent my time. Or with friends going to a movie, you know. That's how I spent my time, and I always thought like everybody else thinks oh-h, I could give this up whenever I wanted, you know? I don't have to use drugs. My will power is strong and all that. That's a lot of crap, like I found out later. I had . . . I'd do the same thing, man, you know. 'Cause like I would use drugs three days in a row, and not use it for a week, you know—like that. That was when I first started. And I recall one time, I caught hepatitis.

S.F. *Was this the same period?*

B. Yeah. And the first few years I caught hepatitis. I caught acute hepatitis and uh . . . the doctor that saw me was, you know, at home, our private doctor and he uh-h-h . . . he took care of it at home. He said it's just beginning so, you know, I could catch it and we'll take care of it at home. . . . I don't know if I was hooked at the time 'cause when I caught the hepatitis I had been using drugs for about a month straight, at least a good month straight, you know. It was a uh . . . towards the middle of 1957, around there. At least a good month straight, I was using drugs, and uh . . . I don't know if the doctor knew, more or less, what it coulda been. . . . I had needle marks, but they were spread out all over my arm, you know . . . here and there. . . . He looked at me all over, you know, at home and he told my mother, "Well, he'll have to stay in bed." You know, a lot of bed rest, and he gave my mother a diet, you know, what to give me and uh . . . he say I would have to stay in bed at least a good month without no kind of strenuous exercises. I did . . . like I said, I don't know if I was hooked 'cause I recall, the first few days, the first few weeks, I couldn't hold no food down. I was vomiting, but I don't know if it was the hepatitis that was causing this condition, you know. Then I didn't realize whether I was hooked or not. I thought it was due to the sickness, you know? But now . . . now I've got a doubt whether it was the hepatitis that caused me to vomit, you know, chills, and all this. . . . I couldn't hold nothin' down, you know, for about a good week, you know. Then I started comin' around, you know, the diet the doctor gave to my mother, you know. He wrote it down on a piece of paper how to cook the food for me . . . and it worked out.

S.F. *How long was it before you became sure you were an addict, hooked during the first year or two?*

B. By the end of '58.

S.F. *The second year? How did you find out?*

B. 'Cause I found that out like this. . . . I was using drugs steadily, steadily, steadily, you know. . . . I didn't stop. Sometimes I wouldn't take off for a day, but no more than a day, and then I would take off again, and uh . . . I found out because uh . . . one time I was feeling lousy, you know? I was feeling bad. I thought I was coming down with a fever or a cold and uh . . . one of my friends that was already on drugs told me, "Well, you take a shot of dope, and all that will go away." And that's how I found out. I took a shot of dope . . . I was feelin' good in a matter of seconds.

S.F. *Well, what did it mean to you then?*

B. Well, it meant to me, every time I got this lousy feeling, a shot of dope would take it away.

S.F. *Did you have any idea that you were hooked?*

B. Yeah . . . I realized then that I had a dependency on drugs. Right, yeah. I realized it, you know? I would wake up and the minute I would sneeze or find a little sweat on my body or chills, I knew like what would take it away right away [Laughs], man, you know? And sometimes . . . I probably even fooled myself, like even if I didn't need it that much, I would say yeah . . . I need it and take off, and you know, and I think maybe I coulda given it up. I don't know, but I found myself depending more and more on drugs.

S.F. *Now, after you found this out, how did it affect your life?*

B. Oh . . . I changed completely. I dropped outta my crowd, you know. I stopped seeing this girl. I still went out with her, but I stopped seeing her. We were seeing each other like every night or every other night, after school, sometimes during school periods. I stopped seeing her. I would see her like once a week, sometimes once every two weeks. I dropped out . . . I started hanging around with drug addicts, you know? Older guys than I was, you know. And like learning the ropes . . . learning the dope game. . . . That's how it affected my life. At first, man, it was like a whole new world—like a new experience to me, you know. It was like exciting, but I look back now, and it doesn't seem so exciting. And it doesn't seem so exciting now, man. . . . It was just 'cause I was young and foolish and it doesn't seem exciting at all, but then I thought it was exciting. I said like hell with these flunkies I was hanging out with. Like they don't know what's happening and all that, y'know? I thought I was Mr. Know-it-all, you know, and uh . . . it didn't pay off in the long run. . . . Got more—more—more involved, deeper and deeper till like I didn't enjoy life unless I was high, you know. Life became very boring to me. I couldn't do anything unless I had that good buzz, that good feeling, you know? That's how it came.

S.F. *This took about two years to happen?*

B. A good two years, right. And still my people, they didn't know I was using drugs until about 1960, and they found out 'cause I got arrested. I told you about that—right? I got arrested acting in concert 'cause I kept up my appearance, you know? As far as clothing was concerned. Even though I was broke, but as far as clothing was concerned like my appearance always looked good, you know?

S.F. *How is it you were able to keep from being arrested all this time? Except that once.*

B. I don't know. I was lucky, I guess. You know uh . . . maybe I didn't look like a drug addict.

S.F. *When you describe yourself when you were using goofballs, you looked like a drug addict then.*

B. Yeah, but that was years later.

S.F. *Well, you haven't been arrested at all except for that one time, right?*

B. Yeah, I have been arrested after that.

S.F. *Oh, when was that?*

B. I have been arrested after that. I don't . . . it's not very clear to me the times I have been arrested, but I recall I got arrested again in '61 for possession of heroin with intent to sell. Uh . . . I got six months on that, and then a few other times I got arrested for disorderly conduct and things like that. You know, and just a few weeks ago I was arrested for 3305. I think it's a 1747B, they call a needle and a dropper, somethin' like that. Yeah, a few weeks ago . . .

S.F. *What happened to the case?*

B. It was dismissed. I recall it because three officers entered the apartment without a search warrant. They had no right at all, and the bags were planted on me.

S.F. *How did you prove that?*

B. I didn't. I didn't prove that. They dismissed the case on the grounds of illegal search and seizure.

S.F. *Ahh! I see. I see.*

B. You know. But I didn't prove that the four bags were planted on me. Even though I said it in court, you know? And the officer acted like he wanted to bust my hands, man. I said—I told—I told the judge, "Your honor, the day I was arrested, they used—they used another party—a friend of mine—to knock on my door, and, you know, I opened the door thinking that he was alone. When I opened the door, these officers just pushed their way into the apartment. And they came up with four bags which I don't know where they came from. They went into the house, and they started searching the apartment, and they came up with four bags and a set of works." I didn't even admit to the set of works being mine.

S.F. *Well, what were they looking for?*

B. They had arrested this other guy downstairs, and he told that he was goin' to my house, where he was to take off. They caught him with three bags.

S.F. *He was going to use your house as a shooting gallery.*

B. Right. It's not a shooting gallery—my house.

S.F. *They thought something was happening there.*

B. Probably, yeah. They said, well, if we go up there, pinch other people or somethin', you know? Or unless they thought he was comin' from my house. They saw him downstairs on the stoop. Now, they don't know if he was comin' in or goin' out, you know? And that's how it worked out and I was sick that day. If I woulda had four bags in the back, do you think I woulda been sick? You know? I tol' that to the officer.

S.F. *Did they think you were a pusher?*

B. I don't know what they thought. They probably—they musta had some kind of idea or somethin' for them to, you know, force this guy . . . they actually forced him to knock on my door, and—and, you know, get me to open the door. So . . . uh that was pretty shitty. I feel pretty bad about that. They took me out handcuffed, out in front of all the people I know, you know. And neighbors and everybody in the street lookin' at me, walkin' out with handcuffs on. I felt pretty embarrassed, very embarrassed, and I recall that day, it was five o'clock in the evening, you know. In the wintertime, it gets dark very early, four—four-thirty, it starts gettin' dark, right? And I recall, that day I had gone to bed very late, around ten o'clock in the morning, and I had slept till around four and then I got up. And I was eatin' some cookies with a glass of milk, and lookin' at the news on television when my boy knocked on the door. And I still had my pajamas on and everything and slippers and what not. I say, "Who is it?" He say, "Robert," you know? I open the door; here they got him handcuffed like this, and then they pulled him in and they came into the apartment. You know? I knew—I knew the minute they walked in, I knew I was gonna go. I just knew, I just had that feeling, you know? 'Cause uh . . . these—these . . . hah, I don't wanta use no bad language—ha—these cocksuckers are not gonna leave till they put somethin' on me, find somethin', you know. Till they find the works at least, you know? And they didn't find the works 'cause the works were behind the curtain on the window sill in the bathroom. They looked under the tub, they opened the medicine cabinet, you know? They looked under the washbasin. They went in the kitchen and opened drawers, and they didn't find the works, you know. When they were pretty disgusted and ready to give up, you know? Like they said, well, we gonna have to take this guy. That's when they came up with four bags and—and this officer got . . . I don't know his religion, but if he swears on a Bible, that's somethin' pretty sacred—right? Like he actually doesn't put his hand on a Bible, but like he raises his right hand almost like it, or somethin' like it, isn't it? Like he raises his right hand and swore to say the truth, nothin' but the truth and what not, and he goes up there and says that he entered the premises on East 116th Street, and the time five-twenty somethin'. And that uh . . . I . . . he asked me for permission to search the house and now, you know, that's a lie and that I gave him permission to search the house, and then he proceeded to search the house with me escorting him through the house. That's another lie 'cause he told me *"Sit* t-h-e-r-e, you know, don't move." And he started searchin' while his buddy watched us. He was searchin' the apartment, and that I escorted him while he searched the house, and that in the bathroom, on top of the medicine cabinet, he found four glassine envelopes containing a white powder which he believed to be heroin, you know? And on the window sill, he found a hypodermic needle with a dropper, a medicine dropper, and a glass of water. When he proceeded to question—they very formal—and he proceeded to question me that I said that I had just finished using the hypodermic with three bags, and that I was cleaning the works when they entered the premises. All this is a pack of lies! Bullshit, you know? But they—they make it look like it's all true, you know? Now, how am I goin' to give him permission to search my apartment knowing I had drugs in there? Or even give him permission to come in. He said that they had . . . to make himself look good, that they had suspected that address for some time. If they had suspicion at that address, they woulda had a search warrant—right? So you know they came in there on just chance, a chance that they were gonna hit somethin' big or somethin' like that. They found me sittin' down drinkin' a glass of milk and eatin' some cookies. . . . I'm no big connection, I'm nobody, you know. [Laughs] My mother took me out on bail though 'cause it was just before Christmas. That's the only reason why. It was only five hundred dollars bail. She took me out on bail and uh . . . we were goin' to court just a coupla weeks later.

[Such stories about police illegality are legion among the addicted, and not all should be accepted at face value. Enough of them occur, however, for an independent observer to be sure that there is merit to some. With respect to a depressed life, however, the effects of such police misintervention are ambiguous. On the one hand, Billie seems to be complaining and adding the police to the list of his woes and sufferings. On the other hand, the startling clarity and even enthusiasm about his narrative leads me to suspect that on one level at least he enjoys getting society out on a limb doing wrong just as he does. These antipolice narratives, in short, are a source of dismal, almost masochistic satisfaction to a man like Billie.]

S.F. *Did you have a private lawyer?*
B. No. We had Legal Aid. He was pretty good. You know, during the hearing, the cop kept tellin' me, why don't you cop out, you know? The arresting officer, why don't you cop out, you know, he'll give you a break. And like if you cop out now, you'll only get six months, you know? You might ask for a hospital or somethin' like that. I says I'm not gonna cop out, man. You didn't catch me right. You didn't catch me with anything. If I lose, I lose, but I'm not gonna

admit to somethin' that wasn't true. I tol' him and I could see on his face he felt like, really, you know, bustin' me in my ass, man. I could see the expression he would put. Because like he—they make arrests but they want to get these things over with as quickly as they can. They don't wanta be goin' back and forth to court, and sittin' all day in court, you know, for just one case. So this last time we went to trial, we were sittin' there from nine-thirty in the morning until two-thirty in the afternoon. We were sittin' in court waiting until they called us and uh . . . he blew the case. He lost because he was a lying cop. . . . I'm glad he lost, man.

S.F. *Have you seen him since then?*

B. Yeah, I seen him after that, and I think he wants to buzz me too. I think he wants to bust me again. And then when, after—after the case got through, he—he walked out of the courtroom real fast, you know, and I walked out after him, and I tol' him, I tol' him, "Was it necessary for you to lie?" And he says, "What do you mean lie? Who lied? Listen, you little cocksucker, don't be sayin' I lied." I say, "You know you lied sayin' I gave you permission to search the apartment, sayin' I escorted you through the apartment—that's a pack of lies, man." I tol' him, "I know you not going to do nuttin' to me in that building, you know me better than that. I know that, so I'm gonna take advantage of the situation now." I'm tellin' him, "You know that's a pack of lies you said, man." And he tol' me, "Listen, you little cock—" but we're talkin' in low tones. He says, "Listen, you little cocksucker, don't be sayin' I lied." You know. Well, I say, "You know you were wrong." He says uh . . . "The only"—this he admitted to me, he says, "The only lie I say was that you escorted me through the apartment, but the four bags and the permission that you gave me permission, and all that, that was true. The only lie I said was that you escorted me through the apartment." I said, "Well, why did you have to say that?" I said that "You say that one lie, man, you—you coulda said a hundred more lies 'cause you were under oath, man." I didn't tell him that you were under oath. That I thought to myself, you know?

S.F. *Are you saying that he actually planted those four bags?*

B. They did! I had no stuff. I was sick. I was waitin' for my mother to come home to give me some money. . . . My mother wasn't even home. She was workin' and when she came home, good thing it was time for her to come home. She gets all upset, you know . . .

Nine years after first becoming involved in drugs, Billie's future appears to him to be as sad and meaningless as he has felt his past life to be. What he seems to look forward to is a continuing round of hospitalization and feeble efforts at therapy. What he fears most seems to be a confrontation with himself and the existential situation that was the matrix of his use of drugs.

Briefly, what Billie has been contending with in the first instance has been an emotional conflict generated by a domineering father and an overprotective, clinging mother, who found a substitute for her husband in her son. The father seems to have crushed him through fear and the mother has swallowed him through love. As a result, Billie has felt anger he dared not express and love that was deep beyond words. Through curbing these basic emotions he developed a life style that was essentially colorless except when broken up by externally and internally generated excitement, the most dramatic of which produced his involvement in drugs. For him, however, as he clearly indicated in his friendship patterns, involvement in gangs was the equivalent of drug use.

Heroin appears to have given him an initial, quite synthetic, experience of what the good life is, but tragically, after being hooked, he has found that the drug life is as chemically depressing as was the underlying life he lived without chemicals.

In contrast, the goofballs or barbiturates that he became hooked on elicited from him some of the rage reactions that he had sought to control by psychological and narcotic techniques. He does not like himself when on pills precisely because they arouse in him not only aggressive, but even masochistic urges that one part of him tells him he should not indulge in.

It is no accident that Billie depended so much upon his family to get money for drugs and that he essentially remains a very petty and vulnerable service person within addict society. His relatively protected early life did not prepare him for the street. He is living the depressed life of a common lower-class person in the ghetto. When he says that he "makes angles" he really means that he makes money by "hustling the hustlers," which involves him in legal risks of a less obvious and hence less threatening nature. Billie never quite plummets to the very, very bottom of the "greasy junkie" level because he always has his mother and his mother's home to fall back upon. In turn, he exploits these as much as he can also to get his minimum money. At this stage in his existence Billie has come to accept the fact that life holds out for him just a minimum, just a minimum. It is as small and as short as he really feels he is.

From one existential point of view, the trouble with Billie's life has been that nothing in it stood out until he became involved in the street and then in drugs. The price of this "standing out" has been the disruption of that life. Least of all did any meaning or purposeful pattern of life and any central values formulated by himself come to the surface. It is understandable, therefore, that the life on drugs, with its cycle of looking for money, buying the heroin, and then using it, has come to have a special value for him. It is a caricature of a kind of life lived by many nonaddicts outside of addict society who live from bill to bill or month to month, and thereby are able to avoid confronting any of the existential questions of contemporary life by losing themselves in smaller units of time.

CAMEO 1

Howie—An Angry Loser

"Howie" is a tall Negro in his thirties who was born in a border state during the Depression.

He was referred to me by the Department of Welfare, which was skeptical about his claim of being off drugs. After several sessions my impression was that he was a man who was almost childishly eager to be sincere and be believed.

He had the feeling that all along fate had been unkind to him. He never knew his father, and apparently was the only illegitimate child and the youngest member of his large family. He emphasizes that as long as he can remember, his other brothers and sisters, acting as a group, excluded and took advantage of him. He found school to be too difficult. When he was nine years old he was already in what he called a reformatory, having been arrested with a group of older boys and accused of having been part of a conspiracy to steal a car. He thought then that he was innocent, and this began a grudge he says he has had against the state. A few years afterwards he was in trouble again, once more accused of a crime he says he had not committed. He came out as a teen-ager, went to work, and this began a series of prison terms for burglaries, most of which he felt he did not deserve.

In his middle twenties, writing from the penitentiary in answer to a lonely hearts column in the Chicago *Defender,* he made contact with a Brooklyn girl and exchanged photographs. While he was in jail his mother died, an event which he found out about much later

158

and which, as he indicated, enormously "shook him up." It was she who had bound him to the town and to the family. This boy, who had wet his bed even as a teen-ager and had night fears, lost the job he had found after leaving prison. This allegedly was through no fault of his own, but the result of a partnership formed in the store he was working at. This persuaded him to go to New York to see his pin-up girl and make his fortune.

Having arrived in New York in the middle 1950's, he got a room, and the very first day was cheated out of some money when he bought a watch from a con man. Soon afterwards he made contact with the girl, apparently struck up a good relationship with her, moved into the rooming house in Brooklyn where she lived, and through her help got a job not too far from the house. Within a month after their meeting she told him she was pregnant and that he was the father, a fact he was not entirely ready to accept. A month after that, apparently concerned about her, about a rival for her affections, and about her alleged pregnancy, he had been drinking. Half-drunk, he had his week's wages stolen from him by two men. Ashamed to go back to the rooming house to tell the story, he went to Manhattan and found a new job as a dishwasher.

Within a year he became involved with a woman who had the same first name as his mother. Living with her, he was enjoying himself for the first time. But trouble dogged him as he took a stranger, whom he had defended, into his home and found that the stranger was trying to "make time" with his woman. This led to fights, and to his being imprisoned and then released on bail. He and his woman then moved up to an area in Manhattan which happened to be an important drug market area.

There he met and fell in love with another girl, who, unknown to him, was a drug addict. Trying to live with two women at the same time, he began unwittingly to support the addict's habit. This led to complications, as his common-law wife, as he called the first woman, objected to his irregular hours.

When he learned he was supporting the drug addict's habit, he insisted upon sharing the drug that he bought for her, and soon became more and more involved, losing his job and his common-law wife. He had been stealing from her and was hoarding some of her property, so she insisted that he leave. This got him more deeply involved in drugs, and after trying to steal, he decided one day, after he had pilfered $46 from a man's wallet, to become a pusher. Aided by his female friend, he pushed for about six months. Early in 1962 he heard rumors of an impending big panic and entrusted over $300 to a man who claimed to have a connection, which proved a fake. In trying to get his money back from this man who had deceived him, he punched him severely, and the next day the man threw lye in his eyes so that one of them was blinded almost entirely and the other was left with limited vision.

A series of eye operations then followed. The doctors tried to convince him that he could not work and ought to be on welfare. This did not prevent him from getting into trouble again, when, with an associate, he tried to burglarize a telephone booth. He was the only one caught. He received a six months' sentence for this. Later he was accused of criminally receiving somebody's stolen coat. The person who stole the coat went free, and Howie, claiming that he didn't know it was stolen, received a year in jail. Lacking in both sight and insight, he found himself lured back into using drugs.

At the time of the interviews Howie was lonely. He acted like and seemed to be a beaten man. Any rage he had at society and the state was tuned out of his voice. Instead, all he seemed to want was to be happy, but it was clear that he wasn't having an easy time of it. At my suggestion he came back several times for counseling and was referred eventually to the Lighthouse. However, he failed to come back for appointments for both myself and the Lighthouse, and eventually disappeared from his home. Nothing more has been heard from him.

Howie's character formation depends on an extremely close relationship to his mother, and on an equally strong rejection of the social order as being unfair to him. Although he became involved in drugs through chance, it is interesting that it was a woman and the disruption of his emotional life that he reported to be the active forces in his involvement. Being on drugs apparently calmed him and gave him the satisfaction of helping others. His use of the drug is an expression not merely of characterological weakness but also of his own sense of worthlessness because of his whole history and the way he feels he has been treated by life itself. His loneliness too, which throughout has encouraged him in making immature or premature decisions, is an expression of his own sense of self-inadequacy and self-insufficiency.

Throughout his life Howie's principal choices have been molded, if not determined, by people other than himself. He has passively let life govern his choices, and then all too often regretted them. This has only inflamed his anger at himself and augmented his self-contempt and his fury at the world outside. This complex of emotions and passivity had prepared him for involvement in drugs. Though one might suppose that his eye condition would be a positive force in helping him to stay off drugs—and this was his own contention—against this is the fact that, having no center within himself and not really struggling to get himself on the way to rehabilitation, the chances are that he has become reinvolved in addict society.

Lilly—Separate, Unequal, and Sad

A Negro woman in her late thirties, Lilly, too, is a client of the Department of Welfare, which insisted that she must be a part of a rehabilitation program in order to get welfare. Throughout most of the interviews I found her hostile and bitter, and she told me frankly that she felt that talking to me was like being on parole.

If there is any theme in Lilly's life it is the persistent one of loss, of being separated from her milieu, and in turn of having fractions of her own life cut away from her. This persistent motif helps explain why, as an adult, she became involved in drugs in an effort to alleviate the depression that she persistently felt.

Her earliest and most vivid memory is that of waving good-by to her mother who was standing at the window, the day she died. Lilly was then five years old. For the next few years she was taken care of by an older sister. Her father was apparently an alcoholic and not so reliable a breadwinner as he might have been, and when she was ten she was dispatched from the New York suburb in which she was living to a Midwestern state to be raised by an aunt. Accompanying her was an older brother who, however, did not stay very long, deciding to make his own way. She stayed behind and endured a harsh regime imposed upon her by her aunt. When she was about sixteen, her aunt wrote to Lilly's sister to have her recalled because she was getting out of hand. Lilly remembers this as meaning that she wanted to go out on dates and parties, and this upset her aunt.

Some time after coming back, Lilly was at a party, became drunk on gin, and was impregnated by one of the partygoers. Her child was born out of wedlock and raised in an orphanage. She herself went to work as a domestic and eventually became the paramour of a gambler who took care of her and her needs. One night she apparently had smoked pot, had drunk liquor, and spent his money unwisely. A fight occurred and, as she sees it, in self-defense she struck and killed him. Eventually she was sent to prison for ten to twenty years, serving part of this time behind bars and part on parole.

It was in jail that she learned about heroin, and within two or three weeks after getting out on parole she had her first snort. She had no friends except those who, knowing her past, would accept her, and these turned out to be people who were in "the life" and used drugs. In the next few years, thanks to parole and its rigorous requirements, she was back in jail on violations and exceedingly depressed because of the regulations about not getting involved with men. This did not prevent her from having a child that was, however, born dead. She turned to prostitution to satisfy her habit, but what is notable about her use of drugs is the high degree of control she exercised over herself. She reports that in most cases she was able to keep from using more than one or two bags in any day if she had to go out and make the money herself. This high degree of control seems to have been bought at the price of persistent sadness.

During these years her son became involved in criminal activities, and she experienced a sense of shame not only about her own life but about the fact that she was unable to do much about his. Just as she herself had the feeling that she was in jail in part unfairly, so too she thinks her son also was unfairly jailed.

One gets the impression of great self-control even in listening to her voice, which is low and almost indistinct. She overtly appears to accept her fate, and yet there are enough signs to show the tremendous resentment and anger that lurk underneath. However, her rigorous self-control has resulted in her feeling depressed. She simply does not allow herself to express her deeper feelings except on extreme provocation, and usually under the influence of liquor. Under drugs she has found a certain degree of relaxation so that she enjoyed the experience even though she was afraid of needles.

Lilly basically is an isolated person. At the time of the interviews she was living in a place occupied by other addicts and simply avoided them all. She spent her time reading or staying in her own room when she was not involved with the Department of Welfare. Though she is relatively passive, she did try to accommodate herself to a parole officer who insisted parodoxically that she reveal to her prospective employers that she had been in jail on a manslaughter charge. As a matter of fact, she had lost a number of jobs precisely because she had to obey this rule.

Lilly makes it plain that she did not relish prostitution and that, in fact, she was involved in a usual vicious circle: she took heroin in order to be able to function as a prostitute and, in turn, the urge to get the drug formed a pressure upon her to go out and prostitute. Money needs and drug needs were reciprocal in her case when she was on drugs. Understandably, also, Lilly experienced prostitution as a loss of status, and it became a reason why she would stay away from her family and her former friends.

In summary, her use of drugs was linked directly and indirectly to her deprivations, which were psychological as well as material in nature, compounded by what she experienced as harsh treatment by life itself and society in particular. Drugs served to alleviate her deep resentment and depression at her unfair treatment.

CAMEO 3

Bert—Divided, He Retreats

Bert, a 26-year-old white man who generally looks tired and harassed, illustrates the situation of the man who turns to drugs to calm and clarify a life that is isolated and chaotic. Heroin serves as a loved retreat where he can be encapsulated safely from the anxiety-provoking conditions of modern life.

As far back as he can remember, Bert's father and mother were always quarreling and acting as an obviously ill-suited couple. Her knowledge of English was so poor, particularly when she was enraged —and she often was—that at times he could hardly understand her. His father, whom Bert described as an intelligent, self-thinking man, died when Bert was not yet a teen-ager. There is an older sister, who as soon as she was able left the home because she could not endure her mother. As a result, for many years Bert was an only child and was given what he wanted materially, but at the price of being humiliated by his dependency upon his raging mother. It is years since he has even spoken to his sister. Sex in general seems to have been an apparent prime source of difficulty for Bert all along, as was foreshadowed in his difficulties with his mother.

In speaking to him over many dozens of hours off and on tape it became clear that he never really fell in love or could let himself fall in love with a woman, and had only one brief sexual transaction with a girl. He started using drugs after he left school. At school, too, he had been relatively isolated although he had a few friends. He found schools to be mildly interesting, and did about average work. But early he felt very guilty about his mother's working and having to support the family. So from the age of about thirteen he was already doing part-time work, giving money to his mother to help pay the rent and the food. This work continued as a pressure on him, and eventually was the pretext for his leaving school. He then secured work as a semiskilled clerical worker and did fairly well there until he started "messing up" because of heroin. Long-standing friends of his had become involved in drugs, and, feeling isolated, he took to the drug life as a "kick."

It is notable that Bert became "a stone addict," that is, rapidly and intensely dependent upon the drug. He stole considerable amounts of money from his mother, went in and out of hospitals ostensibly to detoxify himself, but became rapidly reinvolved once he was outside. As time passed he became more and more of a petty thief, restricting himself to "boosting" supermarkets and then selling the stolen merchandise to candy stores and other local fences. On drugs his life, ordinarily lacking satisfaction, became extremely constricted, concentrated exclusively or almost exclusively upon the getting of money for drugs. When the difficulty of getting money from his mother became too great, he would steal or would shift from heroin to other less costly drugs such as cough medicine.

Thanks to his isolation and his tendency to resolve his confusions by retreating, over the years Bert also developed a tendency to feel that he was a victim of persecution. He was sure that some hospitals, for example, tended to favor Negroes and Puerto Ricans at the expense of the whites. In this belief he was bolstered by his mother, who continually besieged agencies and hospitals to get them to cure her son, and this embarrassment, in turn, led him to be more estranged from her. Pillaging his house gave her the pretext for attacking him, and calling the agencies to attack them, and in general confusing everybody concerned with his life, including of course Bert himself.

To add to his complications, Bert would sometimes take barbiturates and hypnotics, enjoying them at times but not always knowing what he was doing. He had had a certain talent in art and had been given a chance to develop it by his mother, but had not really followed it up. On drugs this, too, was cut out of his life. The main source of contact between Bert's world and the world of reality increasingly has been that of the addict society of which he is a peripheral part. He dissociates himself in his own mind from most addicts around him, but as one watches him in animated conversation with other addicts he seems to have an identity which has helped keep him, somewhat, intact. He might feel that the other addicts think him queer, but this does not contradict his own belief that he knows "what's happening" in the market and among different addicts. As a matter of fact, he is quite proud of being able to stick to "the code" and of never being "a rat." In short, Bert is a man who uses drugs and the drug life as a way of simplifying a complex life and living out a dependent life.

Unlike many other street addicts, Bert prides himself on his literacy and his ability to hold fairly learned discussions with professionals. He dislikes intensely those addicts and nonaddicts who use hip language, feeling that they are putting on a front. However, language appears to give him his own front behind which to retreat from the reality of his being a petty and marginal member of addict society. His analytical cast of mind, which gives him a feeling of being above other addicts, produces in him a continuous process of self-rumination and induces in him the illusion that by this kind of anguished introspection he is not retreating but advancing into life. In short, even his strengths weaken him. The question for the future is: Would he tend to move toward a paranoid style if he kept on using drugs?

Annie—The Prehensile Cat

Among the earliest impressions any adult is likely to get from this teen-age Puerto Rican girl is that for her the world is a boring cage and that any sensible person has a right to do anything to make it more livable. Curiously enough, Annie has a problem of convincing some adults that she is, in fact, completely amoral. Few squares over twenty-one would really believe that this girl, who in certain regards is virginal in her attitude toward sex, would without any compunction exploit them or other teen-agers to get what she wants.

In her time Annie has used a variety of drugs and has a rather strong contempt for their power. She moves from one to the other in the steadfast belief that they cannot control her as long as she can flirt with each one in turn. Her attitude toward drugs parallels her attitudes toward people in that she thinks she can use them and discard them at will.

The phrases "I don't care" and "I don't feel anything" may be heard in any interview with Annie at any time. Both sentiments at times suggest a degree of anxiety, but that is something she carefully conceals. Annie is the youngest of three daughters, and the only one who uses drugs. Early in her life she suffered a traumatic experience in regard to her real father and has been increasingly antiauthoritarian since then. She has no ideology about the Establishment but almost instinctively responds to pressure from above with a negative. This has been true in school, in which she has been something of a problem, as well as in the home. Compounded with this has been a move toward Lesbianism that served partly as a defense against males, partly as an "identity," and partly as another expression of resentment against established authority.

As I have indicated, to get money Annie has exploited others. She steals occasionally, but is more often liable to sponge on people around her, particularly those of her Lesbian friends who have come to depend upon her for what passes for affection.

Though the Exodus House psychologist reports that Annie is, at best, of average intelligence, she shows remarkable proficiency and interest in intrigues of various kinds, and frankly looks at herself as a schemer. She does not find this emphasis on intrigue inconsistent with a highly aggressive, even physical relationship to people. As a "butch," she has been known to strike down not only girls but even boys who have got in her way. However, her contacts with the police have been minimal to the present.

Because of the diverse needs that drugs have filled in Annie's case, we would expect her to get involved in the criminal aspects of the life, and we would be right. With her Lesbian friends and sometimes accompanied by a Negro youth of uncertain sexuality, she has from time to time stolen from stores, pilfered from trucks, and preyed upon available apartments. Sometimes she has done this just for kicks, and at other times, when forced to give an explanation, has tried to adopt a purely hedonistic point of view. These forays into criminality, however, are exciting masquerades of the anguish she feels about an unfulfilled womanhood.

Because she looks innocent she is often given some surprising access up the ladder of the drug hierarchy. It was characteristic in one case that a rather big connection took her to be a "pigeon" (victim) and, sure that she would be flattered by his prestige, offered to "cut her into something pretty big" if she would sleep with him. The poor man found himself blubbering in flustered frustration when she delivered her usual merciless Lesbian tirade at his presumptuousness.

After several months of counseling at Exodus House, her interest in drugs had been reduced considerably, but it was obvious that for her life outside her real self, a pseudo life, is far more desirable than anything she really felt. She has no faith in herself except as an addict and Lesbian, and the two deviations apparently have reinforced each other. Having squashed her most intimate inner feelings and dreading an encounter with her own true life style, this girl has found in drugs a way of narcotizing inner conflicts. How far individual treatments can work with her is a question.

At the time of this writing Annie has left the counseling relationship, using as her pretext that I made light of her Lesbian relationship and allegedly did not think it would last long. She has moved out of her parents' home and in with three other Lesbians. She has formed a tight little circle of her own in which her needs would be satisfied. She has resumed the use of cough medicine and, astonishingly enough, actually believes that she is fooling adult authority in this regard. Whether she will run afoul of the law is certainly a matter of valid conjecture. Annie has "bought" her own fantasies and intends to keep on trying to make the pseudo life a real one.

Portrait of Manny

It is characteristic of this 39-year-old Puerto Rican and the life that he lives that he often invokes the comment "such an intelligent man" from those who listen to him. He sounds so mature, how could he have ever become an addict? And, in fact, listening to one of his tapes one senses that this man who first learned Spanish and then English, and who reads both languages well, marshals his ideas like a general leading his troops in battle.

It so happened that the interviews were held in a small high-ceilinged office lined with books. He commented several times on his own interest in books and later, when the idea was broached, found no objection to having his own life story appear in a book. "It will be an honor, Mr. Fiddle," he said. "It will be an honor."

He is deliberate in speech and movement, and if he is angered he shows it only by the slight contrast between his disturbed state and his ordinary apparent placidity.

In public or private discussions Manny is notable for his critical comments much more than for any large imaginative embracing of public issues. He is analytical and doggedly pursues a topic. I emphasize this intellectual side because I think it corresponds to a general way of life that this man finds most congenial, a life of rules, organization, and structure. I think it no accident that now that he is off drugs, having come to us at Exodus House from a hospital, he continues to complain of what he calls an ulcer. So far the doctors have been unable to establish any physical basis for it, but he does complain from time to time of intense pains in his stomach. Even an amateur psychologist feels inclined to suspect some kind of psychosomatic basis, the ulcer seeming to be a kind of "natural expression" of this man's troubled rigidity. It is equally characteristic of him that he will formulate a theory about himself, and say that he is too mother-dominated or that he is too irresponsible, and then, purely as an experiment, will live with a woman with several children in order to teach himself responsibility. For such a man life has tended to be lived *through* and *in* frames of reference.

(I have deleted references to interruptions and noises that were frequent throughout the several tapes, although it is significant that Manny continued his discussion and dialogue generally with only the slightest allusion to the interruptions. I have made large excisions in the last three of the five tapes that Manny made, because of space limitations.)

SEYMOUR FIDDLE: *Tell me a little bit, if you want to, about your life history as you see it.*

MANNY: Uh . . . going back . . . uh . . . as far as I can remember, recall . . . I start . . . uh when I was beginning to learn the letters, the alphabet . . . as far as I can recall . . . and my uh father like uh. You see, this is something that uh came up the most on my mind. My father, see, because I wasn't raised with him uh and I only knew him for about six years of my life, the first six years, and uh . . . came to New York and uh I was left behind, more or less, and I missed him. I started to—like I was beginning to understand my father in a sense uh was getting used to him and . . . all of a sudden uh I didn't see him any more, and mamma and I were left like by ourselves. That was in P.R., and uh . . .

S.F. *What year were you born?*

M. In 1927, and seems like every time I start thinking back in my past I always get back to the old man. Seems like my father's like a symbol, I don't know, something like uh you can't get away from uh. I'm always going back to the old man. I always come up with that answer like it's a question that really have an intelligent answer to, that I could say uh . . . put my finger on it, maybe this is the reason. Maybe started way back there. My problems, you know, they started

building up, you know, as far as I can see uh figure the only sign I
have, this that I've tried to look for the answer and look, you know,
on my own like uh, well, I'm not qualified, of course. Course, at
K.Y.,* I have seen a psychiatrist at one time when they had uh psychiatrists for the . . . fellows that used to come in from outside.
They was uh doing time, just uh . . . now they don't have that. Before they used to have that, they give you a . . . they send you a
psychiatrist, and you have a session with . . . you, speak to you,
ask you questions, you know . . .

S.F. *What did the psychiatrist tell you there?*

M. Well, he told me that uh . . . the answer lay with me, but uh
. . . he didn't discuss it finally . . . in other words, it was like, it
was my decision. This is the way uh he summed it up now uh that
left me hanging because I didn't know what to think.

S.F. *In general. Well, anyway, how old were you when you got to
New York?*

M. Uh, I was going on ten, I wasn't quite ten. . . . Uh, came I
think it was in October . . . I remember it was my birthday. I was
due for a birthday. [Laughs]

S.F. *Your mother brought you here?*

M. She did, yes.

S.F. *You were an only child?*

M. Yes, at that time. Uh, then over here . . . well, I say I have
to go back to uh P.R. again because you see, so many thing happen.

S.F. *Go ahead.*

M. Mamma uh has always been a woman that uh she doesn't have
that knowledge about uh what's happening in the streets uh like uh
some people call that—it's a figure of speaking—they say like uh
dog eat dog, you know. There's a lot of people that uh wish . . .
others wrong and they *do* others wrong by acting in actions. While
my mother has always been a woman of the house. She uh . . .
that's what she always liked uh home, cooking and sewing and a
regular housewife and uh she was never able to tell me things like
uh this is what's happening out *there*. These things I didn't know anything about. I was—I was a kid and I was—being that I was being
raised by her—I was being raised in the way that uh . . . I was

* United States Public Health Hospital at Lexington, Kentucky.

taught to respect older people—*you* know uh, uh . . . never do anybody any harm, never steal . . . always earn . . . whatever. If I needed a nickel, I have to earn it, you see . . . uh. Nowadays I realize that there was nothing wrong with that upbringing see, but yet . . . I used to see the other kids . . . uh talking about "fa—pop," you know, "my father," you know, and uh I used to see them with their old man and to me it became like an envy. I missed my father and uh it was just always on my mind, you know. Pop. What happened to my father? He's up there, you know, he died or something. I didn't know what to think. Mom told me—

S.F. *You were talking about your father when you were young. Did you try to look for him in any way?*

M. Uh, mom did, uh she uh wrote a few letters to the papers and uh . . . Department of uh . . . Department they have uh . . .

S.F. *Welfare?*

M. No, uh, when somebody disappears.

S.F. *Department of Missing Persons?*

M. Missing Persons Bureau, yes. And uh they never uh did uh find him uh and when I was around seventeen years old uh my aunt, some aunt that I had was living in Fourteenth Street at that time—114th Street? Uh, they came in contact with him. Uh her husband had a shoe repair shop and through her husband, some way or other by talking, he must of happen, just happen to go into the establishment and he started talking and he uh realized that uh she was my aunt and uh through them he got in contact with me and I met him when I was seventeen years old, about seven weeks later. Uh when I first met him, I was confronted with him, I didn't know how to act. I uh it was something like I didn't know what was expected of me, you know? And he didn't act like uh seeing my son, like he was so very happy to see me, so we just kept like uh "Hallo," you know. Just came up with a "Hello," you know. No uh feelings involved more or less. At the time it was just a hello and good-by. We never did really get uh it wasn't a very uh affectionate man in a sense, you know . . . plus then again, so many years passed by and he was just uh seeing me and uh to him it was just "my son," and that's it. He didn't give me uh any more importance uh providing a promise for schooling or uh . . . like uh . . . no interest. Therefore since I was younger,

like I said, uh beginning around since I can remember as far as I can
go backwards, when I was about three years old, he started teaching
me the alphabet uh and uh. . . . He never had any schooling himself. . . . And he was so involved in this like uh he wanted me to
learn the alphabet regardless of the facility of my mental facilities.
You know, I am a three-year-old kid. I am not acquainted with the
letters, you know. He uh bought a board, one of those . . . uh . . .
crayon boards that you teach the kid the first letters and uh specially
made for kids. He . . . tried it out a few times on me like he wanted
me to learn the alphabet, the Spanish alphabet—a,e,i,o,u—and uh
since I couldn't come up with it fully, I couldn't say the whole thing,
I couldn't memorize it, he just batted me over the head with the
board. . . . And after that it seems like I was scared of him.

[The episode of having the alphabet board hit over his head is of
significance to Manny for he has brought it out in other discussions
in public and in private. I take it to be, in the first place, a symbol
of the importance of frames of reference to him. He feels uncom-
fortable, I believe, when things are not routinized and regulated
clearly. Secondly, I take it to be also a symbol of his ambivalence
to his father, and generally to authority which is unjust.]

M.   He was the type of man that he come up to the house, and say
uh if he find me walkin' around like uh kids do in the house and I'm
with mom. Uh, she wouldn't have me in the crib all day, I used to
like I was already walkin', I was just runnin' around the house with
mom, you know, keepin' mom company. And he come up to the
house all of a sudden and uh if he found me outside of the crib, he
wanted me to be sleeping at that time. It was just something that he
set up in his mind, I guess . . . a certain routine that he wanted to
put on me, more or less thinkin' probably that it would benefit me.
I wouldn't say that he had anything harmful in mind, you know.
Probably meant good. He just didn't know how to go about it, probably he was doin' it the rough way . . . uh. He wasn't an educated
man, he never went to school. He was a chief cook; that's all he knew,
how to cook, that was his way of life. I mean that's what he was doin'
in San Juan, and uh like I say, after six years old, I didn't see him

any more. No, I didn't have no affections for him. I was scared of him. So after that it was just mom—everything was mom. Finally, she came over here—1940—she sent for me a year later. During that year, like I was on and off . . . school because my schooling was broken because of this separation between mom and dad. So we went to Mayaguez, another part of Puerto Rico, and there I went to school for a few months and . . . she sent for me a year later, and meantime I am jumpin' from one family to another—my own family . . . umm Mayaguez to San German, San German to Ponce, San German in the hills outside of the town. And this kept on for the whole year, and I am being taken from one place to the other. . . . I'll spend a week over here, week over there, week over there, and kept up for a whole year—out of school, no schooling. And I used to miss mom very much because I am treated like an outsider for certain. Like in Mayaguez, I was treated like an outsider, you know? This uh . . . I don't know, it gave me a complex, it make me feel different. I don't know, it make me feel meaner. . . . I used to like uh I used to like . . . before they used to ask me go over to the movies and find out what's playing, and I used to just go happily. But now since they are treating me this way, I have an animosity towards them or something like I am not being treated right. So . . . they ask me to go and find out what's playing in the movies, and I say no, man, not unless you give me a nickel. In other words, now I'm demanding payment for whatever I do for them.

[Here Manny consciously transformed a situation of friendship into one of payment. The concretion is replaced by the abstraction. Here, too, we have a foreshadowing of a life in which abstractions will have special meaning for him, a special source of security.]

M. During that time that I was there uh I used to go to the beach at night, sometimes by myself . . . and look at the other side. Like you see the sunset and say, like mom is on the other side. I used to miss her so much that I used to cry, and by myself on the beach . . . think that if I could only swim this span of sea, make it to the other side where she was at. I missed her so much, I became so dependent on her. She was my only . . . out, you know, the only person that I could turn to, you know, whenever I—just didn't get anything like that uh my father wasn't there. . . . It was my father and mom, both. I don't know how important that may be in my life, but that has . . . has some—has had something to do with my misguidance or something. . . . The way I have been deviated along the way although I have been told certain things was right and was wrong . . . along the way. . . . And I've been raised like in certain neighborhoods when I was in New York City after that which may have something to do with my deviations, you know? Uh . . . in 1941 to . . . 1945 I was going to school, I took a course learning how to speak English and special class they called the C class. Uh they had kids from all over the world there. I don't know if they still have those classes in public school, but they used to have them at that time. In '45 I wanted to sail. All of a sudden I got a bug, I wanted to sail. A friend of mine was sailin' and he was brought up almost in the same neighborhood for quite a few years, and he started sailing. He was a little older than I was . . . and . . . I wanted to sail. . . . I thought it must be good if he says, you know, and he says you could do this . . . and we see the world. . . and I did. . . . I started talkin' to mom. At that time I was going up to the Bronx P.S. 27 public school, and they had transferred me at just that particular month that I had been geting the bug to start sailing. They had transferred me from C class second year at Morris High School, and they gave me the papers. They gave me all the papers necessary to appear over there, and we sent them so they will admit me in the high school. I got as far as the lobby. And uh . . . the one that was in charge he wasn't in the office, the person in charge. So the principal, I think it was, so I waited around maybe five minutes, and he didn't come in. So I just turned back, turned around. That's the end of school for me . . . now I want to sail. Mom says, "Are you crazy now? Go to school. Finish your schoolin'." Says no, no, and I insisted so much that she gave in. So I took out uh made all the arrangement necessary, and I took out the papers, at that time it was at 45 Broadway. I went over there, I passed the examination; they gave me my seaman papers. And I went and made a trip to the line. They were affiliated with the N.M.U., but at that time they had a separate arm. So I made my first trip as a third cook. I didn't know how to fry an egg . . . so one of the other seamans told me, "Don't worry about it, . . . I'll be on the ship. I'll take care of you." He just so happened to be living in the same building that I was living in. At that time I was living on a Hundred Street. We had moved from the Bronx to a Hundred.

S.F. *What year was that?*

M. Uh . . . '45. Round '45. So I made my first trip as a third cook. I got blackballed on that trip. I got sick, my first trip, I got sick. There was a large group of Spanish guys working there also and they . . . came up with an idea that they didn't feel like they were being treated right. So they stopped work. At sea that's mutiny. It so happens that during that trip some other guys had been helpin' me along because I'd been sick, and I'm getting sick, and I don't know the job. So I'm acquainted with them through this. We'd been working together. But being they mutiny, I get it blamed that I mutiny also because they just consider me a part of the whole, part of the group. And when we land over here we all got blackballed, thrown out of—as a—as a charge that we mutiny on board, and we can't sail with them any more. We can never sail to the whole world any more, see. So, the next best thing that I thought of was the army base. Somebody had told me about the government ships and the transport at that time. Takin' soldiers overseas, bringin' back the sick . . . uh . . . ammunitions, this and that, so it was more or less like a civil service job . . . a civil service employee. You got an I.D. card uh everything was aboveboard uh rules and regulations uh . . . so I got into that. I lasted five years on that.

S.F. *What year?*

M. From '45, same year that I made that trip—that was a thirty-day trip—same year I got into the army base.

S.F. *'Forty-five to '50?*

M. It also happens that between '45 and '46, beginning in '46, I started like smokin' pot.

S.F. *How come?*

M. See, now all this, all this is happening to me uh sort of all at once, and I was with a group around here on a Hundred Street* that uh used to have things that they, like pot once in a while, uh a little

---

* East 100th Street became a most prominent drug market center in the 1950's.

drink, a little bit . . . kicks more or less uh have fun and uh talk, hear music, go to movies, go dancing . . . was big fun, a lot of fun. As for that pot business, usin' a lot, I got acquainted with somebody else that was doin' somethin' besides . . . pot. This guy happened to be . . . usin' cocaine. . . . So he . . . I happened to walk into it. Knock on his door and uh . . . it just so happened that that particular time or moment I knock on his door there was another fellow in there and they were taking off on cocaine. Plain cocaine. It was something new to me. I, you know, "What's this, what are they doin'?" Nobody has told me anything, but my mind is workin'. I'm lookin' at this; they're permitting me to see this. 'Course I know the person so . . . he is askin' me the first time that I have been to his house, and I was bein' respectful, so his doors are open to me, see.

[The words "respect" and "respectful" appear frequently in Manny's discourse, and suggest the importance, to him, of good authoritative frameworks.]

M. So I am looking at this, and they are takin' off and they tellin' me, "Get me a glass of milk or somethin' " like they're petrified after they take coke. They're scared to move. See, so I bring them a glass of milk, they drink it slowly. . . . Two minutes I watch these actions and I wonder, why do they act this way? So they got the best of me, my uh thinkin'. Like I like to find out, inquiring, my mind is inquiring. I'd like to find out what this is. But I got the nerve to ask if they would be nice enough to let me try it. And this I ask. I ask them . . . something new, I want to find out what it is. . . . Says "No, you shouldn't. You know you never done this before. We don't recommend it to you. It's a heck of a kick, but we don't recommend it to you." What is this? "It's a heck of a kick, but we don't recommend it"—you know. That gives me more of a uh a desire. So I insist, I insist. Uh they finally gave me, they gave me a little bit and I got petrified. I didn't know how to act. I got so excited because uh my heart started pumping harder, and that was the first one. It just so happens that I . . . uh . . . just so happened to keep on with them for a while. All of a sudden I find myself that I am not sleeping. I am not eating.

S.F. *Why not?*

M. Because that's the type of—uh—what do you say uh . . .

S.F. *Pattern?*

M. Pattern?

S.F. *Pattern. Way of life.*

M. This is the reaction that you get from using cocaine. It activates you. It makes your heart more . . .

S.F. *Tell me, did you find that using either pot or cocaine had any effects on your sex life?*

M. Cocaine seems to uh kill that urge in the sense that I was getting like weaker. I wasn't sleeping, I wasn't eating like regular. In other words, my like everyday habits of regular habits like eating regular and sleeping regular uh they were being thrown off the axis . . . . It was being changed by using this cocaine. Not pot. Pot has never, as far as I can go back and remember, has never interfered with my sex life. Or my appetite, or my sleeping, but cocaine did.

S.F. *How long did you use cocaine?*

M. Cocaine, I was usin' it for around close to a week and a half before I got introduced to heroin. Heroin was supposed to calm me down. That's how I got into usin' heroin. And it did. It did calm me down. I wanted to sleep so badly and I wanted to relax . . . that uh . . . I tried it and uh it worked that I found myself relaxed. I found myself that I could go to bed and go to sleep. I needed the rest badly. I lost a lot of weight. It was a big change all of a sudden within a week.

S.F. *So that heroin was something that you used to counterbalance the stimulant of cocaine.*

M. Right. At that time.

S.F. *How much were you paying for cocaine?*

M. Umm actually I wasn't paying anything for it. He was giving it to me.

S.F. *How much were you paying for the heroin?*

M. I wasn't payin' anything for it at that time either.

S.F. *You say with heroin, you got involved. Did you vomit the first time?*

M. Yes, I did. The first time I tried it I did, yes. I was sick all night long just about. I tried it with a speedball just after me . . . a speedball . . . that's how come I tried it. I didn't try it alone by itself. It was fixed as a speedball and that's the way I shot it. I never learned how to sniff. In other words, I was introduced into it, the needle. That's the way they were taking that cocaine, that's the way I got introduced into it by asking. I wanted to find out. After I started using that uh speedball, that was another kick. . . . That was horse and cocaine together which gives you a different type of a kick, see? Two stimulants used at the same time, and they're acting as one. In other words, you get both kicks in one. . . . So this is something new. Gee, I like this . . . I seem to like it, I seem to like it. This is what came to my mind. Gee, some kick, ooh.

S.F.   *When you were speedballing, did sometimes one drug come through stronger than the other?*

M.   Sometimes. Yes. I feel the cocaine first and then slowly the cocaine kick will be going down, and then the heroin will be taking hold and then I find myself goofing and going on the nod. In other words, I already vacillated [!] the cocaine, now the . . . I relax now. Cocaine makes you excited. I got at the beginning. Now I'm coolin' down, and now I feel this. Two reactions, you know, one after the other.

S.F.   *Did you ever do the reverse? Heroin first, then cocaine to wake you up?*

M.   No. No, cocaine—heroin will last you longer than cocaine.

S.F.   *So up, and then down.*

M.   Up and down—right. That's one way of explaining it.

S.F.   *Tell me, what was your knowledge about heroin before? Did you hear anything about heroin?*

M.   No, I didn't know anything about heroin. I didn't know . . . uh . . . what the outcome was of usin'. . . . Also I wasn't acquainted with any drug addicts. At that time, anybody who was hooked up or knew anything about it—see the crowd that I was with were clean-cut guys in the sense that they were always clean, guys that work. None of them were guys that knew anything. In fact, I don't think any of them knew anything about drug addicts uh being hooked uh you know, anything about heroin.

S.F.   *Now where did you go to buy it?*

M.   At that time around this part of the neighborhood. Just about anywhere that you could go in this part of the neighborhood you could connect at the time, you know? Even though I didn't know the people who were . . . selling that because I wasn't acquainted with it, like I say. And at that time there wasn't that many guys usin' it openly . . . where people used to pinpoint them as heroin users. It was more conservative, and the old-timers wouldn't bother with the young guys like introducing them into it. Like so happen afterwards uh that the guys didn't care—they didn't care whether the newcomer was a junkie or what. There they is, but at that time uh if a guy was a drug addict it was a drag. It was consider like uh an outsider, an outcast. That's the way the guys that were selling it to them felt about it themselves. A lot of guys were selling and they wasn't using. They just used pot and cocaine.

S.F.   *Are you saying that during those years drug addicts were more invisible?*

M.   They were conservative in the sense that they worked and there was no uh. . . . At that time they could make a dollar better than now. At this present time it's harder to make a dollar in the street than at that particular time during the end of the war. And there was more money being in circulation. So I guess it was easier for them to acquire the money to buy the dope which it was also easy to get at that time—much easier. The laws weren't as hard as now, and no connections were uh . . . visible uh. It was, everything was at hand. It was easier, much easier. To me, it was never a bother, to me. I just never gave it a second thought at that time, see. Being that I didn't know any difference anyway to begin with . . . when it came to that. But before I know it . . . uh . . . I was hooked. Without realizing that I was hooked, without knowing . . . the results.

> [It is characteristic of Manny that he assumed that his experience was universally true. Other addicts from other areas, however, have emphasized that drug addicts during this period were respected. I suspect that at least part of the difference in recollection has to do with Manny's rigid frame of reference. Drug addicts were known to be flashy and big spenders, but Manny sees them as conservative businessmen.]

S.F.   *How did you find out?*

M.   Well, one day, I uh . . . it just so happens that I didn't use anything. I was using for almost three weeks steady. See.

S.F.   *What happened then?*

M.   I found myself in that position that I could use it for almost three weeks steady . . . and then . . . all of a sudden . . . uh— stop. That night I started getting sweating and yawning and crying and got diarrhea, and felt like vomiting. . . . I thought I had a cold or something, a fever. I thought I was sick. I didn't think it was, you know . . . the result of that. So that night I stayed home. I got the chills and my mother covered me very well with blankets, and she gave me a rubdown with acqualon and so forth like if I was just uh catching the flu or something. That's what I thought I had, see? Then as I spent about three days at the house sick that I realizin' what was wrong with me. She even called the doctor for me, and he came up and give me an injection of penicillin.

S.F.   *Do you think, in general, people act pretty cool or cold to drug addicts as patients?*

M.   At that time, like I said, at that time they were considered out-casts. Even around this part of the neighborhood. It was like dirt. That's the way they considered a drug addict . . . at that time. Most of them guys that did consider a drug addict that way, in later years, they became drug addicts themselves . . .

S.F.   *You said that pot did not have any bad effects. How did heroin affect you?*

M.   Well, heroin, like I said, it seemed to take a hold of me in the sense that uh . . . after that happened I was off it because I was sailing, of course. At that time, like I told you, I went on a boat. I felt like I was recovering from the flu, which happened to be the habit that I was getting. I didn't realize it. I didn't fully realize it. I went on a trip, and uh—twenty-one-day trip to Germany—came back. I went lookin' for it. Seems like when I came back, when already I had that in mind, I had to take off. I felt like I wanted to take off.

S.F.   *What was your position on the boat?*

M.   I was working at that time as uh janitor, just cleaning rooms and . . . hallways and showers and crew's quarters at that time. When I first hit New York that night, everybody showers and uh hardly any-body sleeps when we pass the Statue of Liberty.

S.F. *Where'd you go to buy? Around your old neighborhood?*

M. Around the same neighborhood. I found out who have something and I just went ahead and got me a couple cocaine and a couple horse and I mixed them and I had me a speedball. I didn't really take the whole thing because at that time the stuff was much stronger. So I shared what I bought with somebody else that was hooked. Happened to go to the shooting gallery where they were selling it. I took off right there! So . . . I went back home.

S.F. *When was the first time you were arrested?*

M. Nineteen-fifty . . . the end of '50, going on '51. I happened to do a favor. I came from the army base. I got up on 103rd Street and found me a person that wanted to connect. And he asked me, "Will you please go over and get me somethin' and bring it home because I can't do it now. I have someplace to go, and by the time you get back, I'll be home." I was just coming out of the train and I happened to have my works with me. I was also usin' something, but I wasn't really hooked then. I was like goin', tryin' to get a ship, a boat. But I still had a set of works anyway. And uh . . . I told him, "Will you please take the works that I have here with you? Take them home and that way I don't have to carry works." He says, "No, uh, you carry them because I don't want to. I got to make a stop before I go up to the house. Shouldn't take you long to get over there and get back anyway," he says. So I said, "All right, fine." I made it and I went on to cop and when I was coppin', when I come out of the buildin', the detectives—uh four detectives—were in a car and they were . . . They seen me when I went one way and another boy that went up the house with me went another way. So they just sort of figure something funny there. "Let's stop these guys." So they stopped us. . . . They made me go back from across the street all the way back to the hallway, and they searched us and they found the bag that I had and the works. That was a 422 at that time . . . the bag. . . . I got me a suspended sentence. That was my first . . . run-in with the law.

S.F. *And what was the next time?*

M. Next time wasn't too far behind . . . [Laughs]

S.F. *Same year?*

M. Seems like I found a way.

S.F.   *A way to what?*

M.   A way to go to jail. I got acquainted with that, so . . . not too long after . . . '50 . . . was '52 or . . . I went to jail for . . . a burglary. I got really hooked after that uh . . . and then I started . . .

S.F.   *How were you supporting yourself?*

M.   Odds and ends uh throwin' rocks like they say. Uh I didn't know how to—I didn't know how to make a dollar in the street. I didn't know anything about it because I was workin', I was used to workin' so now—since I got a habit—and I have learned what it is looking for a way to make a dollar without workin' because it seems like a, like a handicap 'cause all of a sudden I can't go to work. I didn't know how to cope with it. Like I wasn't acquainted with the way to make a dollar in the streets. I had to find a way of learning in order to survive and keep up with the habit. Uh being that I wanted to keep up with the habit, I imagine it just seems like I didn't want to quit the habit at that time. . . . I went around the neighborhood checking what was happening and . . . found a few guys that were also in the same boat. . . . Put our heads together and . . . they were crooks. They seemed to like to steal. That was one way of making a dollar. . . . I went out with them. . . . Seems that at that time it was—I felt that it was as good a way as any of makin' a dollar. They seemed to be doin' it, so . . . let me try it and see what happens. . . . So, my first—the first chance that I took from that uh happen I get busted; very unfortunate. . . . I uh there was a . . . nothing there for me. I didn't make anything on the deal.

[In the ordinary evolution of the sort of life style of a man like Manny, stealing is not a compatible way of self-maintenance. He has to learn from the street, which means breaking with his conventionalized frames of reference. In Manny's case, as we shall see, stealing proved only to be an abortive method and he gave it up.]

S.F.   *What did you get in the way of punishment?*

M.   I got uh pen indef—Riker's Island indefinite sentence, one to three years. . . . I got out of that in twelve months . . . and I'm out maybe two, three months and . . . I hung up on the parole. I got hooked again. . . . Um-mm . . . let's see, two months later,

which would make it five months out on the streets, I'm busted again.
. . . Another burglary. Gave it another try. Didn't succeed either.
Didn't know how to steal. . . . I went to jail again.

S.F. *What year was that now?*

M. That was goin' on . . . '53, '53, I believe. And uh I got another pen indef out of that . . . killing my old pen indef the time
that I owe. One indefinite sentence kills the other. . . . I was recommended not to do more than one year by . . . uh . . .

S.F. *A judge.*

M. A judge. I didn't do no more than one year and got out of that
on parole. City parole. Stay off for a while, workin'. Seems like my
mind was getting kind of settled; seems like I was failing at everything
that I was doing, and uh like stealing uh seems like I couldn't steal.
It wasn't, it wasn't the way to look for a dollar. Uh . . . stayed out
for a while and I hung it up again because I got hooked again. I
stopped reporting . . . had a wonderful parole officer, but I didn't
know any better. I didn't seem to realize what I was doin'. I was just
. . . uh . . . doin' things uh for the heck of it, for the heck of it.
No aim . . . stay out awhile until I got violated because I went to
visit some guy uh. . . . Just so happened that he was down for a
bust and unfortunately I happen to knock on the door at the wrong
time. . . . Officers were there, and of course, being that they had
him uh pinned uh automatically search me. They don't find anything
but they want to take me for investigation. Being that I had jumped
parole, there is a warrant out for me. They find this out. . . . Next
day I am on my way to Riker's Island, with the habit, sick. Kickin'
my habit in the pen, I started gettin' sick and throwing up and . . . a
mess. Made it to Riker's Island, started that time, my violation, three
months, my first violation. Got out of my three months' violation . . .
went back to it again. Seems like there was no sense up there . . .
[pointing to head] I went back to it, got hooked again. Got violated
again. . . . Went back again. They gave me B.O.T.—balance of
time—finish my time, came out and I'm thinkin' . . . gee, I can't
keep this up. Now I'm realizin' that this in and out isn't doin' me any
good—there's somethin' wrong somewhere. I need help, but I don't
realize it. What type of help do I need? I'm goin' into books now. I

want to go into books. I want to learn. I want to see what's happenin',
what's wrong with me.

[It is characteristic of his perspective and outlook that Manny turns
to books to find out what is wrong and how to help himself. It is
also a sad reflection on the state of prisons that he could find no
significant help from psychiatrists on a long-term basis even though
he was in jail for some time.]

M.   Let me check those psychiatry books uh let me read a little
Freud uh a little Dewey uh evolution. Uh I'm reading anything, you
know, I'm tryin' to get a hold of somethin'. Maybe I can find somethin' in a book that will help me. . . . I read and read and read, and
I don't find the answer. Books that I didn't even understand half of
the words sometimes. I finally got acquainted with quite a few and
. . . still didn't come up with the answer. All I could see was . . .
was for me to decide whether to keep up with it or to . . . not to
keep up with it. No sooner I decided to stay awhile, that I'm not
messin' around, before I know it, I deviate again. Some pretense or
another. So I got a few other busts like . . . uh possession of narcotics. . . . Got busted for possession of narcotics, goin' and do six
months. Come out . . . back to the grind again, work for a while on
shore. Seems like I couldn't get used to workin' on shore because I
was so used to sailing for five years, and uh that was all I knew, how
to work at sea. That type of work, routine that I like. And now I find
myself working eight hours a day, over here, and the demand on me
was so strong, and uh I wasn't getting paid enough money and uh
didn't see no consideration from the bosses. Maybe I was workin' for
the wrong people, I don't know. Anyway, at that time uh if you're
Spanish and uh . . . there's a job open for you uh you're supposed
to work to the bone—the fingers to the bone without no consideration
uh like if you was a work dog or work horse or somethin'. And I
noticed this attitude and uh being that uh my fellow . . . fellow
uh . . .
S.F.   *Employees?*
M.   Fellow citizens uh [Laughs] my own uh Spanish-speaking peo-

ple, we were being treated in such a way uh they couldn't say "boo" because they didn't even know the language, and uh it just so happens that I worked for quite a few factories that uh they had uh people that came from P.R. and different places. And didn't speak English at all, and they were workin' for few dollars uh they wasn't getting paid. Actually the uh type of product that they came up with, they uh . . . wasn't getting paid as they should—I didn't think it was fair.

[Two frames of reference are expressed in the phrase "getting paid as they should." First, there is a generalized conception of natural justice by whose canons he and other Puerto Ricans were underpaid. Second, there is his own personal experience, the ship frame of reference, in terms of which shore jobs lack both prestige and work. The second lingers on for many years and colors his view of life in the city. Both together give him the emotional basis, i.e., the frustration, which makes it understandable to him that he gets involved with drugs.]

M. I'm not used to working like this, eight hours and not makin' enough money. On board ship I was makin' enough money; I wasn't workin' eight hours. It wasn't demanded of me to work eight hours, I didn't have to work eight hours . . . I was getting consideration and I was . . . I even had retirement. I could foresee retirement if I had stayed on at uh twenty years, just like other civil working employees. I had those uh benefits or somethin' . . . and now I find myself that I messed up my record. I uh can't go back to sea; the army base didn't want me. I sent an application when I came out of Riker's Island the last time, and they uh send it back uh "Sorry, we don't have any place open—position open for you, uh your type of work. Uh please try uh find employment someplace else." Politely they told me—they didn't want me and they marked down on the application, 'round it, marked a circle around uh the question that says have you been arrested, and they say I was arrested, on the application. . . . So they didn't take me any more . . . it's out, the government is out; I took my retirement pay . . . which I had there . . . and that did it. I'm not connected any longer with the army base. Now I have to shift over here, with the city and I have to cope with the city life.

Huh . . . you been here in the city a long time. You imagine more or less uh what a person could make uh that doesn't have an education. Uh he's just a laborer and he works at any job like . . . delivery jobs and messenger, handy man, stuff like that uh . . . factories. I used to get an attitude every time and used to like . . . go from one job to the other. If I was makin' it uh at a delivery job, and they send me out . . . it was raining, I tell the boss I uh wait until it stop raining. He tell me no, we pay you to . . . deliver whether it rains or shines. Well, give me my pay because I'm not goin' to go and get wet and that was that. That's the type of attitude that I had and I kept on jumping from one job to the other.

S.F.   *Were you using drugs then?*

M.   No, not when I was workin' there in those places. Uh it just so happens that uh every time that I have been workin' I haven't been hooked . . . but la—later on I got hooked and uh there goes the job. Before they fire me because I can't keep up the responsibility as much as I like to. See I feel that uh . . . instead of getting kicked out of a job, I would rather quit being that uh by using drugs I can't keep up with the responsibility because today, I may have, tomorrow, I might not have, or tomorrow I might wake up sick, uh like that happen so many times already. And I have to call down the job, and tell them a lie . . . something came up very important uh. . . . I try on being in in the afternoon or could I get the day off or this and that—or asking for money on the job. Uh it became so difficult uh at times that I just felt that I wasn't keeping up with the responsibility that was uh . . . that I was supposed to keep up with.

[Here is the other side of the coin. Once he gets involved in drugs, more and more he is unable to perform according to his own standards of excellence, and he finds it necessary to quit work because he cannot perform his responsibilities. This, in turn, guarantees that he gets hooked and remains so.]

S.F.   *What happened then?*

M.   After I quit uh I go back to the streets . . . and . . . shift . . . hustle the dollar like they say . . . in our lingo . . . till something happens, till I decide that to go to K.Y. like I went there a couple of times, decide to go to the Tombs* and kick the habit like I did. And I went to Riker's Island and kick another habit. They had at that time, they send you to Riker's Island for twenty-nine days, something like that. I went there one time . . . seems like I was trying to . . . kick the habit. . . . Seems like I was trying to . . . do something about it, but seems like I could never do anything about it. Seems like uh . . . I was stuck with it. Uh I don't know why . . . uh couldn't realize it. I knew I needed help, but I didn't know who to ask for it. At that time, there wasn't many doors open for a drug addict to go and knock on and ask help outside of K.Y. . . . K.Y. was givin' up also . . . in the sense that they no longer had any . . . more psychiatrists for the, for the fellows that check in . . . just to kick the habit. They were more or less concentrating on the guys doing time. They came up with this answer, I guess that's what they decided that was best . . . for the institution. So we no longer had any doors to knock on . . . couldn't knock on the . . . Police Department. They put you in jail if they caught you with somethin'. . . . Couldn't knock on anybody's . . . couldn't go to the hospital and then say, "Uh, well, I'm a drug addict. I'm sick. Uh I want to kick this habit." Uh, they tell you go to K.Y. . . . At that time you couldn't even get the welfare to pay your way. That started afterwards. All this started happenin' at once, see. The first time I went to K.Y., they give me a psychiatrist, a doctor.

S.F. *Did he help you?*

M. Uh . . . we used to speak, uh he'd ask me questions. I'd answer him. I tried to be as sincere as I possibly could. . . . Uh I couldn't think as straight probably as I can now . . . in the sense that I can see more clearly my faults, and I can admit them. . . . At that time I used to hold back a whole lot. I was younger, of course, and I don't know my mind was all clouded up. . . . Lack of experience. I don't know what to—

S.F. *Do you sometimes feel that being on drugs is like a dream—a bad dream?*

M. Uh . . . yes, I feel it is uh . . . I'm on a different . . . I'm like uh by myself.

* The Tombs—Men's House of Detention in New York City.

[Many addicts of different types of life style refer to the feeling of isolation. However, for a person like Manny there is a poignancy that is special. His own boundaries become a frame of reference through which he looks at the world. The boundaries are quite sharply defined in general and give him a feeling of loneliness and stasis. Things are outside him and he is unable to move, imprisoned by his own frame of reference.]

M.   Yes, uh when I'm usin' drugs I find myself like everything's goin' by . . . and I'm just standin' in one spot, watchin' the world go by. And everything is happening and there's nothin' happening to me at all. I'm not doin' anything for a while. I'm just like stopping in water. . . . After I kick the habit I start seein' things different, and I feel like another person altogether . . .

S.F.   *What was the next time you were in prison after the time you just described?*

M.   After . . . uh I went on a few 330's for possession, in and out, in and out. Uh and I never did get another—another big bit until . . . 1961. Two which I got six years.

S.F.   *For what?*

M.   For . . . 1751—sales—sales of narcotics.

S.F.   *How did it happen?*

M.   Well, I was . . . taking care of my habit uh. . . . Since I can't steal because it just so happens that I don't . . . know how to steal . . . I don't know how to pick pockets, I don't know how to . . . I don't have the heart . . . or the inclination or the desire to hold up anybody or to hurt anyone—handling someone or some person to take their money away from them. . . . Never been able to do that. . . . My conscience had never . . . permitted it . . . although I've been hooked . . . that part of me has always been functioning.

[What Manny refers to as his conscience is equivalent to what we have been referring to as a frame of reference.]

M.   I've never been able to do it, just have to, that's the way it is. Uh the next best thing that I could do, the only thing that I could possibly do in order to . . . manage . . . was to sell . . . a few bags

. . . in order to . . . to take care of my habit, support my habit. So I don't have to . . . take a chance on stealing . . . although it was against my wishes, but if I was forced enough to do it uh . . . I would take a chance on it, and I didn't want to do that. . . . I just uh sold a few bags and it so happens that I sold to a secret agent—uh, undercover man.

S.F. *Do you remember doing it?*

M. I made two sales uh. I remember one individual . . . and uh that individual . . . has to be . . . the agent. Now, I was never confronted with the agent; I never fought the case. I never said I didn't sell although . . . it wasn't no big sale, big seller or anything. I was just trying to support my habit, but nevertheless, that I did make the sales . . . and uh that got me a . . . six-year bit—three to six. That got me a six-year bit, which is the parole that I'm on now.

S.F. *How much more time do you have?*

M. Uh . . . time finishes . . . uh . . . March of '68.

S.F. *Two more years to go.*

M Yeah, uh brought that down I got around '63 . . . '63, '62, the end of '62, somewhere around there.

S.F. *Which prison did you go to?*

M. I went to Sing Sing first . . . receivin' uh stayed there a few months. Uh then they sent me to uh . . . Auburn Prison uh . . . because when I was in Sing Sing uh they told us that they had a new program at Auburn. They had opened a school . . . and I was interested. Uh . . . I filed an application . . . asking to be permitted to go over there . . . and . . . they sent me over there. Right to the school. I uh . . . didn't have my uh high school diploma because, like I said, I uh dropped out of school. And uh . . . I uh . . . acquired a high school equivalency at Auburn. I uh went to another class that tried to take up uh commercial artists' course, but I didn't stay long enough at Auburn and I got released before I could really get into the commercial artist uh deal . . . until now. Ever since I got released, as soon as I came out, the same week I uh got a job, as a messenger with the 54th Street Employment Agency. And I worked at that job uh . . . seven months. In between I got me another job . . . at a stationery . . . and uh . . . that was two jobs

I had, and it just so happened they were too much for me because I wasn't getting enough rest.

[Manny is an anxious person and once outside of prison walls he overconforms. One job won't do. He needs two jobs. The pretext may be money, but close inspection reveals that he really wants to have instant acceptance, instant rehabilitation, in short, instant passing as a square. Hence, two jobs are needed, not one. In turn, however, this sets up its own dynamics and tensions, and eventually he falls back into drugs.]

M.   So I got sick, got a pain in the stomach. Maybe it was the change of diet uh I uh got no exact time to eat. I was uh on the messenger job. It was in and out. . . . It was a painting concern, and it was just in and out. It was very busy and . . . always eight hours, sometimes nine. I get out of there around seven o'clock at night, sometimes eight, sometimes nine, all depending how many hours they want me to work. And uh . . . the other job, I start at uh . . . six o'clock in the morning at the stationery, which I have to open the stationery until the other man come in . . . at nine o'clock—eight-thirty or nine, the other man come in. And uh . . . he take over. It was a part-time job . . . see . . . workin' five hours or more . . .

S.F.   *And it was money you wanted? Was that the reason you took both jobs?*

M.   In a sense. I wasn't getting enough in the . . . messenger work uh being that I just come out of prison, I needed a lot of things like clothes and a watch to tell time with uh by. I needed . . . uh to have a few dollars in my pocket to travel and so forth. I always like to look presentable. . . . I believe that cleanliness is very important in the individual in a sense that uh . . . some persons, like they say uh . . . like to look presentable. Others don't care . . . and it so happens that I care, and if I can afford it . . . I can do it. . . . I can be dependent on no one because I am a man already. If I uh in order for me to acquire that I have to work for it. . . . Uh . . . being that I was also on parole, that was another thing that uh . . . I had to work anyway—rules and regulations. Although I would have still worked anyway in the state of mind that I came out of prison, without being told to . . . and . . . I wasn't making enough on the messenger job, so I got me another job. All right so now I was makin' a little more. . . . I was harming my health because—my P.O. told me he didn't know how long I was goin' to last with that routine because he figured it was too much for me. I told him uh well, we'll see. And I uh lasted a few months but uh I had to give up one job. I gave up the messenger job. I stayed with the stationery job which was lighter . . . less hours . . . and I went over to the————* Hospital, and they're doing some stomach tests on me, and they beginning to put me on a diet, thinking it was . . .

S.F. *Ulcers?*

M. Ulcers, yes. Bland diet. So they check the X rays, and they find out that uh . . . they couldn't find any uh ulcers. Uh my pain went away anyway. I uh got rid of that, I started restin'. . . . I stood away from uh drugs altogether while being on parole.

S.F. *How long?*

M. About eleven to twelve months. From eleven to twelve months without touchin' it at all.

S.F. *What caused you to relapse?*

M. Well, now, that's a question that I'd like to answer—if I could. But I don't find the answer. Uh . . . I got out of the stationery one day . . . around this part of the neighborhood also. [Laughs] It seems like uh, we sometimes go back to the beginning . . . you know? Automatically, we always seem to uh have a big desire of going back to where we came from.

> [Manny is full of generalizations, homilies, and wise saws. This proverbial content seems to give him a certain degree of emotional security.]

M. I uh . . . come out of the job and the stationery which is on Ninety-sixth Street . . . and Madison . . . and I walk down to Second Avenue. I want to find out what's happening around a Hundred Street. I haven't been around a Hundred Street for years. I come

---

*Refers to a city hospital.

around a Hundred. It just so happens that I am with someone that I know, and there happened to be something by . . . so uh like all of a sudden I am interested. . . . I'm the feeblest guy. Eleven, twelve months I haven't used anything . . . uh. . . . I know who got a good bag, blah, blah. I says, "You do?" I got money, of course. I been workin', I been workin' so long I gotta have some money in my pocket. Uh . . . not wasting my money, not throwing it away. I am buying things. I have something to show for, but uh . . . seems like I don't appreciate it any more or somethin'. Seems like I'm workin' and I'm not making enough money, but I'm making some, which is better than none, which I realize that now, and be satisfied with the money I'm making. But yet I know that I have to do it . . . it's the best thing that I can do. I uh . . . tell the guy uh, "I'll tell you what. Get a bag; I don't have any habit and uh I'll take a little. You take the rest." Just like that. And I did.

S.F. *Did you enjoy it?*

M. Uh . . . I don't even remember what type of a kick I got out of it, so I don't think it was worthwhile. I realize that now.

[Manny described some of his feelings and his difficulties in entering a hospital to kick his habit while on parole.]

M. I got admitted into the hospital, and that's when I find out about Exodus House . . . from two fellows that had dropped out . . . and I started thinkin' about it, and they started splainin' this and that. Exodus House requires this of you, and perhaps might be some opportunities there for you. . . . They seem to help quite a few guys . . . if you are sincere. I . . . thought about it for a while. I got out of the hospital. . . . I never forgot the address they had given me, the directions . . . about four, five days after I got out of the hospital, I came over to Exodus House, and I knock on the door . . . and I ask for help . . . and I was received.

S.F. *Let me ask you, as you look back on it, do you have any theory to explain why you kept on using drugs?*

M. Uh way I look at it uh . . . insecurity might have something to do with it in a sense. . . . Once I got acquainted with uh . . . drug addiction, with the kick of . . . uh . . . heroin seems to kill your feelings, like deaden them. Like you take off umm . . . except uh it changes your whole mode of uh thinkin' and desires and . . . anxieties. . . . Seems to just calm you down altogether. Seems to stop you in your tracks, which is the reason why I figure that uh seems like the world . . . was goin' by. I was just . . . stagnant.

[The insecurities and anxieties to which Manny refers are those, I believe, generated by his feeling of failing to conform to his own aspiration level and frame of reference. He also experiences the chill of a frozen future.]

S.F.   *Let me ask you another question: When you think about your-self, and I'm sure you do, you're an intelligent person, what are your most prominent characteristics as a person?*

M.   As a person, respect is one—

S.F.   *You're thinking of yourself as a person, right? Now, how would you describe yourself? What's your most prominent characteristic, your actions, your way of thinking?*

M.   Being hooked or being in my state of mind now?

S.F.   *First normal, then hooked.*

M.   First normal, then hooked. My actions, my way of thinking?

S.F.   *The way you do things, the style you have, and so on.*

M.   Well, uh . . . I like to work is one thing. I like to get paid for workin' . . . my work. Uh . . . doesn't always happen that . . . one gets what one wants anyway, plus uh . . I have never been qualified in . . . having a trade that I could ask for a certain amount. . . . Therefore, I have come to the conclusion that uh . . . until I do learn a trade I won't be able to . . . get that amount, a certain amount, but uh. . . .

S.F.   *May I ask you this question: Have you ever been married?*

M.   No, I never have.

S.F.   *Why not?*

M.   Because of the drug addiction. I didn't want to make anybody more miserable, as miserable as I was in the sense that uh . . . mar-riage, to me, is . . . kind of sacred. Like uh . . . requires a certain amount of responsibilities, especially when you get married, you ex-pected to have kids, build a family. You expected to provide and I don't consider myself a provider. I never have uh . . . because I have been in and out . . . uh . . . on and off. In other words, I have not been . . . uh . . . a steady worker. Uh . . . I have never been doing somethin' outside of . . . uh . . . messin' around with my own life, playing with it like if it was a pogo stick.

[I do not know whether Manny's comparison of his conduct on drugs to playing with his life as though it were a pogo stick is his own idea, but it is a highly imaginative figure of speech. Not only does it give the image of the highs and lows of the drug addict's life, the moods, but also it shows that he is aware of the existential changes that take place within him on drugs, the feeling that fractions of his life can be thrown away as though in a game.]

M. And uh . . . I felt myself that I wasn't ready to get married . . . to meet up with any responsibility that they call for. And since I felt that way about it, the chances and the opportunities that I have had, which I have had, with quite a few girls . . . I have let them go by because of that. I realized that I couldn't meet up with the responsibilities that uh were required of me . . . and one thing that I would try to always avoid . . . would be . . . like uh beginning a home, a family uh and then abandoning them. That's one thing that uh being that it happened to me, it's always on my mind that I wouldn't like to act like the old man acts—acted. He did that uh and I find that it was a great error on his part. . . . Although I don't know the circumstances, maybe he and my mom didn't get along any longer . . . this I don't know. I have never been told this; uh mom never talks about it. I never bothered to ask because I figured if she wanted me to know she would tell me about it. . . . I will give her that respect . . . her personal life . . .
S.F. *Did you ever have any kind of ambition to be some kind of professional, do anything at all when you were younger?*
M. When I was younger . . . I wanted to be a policeman with a helmet. In my family in P.R., quite a few of them that . . . like uncles, and . . . grandfather, and they have all been cops, policemen. They have had that as a career. They retired from it. I have great admiration for my grandfather.

[Manny's professed adolescent desire to be a policeman sounds almost too pat, too characteristic, to be true. However, what gives it plausibility is his own statement of the number of people who have been policemen in his family.]

S.F. *This is on your father's side?*

M. No, my mother's side. My father's side, I have never met his family.

S.F. *No? Not even your uncles, his brothers?*

M. No, I never met them. . . . I don't know who's who on my father's side. Like he died in '56 and . . . I didn't even know he had died.

S.F. *Your father?*

M. My father. I was in jail at the time, I think, and my mother wasn't in contact with him, so—we didn't know. He died a natural death.

S.F. *How old was he when he died?*

M. Let's see, he was, he was in his seventies. He was old . . . oh . . . Yeah, I had those ambitions. I wanted to be a policeman, and like I said I had a great admiration for my grandfather, who has died, and I didn't get to see him because he died in P.R. He never came over here. That I had as a kid, of course, then as I grew up, like I said, a different environment, different actions, uh different happenings, uh changed my views in some ways and circumstances brought me to—or kept me from uh . . . thinkin' that way any longer. My thinking was changed. Maybe because of the circumstances that surround me, the environment which is just about the same thing . . . uh . . . lack of education because I dropped out of school, not had certain requirements, this certain such and such a thing. Then when I finally got in trouble, and that was the end of my plans.

S.F. *At this point, what are your plans?*

M. At this point my plans are trying to find a trade, of some type.

S.F. *Do you have any particular preference?*

M. Preference . . . I seem to have a preference for clerkin', a clerk job.

S.F. *Can you type?*

M. No, I can't type. I have to . . . learn typing.

S.F. *You're interested in that kind of thing?*

M. Yeah, I am interested.

S.F. *What kind of work did you do in jail?*

M. I uh . . . worked in just about anything . . . outside of uh, like I said, in offices. In the office I can't work, but if I have to work in the library, checkin' books and so forth, that I can do. Uh . . . switch . . . to be a porter, work on different type of jobs in prison uh . . . dishwasher, and uh . . . tailor shop, in the laundry, cabinet shop, which they teach you these things, uh like the cabinet shop.

S.F. *How did you adjust to prison?*

M. Uh . . . I believe I adjust, sensibly. . . . I usually follow rules and regulations, as close as I am able to . . . uh. . . . I always begin like that when I go to jail . . . rules and regulations, and then getting acquainted with—with my surroundings. . . . I mean beginning with the other persons around me, near me. People that I come in contact with day in and day out uh. . . . I would be studying them, and of course, they'd be studying my actions, and I studied theirs. They'd get—they'd pass some judgment on me, whether . . . I'm decent, that type of person, or easy to get along with or hard to get along with or cranky person, person of moods; different individuals come up with a different conclusion. This is the way I do it. My way is to watch everyone . . . not overstep myself, respect everyone because I expect to be respected also. By my actions, not because . . . I'm meaner than anybody else but because . . . by giving respect . . . that person would feel that I deserve . . .

S.F. *Were you ever in the "bing" in jail?*

M. No. Never got in trouble in all the time that I had . . . just didn't happen. I don't know—seems that I get along. Mind my business, be sociable.

S.F. *What's your reputation on the street among drug addicts? What do they think about you?*

M. I don't have a reputation.

S.F. *What do you mean by that?*

M. I'm just uh—just an average Joe uh. . . . Just uh "Manny." Uh that's it—Manny's just a name. Nickname, call it that. Some guys will call me blackball uh like that you know, different names . . . call me shmo, anything. But uh like I said, give me a certain respect, like I said. I carry myself like a man. They respect me as a man. Now, I am not—I have no fame.

S.F.   *You're not a fighting man?*

M.   I'm not a fighting man, I am not violent. Uh I don't abuse anyone, and I don't expect to be abused because . . . it's beyond me to permit someone to step on me if I treat that person decent . . . and . . . I don't ask from no one uh any more than I give them.

S.F.   *Were you ever taken by a take-off artist? Did a mugger ever steal your stuff?*

M.   I have . . . been taken, yes. Uh money has been taken.

S.F.   *By other addicts?*

M.   Yes, . . . and stuff has been taken. Guys that has my confidence. He tell me a lie, and I believe him . . . give me so much and I pay you a little later uh . . . he'll take it and . . . that's it . . . and maybe I see him in jail. But I have never done any harm to the guys that have done it. I have been mad, of course uh . . . for the moment. . . . Then it just . . . goes by, and I say it was just one of those things that's to be expected in this type of life that I'm leading.

S.F.   *Did it happen to you very often or just occasionally?*

M.   No . . . it has happened a couple of times uh not often. Just one time I think I could say; you could say I was mugged with four guys with knives . . . uh . . . guys—Spanish-speaking guys—but that's all. That's the only time that has happened that they have used . . . they have come to nearly . . . do some violence. They have come close to violence, and that's the only time, and no violence was used. They just . . . took what I had, that's all.

S.F.   *Okay. Now, we've had enough for the first hour and a half.*

[Second interview with Manny.]

S.F.   *O.K. I have listened to your tape very carefully and I have lots of questions. You mentioned your mother, and you said you were an only child at that time. Does that mean that she has had children since then?*

M.   She did uh. . . . I have another sister, stepsister . . . when I was . . . eleven. About a year after I was here at the United States. She uh . . .

S.F. *Had a child.*

M. Had a child, yes, uh which is my stepsister, which is the only sister which I do have.

S.F. *Did your stepsister's father adopt you?*

M. My stepfather, yes. I knew him for a few years. Anyways, he have . . . raised me.

S.F. *How do you feel about him as a father: Did you like him?*

M. Frankly speakin' uh . . .

S.F. *No?*

M. No.

S.F. *What was the matter?*

M. I was never satisfied with him . . . unfortunate to say now that I realize these things. Uh . . . he's a man that likes to drink a whole lot . . . uh. . . . He got his own set ways in life. Uh . . he was an elderly man at the time anyway. Uh he's still alive and he still has the same ways. . . . It's always been like uh . . . ever since we met him . . . my mother met him, a workin' man, but . . . a man that drinks . . . in excess . . . and . . . to me he was a letdown. Like I couldn't . . . I didn't have the type of home that I could . . . be so . . . uh feel happy and contented just goin' back up the house. A lot of times I used to just . . . go out with my friends in the streets, you know. School friends uh . . . anyway uh . . . I was never satisfied going home. Not on my mother's account. She has always been a person like I said, that doesn't have any . . . she didn't have no experience about the outside world, everything happening around her, and she didn't know any better . . . but . . . always been a person that would like uh . . . to respect, you know, I mentioned that before, elderly persons and . . .

S.F. *Your father was also rather elderly, wasn't he?*

M. My father was, my father was older than my mother. He was forty-nine when they got married, and uh my mother was . . . I recall her telling me . . .

S.F. *In her thirties?*

M. Uh . . . *no* . . . going on sixteen.

S.F. *Oh, very young.*

M. Very young, very young. She didn't have no . . . experience whatsoever outside of the home, cooking and the house. And she was brought up by uh my uh godmother, which happened to be her . . . aunt—my mother's aunt. She wasn't . . . brought up by her father and mother. My mother's mother—my grandmother—she came over here to this country. My mother was raised over there. She wasn't raised with my uh grandfather because he remarried. . . . They also separated. In other words, it's like a cycle [Laughs] the way I look at it, it is like this, what's this, everybody's doin' the same thing uh to me. . . . It leaves that type of impression like uh . . . it's the destiny or somethin' which is set. Now I don't—I hate to buy that, you know.

[The concept of destiny comes easily to Manny's lips; he's used it in discussions, public and private, outside of this interview. It serves as an ultimate frame of reference for his future, and therefore, also as a source of security for him.

At this point, Manny went on for some time examining his own introspective processes and preferences for and against older and younger women.]

S.F. *What about yourself? When you observe yourself, what do you see?*
M. I see a person who is looking for an answer when I observe myself. Looking for a certain perfection. Because . . . he doesn't want to make the same errors that his fathers have made in a sense . . . and other people, acquaintances that have made the same errors also, or similar ones. . . . But they have broken homes and so forth; in life they have, you say like make a comparison . . . the husband and wife, they get married.

[Manny's view of himself as someone looking for certain perfection shows how rigidly he looks at his own life, and he really means it when he says that he benefits by others' errors. He really sets up impossible standards for himself that are guaranteed to produce underlying frustration, depression at times, and the kick from heroin. His idealistic view of marriage also serves as a rationalization for his not getting married as well as a weapon to thrust at his own family and its "inadequacies."]

S.F. *Have you ever been very close to marrying anybody?*

M. I have. I have gone as far as pickin' the . . . veil and the wedding dress.

S.F. *When was this?*

M. Around . . . ten years ago.

S.F. *Was the girl somebody you had just met? Or did you know her from before?*

M. Uh, she came from P.R., and I met her—she was close to the family in a sense that uh . . . my sister's godmother was her aunt. This particular one. It happened . . . another time also. Uh . . . about two years before I met this other girl, it happened also. And uh . . . I just . . . Well, at that time I was, I was, like I said, I wasn't really uh ready to settle down. I didn't feel like it. Some young guys they get married and uh . . . the moment they get married and settle down they uh . . . jump into it, like I said. But uh . . . I . . . wasn't ready. I had another girl in the Bronx, and we used to go out. We used to look at the furniture in the store windows and . . . make plans. At that time, when I was sailing. I was sailing when this happen—this other incident.

S.F. *Were you using drugs?*

M. Uh . . . I wasn't hooked.

S.F. *You were using, but you weren't hooked.*

M. I wasn't. I had chippie, you know. But I wasn't, I really wasn't hooked.

S.F. *Why did you pick that particular girl? What did you find attractive?*

M. Well . . . this girl I met through uh . . . say uh . . . by chance, they say. New Year's Eve I went to a dance at the Diplomat, a dancing hall on Forty-third Street, between Sixth and Seventh Avenues—Hotel Diplomat. And . . . came close to twelve o'clock, I met this girl, and she was with three other girls, sitting on a table. They was four of them altogether. I uh there was another guy uh . . . merchant seaman. He from—he was from Nicaragua, see, and I met him also, and we got acquainted—uh started talkin'. He was by himself also. He hadn't brought a girl to the dance. And he was looking for friendship and was . . . socializin', trying to socialize. I was also, so came to there, and . . . we started talkin', and he said, "Well, what about those girls over there?" So we went and talked to them, and they were very nice and sociable. So we got acquainted. We got introduced. Came twelve o'clock, we had already danced one or two dances, and came twelve o'clock we hug each other uh everything respectfully and not . . . way out, like they say. You know, no disrespect. And we left together. That's how I got acquainted with her. I gave her my address, she gave me hers. We wrote a few letters, and then we went on dates. A very uh . . . nice person in a sense, you know, her character, her way of acting, and she was very nice. Not a girl to be disrespected. Uh I'd say uh . . . she would never have a uh lousy word. Uh educated girl. She was going to school. Had intentions of going to college, taking up nursing. She had intentions—in other words, she was looking forward to her future. She liked me, and I liked her. We understood our characters.

S.F. *How old was she?*

M. At that time she was eighteen, going on nineteen. I was a little older than her. I was twenty-two.

S.F. *That's more than ten years ago.*

M. More . . . fifteen. Well, you know, in that span if you make an error in the years. Couple of years difference. She uh was living with her mother at the Bronx and she had a kid brother which she used to bring out on dates with us. We used to take him, we go to the movies, you know, and everything. And like I said, we used to stop by, and—she was a serious girl. Very serious, you know? But she had a good sense of humor. I was—to me, she was kinda perfect, in the sense that I liked her enough to marry her. But not enough to settle down. [Laughs] You understand?

[Manny seems to see his dilemma this time as a conflict between two perfections. On the one hand, the perfect woman who would make the perfect wife attracts him, but he himself falls far short of being the perfect husband who could be responsible. Ergo, no marriage.]

S.F. *What happened that you backed away?*

M. We were getting so serious . . . so serious that she was . . . looking forward to a set date. I wasn't in that state of mind.

S.F.   *Were you working then?*

M.   I was sailing. I was sailing, yes. So what I did was, I shied away from her. 'Cause the day was like . . . so . . . so near. I could see it, and I really didn't feel like it was the proper time for me to settle down. I didn't have enough experience. In fact, . . . I couldn't see forward to married life and settling down and having family, and having a house, otherwise responsibilities. I was more or less happy-go-lucky, a happy-go-lucky guy. Uh . . . go out, and go dancin', this and that. I figured she might tie me down because I have seen other friends of mine which did get married during that time. Were happy-go-lucky; they settle down, and they are very unhappy.

[Manny characterizes himself as having been happy-go-lucky. We have to interpret this in the light of his rigid perspective as well as his tendency not to see or feel his rigidity. He has said on other occasions that he was a very flexible fellow, which is another illustration of the same tendency.]

S.F.   *Let me ask you, Manny, what are the most important differences in the way you are on drugs and the way you are off drugs? In the way you act, the way you feel?*

M.   Well, my feelings . . . all uh . . . it's the difference between night and day.

S.F.   *Tell me how.*

M.   When I'm on drugs uh my feelings, my views are changed to the extent that I can *feel* all this happening to me, and can—and can do nothing about it. I cannot stop myself like when I'm on drugs from . . . thinking of where my next fix is going to come from. . . . And doing things outside of the law . . . which, I can realize, the result will be . . . will be . . . lousy ones uh . . . like I will get punished for them, should I get caught. Uh if I am caught doing them, I'm going to go to jail. Uh . . . my family's going to suffer, people that care. Because there are people that care although I have been an addict and so forth. There are people that respect me, yet I have always . . . been able to maintain these two different lives. . . . See, I'm without prejudice to the other type of life that I was living when I wasn't hooked and the one that I live when I'm hooked. See, I change my friendships and everything. In other words, when I'm not hooked I'm with a different circle of people.

S.F. *Do you have an actual circle of people now?*

M. Yes, I do have it . . . with . . . I haven't knocked on the doors, but I do have it.

S.F. *Potentially?*

M. Potentially. I mean they are there. They *are* there, and when I do knock they open their doors and receive me with kisses. They embrace me.

S.F. *Who are these people? Your relatives?*

M. Some of them are, and others are just friends. And some relatives, and so forth. . . . It's quite a big circle. Uh . . . they admit me as one of them because I have proven myself to them when I am not hooked. When I am hooked I shy away from all the circle altogether. Outside my immediate . . . family, which I have to come in contact with every day, because my mother, like I said, she doesn't have any husband, and there's just my mother and my sister—two womans. Those two persons I have to constantly keep check on because of anything that could happen to them, because . . . being that I am a man I could always . . . perhaps do something for them.

[Manny continues the discussion of his sister and his "responsibilities" to her.]

S.F. *I'd like to ask you another question. You control your attitude towards sex, do you also control your temper? Are you a man who is easily made angry, or do you control it?*

M. It varies. Sometimes I am in a state of mind that uh . . . I could become emotionally involved at the spur of the moment but . . . I try always to be very aware of this and control it to the extent that it doesn't get out of hand. . . . Now, these later years, I have been able to do this. Years back uh it wasn't so.

S.F. *No?*

M. No. Years back uh I was very emotionally unstable and—

S.F. *This was before you were on drugs?*

M. Before, yes. Before I was on drugs, and after I got in drugs, and . . . this different type of life, altogether. Like I said, night and day uh my character changed when I am hooked . . . uh . . .

S.F. *When you were young, how did you show this emotional instability?*

M. . . . Far as I can go back I used to like . . . fight with other kids. Used to have a group . . . friends.

S.F. *This is in P.R.?*

M. P.R., yes. And we used to fight with other kids from *another* part of the neighborhood. Uh over there . . . you belong to one neighborhood, there is uh usually a group that is supposed to be rough in that part of the neighborhood. We, in turn, had our own group that is . . . also rough in this part of the neighborhood. Uh sometimes we used to get together and when we didn't see eye to eye, well, . . . let's talk about it, let's fight about it. And then we come up and say we friends after we fight. This was the way you was over there. . . . There it was like . . . I dare you to hit me. It was that way uh . . . and this is the way we were brought up. I was brought up that way anyway. That part of the neighborhood I was livin' in at the time a kid will spit and say, "I dare you to step on that spit." You step on it, and he will throw a punch at you. And that's it—you started rumbling, you started fighting. He put a little piece of wood on his shoulder and say, "I dare you to knock it off." You knock it off, and he'll hit you. It's like that. It's a dare. I dare you to do this. We dare each other.

[Notice that, although Manny is trying to make the point that he was emotionally unstable as a young man, his illustration is in the obsessional style. That is, he presents a frame of reference which is that of the "dare," a situation which is traditionalistic, even ritualistic, between children. It is a question whether the instability to which he refers is not due here to the rigid standards he placed upon himself and the frustrations resulting therefrom.]

S.F. *What town was this?*

M. Mayaguez.

S.F. *When you were young, was there any problem with drug addiction?*

M. No, sir, I didn't know anything about drug addiction till I uh started on this uh myself . . . actually. And then uh . . . I didn't, I didn't know anything about it, like I mentioned before, I didn't know the results of it. I was living in a Hundred Street, I still didn't know anything about it.

[At this point, Manny speaks about the strictness of schooling in Puerto Rico.]

S.F. *Did you play hooky from school?*
M. No . . . not much. I did once in a while but not much. Every time I did I paid for it. I got punished for it. Uh . . . first of all I couldn't go back to school. Once you miss a class you don't go back to school without your parents. . . . That is to say, your parents have to go with you. They have to say—give the reason why you was absent. Excuse me. . . . Oh, that's right, you don't smoke. And uh every time my parents have to go to school because I couldn't go by myself, they won't permit me to go in the classroom without my parents. And uh . . . then my parents would go over there the times that I did miss and . . . I would pay the consequences afterwards. See like uh my parents wouldn't hit me, to hurt me in the sense that they would damage me physically. I would get probably spanked a few times very hard with somethin' . . . like a belt, and then if I was going to the movies Saturday, and it is Friday, there wouldn't be any movies for me on Saturday. . . . No matter how I cry about it, there wouldn't be any movies for me. That's punishments like this uh . . . I wouldn't say they work with everyone. I wouldn't say they worked with me.
S.F. *In this kind of gang you had in Mayaguez, did you do any drinking or smoking?*
M. . . . One time of each. Only once of each.
S.F. *Not really a pattern. You were fighting. Did you also do any stealing when you were there?*
M. One time.
S.F. *Do you have any idea why your father married so late?*
M. I never got to know him that good, and my mother—I don't believe she got to know him that good. She didn't have no experience.

She couldn't go into detail with him; he would be probably the one to teach her. If anything. And he wouldn't stand for all that questions and answers and he had more experience, and therefore he was the one that would lead her, in a sense. Uh that might be the reason for it, uh . . .

S.F. *How old were you when you first had sex with a woman, with a girl?*

M. The first time uh that I had an idea what that was for . . . about seven, seven years old.

S.F. *What happened?*

M. First *idea.* Well uh we were playing bingo . . . underneath the house, two girls and I—neighbors. Just like kids playing Mom and Dad and . . . Spin the Bottle, and . . . we were playing bingo. I don't know exactly who came up with this idea. . . . I was—one of the girls was about my same age, nine, and the other one was about eight. About a year's younger difference. Uh we came up with the idea that uh . . . playing bingo, let's play bingo for somethin'. . . . Uh we came up to with the agreement that I would play her. If I won, she would lay down under me, underneath me, and if I lost, she would lay on top of me. I came up with the . . . although I was a kid I said I can't lose in this [Laughs]—either way. I didn't have much experience, but this I could realize—I don't know the reason for it. So anyway, I agreed, and the three of us agreed. Two girls and one boy. I can lose either way. Now, this is uh . . . kids anyway.

S.F. *What happened?*

M. We didn't have each other actually, in the sense that we had sex, outside of mentally perhaps. Uh I can't say—I'm not qualified to say this. But this is the first experience that I had.

[Manny then refers to his first sexual experience at the age of sixteen with an older woman, and his preference for older women.]

S.F. *Did you ever have any close tie to any of these women?*

M. Yes. . . . More than one.

S.F. *More than one. Did you have to pay for it?*

M. No, it seems like I had never to pay for it after that.

S.F. *Women who had their own apartments?*

M. Yes. They work. Younger man. Seems like I met quite a few like that. But I could never stay with them . . . steady.

S.F. *Why not?*

M. I could never do it. Uh I just wasn't, I didn't know what getting tied down was. And seems like I didn't like it. I didn't like for a woman to be telling me, do this, do that, and expect for me to be there every day when I was still a kid anyway, and uh to me uh I wasn't doin' like, always want to go into the parks—still like to go into the park and swimming with the other kids, and so forth and participating—as kid. Once in a while, have a day away, have a piece away, and this is what I wanted. But when I seen that they were trying to embrace me and say like uh . . . "Stay with me," and demanding of me, I resented that. I didn't want . . . I didn't want it to be that serious.

[Manny here reveals a characteristic conflict. On the one hand, he wants adult women. On the other hand, as a younger man, he prefers "to play the field." Two ideals are in conflict, and he therefore goes through a period of oscillation or cycles in which he is attracted to and then repelled by these women all the time.]

S.F. *What did your mother think about all this? Did she know about it?*

M. No, sir. No, uhhh, no uh . . . I wouldn't tell her about those things uh at that time. Later on in years uh whenever I do have uh a woman that we live together and try to understand each other, try to see if we can make it together, she has gotten to meet . . . a couple of them. Now . . . later in life, now, that I can vouch for myself in that sense.

S.F. *What have her reactions been to the older woman?*

M. Her reactions have been that uh we should get married. Uh the right way, the correct way. You shouldn't . . . be with a woman, like have kids like that, you know. I met a couple that have kids and . . . I tried it with them . . . and . . . when my mom got to hear, when she find out and . . .

S.F. *Let me ask you a question: Do you think there's any kind of pattern in your life that keeps on coming up over the years? Any pattern in common to your youth, your middle and later years? Any law of logic to your life?*

M. . . . Before?

S.F. *Things that keep repeating.*

M. The need to advance myself.

S.F. *That keeps repeating?*

M. That I can't make headways.

S.F. *That keeps repeating. Failures?*

M. Failures? That seems to keep repeating. And . . . it seems to be taking me quite a while to find a state in life.

S.F. *Let me ask you another question about drugs. Have you ever used pills?*

M. Goofballs? Uh . . . yes.

S.F. *Which ones?*

M. Tuinols.

S.F. *Tuinols? How many?*

M. Never too many. Not more than three. I have never been able to . . . use them too well.

S.F. *What were your reactions?*

M. My reactions? Let's see. I remember the last time that I took them, I took about three of them, and I even lost my uh balance. My sense of balance. In fact, I uh I got knocked out.

S.F. *Really? Just tuinols alone?*

M. Tuinols.

S.F. *Plus heroin?*

M. Plus heroin, yeah.

S.F. *Have an O.D.?*

M. It might—it was an O.D. because I lost my sense and uh I woke up, I woke up out of it but . . . on my own, but I did uh lose my sense of balance. I was walkin' before I remember, I got knocked out. I was walkin' back a ways. . . . The only thing I wasn't doin' was crawlin'. . . . I didn't like it at all. I have never been a pill user. I have had a little experience with it, but I have never liked the reactions.

S.F. *How about the bombitas?*

M. Bombitas, I have never liked the reaction. I have used them.

. . . I don't like it. There's no—I don't find anything with them.

S.F. *What happens?*

M. I tell you . . . nothing happens behind the bombitas to me outside of a little reaction that uh you get a little nervous. Find it hard to go to sleep. They pep me up a little bit, you know like . . . getting one and . . . instead of just getting the horse uh by itself and going on the nod all the time, it gives me a little energy a little bit, the reaction mentally. Uh . . . some guys may find it similar to cocaine. I don't—I don't find it anything at all like cocaine. I find it is like someplace you could do without. Something I have no use for. In other words, I'm lousy enough uh shooting heroin without usin' somethin' else which I don't think is any good for me. Uh which I'm not getting any benefit from it anyway. Uh if I want to get high, you know, in the sense . . . high sense . . . is no kicks to it.

S.F. *No?*

M. No. I don't find it so. This is my estimate of it. Other guys will shoot a bombita, and jump and climb the walls. Uh my reaction to it is just . . . I have no use for it. Never have.

S.F. *When you were on pills, you didn't associate much construc-tively with other pillheads. You were by yourself most of the time? Did you form any kind of deals or ventures with other guys using pills?*

M. I was with guys that were usin' part-time . . . usin' bombitas, . . . maybe taking one pill. Because they were doing this only be-cause uh . . . the heroin they had is very weak.

S.F. *Could you talk to someone else on pills? Rap with them like?*

M. Partly so, partly so, yes. The conversation is very limited. Pills tend to uh make a person lose the sense of balance, the sense of speaks. It seems to like muffle your speech. You be talkin' and uaugh —uaugh—uaugh, and so forth. Ever seen a drunk speak? They eat their words, and so forth. They come out with . . . part words and sometimes you don't realize what they're saying. To them, they just expressing themself accordingly, but they're not actually. They're just high. This happens with these persons. They go on a goof and they come up with anything they could come up with anything. It's like a dream uh. They talk about anything . . . they talking about . . .

S.F. *Do you have any fears when you're under these pills? Any dreads, any anxieties?*

M. Not that I can recall. I haven't been on them that often. I have never been on them steady like uh . . .

S.F. *You said also that you used to have a bit of a temper, but as the years went by it became less and less. Is this because of the heroin? Would you use heroin often when you got mad?*

M. . . . I wouldn't say uh that just because I got mad I used heroin, no. I have never been able to put that together. So far . . . perhaps as I don't know.

S.F. *When you were using drugs, going out in the street to get them, did you find any pleasure in the street scene?*

[Manny's relationship to the street involved more than just the getting of heroin. This is a whole way of life, one which contrasts markedly in its excitement and motility with the rigid frames of reference that he carries around with him. The street and the addict culture generally serve to release and relieve him from his inner bondage to the obsessional style.]

M. Yes. Very exciting. Very exciting in the sense that uh . . . here is somethin' new, uh like uh "Hi, Joe. Howya doin'? What's happenin'? Anything new? What's on the set? So-and-so is on the set. Uh somethin' good over there—something lousy here. Know what happen last night?" Come up with a story. Uh something's going on in that uh type of life constantly. With the other uh type of life, the everyday life, there's a lot of things goin' on, of course, . . . but the pattern is so different that it could become boring because the excitement is different. The excitement is something which is very real which—that also is very real. But this type of life is a pattern which is everyday. You have to meet up with this responsibility, and the other, the other—the responsibility that you have to have in that other type of life is very irresponsible. . . . It doesn't have a pattern that everyday life, I make uh comparison so it can become a little clearer. The way I have seen this . . . I work every day, I get up a certain time. I have to be at the job a certain time. Punch my card, I work. Coffee time—ten o'clock, go out for lunch uh . . . come back within the half hour or the hour, according to the type of rules and regulations they have at the factory or whatev—whichever type of place I'm workin' at. . . . This . . . four o'clock, five o'clock I'm out. Punch my clock out. The pattern that I'm living here, from the job, I go back to the house, let's say. Okay, let's say I want a little sandwich before I get to the house. I want to stop by the bar, maybe and have a drink with Tom, Dick and Harry, which are from the neighborhood. They are also working, see . . . but they have a beer or two and . . . rap a little bit uh change of scenery. Now, if I have a wife, say I go back—I go up the house. I report home. Right? This . . . this is the pattern. I go up the house. "Hi." O.K. They receive me kindly with a smile . . . uh perhaps she receives me with a face. I uh it changes I imagine [Laughs] uh . . . we had a spat last night or somethin'. Well, anyway, this is the pattern that I'm living. I go up to the house. I stay home. I take a show, I eat, I relax, stay with the wife. Whether we happy or unhappy together doesn't matter. Say I decide to . . . see something that I'm doing every day now. The responsibilities that cover this. I can take care by just going to work every day . . . coming back and maybe stoppin' at the bar and have a beer, and maybe say, "Hello there, Joe. How are you, Pete? See you later, probably on the weekend." My day off, I come down, watch the game in the summertime, have a few beers. My wife knows I am over there in the corner bar. This is—this is a pattern which is a tight pattern—an everyday deal. Now my responsibilities could be the life insurance of the kids, which is one, got to eat every day. Well-balanced diet for the kids and myself and the wife, of course. The doctor bills, if any, uh health program. The rent has to be paid. Telephone has to be paid. But I'm workin' and staying in good health, and praying that I remain in good health . . . to accomplish all my responsibilities and keep up with this and give my kids an education, and so forth . . . whatever I can afford, of course. And with—there's a lot of help I could probably receive from the city in my kids' education. City College is opened up for them in the later years. Perhaps they go into the service or somethin'. This is somethin' to look forward to, this is for the future. Right? So, in the event that I am looking for this future for them I have to cope with the present, present-day life. This responsibility requires a certain amount of energy on my part, and thinkin' . . . the sacrifices that it requires of me, I have to look at it intelligently. Everybody doesn't or, to their own estimate, perhaps they do. Some fail, some manage to make it. Some persons manage to give their kids an education. A wife and a man may live twenty years together, fifty, a hundred perhaps. Some of them don't manage to live six months after they get married. This is a different pattern than the other one.

S.F. *How does the drug addict pattern go?*

M. Drug addict is, like I said, "Hi, Joe. Howya doin'?" This is the guy on the corner. This is not the guy any longer that's . . . in the bar. . . . Guy in the bar is always there unless he get sick. He's following that responsibility that he's the bartender. The guy on the corner, he might get picked up ten minutes after you speak to him . . . uh you won't see him for six months. Maybe ten years. And he knows whatever is happening around the neighborhood . . . and here I am stepping from one circle into the other. From night—I mean, from day to night, from light to darkness. I'm getting acquainted with the night like they call . . . two, three, four o'clock in the morning—there's no hours set there. It's not set there. I'm being introduced into an irresponsible life . . . which is the irresponsible life of no hours. No steady pattern in the sense that it variates so much from one corner to the other. Let's see who's got somethin', let's buy somethin', let's get together and get high. After we get high, let's just walk around and . . . I'll pass my kicks according to the way I feel I should. If I want to stand and look at the sea, I look at the sea, I look at the East River. If I feel like taking some air . . . if I feel like going into the park, I go into the park and enjoy my high. . . . It varies with different guys. Some guys feel like they want to drink coffee. Some guys feel like they want to eat candy, some guys feel like they wanta go to the movies. It variates so much in the individual. Some guys want to share their moment with each other, and they just go into a pair and just goof. Some guys want to listen to music . . . even though they might fall asleep in the middle of the record, at the beginning. Like guys go to the movies; they goof. They go to sleep. When they wake up, the movie's over. All right, so that's their kicks. It variates in uh myself also. . . . I uh feel very irresponsible when I'm hooked. I feel—I have noticed this—I have looked at it. The way I am explaining it to you is the way I see it. This is my experience. I evaluate one life and I evaluate the other. I put myself in the middle and I put myself on both sides because I have been there. . . . So the evaluation I get from the night life, meaning drug addiction and pot smokin' and throwin' bricks, and doing things against the law, is very exciting. In the sense that you are doin' something which is out of the . . . regular rules and regulations which are set . . . by society . . . and which have set through trial and errors in the past, past generations, and . . . get set with the aim that individual himself, law-abiding citizen should abide by the law according to the rules and regulations. Even if he is dissatisfied. There are some other channels that he could go and take his . . . complaints to a representative of the law or whatever. Go into politics.

S.F. *Let me ask you a question. Why do you suppose you found it necessary to go into a life that was exciting? Wasn't your life exciting to you?*

M. Not really. Not really because I couldn't see it. I couldn't see it. It was monotonous. I found it so. It was boring. I couldn't settle down. I was full of energy, ready to spend it. I didn't know how to spend it. Instead of doing the wrong things, I could have been using that energy for the right things; I would have perhaps accomplished something. In fact, there is no doubt in my mind that I would have accomplished something which . . . nowdays I could look back and say . . .

S.F. *Do you ever feel like Jekyll and Hyde?*

M. Yes, uh . . . Jekyll and Hyde is more than two, more than two personalities involved. Uh different makeup every so often. Like I've come to the conclusion that within, say within myself at least, there has been quite a number of personalities involved. More than two. I couldn't, I couldn't say yes like there has been—there only has been two personalities in me. A yes and a no. It hasn't been that simple. I find a numerous amount of personalities at different times. My makeup has changed . . . so often, and one personality, like I say . . . speaking to the other one, and conflict between personalities, and . . . it's been like in a . . . a meeting with a numerous amount of people, all individuals, each has a different view . . . and yet there's one that stands out—that's supposed to be in the middle. He's directing. This is the way I have felt. That I have one . . . special personality which is trying to overcome all these other ones. . . . And I've felt that if that particular personality accomplishes to become the leader—in other words, to conquer this conflict, the group. In other words, to come to an understanding with the whole group. I come to the conclusion that I'm going to be the leader. Until then I haven't work out my problem. In other words, I just . . . fortitude that I am looking for. This personality in particular which I think is very good in my makeup uh . . . is always there . . . and is the strongest that I do have. Because I have been in quite a few deals that if that personality wasn't present, anything could happen to me. Things that uh I couldn't even see uh that all I could do is think perhaps it's going to happen to me.

S.F. *For example.*

M. For example uh times that I have been uh in a position that I could do . . . a lot of harm.

[Manny has observed and intuited that the central personality, as he calls it, the directing personality is a highly moral, even rigid life form. He senses that the multiple personalities that have operated in his life in response to drugs are given a frame of reference by his own ingrained morality. It is the same reference which he is saying has led him at times even against the will of his peer group. There is a certain strength in this rigid frame of reference that only diminishes when, as happened to Manny at times through drug dependency, he experiences a conflict between the conventionalized and criminal frames in which the former is weakened.]

M. Harm, like uh the use of a gun. Different uses, position to harm another individual that I have been in a crowd with and want to do harm. Before that crowd becomes a wolf I come to the conclusion that this shouldn't be done. Somethin' within me. I been with the pack and I have almost went along with the pack, but I have been able to step out . . . and see why it shouldn't be done. It wouldn't be humane; it wouldn't be correct. Everything is against the doers. It shouldn't be done. And I have said it. There have been times that they have gone ahead and done it. I have stepped out. I have uh no use for that. This is the way I have felt, see, like you guys go ahead and do whatever you wish, but I tell you this is this, and this is that, and this is the way I see it. . . . If you care to go ahead, and you can't reason now, at this moment, well, . . . can't take time out to reason is . . . you gonna pay for it one way or the other. I'm not gonna go with it. And I've done this. I've stopped them. Sometimes I have been able to pull one or two guys from doin' . . . such . . . and I don't pinpoint anything because the variation is so large, and that night life, like I said, from one block to the other, the scene changes so much. Incidents. Like I explained before, comin' out of the house down there on the stoop, so, see, things just happen this way. There's always somethin' goin' on . . . keeps on goin', and it seems to make it interesting which . . . yes, but . . . is no good. Uh seems like since I was a kid uh perhaps it was the way I was brought up . . . uh my family, they—the ones that I came in contact with when I was younger—my mother included—they have a high sense of . . . morality, although it may not seem so in certain incidents, . . . and . . . they uh have always been very strict in that all of my family, which is very large, there has never been . . . anybody that has gone to jail, that has been a crook or . . . They have all been working people, responsible persons; they have had their ups and downs, of course, uh. Personally, like misunderstandings between each other and so forth, but uh outside of that there has never been anyone that has started before goin'—like becoming a crook or so forth. Now, this is something that I have, that I am carrying with me like the black sheep of the family, they say. But . . . since I was brought up, I always been brought up with that sense that I should earn . . . what I make . . . all my needs. When I was a kid, they used to, like I say, "I want to go to movies." "Well, you go to movies, you earn the price of the movie." My godmother she used to tell me, "Will you bring me some buttons—shirt buttons, and I'll buy them from you." She used to sew with them. Now, where am I goin' to get buttons? I'm a kid. Now, my intelligence—a kid's intelligence, mine worked this way. I'll go around the neighborhood, and I couldn't find any buttons. . . . I wind up taking the buttons from my shirts, my clothes, and selling them to her. Now, she will have to put them back on when she find out, of course. And she reprimand me, but uh . . . she get very mad. Because what I did right there was like lying, you know. But then to me it was, you know, I want to go to movies anyway, regardless. You know, I was a kid. That's all I had in mind; the movies, the chapters. I didn't want to miss one chapter. It was very important. So I did that with the buttons. But I kept that in mind that they were trying to direct me correctly. Later on in years I realize that. And until the time that I started using drugs. I had always been a person that . . . you could leave a million dollars anywhere. . . . Say I'm in your house visiting, and so forth. Well, from the moment I am in your house, I have high respect for you . . . for the whole family, anybody that is present. And your home I respect very much. Uh I would never take gran—for granted the friendship that I may have with another person. See uh, in other words, I wouldn't abuse, see, I wouldn't abuse the . . . the doors that are open to me, and uh . . . you have open arms, and you offer me the hospitality of your home. It could be very friendly, it could be uh . . . just another of the guys, in fact. Uh and I go over to his room or something, but I have a respect. To me that's sacred. A home is sacred. That's part of my makeup that I have been brought up that I always have this in mind. I'm very self-conscious of this uh ways of acting in life uh which are supposed to be very important, and I find that they are. I came to the conclusion that they are good. That there is nothing wrong with them, to respect not just the person but whatever belongs to the person also. Now, when I got into the drugs deal . . . my life had started changing and I found myself thinking very wrong . . . all the opposite of the way that it uh I was used to acting, and the way that I was brought up, and respect the things of others, and so forth. And I came in contact with so many different type of characters that were involved with this . . . drug deal, conniving and thinking about this . . . stealing. Guys that would just steal, every day, just for the heck of it, like there's . . . nothing else to do. They can't do for a dollar any other way. And to me that was very wrong, and I was very self-conscious of it. I just wouldn't go for it. I couldn't make myself do it. I always used to look for other outs like borrowing, and—I told you that before—borrowing and paying my debts.

And . . . sometimes when you're in the drug deal you spend a tremendous amount of money. See . . . for a person that never been in it it's very hard to even realize the tremendous amount of money that a drug addict spends . . . at times . . .

[Manny then devoted a considerable amount of time in tracing out his life history, again this time in the form of stages from the time when he was fighting the drug to the time in which he was becoming progressively more involved to the point that he couldn't work, to the stage then where he accepted his situation as a drug addict and sought to make it easy on himself by becoming a pusher.]

S.F. *Was it—that is, pushing—secure?*
M. There was a security in it, according to the life that I was leading. . . . That's what I can say was pleasant, you see, because I was at a stage where I wasn't completely successful . . . but I was very far from failure . . . which . . . had always been constantly on my mind. Failure, failure. I have always wanted somethin' out of life. I have had that desire since I was a kid, to accomplish somethin'. There were people that I admire in my own family. I believe that I mentioned that to you in the . . . session that we had a couple of policemans in the family that are detectives in P.R. Career men. And . . . there was the first people that I came in contact with when I came into this world. Now this is where my constant . . . constant . . . images that I remember since I was growing up. Outside of my old man . . . my old man. But these other ones were . . . I made them my ideals. I used to have great admiration when I used to see my uncle come home in Mayaguez and visit us from his home town. He used to get out of his car with his wife in a white uniform. He was an official . . . of the police department, see. Everybody used to look at him. Umm, the kids that I was playing with would look and say, "Oh, who is he? Who is he? Who is he?" And I used to get a kick out of saying, "He's my uncle—he's my uncle." [Laughs] I used to run up to him and hug him. He was very affectionate. A very serious person, but very affectionate. And he always used to give me a quarter. I remember, every time he used to come to visit he used to give me a quarter. And his wife was a very beautiful woman. Blanca

. . . blanca is white, you know? . . . And uh these remembrances that I have like and then later on in years, I seen myself like I wasn't accomplishin' anything worthwhile. My life was just like a . . . gyp. It wasn't leading to anything . . . uh was all mixed up. And by . . . goin' into this business of the drug dealings and . . . identifying myself, by acquiring another personality . . . and . . . building that personality to—to the extent that I felt at ease with it, that I belonged . . . that this was a world that was there. It was another way of life. Realizing that it was still against the law, and that it was not correct, according to society, but according to the . . . morals of the under . . . world, I say that it was correct. . . . This other personality accepted that, went along with it. I just took it, like I said, one half of me, and went into it. . . . I built up this personality where I was just a wrongdoer. But to me I wasn't doin' wrong, really. Uh . . . society just doesn't see it my way. That time, this is the way I felt. And the guys that I used to talk to about it were guys that were in the same deal and they also . . . were dissatisfied with society. They probably had the same ups and downs that I had, similar attitudes that they were forced to—they came from poor families. Some of them from working family also. That's why the variation is so uh extensive. That uh is hard to pinpoint the reason from one guy to the other. But yet they don't seem to identify—used to identify each other with that type of life and uh . . . seems like we live from one day to the other, twenty-four hours a day. Seems like every hour meant somethin' to us, every moment we were thinkin' about somethin'—we could bring us a dollar. Seems like the dollar sign meant a whole lot there. And then the result, what you get with the dollar sign, once you acquire that sign, seems like you could go anywhere and be accepted. It was an acceptance deal there, where if I didn't have enough money I couldn't go, but if I'm . . . didn't know how to carry myself, I couldn't go. Uh if I didn't know the right people I couldn't go. In this life I kept meeting . . . all types of people, people outside of the circle, and invitations were made and . . . educated people were on the scene, so we used to have little sessions. Little things that I would pick up here and there. And I would compare them and say uh this guy is . . . so high, an educated man, and he is dependent on me. He gotta come down to my way of life.

[We might call Manny's emotional gratification a result of a fortunate juxtaposition of two frames of reference. Experiencing himself as a pusher coming from humble origins, he notices that because of his market role he is kowtowed to by someone, who in the legitimate society has a much higher position. This meeting of two hierarchies with one yielding to the other, if only temporarily, gives him a definite mixed pleasure. Here there are elements, I would imagine, of vicarious enjoyment of the other's anguish. The dependency of the professional man, the model, the actor, the interior decorator, or whatever customers who are compelled to make use of Manny's services under the stress and pressure of drug addiction may well fit into some well-concealed aggressive urges that are not inconsistent with the obsessional style of life.]

M. He gotta give me that importance because he needs somethin' from me. . . . He's forced to do this and he, in turn, has a choice, that he can come to me, and I won't pull the covers off on him. In other words, nobody on his other side would know about it. . . . So he feels that he can trust me, so he's coming down from that pl—from that pedestal that he is on, the highest degree, and, like they say, category. He was from, they say, the upper brackets, and he comes to a legitimate living. He is within the law, doing everything within the law, but . . . he also is handicapped in the sense that he is using drugs. And he is an intelligent man, and I came in contact with quite a few of them . . . personalities . . . which I say that I have learned a few things from them, and they have made me aware that other categories in life exist . . . that a person could better himself by studying, by going to school. And the amount of sacrifice that they have put in it, to what it appears I used to just look at it, like an outsider does. . . . 'Cause then, when we used to share with each other, came in contact with each other, it was a different thing 'cause we'd be taking off together. We'd be dealing together like . . . you need this, I have this, blah, blah, blah, like let's share a few moments together. Making plans for the next time. All this left an impression on me, but I was . . . like they need me, and I need the business. . . . That happen for a while; that was when I lost that uh . . . reasoning that I had, that I could look back. I believe there's very few drug addicts that don't think about the other way of life, the one that they had a chance to . . . to act upon, and instead they chose this one which became a habit. Habit forming, detrimental to his health, and somethin' that he couldn't do without, that he couldn't function rightly, correctly without . . . dependin' upon the drugs. And . . . by him having chosen the wrong one . . . he feels guilty. I know I have felt guilty, and I'm talking about myself. . . . This is . . . I . . . of course, cannot say what another person will be thinkin', but I have heard these complaints, different times. We have gotten high; we have talked about it, and I have found that they're very dissatisfied with the type of life they're leading. But yet they can't get out of it because there's something that keeps them there . . . somethin' that they can't find out themselves. Some do, like I am trying now. . . . I am trying very hard. I am sincere about it, and I do want to get out of that type of life because . . . there's actually nothing there that I can see that's worthwhile. This is a picture in the world for me. This I can see that uh . . . ruined many chances, good chances that I have had, finishin' my education for one. Even my family life, my immediate family life uh they are not satisfied with the years that I have wasted . . . wasted in the sense that I could have accomplished something during those years, which I haven't. I have nothing to show for them, but an experience, which is very important, of course, . . . that's all I have. But being that I have that, at least, I am trying to do something worthwhile with that experience. I can accomplish this. I can use that experience to better myself, and help others, see. . . . Then I believe that I could feel satisfied that I have accomplished something, that my life has . . .

S.F. *Let me go back to that topic that we were talking about, pressure. Were there times you found the pressure too much to take?*

M. Surely. There are times when uh . . . you just don't uh . . . you tire. You tire of staying up twenty-four hours a day, perhaps even staying away from home if you have a home . . . and even staying in different guys' rooms. Uh . . . just not sleeping, staying in cafeterias and bars till they close the bars, just tryin' to make a dollar. Not necessarily so, you don't have to do this but . . . it's a must because you're dependent on the drug. You can't get it. The only way you can get it is by conniving, and like they call a hustler, you have to hustle. Now, to hustle you have to go out there and try and be smarter than the other hustler—a step ahead—beat him to the . . . to the opportunity. Whatever that may be. . . . Some guys go for stealing, and some guys go for other things; some guys put their minds together. They don't have to steal, they don't have to mug nobody. They do it . . . even from the other drug addict, from the one that steals, from the one that connives to do harm, even if they have to get a dollar which it variates. All drug addicts are not killers. All drug addicts are not lousy. . . . All drug addicts don't like to harm anyone, but there are exceptions. just like there are exceptions in the other way of life.

S.F.   *But you were known by all these different groups.*

M.   Yes. I have gotten acquainted with them.

S.F.   *So you knew boosters from Queens.*

M.   Yes. We have been in jail together, and uh when you go to jail, you met a whole lot of guys from different boroughs, become acquainted with them. All right. So in jail you're all right. Guys in jail thinking, guys are talkin' about, "I'm going to stay away from this," and give a lot of advice to each other. I, for one, gave a lot of advice. Although I have been unable to take it in the past, I have always been a very good adviser. The guys who have seen me hooked afterwards would say, "I thought if there was one guy was gonna make it, was *you,* and here we are, taking off together." I tell them, "Well, I tried. . . . I am very good at giving advices, but seems like I can't take them." It's that simple. Some setup. I have really been unable to take my own advice. I have seen . . . and I have given advice on this and that. Things that are reasonable but yet I have not taken them. That's where the problem is. . . .

S.F.   *You know, I have the impression that for drug addicts every day is a brand-new world. Right? Brand-new life. Like in a sense that every day has its own characteristic mood, its own characteristic problem. And you have to worry about that particular mood and that particular problem that day. Tomorrow is another mood and another problem. Yesterday was bad, but today is good. But tomorrow is worse or whatever it is.*

M.   Yes, there's more than one daily though. Like I say, it changes from block to block. You meet up with one problem here before you solve that one. No sooner you solve that one, there's another one there.

S.F. *Can you give me a typical, I mean a more concrete example of what you mean by that—taken from your own life?*

M. I go outta my house. I leave my house. I stand on the stoop, and I look around.

S.F. *O.K. Go ahead.*

M. I stand on the stoop and I look aroun'. I don't have a penny in my pocket, and I have need of getting a fix.

S.F. *Right.*

M. Or I'm fixed, and I'm lookin' forward to the next fix which I must have.

S.F. *Right. Go ahead.*

M. Now this, I'm calculating through experiences I'm goin' through the process of elimination in my mind what I have to do and what I must do. What I should do, the chances of doing this, and doing that other thing. Standing on the stoop I will see the sun glaring in my eyes, if it's early enough and the day looks very clear. Like I was in a cave, and I just came outa the cave. It's very clear. It might be a summer day; there are people going back and forth. My problem now is I'm watchin' all the scene—people goin' back and forth. They all seem to be going some particular place, and I'm seeing this, and it's very strange, but the most important thing on my mind is what am I gonna do, which way am I gonna go? Shall I go over to a Hundred Street and somethin' or shall I go over to Ninetieth and somethin'? Should I go downtown or should I go uptown or crosstown? Now, I weighing my chances what my next move is gonna be. So I decide to go to 96th Street and take the bus over to the West Side. I'm on the East Side. This is where I live, you might say. I start walkin' towards 96th Street; I made a decision. Right? I'm goin' to 96th Street, and I walk maybe a half a block. "Manny! I got fifty dollars."

S.F. *This is a friend of yours?*

M. This is somebody—an acquaintance. An acquaintance. I wouldn't say friend I say an acquaintance. And he knows that I know about the neighborhood more than he does. Therefore, I have a better chance of connecting something better than he can, plus he believes that I'm not gonna beat him for his money because he has had this experience with me before. Because I have perhaps shared with the guy. Maybe he's been sick and I have given him a fix. He's been up tight. Maybe he had two dollars, and I say, "Don't worry about it. Let me have the two dollars," and I put maybe ten or fifteen dollars, and I buy enough stuff, and then I say, "Look, c'mon," and I give him way more than his two dollars are worth. Or I give him his two dollars' worth, three or four dollars' worth, *plus* I fix him. Now this guy comes with fifty dollars. I made a decision to go across town already. He stop me a half block now. I didn't even go a whole block. "Fifty dollars I have— What do you want?" I don't got anything good— what do you think? Now I start thinking; I stop in my tracks, right? I'm thinkin', well, let me see—geez, so and such, there may be something up there, uptown. There may be somethin' a little further downtown. There may be somethin' around the corner. Now, there's money now. There's fifty dollars. Now I'm thinkin' about who's got the stuff. I probably know less than the guy too, who's got it [the money] now. Apparently he thinks that just because I happen to be around the neighborhood, and by chance another time I been able to connect, he's—he believes that I can do it again. I'm gonna do it again, of course. If we have to walk fifty blocks, I'm gonna do it again; I'm not gonna try and let him go with fifty dollars. Because this is the man I need now; I'm gonna get something here, see? There goes 96th Street. I changed my mind there. That's one incident. That already happened this day, this particular day.

S.F. *How do you protect yourself from being accused of selling? Because if you get the stuff and give it to him, that's a sale. So how do you protect yourself?*

M. You just . . . uh take your chances. Different guys act differently, of course. When you going to connect, some guys act nervous, some guys act natural, some guys walk fifty blocks in order to connect, and they go past the block they gonna connect. They got different ways of doing things. It's like I say—hide and seek—you're always aware of the bulls.

[Manny has just illustrated one of the numerous interstitial roles generated by the market economy. A man does not have to steal. If he does have the kind of concern and life style that Manny exhibits, then it is likely that he will feel more comfortable in doing the sort of services he has just described. Some estimates of the amount of larceny committed by addicts are inflated because these roles are not taken into account.]

S.F.   *I wondered whether you thought that drug addicts are under more pressure than people who are not drug addicts.*
M.   Yes. Sure! There's more pressure, but there's a compen—there's a compensation here that . . . that's when you take off. This is the —that's the clitch—this is what keeps you in this.
S.F.   *The fact that you can always get the pressure off you? Temporarily?*
M.   Temporarily. When you take off. That's why most drug addicts, if they have enough stuff, they won't go out. You won't see them on the avenue. If you see them on the avenue, it's just like uh "Hi. How are you? What's happening? I'm—I—you got some money? Here, how about a—you don't got anything good?" This guy got somethin' for himself. He's got enough—for himself. You know what he says to the other guy? "Gee, man, I don't know who got anything." Now, if it was the other way around, like that incident that I said the guy is sick, he doesn't have enough stuff there for his fix. And he's thinkin' to the next fix, and this guy comes over and says here I got a certain amount of money, and you know who got anything good? "Yeah, Jim; I know who's got the best thing around here." See the difference between having and not having? A guy has, and he stays home, and he comes around the neighborhood and he don't wanna do nothin'. He don't wanna take a chance on buying a bag from anyone—jus' because he has his fix. He has enough to keep him maybe two days. Them two days he's gonna relax in the sense that he doesn't want any part of the deal altogether. All he want to do is take off and take it easy and to walk around the block and—"Hi, there—hi!" Probably clean that day. If he's a guy that just clean once in a while he's probably went to the dry cleaner, took out his clothes, you know, and when he changes, he comes around the neighborhood clean and fixed and like uh he's playin' another part now. He's playin' another part. Another mask, and the same deal though, but it's another mask anyway, and that way he's lyin' to himself again. [Laughs] He's still lyin'

to himself. He's playin' a part that makes him feel good. He can't go anywhere 'cause he's hooked anyway, so he's playing a part around that neighborhood anyway, the same neighborhood.

S.F. *How would you call that part?*

M. Say, he's doin' it for his ego.

[Manny has indicated previously, and now reiterates in another way, his feeling that when he is on drugs his life style runs into conflict with the familiar addict pattern of playing roles, of conning, of deceiving, of lying, of acting like somebody else. For a man so rigid as he, the experience of addiction highlights his own negative perception of a life style that is characteristic of addict society. Since he tends to think and act in terms of rigid frames of reference, at certain phases of his existence as an addict he borrows the framework of the artificial synthetic life. In other words, he accepts, as temporarily real, the necessity to engage in make-believe. However, after a man stays on drugs for fifteen to twenty years, role-playing threatens to become a kind of second nature, challenging his fundamental nature. Two life styles as radically different as these produce conflict whose outcome may not be easily predicted.]

M. He gets a kick out of it because there's no other way of doin' it. So he can't do anything like going out of the circle and come into that other circle up there for one or two days 'cause he's been away from the circle altogether. Probably his own family circle—his immediate family. He's become a stranger to his immediate family by his actions. He's a stranger actually in his home. I have felt this way in my home.

S.F. *Really?*

M. I have felt like a stranger with my own mother. My sister. Because I'm doing things—I'm doing things which they don't know anything about. They are not acquainted with. I'm comin' in the house, and maybe I take a shower, somethin', and I change clothes and I don't even eat. Now, mom realized that I'm hooked already because she knows that when I go up the house—when I'm not fooling around —I'm very affectionate with her. I'm very affectionate. When I'm hooked, there's no affections—I lose all that because I'm displeased with myself. Actually I'm so displeased with myself that I just don't —I lose all those affections that I could give somebody else because I'm—I feel rotten—to the core. But I'm hooked nevertheless, and I have to keep going forward, and I'm gonna get that next fix and I go on the avenue. That's where I can get it. And this is what I do, and where I felt like an outsider in my own home. And my mother, which I know since I was—since I came to this world—if I can feel that way towards her, it's quite a change has been made on myself. Some change—some process that uh . . . is very detrimental to me.

S.F. *You mean you are unable to talk about these things to your mother at all? About what you do?*

M. Some . . . some, but she's very hard in understanding. She doesn't realize a lotta things that . . . Now she understands more than before, but it always hasn't been this way. I have spoken to her, I have explained to her, I've explained to her what to expect of me when I'm hooked, see? I've told my experiences to my sister, so they know, they realize just what I'm going through. Now, this has been going on for years, and uh it has been a slow process, and finally they're more understandable nowadays than years back, see?

S.F. *You feel more at home now than you used to.*

M. More at home. Yes, of course. More at ease. I can talk problems with them nowadays that I couldn't before.

S.F. *Just what do you feel, what ideas do you have about religion? How do you think they affected you in the past? Off and on drugs?*

M. I don't know much about religion actually . . . not enough to . . . talk about it or how much it affected me. My family have always been . . . churchgoers and every Sunday, and so forth. We had one particular . . . my grandfather's sister which was—she never got married, and she was a very dedicated uh . . . to praying and going to church at some convents and asylums and . . . doing work for them, you know. Uh . . . in her particular . . . I grew up with a sense of, a sense of Christianity, let's say . . . and very conscious of not going to church. When I didn't go to church it bothered me. So, as far as having anything . . . had any uh . . . how should I say it . . . impression . . .

S.F. *What about specific types of people? Were there any priests or other spiritual leaders affecting you?*

M. Not really. No. Not outside of having a very high respect for—

not just Catholic religion but all religions. In other words, I don't have much to say one way or the other.

S.F. *Many Puerto Ricans have told me that they've been affected by spiritualists, mediums, and such. Have you had any—*

M. I've been to a spiritualist a few times. And uh . . . they have gone through the rituals that they do . . . according to what *I* have been to them for—whatever cause I have been to them.

S.F. *You have been there several times?*

M. Yes, I have been about three or four times.

S.F. *When was this?*

M. Last year I went to one which is the last one that I went to.

S.F. *What reason did you have to go there?*

M. Uh . . . my reason was to see whether . . . she could find a cause for me—something wrong with me. In other words, I wouldn't tell her my problems. I'm not supposed to. If she's a good spiritualist, I don't have to. 'Cause if I go and tell her my problems, I'm . . . I'm telling her what's wrong. In this way, she can talk to me, and without me saying anything she's supposed to come up with something. If it make sense to me . . . I'll give her the benefit of the doubt. Because what she is going to do is help me . . . in the sense that, if I have, like they say, a bad spirit on me . . . it could be possible. I can't say—I can't just say, it *is* so because I haven't had that experience yet. But nevertheless, being that I respect that type of religion also . . . whatever you want to call it. It's a belief anyway. I went to one, and I've been to a couple other ones, and this one in particular, she went through some ritual like taking the spirit out of myself—a bad spirit—a woman spirit. A woman that wouldn't . . . let me get married, that she was very jealous of me, and that uh . . . every time that I had some dealings with a woman she would intervene. In other words, she wouldn't let me get ahead—be at ease with this woman. She would always come in between. Now, this is what this woman said. Now, I can't swear to it because I don't know that much about it. See, but anyway I went to it, but uh outside of that, that's where I left it. I left the house.

[It is peculiarly symbolical that Manny goes to the spiritualist to wrestle with the problem of an obtrusive and persistent internalized authority in the form of a woman whom he blames for his inability to get married, and so on. It is as though he were trying to pull out from the roots some obsessive and inhibiting frame of reference. It is as though he were seeking help in exorcising an excessive moralism.]

M. My reactions were that if it was so . . . if it was so like she said, well, then I appreciated what she did for me. In other words, certain trust in the woman were a trust that uh . . . is not based on that I know anything about this . . . but a trust that I believe she knows. *I* don't know—*she* knows. In other words, if it is like she said, then I'm just going through the right thing. I'm doing the right thing by . . . coming to the woman. If it isn't so, I don't lose anything by it.

S.F. *How did you feel after it was over?*

M. Well, in a sense I feel relieved. I mean, it did alleviate me in a sense that I did something for it . . . and I no longer have that feeling that . . . like there was something that went away. But it's not something that I'm sure of, see, but nevertheless I put a certain amount of belief on the woman. We have to believe in something, I believe, and . . . I repeat myself I believe because . . .

S.F. *Now let me ask another question, not about religion, but another structure. You weren't too involved in religion as such, but you were involved in drugs, and I was wondering just what feelings you had when you were on "stuff" about the fact that there was a giant structure over you. You know, people were investing money—large amounts of money—in heroin. They had a vast traffic. Just what feelings did you have about the people on top whom you never saw?*

M. The people on top that I never saw? Uh . . . well, actually, I never gave that much thought.

S.F. *You didn't?*

M. To me the people on top have always been like unreachable to my way of thinking.

S.F. *What do you mean by that?*

M. Unreachable, at least to me as an individual. I've never been in it so deep that . . . I have never met so many characters that are into something like uh . . . even halfway to the top, what is considered the top. . . . I have never known any big connections. All I know—have known is like from the neighborhood, my neighborhood, guys like I.

S.F. *Well, how did you feel when you'd read in the paper, let's say "Twenty Kilograms Have Been Seized" or "A Hundred Kilograms Have Been Seized"?*

M. Well, I would say "What a shame." This is what would come to my mind if I was hooked. "Gee, what a shame. The stuff around here is no good, and look at that. Such a big amount . . . and it was taken." See, I felt that way about that much anyway.

S.F. *What about the ambassador who was arrested? Remember?*

M. Oh, the ambassador. Yes, that was in that connection, Paris, France, and so on—international. Well . . . it was a shame. That's like I said—

S.F. *You regretted it. It was a regret.*

M. A regret. Yes. Right. A regret that—

S.F. *But did you think at all about the fact that these people could afford losing that money to the racketeers?*

M. I never thought about it that way. No. I just know that man is going to go to jail and . . . just like I have gone to jail, and . . . and uh . . . if that's what he's doing and he goes to jail, . . . well, that's it. I never thought about it the other way. I always thought that if you're doing wrong, and the time comes when you have to go to jail, you're just supposed to go to jail.

S.F. *What are your feelings about the people who were investing their money? Do you have any feelings at all about that?*

M. No, I never been . . . I never looked at it uh . . . as I have something against them or anything.

S.F. *No?*

M. I never looked at it that way. No.

S.F. *You never felt exploited by people? Exploited in the sense that you had to do all this running around?*

M. No. I felt . . . that I'd been exploiting myself. Not that anybody else had been exploiting me. Exploiting myself, knowing the outcome of this where I walk. I have gone into it, and then I have found myself . . . thinking and trying to make a dollar twenty-four hours a day, and having a rough way of acquiring it. And staying like out uh . . . twenty-four hours out of twenty-four hours. Sometimes without sleep, and so forth, just because I had to have my fix, and I'm going to get sick, and I'm going to need it. See? So maybe my way for looking for a dollar takes longer for the average guy 'cause he probably goes and breaks anybody's door, takes a lot of unnecessary chances which I refuse to take because I uh . . . don't like to steal. This is . . . this is my way of looking at it, and when you go out stealing you're liable to run into anyone. You never know who's going to walk into you. The other day a guy got killed. He got shot by the owner of the apartment came in . . . found him inside. Just lately a Spanish guy got killed, twenty something years old, I think. And uh . . . the guy had a rifle, a carbine. . . . Went and got it and said, "Don't move." The guy starting running for the window, and he shot him . . . five times. That's it. These things, it could've been the other way around. He could've killed the guy. So, these things I look at them that way, and the other way that I look for a dollar, well, my chances are much better. Because I'll be making a dollar out of the hustling . . . like me. He'll be getting what he's looking for and I get what I look for. That's the way that I've done it because that's the simplest way that I've found . . . that I could do it, and still be close to what I need, which is the drugs. And yet I'm not a pusher, I'm not a big man, I'm not . . . anything. I'm not into anything, more or less. I'm just . . . making a fool out of myself. I'm hustling *myself*. In other words, nobody's using me—I'm using myself. That's the way I felt.

S.F. *You felt but, of course, it wasn't entirely true. Obviously, you're exploiting yourself—*

M. Exploiting myself.

S.F. *On behalf of some other people. Somebody was making money out of it.*

M. I don't see it. Uh . . . I don't—this is what I don't see because that's available.

[One would expect Manny to be peculiarly conscious of the hierarchical illegal structure above him, and also in some way would respond to its pressure. In fact, we notice that he professes no jealousy or indignation at being exploited, and claims to have experienced none. In part this is because, if he were to experience what really happens to him, it would hurt him, but in part also it is because his style of life gives a special legitimacy and worth to structures as such. He finds justification for the illegal bureaucracy in the risks taken by the illegal suppliers of capital and heroin. Moralism turned inwardly, as it were, serves to make him feel that the only person who is exploited by himself is himself. He is conscious of the bureaucracy but he does not feel punished or hurt by it.]

S.F. *What's available?*

M. That's available just like uh . . . everything else is available. It's a business.

S.F. *What's that? Now, what are you referring to?*

M. Well, like you say, the big man. The ones that control it—the international connections. They smuggle in and out. To me this is just a business. Just like smuggling diamonds.

S.F. *All right. Good. But somebody is making money. Right?*

M. Somebody has to.

S.F. *All right, but you weren't.*

M. I wasn't.

S.F. *Therefore, you were being exploited not only by yourself but by people who were making the money. Right?*

M. But I was making enough for my fix—what *I* wanted. That's all I wanted.

S.F. *Right, but somebody was benefiting by your self-exploitation.*

M. But they're taking—in bigger terms than I am—they're taking bigger chances than I am. Now, this is—this is what they deserve.

S.F. *You feel they deserve it?*

M. I—I believe they do.

S.F. *That's what I want to find out. Whether you feel that—*

M. Now, looking at it the other way now. . . . Like uh the point that you're probably trying to get at is what I think is a very humane thing. To even touch that, I don't think it is. I think it's very harmful to the user. Not only of the United States, but of any place. Just like it was harmful to me, but when I was on the hustle, and I was trying to make a dollar, those people were not exploiting me. I was exploiting myself. See . . . I'm taking my chances—my little, little chances, and when the police make a bust, and they—they get me on this little chances that I'm taking I'm the one that goes to jail . . . but I'm paying for something I'm doing. . . . They don't blame that guy up there. They blame me. Because they can't do anything about that guy unless they catch him. Right? . . . So, I'm responsible for my own actions.

S.F. *Suppose you had known these connections. Do you think you would ever have turned them in?*

M. I don't believe so, frankly speaking. No. Just like I . . . I don't believe if I was up in the front, and I got captured, they wouldn't break me unless they kill me.

[As we would expect, Manny with his background and style of life feels that the police are carrying out their work in terms of rules and regulations that do not in any degree exploit him.]

M. I'd probably wind up killing myself thinking that I might break, but I won't give them the opportunity to. In other words, I believe . . . I believe in being real about things, and being that I'm not a policeman, that is not my job. And I am considered to be a citizen. Not right now perhaps . . . perhaps in the future. Now, citizens are expected to do a lot of things that they never do, and sometimes that they have done, they have harmed themselves and their families. See? And they have not been able to do anything about it—the law.

S.F. *Are you talking about the way in which sometimes citizens—*

M. The law some—the law is . . . to me the law is a balance.

S.F. *Balance between what?*

M. It's a balance . . . but the one that's holding the balance is very blind. . . . I believe, you know that justice—the Justice Department, they have the statue with the balance. There's a blind on the lady.

[Manny was asked what he would do if he were told that he would die at a fixed date six years from the day of the interview and among the things that he said were that he would try to get a trade, raise a family, and in that connection he said that he would like to have a family because it would keep up the family line.]

S.F. *Why is that important to you?*
M. Oh, it's very important to leave somebody behind because—at least according to the Bible.
S.F. *No, according to you.*
M. I'm going by the Bible because that's the way it quote—the things that we quote automatically.
S.F. *What do you believe?*
M. With me, I believe that is right. It's correct that in leaving kids behind you're leaving a part of you behind . . . that will keep going. It won't be a complete failure, your life. In other words, this is something that is considered normal to accomplish in life, and if you haven't accomplished this, when you leave, you don't leave anything but a memory. Memories are forgetfulness. They're forgetful. The people will forget you eventually as years go by. Maybe once in a while you creep up into somebody's mind.
S.F. *Is this important, do you think? To be remembered?*
M. I believe so. It is to leave kids behind, but in those five years I'd try and provide for them and . . . leave something set up for them. In other words, my sacrifice would be *more* of a sacrifice then . . . because I would try and leave everything to them.

[I next omit the topic of Manny's supposed remaining years, which runs into a discussion of humor while using drugs and cheating other addicts out of money.]

S.F. *Well, frankly, did you ever beat anybody?*
M. I have also . . . yes.
S.F. *Often?*
M. No, not often. Not often. Just . . . certain locations where . . . I felt that I could beat the person—that he called for that. There are certain incidents where it happened like that I have had a certain amount of money in my hand and I have seen where . . . if I don't beat this person . . . something else will happen to me.

S.F. *Tell me what. How does that happen, that kind of circumstance?*

M. Circumstances like . . . like I could see where I could be making a sale which might come something . . . the outcome would be like the time I make the sale to the undercover man. Now, this has happened a couple of times to me, and, thanks God, I've been able to keep away from the bust. And uh . . . I have taken the money. This is—my experience has told me that *this* time I shouldn't do it. I shouldn't go through with it. See? Now, this is the way it has been. That person has been brought to me . . . and I have gone as far as taking the money without telling the person that I'm the one that's going to give him anything or whether somebody else is going to give me it or anything. Just taking their money and saying "Well, where you . . . this and that. . . . All right." Now, this person to my way of thinking . . . is an in-between man. If I get to him, somebody else will come up, and . . . and I know, for me to do this and put myself in this position when I'm nobody, when I'm not a big seller, when I'm not into anything. I'm—this is—this is just for *my* habit, taking care of my habit. If I put myself in this position, like I did the time that I got the six years . . . the outcome will be six—not six, maybe more. . . . That's what I will get out of it. See? So I have taken their money.

S.F. *In other words, when something told you that you were dealing with a possible intermediary to an agent, you took the money and—*

M. Took the money and that's it.

S.F. *What happened then? Did they go after you?*

M. Change your neighborhood.

S.F. *You changed neighborhoods?*

M. Yes . . . sure.

S.F. *That's a way to avoid complications?*

M. Well, I believe so. And . . . it works to an extent. It has worked for me to an extent. And I have met the guys years later perhaps. Perhaps months after this.

S.F. *And what happened?*

M. Nothing. . . . It seems that I was right.

S.F. *Really?*

M. It seems that I was right. One is not right all the time now. I could have made a big error too, and beat the wrong guy. You understand? I could have done an injustice to the guy by taking his money.

[At the time of the interview Manny is off drugs, and does not feel the pressure therefore of having to make money illegally. He is also experiencing more and more the characteristic tendency toward overconformity found among those who are trying to stay off drugs. He therefore gives an example of cheating someone which leaves him in the most favorable light, namely, where he is cheating an agent or informer. It is likely, however, that he actually did connive to beat people on some other occasions.]

S.F.   *Every so often, do you hear So-and-so is dead? Get a wire like that, and then it turns out, he wasn't dead at all?*

M.   He wasn't dead at all.

S.F.   *Is that common to you?*

M.   Well, I have seen it happen. I have seen the person afterwards, believing he was dead or she was dead, and I ask—in fact, it happened to me!

S.F.   *Really?*

M.   Yes! I met—one day I was standing on the stoop of my house— the building on a Hundred Street, and here comes two very dear friends, two girls, and . . . they were sisters of a very good friend of mine. Another fellow that used to sail with me. And they were coming on the way to go up in my house with bouquets of flowers. Somebody had told them I was dead. . . . They found me in a bathtub. . . . They actually believed it, and when they walked in, and seen me on the stoop, they couldn't believe it. I had to pinch them in order for them to believe it. They were flabbergasted . . . like amazed. "What happened? Gee, they told us you was dead." Now, had I not been there, they would have gone up to the house, and met my mother, and everything, and tell, "Well, your son is dead. Gee, I'm very sorry." You know, and go through all the processes of condolences. They actually believed that I was dead. And there I was. Had I—

S.F.   *Did they say how you died?*

M.   Yeah, they told them that they found me in the bathtub.

S.F.   *Yes, but died of what?*

M. Of a . . . overdose of narcotics.

[It is no accident that the rumor about Manny takes the form it does. It describes him as overdoing one of the ritualistic acts of the addict, namely, injecting the heroin. But having injected himself, he has received an overdose. Presumably, according to the rumor-mongers, his friends had tried to restore him to life by throwing him in a bathtub of cold water. And again, presumably, this failed, so he died. The picture is of someone who is trusted and well liked, but also someone who would be expected to sacrifice himself for others. He doesn't hurt someone else, but he does hurt himself. But in another way, this is another example of self-punishment for his guilt feelings.]

S.F. *If you talk about your sister or talk about your mother, I see no difference between your mother and your sister—in your mind, that is.*

M. They're very similar.

S.F. *They are. To you they are.*

M. To me they're very similar . . . as far as it goes with me at least.

S.F. *Don't they have any imperfections? What's wrong with them?*

M. Oh, faults you mean?

S.F. *No. What's wrong with them?*

M. They have their faults . . .

S.F. *Namely, what are they? Take your mother. What are her faults?*

M. She makes errors and . . . decisions and so forth . . .

S.F. *How does she bug you? In what way?*

M. With me? She's very nice. There's nothing I can say wrong of her because the faults that she does have . . . I don't think about it too much because she sacrifices in other ways . . . to compensate for her misunderstanding of certain things.

S.F. *How about your sister? How does she bug you?*

M. My sister . . . according to what she has shown me within herself, I can't vouch for her thinking or other actions which I don't know about, but in front of me . . . she has always been very understanding. She has always listened to what I have to say, and very few times we have come to any misunderstandings . . . and very few times that I have noticed that she has gotten mad about any particular subject or action perhaps that I have committed or said. And I have high respect for the two of them. And that's about all that I can say about them that I find that I can say about them. I don't know in the future, but at the present time—this is the estimate I have.

S.F. *All that means, Manny, is that you really have not examined them as people.*

M. I have examined them. It's just that—

S.F. *It's an empty picture you have there . . . an empty picture.*

M. When it comes to that, I have to be automatically . . . they have been so nice to me, and I don't deserve it. You see, I feel that I do not.

S.F. *You feel.*

M. I feel that I do not. I feel that I have not earned it. Therefore, being that I have been close to them in a sense, and away from them in other sense, because I have not shared with them, like I say. I haven't been with them—out of ten years, I haven't been with them ten years, sharing every day, day in and day out. Say half of them, I have been in jail and half of them I have been in the streets.

Here is a 39-year-old man whose life style has progressively, if not continuously, tended toward more and more dependence on sharply defined frames of reference, one of which was the addict culture. As far back as he can remember he was searching for what he thought to be his father, and what we may translate as a dependence on authoritative frames. Paradoxically, the very quest for the father as well as for these frames of reference was at best ambiguous, and at worst a source of emptiness and frustration. In the scene in which he describes a remeeting with his father, and then failing to experience what he thought he should and rightfully should have experienced from a father, we see a symbol of the promise and the failure of the authoritative frames of reference that he thought he needed and sought.

One would expect that his love for his mother and the sensitivity he experiences toward her, as toward his sister, would, in some measure, leaven the rigidity and the obsessiveness of his life style. To some extent this may be true. However, we notice, too, that in his manner of speaking about both his mother and his sister there is a stereotype quality characteristic of the adolescent's placing a woman on a pedestal. One suspects that these platonic beings were at once norms for judging other women and also persistent annoyances, negative models, that made him feel that he was a gnawing, miserable, and incomplete wretch. There is some indirect and external evidence of a drastic childhood homosexual encounter. His relative shyness in the sexual sphere suggests that during his pre-teens and teens he was very anxious about his manliness.

Under these circumstances, when his family moved to East Harlem's 100th Street, which was then becoming "the Fifth Avenue of Addiction," this young man was ready for some kind of excitement, some source of external stimulation which would alleviate the burden of trying to live up to implacable ideals. This he found in street life, in cocaine, and then in heroin. The fact that one is a stimulant and the other a depressant is existentially irrelevant. For a man in need of relaxation and diversion, the addict culture formed an appropriate context within which he could for a time safely and cheaply meet his needs.

However, even within addict society Manny's life style helped shape the roles he could play most conveniently, and the ones that he tended to choose if he had options. It is no accident that he was a failure as a thief and that he preferred interstitial and service roles. These latter he could more easily accommodate within his rigid orientation.

Still, in the long run, given a chance, a man like Manny would persistently try to re-establish himself within a traditional or conservative framework. It is no accident, therefore, that he used his prison time, in part, to read books on psychiatry and society. He tried to stay off by himself for eleven months, and when offered a chance he entered the Exodus House program, where he has done very well. At the age of thirty-nine, he found himself to be a useful and respected member of a program where his strength would be noticed and contribute to the rehabilitation of others as well as himself. A prognosis for a man like Manny would seem to be good, but of course would depend on his chances for achieving a balance between the rigid frames of reference of a rehabilitation program and the exigencies of family life which might cause him to return to drugs.

Johnny—Sluggard and Victim

Although Johnny is not an overt homosexual, many things in his life have eviscerated his drive, and to a degree have rendered him vulnerable to the kind of street life to which he has been exposed since he came from Puerto Rico in his very early teens. He had great difficulty learning English, and the net impression one gets after knowing him for a number of years is that he never really has become lucid in his understanding of the American scene. He tends to fall asleep when things get too complicated for him, as they easily do. Though he went to high school, he can barely read English and cannot read Spanish at all.

One of my most vivid memories is of hearing Johnny getting a lecture from two older addicts about their insistence that he stop using drugs because he just didn't have the caliber to be an addict. He just was too stupid, too weak, too cowardly, they informed him in no uncertain terms, and they argued that these were ample reasons for anyone with any sense to stop using drugs. Johnny is the sort of person who will get a job, and work, and when he comes home with the pay on Friday night will be jumped by addicts and forced to give up part or all of his money. If he happens to float into pushing through connections that he has picked up, it is likely that one or more of the "take-off artists" will manhandle him and take away his heroin. He will bluster and threaten, but no one will take him seriously, least of all himself.

At home Johnny finds that his father is down on him and scornfully regards his son as an inept nuisance who may steal the family tape recorder or his father's watch and pawn them rather than steal on the outside where the chances of being arrested are much greater. The father will rant and rage and threaten to have him arrested, but in the last analysis will be dissuaded by Johnny's mother who has "spoiled" him (as he says) ever since he was young. Johnny's two sisters also play a role here and it is characteristic of his insularity that incestuous fancies and gestures also mark his life in the family.

It is equally characteristic that Johnny describes the process of becoming an addict as one of a person being gulled into a pattern he knew nothing about by someone who played upon his desire to be important. Nobody thinks Johnny is important and he has found that, at most, he can get a measure of respect from a girl through using his good looks. However, here, too, in the past he has gotten in trouble through an unexpected pregnancy, and the fact that the mother of the girl he was involved with did not like his dark color. This dark Puerto Rican finds that the light Puerto Rican resents him.

On the other hand, Johnny's very plasticity and passivity may, in the long run, prove to be his salvation. Once pointed in the right direction, given ample supports, protected from temptations, a fellow like Johnny can stay off drugs indefinitely. As a matter of fact, after a number of tries Johnny stayed off drugs for several months, first under the pressure of the law and later under the influence of a girl friend. Whether he could continue to do so depended on the continuation of favorable circumstances: a job, his girl friend, and a family. Characteristically, when his girl friend left him, he ended his period of abstinence and started the downward spiral again.

Joseph—Between Anger and Sadness

Whether Joseph is trying to recall his childhood or recollecting events in his most recent present, he is likely to express anger, if not outright rage. Joseph, who is a 30-year-old Negro, was born in the South and came to New York City when he was a pre-teen-ager. Even before that event he had a feeling of being deprived of his most essential nature, of his identity. In words and in action, his father as much as told him that he did not think Joseph was his son. Much earlier than that Joseph remembers receiving a gift and having it taken from him by his uncle, his father's brother. He recalls a violent quarrel in which his father, suspicious of his mother's attention to another man, beat her and him and then told her she could stay but that he, the son, would have to go. There was much ado in his early years about his birth certificate, and what it said, which created much confusion in his own mind. When he was thirteen and intervened on behalf of his mother, his father told him again that he was not his son, and he was told that when he was twenty-one years old he would learn his true identity. This business haunted him into his adolescence, which he spent in New York.

Joseph is the oldest of three brothers, one of whom became a drug addict, the other an alcoholic. This combination duplicated the situation in his father's own family, for *his* father was an alcoholic, and his two brothers became drug addicts. (His father has served a term in a New York prison, under conviction for manslaughter.)

The only person in his family to whom Joseph had related with any positive feelings was his mother. And to her, almost by contrast, he responded with exaggerated attention and affection. It was she to whom he would come with his problems and whose advice he generally followed. He was not a good student at school. In the South he played hooky and to some extent he did the same in New York. He started using pot when he was twelve, though his friends took to heroin. For reasons not clear to him he did not at first ingest heroin. As a matter of fact, though he was jailed when he was nineteen for possession of a gun and had drugs available to him at all times through family friends with connections, he did not use until the year after his mother died. He took her death very hard, not only because of what he thought of her but what he felt were his responsibilities for his brothers. His mother, he said, had given him to believe that it was his job to look after his brothers, and he found that this was too much of a burden. Within a year after her death he felt that meaning had dropped out of life, and he did not care about anything. He turned to drugs as an expression of this depression. His life on drugs was one of sadness about his situation, accompanied or interspersed with anger and expressions of violence toward those who upset him. Joseph reports that he has always tended to be on the side of the underdog and will go out of his way to pick a fight with anybody he thinks is taking advantage of anybody, including himself. Ironically, drugs have not always given him a sense of calm; in fact at times they have stimulated him to go out looking for action and for opportunities to commit aggressive acts.

Joseph says that he looks like his father and has his ways. When he was twenty-one he approached his father to unravel the mystery of his identity, but his father shrugged off the question by saying that it was not at all what he said it was. His father's answer left him nonplussed, but he wants to believe that he really is his father's son. His two brothers in turn have played upon the same motif, making him feel less wanted. In order to secure their affection from time to time he has to hold out gifts of money and property. He says that in general he has a hard time saying no to people and is conscious of the fact that he is manipulated. What he does not seem to understand is that this mixture of depressed and paranoid styles is self-combustible in that the more angry he gets the more depressed he gets and the more depressed he gets the more liable he is to seek violent action.

Over the years Joseph has noted a declining sexual interest, thanks to the use of heroin. However, he has fathered one child out of wedlock, who he says reminds him of his own situation in that this child too is not certain who his father is. This also makes him feel very sad. He has married another woman, has children by her, and reports that gradually she has come to understand him very well and has sought to help him organize his life somewhat better. In talking about his life Joseph burst out into tears very often and it was clear that these were as much expression of his pent-up anger as of sadness. After his last stay at Riker's Island he came out feeling extreme puzzlement. "I was lost." It was in this situation that he heard of Exodus House and decided to try this program out. Joseph has done very well and at thirty years of age seems to have both the motivation and the strength of character to be willing to stick to a difficult and demanding program. The accuracy of this prognosis would also depend upon the extent to which his old feelings of being deprived and persecuted would be elicited by some of the typical events that belong to a program such as Exodus House would entail, e.g., his restiveness at not being advanced as fast as he would like to be.

Artie—A Man Beside Himself

When Artie was asked what characteristic he most disliked about himself, he said it was that he always took advantage of people. Give him a hand and he wants the whole arm. For example, he would con women by sweet-talking them; he would steal their keys and burglarize their homes. He is especially predatory when on heroin. Since he began to use drugs, around 1960, this 26-year-old white man has only infrequently been off drugs and at those times has experienced great anxiety. On drugs he becomes a manipulator, but off drugs he is a terrified child.

Trying to account for his use of drugs Artie inclines to stress the role of frustration. He cannot remember when he did not feel frustrated. It was not that he was deprived but that he practiced the principle of "I want what I want when I want it." And he offers many anecdotes which illustrate this. He admits freely to having been spoiled by his parents but goes further and implies that he fulfilled his part of the bargain by being a good student and graduating from high school. He took civil service tests, following in his father's footsteps, and passed conspicuously, he says, for positions in critically needed municipal jobs. In fact he held one of these jobs at a lower level and was about to complete his probationary period when his use of drugs was accidentally detected. He is especially proud of having been the only junkie ever to have worked in this civil service post.

In telling his own story he stresses his navy experience, which was for him one wild sowing of oats, leading him when he was tired of ordinary kicks to get involved with Turkish hashish and eventually with a variety of other drugs. After having been discharged honorably he speedily became a pusher to meet his considerable habit.

As his story indicates, he is not one of those addicts who stick exclusively or primarily to heroin; he has tried everything, including LSD, preferring the stimulants and the hallucinogens to the opiates. He pays the price in sleepless, anxiety-ridden nights and toxic nightmares.

He confesses—and is ashamed of—his tendency to lie and also professes to want help to stop this pattern. Surprisingly he expresses both unconsciously and consciously much guilt about his past. For instance, he reports dreams which reveal anguish and anxiety about having brought a disease to his child. (He is now separated from his wife.) He expresses a certain degree of contrition about his failure to be a good husband.

In the main, however, this is a picture of a man who has preferred to live outside himself and to fill himself with drugs that give him a sense of a synthetic life. His relationships to people tend to be superficial and manipulative even to the extent, I suspected, of using the interview as one more ploy in influencing the Exodus House staff opinion of him. He professed a great desire to revolutionize himself and during the interview showed pride in having been off drugs some nine days after having left jail. Shortly after that, however, he dropped out of the candidacy stage of the Exodus House program and has not been heard of since.

Artie found it difficult to adjust to the Exodus House program because his style of life made it hard for him to take rehabilitation seriously. He was undergoing a ritual drama in which he apparently did not know his lines, but there he felt it would seem that everyone around him was as phony as he. He confidently informed me that he was going to "make it" with one of the females whom he saw at Exodus House, and when he had no success, this failure seemed to warrant his taking a shot. In sum, Artie is one of those men who transfer their own responsibilities for making a life of their own on to the existential drugs, and these through their action shape his life despite himself.

Ronnie—The Would-Be Master of His Fate

If there is any motif running through Ronnie's story of his life it is this 24-year-old Negro's persistent, even frenetic, search to control the conditions of his life and the reactions to his success and failure. In trying to recall his earliest experiences he significantly makes the point that after his mother died, when he was three, he was shunted around from hand to hand. His father at that time was in the army and he reports that he was eventually taken back by his father, who told him later that he had not known what was happening to his own son. His recollections of his mother emphasize the fact that he sees her in the light of her quarrels with his father. There are shadows that he sees, not people, around this period of time; but the whole set of recollections indicates great anxiety about not being able to know and control what was happening.

Ronnie is the youngest of a large family, in which smoking pot and drinking liquor were common. He was raised by an aunt whom he calls his mother. Even though his father made a good living, Ronnie very early got a newspaper route and also sold ices. In the latter he was so successful that, he says, he had a couple of assistants. He made contact with heroin through a friend who was in school who would deliver heroin. He took up a trade and even worked at it, he says, quite successfully, but found himself involved in drugs and even pushed them. For two years he says he was a drug addict and then for three more years he tried to get rid of the habit. When he could not function any more in his trade he turned back to his street connections, became involved in numbers, and characteristically after a while had his own bank and his own runners. But he lost this too when he became a victim. At the age of twenty-four Ronnie shows great drive to make use of what abilities he has. It is understandable that having had access to the Exodus House program he has taken full advantage of it. Everyone in the program with whom he comes in contact sooner or later becomes impressed with his interest in rehabilitation. At the same time, paradoxically, he can be diverted from his rehabilitation program by getting into other habits. For example, during the period of time that he has been in Exodus House his problem has not been drugs so much as liquor. He easily lets himself drink large quantities of alcohol and then cheerfully sets about trying to control it.

In summary Ronnie's history shows an apparent aggressive desire to control his fate along with a persistent undercurrent of a desire to be controlled by something or someone outside himself. This life style found its expression, it would seem, in his use of drugs.

It is significant for our understanding of this young man that at first the Exodus House staff had some reluctance about accepting him. What struck us first prominently was not his drive but the inner chaos that "shook him up." Could we expect that such fragile bric-a-brac could endure the tremendous pressure of testing and retesting that goes on in our program? And, in fact, before he was accepted he had more than one slip back into heroin. The pressure was taking its toll. Then suddenly, showing how hazardous is prognosis in this field, he seemed to "straighten up." He had "bought the program," and it was as if he was harnessing all his life energies to achieve this primary goal. He was then accepted into candidacy and from that time to the present writing, some ten months later, has not had a single slip.

The drive to succeed appears to have mobilized the scattering energies within this anxious man and through this simplification he has barreled ahead. The psychiatrist reports that he takes the initiative in therapy sessions and obviously is operating on a peak level of performance. Not content with group therapy, he has from time to time approached me for individual counseling. The man with a disorganized style of life is moving with great zest to a healthier style, and his future depends upon the continuation of favorable circumstances which will reward his average abilities in a way that gives him continuous satisfaction.

Portrait of Justis

These tapes, like Manny's, were part of a screening process but were made in a basement apartment where we both could hear and see boys and girls playing games outside in the street. Justis' manner throughout was one of almost excessive adulation to me, and I had to interrupt him from time to time in the midst of unctuous praise. His first tape, however, was marked by considerable latent anxiety because he wanted me to give him questions to answer. He also sensed that he was being tested, and this was an independent source of anxiety.

I first met the short, 33-year-old Negro I call Justis in Metropolitan Hospital where he had a reputation as an artist, a teller of tales, and a maker of poems. I have subsequently learned that he was known to the Rev. Norman C. Eddy as far back as 1951. As he got to know me he was reluctant to talk on tape, although he was very polite about refusing. He did talk about himself and as a matter of fact at one point formed part of a group that entertained themselves with my tape recorder. He dropped out of sight, and then through the grapevine I heard that he had been killed. More precisely, the rumor had it that he had been shot by a policeman while in the act of robbing a liquor store.

It was therefore much to my surprise that I met him while on a trip to Riker's Island. He, too, had heard the rumor, but was eager, as he put it, "to deny its truth."

Justis eagerly came to the Exodus House meetings in Riker's and continued his interest on leaving the prison. At the time of this writing, late in 1966, he has been off drugs for many months, and in his own way is trying to wrestle with the problems of emotional growth.

The following tapes were a part of the screening program used in Exodus House. After they were over I asked Justis if he would object to having them incorporated, in part, in a book and he agreed wholeheartedly. His manner is rambling and discursive, but, as I think will become clear, the very language is one more clue to his life style.

SEYMOUR FIDDLE.   *Tell me the story of your life as you see it.*
JUSTIS.   Well . . . I would like to give you first . . . from the time that I started usin' drugs and uh perhaps after that, I would be delighted to go from the time up until I started usin' drugs which would maybe would be able to—some of the questions would be self-explanatory. In 1949 . . . I . . . was havin' some of the problems . . . and it was a problem bein' in New York City without adequate livin' conditions . . . money . . . bein' able to get some of the things that seemed to fascinate me that I wasn't able to have just comin' from the South. And actually New York City was the only city that I had ever been in and my . . . parents wasn't very much educated, so . . . there was not very much unity there. And so every time that I would seek help of any type I would have to leave home to seek it.

[From the very outset Justis represents himself as a victim of circumstances beyond his control. He had problems of inadequate living and of domestic pressure with no adults except the mother of an addict to give him help. He is suggesting that ironically the very source of help and strength was the means by which he became involved in drugs. Later on in other tapes he modifies this interpretation of the precise way he got involved in drugs but the rambling and at times unconnected discussion serves to point up a thematic motif of his life style. It should be added that his discussion about poverty and so on is not merely a reflection of material values but an expression of a need to protect his pride. What this implies will become clearer as the tapes proceed.]

J.   There wasn't very much love there. Any time I wanted to . . .

some condolence or someone I had to go out to see the lady next door. She too was somewhat like my parents—not very much educated, and she had sons was wounded in the service, and he was usin' drugs. And durin' that time drugs was—drugs, I suppose—but not very much detrimental. There was not too much chemicals in it in the way of this destructiveness, and he would see that I was upset. And not knowin' what it really were himself, he offered me some. It seemed to be givin' him the same amount of relief . . . Takin' away the stigma in his family. It was replacin' the ignorance there and no understandin'. And I started with him. And for the first time in my life I could find something that would relieve me of all anxiety . . . not havin' had adequate clothing to go out to dances . . . not havin' money in my pocket. I found out that if I hear my father and mother . . . in a—I would say a debate. Now I would say a debate, I would know how to handle it by goin' out and gettin' me some junk. And I couldn't very well let it disturb me because I would somewhat be in another world. And I was goin' to school . . . and durin' this time I'm havin' to fight in school, and I was kicked out after the second year of high school. And, as you know, from that, I didn't have very much education. And, you know, my parents, they had much less than that. And psychology or anything like that . . . spiritual guidance, we—we never had. We had, down South, we had very funny ministers, you know? I—I always use this because it's a joke to me now. They would come to your house and they would eat chicken. We had to fry chicken for them, you know? And uh . . . that would be that. Now, I was baptized when I was twelve years old and I remember it as if it were yesterday. But the only thing happened is I was baptized . . . the next Sunday the minister came to the house and ate chicken. And it was a long time before I even seen him again, you know.

[It is not clear why in view of later discussions showing how he admired the church down South Justis chooses to mock the minister's habits. However it would seem that in view of his focusing upon himself as being a victim he felt a need to show that even ministers were not very helpful to him.]

J.   And he didn't know who I was really, and, you know, that's somethin' that bugs me now, you know, to find out that why couldn't there have been some type of spiritual guidance, you know, to hold a family. In the South they don't have that, you know? And everybody come from the South is *completely* ignorant, especially back then. Now it's very much different. People comin' from the South now are very much educated . . . and not havin' all this benefits of understandin', unity, spiritual guidance, after I was kicked out of school I was like in the street. I was in the street with junk because it was an escape . . . I didn't need a lot of money in my pockets . . . drugs was plentiful . . . and there was no one who could orientate me on this . . . could explain the bad points about drugs. Very few people were usin' naturally compared to what it is now and . . . it was usually with one or two chemicals. Now it's more than a dozen in it. Everybody's had their hands in it. It's . . . not heroin you're usin' today. It's everything but that. Usually one percent is heroin with four, five chemicals makes it very detrimental. If it's somethin' that you're allergic to you're in a lot of trouble, you know? You take a shot of dope and the first thing you got to do . . . is be excused, you know, it's diarrhea or somethin', you know. It's all these chemicals started workin'.

[When the addicted use the term "chemical" it is meant as a derogatory term and excludes heroin, which in some way is deemed to be a natural product as opposed to the synthetics and fillers used to make a bag hold up or feel heavy.]

J.   So . . . bein' wild, and not knowin' anything . . . I just used every single thing that I know, and bein' fifteen and a half years old, I was—we grew up together. And uh . . . and I'll jump ahead for a moment. Bein' sentenced three times, I've been sentenced to eleven years.

[The sudden jump by Justis into a discussion of his lengthy prison career also seems designed to impress us with his victimization.]

J.   And every time that I would come out it would be just . . .

tune up, comin' out to use drugs again. 'Cause I couldn't find *no* therapy nowhere. No one could . . . could, you know, give me the key word. Uh . . . wake me up to what was really happenin'. And I went so far as to stop usin' and actually that was all I was doin'— just stopped usin'. I was completely lost, you know, nervous wreck. I had kicked one time . . . and I started drinkin', you know, and I would drink until I would get drunk and I, you know, would try to drink even more than that, you know. And I'd wake up, and it would be the same thing. And . . . finally I would say I was better off usin' junk. And I would go back and start usin', but durin' all this time I started to workin' up in a way where I would be doin' so much to other people, not so much to myself, I was losin' all the respect I had for people . . . And a lot of these people would keep tellin' me that someday I would—I would change because I always I carried somethin' with me that they was always proud of.

[Here we have what turns out to be perhaps the first of many self-alluding, self-aggrandizing statements made by Justis. In the strict Freudian sense he is narcissistic when he is off drugs in that he acts in the light of an idealized image of what he thinks people think of him. As will become evident, two trends strive with each other: a highly verbal narcissistic pattern is in continual conflict with a raging hostile self-victimized trend. This long rambling preamble shows how he moves from one to the other through time, events from different epochs in his life colliding with each other.]

J.   They said that I seemed to have a special love for babies—children, you know. And I used to get high, and I used to take all these kids from the block . . . and take 'em to stores and their mothers would be lookin' for them, and she would find out that I was with them. And they say "Well, they all right because we know what happened. He carried them to the store . . . and bought them somethin'." With that, people always . . . tellin' me that they know I would change. They would give me encouragin' words that I might be a preacher someday. That's because I had so much love for kids, they wondered why I couldn't, you know, associate with adults the same way and . . . Once I had a somewhat . . . a nervous breakdown they called it then, so I would call it that, and after it happened—

S.F. *How old were you then?*

J. Uh . . . I was . . . seventeen. And I was with some doctors in the hospital and . . . they told me I were somewhat mechanical inclined. I used to wonder I said, "mechanical inclined"? What do you mean I'm "mechanical inclined"? So . . . they told me that they would give me some tests and . . . and prove to me that I was somewhat mechanical inclined, that I was able to do a lot of things with my hands. That I was able to . . . to recognize things and put them together. My hands would tell somethin', you know, unverbally. It would tell somethin'. They would give it to me, and I would do these things and . . . I could see somethin' was there but it didn't go any farther than that. I felt as though they were . . . you know, just tellin' me that I was all right 'cause I couldn't see what they were tryin' to do. I was a drug addict and none of them were . . . and we just didn't have the same outlooks. So over the years . . . I've tried my hand at doin' these particular things . . . and I could see where I could do things like that. But I knew there was somethin' missin' . . . but I just didn't have no idea what it were. I . . . had a lot of excuses . . . I didn't have much education . . . and the family was so erected there, you know, no unity, no understandin' in the family (and) my father would do a lot of drinkin' . . . and he would use a lot of profanity in the family. And I . . . with that, I seemed to have more love for mother than I did my father, you know? And to me it seemed as though he were a little too . . . too rough, you know, on us. And . . . that I had to always run to her for, you know, consolation, that I couldn't go to him for it. I remember when I was a kid if I wanted any money I couldn't ask him. I had to ask her for it, you know? Because I was expectin' somethin' from him and I would get it if I asked him for the money. He'd shout . . . and do this, and right away I'd get a shock, you know? And I'd get very angry . . . and I would go out and I would go out and I would get me some junk. And with that, I started to growin' a lot of hate . . . it was normal then. I mean, I had a right to . . . grow that hate because it's nothin' there in the family.

[In view of his later references to the Bible and interest in becoming a minister this discussion of "a right to hate" sounds incongruous. However, this inconsistency merely points to the division within Justis: on the one hand, toward vindictiveness and, on the other hand, toward narcissism and manipulation.]

J. I visited all of the gymnasiums in New York and . . . I . . . met a lot of people . . . professional fighters, ex-fighters, who never made it to their profession, but were very good fighters. And I associated with these people and I found out that I wanted to fight because I was misused, you know, I wasn't treated right, and I've got to be able to push this off on somebody for what I called abusiveness that I had from, you know, the father there in the family. And . . . I . . . always was ready to accuse him for anything that happened to me. It was his fault that he didn't give me what a father should give a child. By the way, that's one reason why I never got married and raised a family because . . . I knew that I wasn't capable of . . . givin' a family what a family is supposed to have. I—I always believed the family was supposed to have had more than . . . I had. I always had a strange idea if a person wasn't born rich, he should've been born educated or someone in the family should've had some education. And . . . they would have been able to give him somethin' —not money, but a little understandin' . . . education or whatever, and it was no such thing as a chip off the old block in the family. My father was an alcoholic, and I turned out to be a drug addict, and it certainly was no chip off the old block 'cause I didn't do anything like he doin'. We had no . . . no concepts the same whatsoever. And I remember when I was a child somethin' else that . . . hurt me a whole lot is that I used to like to go to church when I was a kid. And one Sunday I was waitin' to go, and it was rainin', and I couldn't go unless he was there with the car to carry us to church. And he didn't get there. And . . . it was the last minute that I left anyway, and he didn't like the idea because I left and went to church because what had happened, he had bought me new shoes, and I really goofed the shoes off in the mud. I say, "I'm not goin' to stay any longer. I'm goin'. I'm goin' to walk." And . . . but it was in the summertime, and when I had came back I took the shoes off, you know? And I rolled my pants up, and I walkin' in my bare feet when I got home, and by that time he had got home and slept off his drunk. And he . . . really had it for me, you know. Just like he had a hangover and when I walked in, and he found out what I had done, he really gave me a shellackin', you know?

[This episode of the muddy shoes Justis describes again later in material that cannot be reproduced here because of its length. The episode involves a "double bind" in that Justis was damned if he did go to church because he was given a shellacking and damned if he didn't because then he would not be gratifying certain proud impulses. At the church he would give recitations, as he says later on. The effect of the episode is to make his father look like an ogre and himself as the child victim.]

J. And . . . it caused so much friction in the family until I say "This is it. I can't see eye to eye with him no longer because that's the only thing that I really wanted to do was go to church. Especially this particular day like Easter Sunday. I never could miss anything like that, and I had a poem that I had to recite that particular day . . . and somethin' that was very important to me. I used to stay up late nights learnin' it. And . . . it was the little things like that that made me proud of myself, but I wasn't able to step out of there, no further than that. If I would've had somebody . . . I would come through with one of the poems . . . what we used to call recitations. I suppose you still do. Is that right? And . . . that's as far as it would go. When I'd get back home I couldn't get anything there. It didn't seem to do anything for them. The people in the church would clap, and would . . . give me a lot of pats and it was terrific . . . but when I'd get home, it would be somethin' different. Didn't seem to amuse them any. And I would often wonder why did these two people have to make mother and father. And I used to ask my mother, and she used to—be very religious. And . . . I suppose I understand now why she still have him all these years—thirty somethin' odd years—is that the love and understandin' in her . . . that holds them together. I told her plenty of times "You couldn't have loved him." I told her plenty of times, "You couldn't have love this guy and go through this shit that he puts down," you know. And he went so until now the doctors say he has cirrhosis of the liver. You know from alcohol. And . . . he doesn't stop. The doctor told him a few years ago not to drink any more, but he keeps it up, and he becomin' aware now of what it is. And . . . he seemed to get some education through *me* . . . you know? See what I've been doin' . . . is I've been goin' to prison a lot, and bein' incarcerated, I'm— I'm findin' I'm creatin' different types of art as such . . . that tells you the things that I'm not able to express verbally. I've been able to create some type of art, and it's somewhat associated with what I used to do with the little kids, you know?

[Children and childhood, on the one hand, and art, on the other, are two frequent and intersecting themes in Justis' thought. The multiple connections between them would, I suspect, challenge the most gifted psychiatrists.]

J.   I used to take them out. It was somethin' that I was tryin' to do, and this is the only way that I could express it by action. . . . And when the doctors had told me that I was somewhat mechanically inclined . . . they just told me that I was mechanically inclined . . . that wasn't anything else wrong with me and that I should go and stretch my head out or somethin' like that. I should fight, I should play music, I should create art, I should be a carpenter, I should be a writer, and that's somethin' I was never very good at—writin'. I have a very poor handwritin', you know, and it bothers me sometimes not to be able to . . . to write where I could use the same hands and . . . somewhat express myself which I think that very important that I should be able to express what's on my mind before I create somethin'. Because after I create somethin' I can easily express myself. I would . . . I carved a head once of Abraham Lincoln and I couldn't even express no desire or anything before I done it, and after I done it I was proud to show it. And I was on the subway and a lady asked me, "Excuse me. Is that Abe Lincoln?" And I laughed and I told her "No. This is a friend of mine. His name is George and we went to school together." And there was quite a few people chuckled, you know. They laughed there on the train, and I was able to express it to them people who asked me about it, and I was able to express it.

[Wood carving is one of Justis' favorite pastimes and while in the hospital he made and sold some statuettes. I think it is no accident that in talking about the carving of Abraham Lincoln the point is indirectly to "put down" the person in the subway. There is an aggressive element about his wood carving that fits in with his total life style.]

J. And then I done another piece . . . that I didn't put any eyes in it. And I guess for the hell of it without actually analyzing it I'd named it Blindness. And I'm able to express this to people, explain it—my ideas—but I couldn't do any of that before. If they had asked me anything . . . I couldn't express it, but after I created these particular things I found out that I could express what I just created. Showin' it, you know? Havin' the object before him, and I believe if the doctors at the time would have gave me a little somethin' else to work on I would've found out long ago what bein' mechanically inclined meant, if I'd have had somethin' to work with. I was told that I was mechanically inclined and . . . that's that. I got to go out of the hospital. I got to leave the doctor . . . I got to go back to the family . . . there's nothin' but problems there. . . . Somethin' happened once in my family also that wake me a whole lot, that told me that I didn't never want to even try to understand anything after somethin' that I had seen. . . . I've, you know . . . seen my father once with another woman. It burnt me up, you know. Couldn't nothin' . . . nothin' calm me down when I seen this. And the only thing I could think of at the time was that he had a wife that was so faithful to him . . . that had bore him seven childrens and he had the gall to be layin' up with another woman.

[Justis identifies so much with his mother that he feels his father's peccadillo as an insult to his own pride as well as hers.]

S.F. *How old were you then?*
J. Uh . . . I don't remember, but it wasn't too many years ago. It

was maybe eight or ten years ago. And . . . course you know I'll be thirty-four soon. And that really, really, really burnt me, you know? I say "What kind of guy is this?" And I could never have any kind of respect for him. I would never let him even see me drink, you know. He used to carry me out to the bar with him and say "Let's go have a drink." We hang out. I went with him, but he found out he has to leave for a moment, he'd come back and he'd find a glass empty. It's . . . a certain amount of respect that I *did* have for him, but the only thing that was missin' was the understandin'. Never—I must say this over and over again—there was never no reunion, never no togetherness there. We never ate at the table the same time. Some-one was always eatin' later. . . . We could eat, and everybody could eat *but* him because he was never there. . . . And I had somewhat given up hope of ever findin' anything. . . . I definitely couldn't go back to school . . . and no one seemed to be able to give me an answer. Everyone was always understandin' enough to say they know that I would make it someday. They still had confidence in me . . . but could no one help me at all. A funny thing happened to me though a few years ago as when I met you in the hospital . . . over there. And it bugged me a lot, you know. You sat down and you had the tape recorder. I was on medication at the time and I didn't feel too good that time. And you told me you'd come back the next night, and I said, "All right, come back." Now the next night I didn't feel like it either, but I wanted to so bad and I say, "Now I can *feel* these things. I can *see* these things, but why can't I get the shock?" You know? So . . . finally when I wind up in Riker's last year . . . I was tellin' a boy about a fellow I know. I say, "You know, I would like to see him now. You know, I feel like I can talk to him now. I feel like I can get the answer." So he say, "Who is it?" I say "It's Mr. Fiddle from Exodus House." "What! What do you mean, Fiddle from Exodus House?" He say, "I go to see him every two weeks. He comes over here." So . . . right away, you know, I started to feelin' differ-ent. I say "Yeah, I want to see him. Please. Take my name and num-ber and tell him, there's a guy here who'd like to see him." And . . . when I started to seein' you I started to gettin' a shock, you know? Everything seemed to have been comin' realistically then. So I told him that before I was arrested I had stopped usin' junk, but that's all.

I wasn't goin' no place. I was . . . at a standstill. Had stopped usin' junk. That wasn't no problem . . . not usin', but the other things that I was doin'. And . . . I told him, I say, "I believe I understand what it is. My mind has got to be free enough . . . to know that I need help, to understand I need help, and to say I believe he can help me if I just open up and say I need help.

[For a man like Justis to admit even in words alone that he really needed help was truly evidence of a change. It meant a partial lowering of the pride and even arrogance (in the etymological sense) that bedeviled him over the years.]

J.   If I say, well, why are they, you know, comin' to me? Why they admittin' they willin' to help me if they're not. . . . And I began to understand, I haven't been allowin' them to help me. I remember the first night you came into the hospital to see me, and I could have allowed you to help me that night, but that was somethin' that . . . would admit everything needed help. Even though I was in a position where—in a place where I was bein' detoxified, but as definite proof, I just wouldn't admit that I need help and . . . would open up and allow myself to be helped. I have a little—in my pocket, I have a little passage I read durin' that time just before I met you in Riker's. . . . It was in the Christian Science . . . paper. It was somethin' that . . . Dr. Martin Luther wrote years ago, and it said . . . the topic was about "Where Do I Stand?" You know? And down underneath it had somethin' he had said. Dr. Martin Luther, he say, "Here I stand. I can do no otherwise. So help me God." You know, and I started thinkin' . . . I got to do this. I got to say, well . . . I have nothin' . . . I know nothin' . . . would you help me? I—I can't give you nothin' but my attention, my open mind. I wanted you to try to get me. I'm goin' to allow you to. I know you've been tryin', but I have been holdin' back. I got to try to get to you like we say and I opened up. This don't—what happened, a certain thing comes all of a sudden, but it just comes to a point where it'll always keep you in suspense. It looks good, that little bit, and you have to try just a little more and a little better and uh . . . you keep on doin' so. I was tellin' the guy . . . today, this mornin' while we was paintin' over there about—he had asked me why was I comin' here. And I told him in time I would be able to explain this more to him. That . . . there is no law against [here he means favoring] ignorance, and that's why I'm here, you know? I'm admittin' to bein' ignorant and missin' a whole lot, and it's because that I think the people can help me. So he said, "Well, lot of people come here expectin' help, you know, one hundred percent." So I told him, "Just to put you on the right track . . . it's only one hundred percent thing and that I have fifty percent myself. And that fifty percent that I have is . . . allowin' someone to help me. I've admitted that I need help, and I committed myself to this particular thing. And that is fifty percent comin' from you that your fifty percent is willingness to help me and my fifty is allowin' you to help me. See? I'm aware fifty percent that . . . you can and you have . . . gave me a shock. When I say a shock I mean wakin' me up. Really. And made me realize that I can be very important because I figured that respect, particularly things like ego, I've argued that point with Vic* a lot about ego. I didn't seem to think I had any ego when I was running with that junk out there. I told him that . . . things in my—my mind is used on a high level when I speak of respect and ego. I say, "Well, I don't have any of that particular thing." Not that I'm, you know, goin' through what I'm goin' through, but he gave me the idea that I was wrong . . . and everything that I would bring to him he would tell me that I was wrong. "There's one thing wrong with you," he said. "You . . . you have a false concept of everything. Your outlook on everything is completely false." He say, "You have channels here, you know? And you've just been put on the wrong one, and no one's been able to shock you and wake you up and get you out." So he said that "You understand that you have to admit that you need help before anyone can help you."

[The first interview ended abruptly when Justis had to leave to make an appointment. The second interview began with a lengthy discussion by Justis of a complaint that he had of having been wronged. He denied the validity of a laboratory report which suggested that he had in fact taken a shot of heroin.]

* Vic: Victor Biondo formerly of Exodus House, now special assistant to Dr. Efren Ramirez, the New York City Narcotics Coordinator.

S.F. *Did your older brother use before you?*

J. Uh . . . about the same time.

S.F. *Is there any connection between the two of you using, do you think? Did he affect you or you him?*

J. Well . . . I believe so. I could say so.

S.F. *In what way?*

J. Well . . . he and I were always very very close and uh . . .

S.F. *How much older is he than you?*

J. He's almost two years older. I was born January of '33. Just a little over a year older. Uh . . . I used to have to fight his battles for him . . . you know? And he used to always seem to take a lot of pride in me. If anybody was misusin' him, he would uh . . . go get his brother, you know? And uh . . . usually when uh we would get there . . . he would tell them, "Now my brother's here." And he was bigger than me, you know. Maybe that, you know, always made us feel close to each other, you know, but . . . no matter . . . uh . . . what, you know, how we disagreed on somethin', it was always the fact remained that uh we was blood brothers, you know? We could be ready to fight each other, but if somebody come and try to misuse the other one . . . we would just . . . you know, do opposite, you know. We'd forget uh we was havin' disagreement ourselves and uh . . . work together as brothers. I believe though that uh I could get him to go like me, you know. And uh we—my mother always had pride in us because uh up until we got a certain alike and people used to think we were twins, you know? And uh that knitted us pretty close together, you know? After we reached about twelve years old he grew taller than I.

[Justis himself points out that his brother outgrew him, but this statement is made in a larger context of his always having been his brother's defender in street fighting and elsewhere. The implication he wishes us to draw is that he was able to make up for his height with his fists.]

S.F. *But you think he used first or about the same time?*

J. About the same time. Uh . . . yes, about the same time. I believe he used it a little before I did. Yes.

S.F. *Were you aware of that fact, that he was using before you? I mean at the time?*

J. Well . . . yes . . . but I knew that he had used something, but, you know, I didn't know what it was or anything like that.

S.F. *How could you tell he was using?*

J. How could I tell?

S.F. *Do you remember something about his conduct?*

J. Yes. Uh . . . we were snortin' it, you know? And it would make you uh . . . vomit when you snorted, you know? You have to bring it up. And uh I asked him, "What are you doin'? What's wrong?" So he told me, you know. And the guy that gave it to him . . . had served some time in the army, and uh . . . was injured, you know? And uh . . . he came home an addict, you know? He was much older than we were, and uh my brother had told me, that's uh . . . where he got it. But I never heard of any and most certainly didn't hear any evils of it and he told me about that particular thing and what it does to you was never a mystery. I don't know why. I . . . it would do something nice uh I thought, but it was never a mystery to me, you know. I didn't even question it as bein' somethin' out of the ordinary. And with that . . . I started too and uh . . . I'd stay where it was the days when we were leavin' school [that is, after school hours] that uh instead of goin' home and goin' upstairs and acceptin' the family and the situation I, you know, would be able to be out in the street, you know. I couldn't even—didn't even have to think about the family, you know. When I'd go home I uh would be in another world and, you know, wouldn't have to listen to it.

S.F. *What particularly bugged you about your family? Then.*

J. Well . . . uh the relationship between father and mother . . . uh . . . my father uh . . . I remember as a kid uh, well, he used to drink a lot . . . and uh after his mother died, my mother told me that uh . . . you know, he just started drinkin' himself to death really, you know.

S.F. *How old were you then?*

J. Uh . . . about fifteen or fourteen. No, I was about twelve or thirteen. That was uh . . . the early forties. Now . . . she said that uh he was so attached to his mother . . . that she believed he was goin' to drink himself to death, but ever since I can remember him he was a terrible drinker, and he would get very violent, you know, when he'd drink. And uh . . . I—I—I somehow resented him because I could never . . . uh accept him arguing with mother. And uh I remember a terrible experience whenever it was about 1940 or . . . 1941—something like that. He had came home drunk . . . and uh . . . he hit her, you know. And uh . . . I could—I could never accept that. I remember I was so angry that I . . . I felt . . . like . . . Well, a child always says things, but I say, I felt like killin' him. Really! As—as a child, you know, just sayin', nobody in the world could hit my mother. You kiddin'. And I don't know, you know, about father and mother. I could say the same thing about father . . . but uh these things started to grow stronger over the years, you know. I couldn't . . . never find any fatherly love from him, and I always said I needed a father. And—

S.F. *Was this something you said after you started talking to the doctors in the hospital or did you have this feeling before?*

J. No. I had this feeling before . . . uh . . . well, it happened I had another experience uh . . . along after I was usin' drugs . . . maybe a year . . . that I—my mind got so twisted around seein' him argue with her, you know, and uh . . . I had to stop him, you know, and tell him, you know, and uh . . . I couldn't take it, you know. I said, "Wait a minute! You know, this is—this is no family at all. You a drunk and you—you—you're cursing mother and she's cryin' and uh other kids is here, and you're just yellin', you're just cursin', you know. Like what kind of dad are you? Why can't I grow up, you understand, and be a man that I could straighten you out. Really!" So I said, "I'd like to sock you right in your jaw. You know, I—I— I'm at—at the end of the line." So . . . he uh . . . I was about fourteen or fifteen then, I believe, and he get up and he smacks me across the face. And uh . . . I told him, I said, "Now . . . I'm goin' to always respect you as a father to a certain extent because you know I wouldn't strike you, but this is the line. I won't allow you to strike me no more." And uh . . . I held him by the arms and I pushed him back on the bed. I say, "Now . . . I won't uh allow you ever in life to strike me again because I've had enough of you." Uh and he shouted toward her, "I predicted!" So this is the time he told me to uh . . . leave, you know, and uh . . . uh . . . never come in his house again. And I was gone for a few weeks—

[Notice that in this Harlem version of the Freudian triangle, mother, father and child, the child defending the mother appears as a knight and the father as one whose strength lies finally not in his physical constitution but in his formal role as paterfamilias. Unlike the Freudian myth of the son killing the father, here the son is forced to leave the home and become more and more involved in the street life and hence ultimately in addiction. The son in this case plays upon the mother's love for him and upon the father's dependence upon the mother to get at the father through the mother and her illness. Thanks to the intervention of his mother's friend, as we shall see, he has his initial confrontation with a psychiatrist around the question of his relationship to his father. In the end, as he recounts the story, he returns triumphant. The arrogance and vindictiveness which might be objectively seen here are experienced by Justis subjectively as right and noble conduct. The concern with triumph over his father appears to him as love for his mother.]

S.F. *Where did you go?*
J. . . . Livin' in the street . . . movie houses . . . and about three weeks later I seen my brother . . .
S.F. *That was during the summertime or during the school year?*
J. Yeah, durin' the summertime. And I seen him and he told me that uh . . . he had been lookin' all over for me, you know. Uh . . . that mother was . . . uh—had became very ill, you know, very emotional upset because they couldn't find me, you know, and uh . . . bring me back. So . . . I thought and say, "Well, he told me nev—never to come back in his house again, and—and I won't go in his house again because I don't feel like I belong there." So . . . I refused to go back. So . . . he say, "Well, I'm goin' back and see mother and I'll let her know you was all right." You know? So he told her what I said, but I told him—he asked me, "Where you goin' to be?" I said, "I'm goin' to be at this movie all day." And when I

decided to leave . . . I didn't stay all day. I don't know which way I was goin', but I decided to leave and when I get outside they's there in the car, you know, a friend of theirs car what had came and uh . . . she told me that uh, you know, she wanted to take me to a doctor. So I told her all right. And we get to the doctor . . . and . . . she had told the doctor that the relationship that we have had, you know, how we was gettin' along, you know, that uh she knew that I felt that I needed another father. That I couldn't accept this as bein' my real father. So the doctor went through the routine of, you know, askin' me "Who is this?" I say, "That's my friend James." And "Who is this?" "That's my mother." "What's her name?" And he say, "Who is this?" I say, "That's my father." He say, "What's his name?" So, you know, he asked me, "Are you sure that's your father?" You know. So . . . at that particular point I got very upset, you know. And uh . . . I couldn't accept the fact of him askin' me was I sure that was my father, you know? And I told him, I said, "That's why I been havin' so much difficulty . . . I've got to stand here and say that's my father and down in my heart I don't believe it." So, I left them there at the hospital, but when I get out I walked and came to the house anyway, you know, and she had got there, and uh . . . he told me, daddy told me, he say, "I want you to know that I was drunk that night and uh . . . I don't know what I was doin' you know?" So, I would say, "I want, you know, to stay here—stay home, you know?" So I said, "Okay, but I'm only goin' to do it because mother's here. That's the only reason I'm goin' to stay here because mother's here." And we were livin' in the same house . . . and sometimes for two or three weeks at a time we wouldn't even see each other. I would make it my business to wait till he be goin' out before I'd come in, you know, because I just couldn't meet him. And . . . we met on the street one night . . . and uh I know he had seen me, and he didn't say anything to me, you know. Well, I was so burnt up over that, and I went and told mother that I met him on the street and he refused to speak to me, you know? She asked me uh . . . well, she actually told me that I should talk more with the doctor—the psychiatrist, you know, I shouldn't be wary of the psychiatrist. And that uh . . . they thought that the dope I was usin' was doin' this, you know? These

particular things, they existed long before I . . . even knew anything about dope, you know. And we—we—we built up a relationship
as somewhat like strangers . . . you know? And . . . what we used
to argue about all the time, he used to—he wouldn't—like I couldn't
get no conversation of him. A lot of times I'd want to talk, you know.
Like I want to know my problem and uh . . . I could never get him
to talk until he would start drinkin'. And uh then he would want to
give me advices, you know. I used to, right away, I used to revolt
against that quick, you know. "How can you tell me anything—any
advice?"

S.F. *Did you find that taking a shot in any way permitted you to
endure your father more or to feel better about him or some way different about him?*

J. Yeah, well it done somethin'. It taught me that uh . . . when I
take a shot that uh . . . I could uh take his bullshit . . . because I
was in a different uh channel—a different world, you know? And uh
why I would say to him, "How—how you goin' tell me anything?
You—you're half drunk, you know? How you goin' to give me any
advice?" And I would feel better when I'd go and take a shot, you
know, and uh he would start tellin' it, and I—I'd tell him right away
"Bullshit!" You know. And I would feel stronger bein' able to face
him like uh . . . "I don't—I don't feel like listenin' to what you're
sayin' because you're drunk and you're in one world and I'm in another world."

[At a time in his life when relationships with his father were still
ambiguous and Justis existentially was overresponsive to his father's words, heroin served as an artificial insulator desensitizing
him to conflicts between his father and mother as well as between
his father and himself.]

S.F. *It gave you a kind of courage to tell him directly what you
thought of him?*

J. Right. Right. And it gave me the courage to tell him . . . that
he had never treated like a—like a son—like my father. I used to ask
him, "Am I really your son?" He used to take uh . . . the other kids

out—he used to take them out to town on Saturday and leave me home.

S.F. *When did this happen?*

J. When I was a kid down South. But my older brother, it didn't seem to affect him, but he was older than me and he was able to drive the family car—take the car out, but I was never able to drive the car. I had a license, so it always affected me and uh I definitely could see as a child him takin' the other kids to town and he wouldn't never seem to take me. He could find time to play with them uh and uh . . . but I could never get that same time.

S.F. *Did you ever ask him why he did it?*

J. Plenty of times. He couldn't give me no uh no explanation.

S.F. *These were friends or—*

J. Yeah, well, these were friends uh but uh . . . the idea was he would take them out and he would play them, and I couldn't get the same . . . thing from my father.

S.F. *Was he paid to do this?*

J. Was he paid to do that? No. No. You know. And that's why there was *never* any understanding in—in—in my family then.

S.F. *When you look back on the period of the South is it all melancholy or did you have happy times also?*

J. I had happy times—happy times, and it was a funny thing, the happiest times I had was when he was away from home drunk. He used to go—be gone off for days. And those are the happiest times I knew when father wasn't there.

S.F. *What would you do in his absence?*

J. I—I would be free to do anything. Uh even if we—we—we'd do somethin' wrong, and mother would give us a spankin', she would give us a love-spankin'. Where it would hurt her to hurt us. You know? And uh I would enjoy a spankin' from mother because she would give me a love-spankin'.

S.F. *Is this what she called it?*

J. Yeah, well . . . you could see that it hurt her more than it hurt you.

[Justis' stress on the fact that it hurt his mother more than it hurt the son when she spanked him, I think should be taken as expressive of the "symbiosis" between mother and child found so often in cases of addiction. I do not think we can exaggerate the manner in which this physiological empathy manifests itself also in the case of addicts who can feel what each other feels when going through "changes" due to lack of drugs. Reverting to the mother-child relationship, it is not chance that so often an addict reports that the mother understands him without using any words and that the mother feels a comparable response to her son. This kind of mutual absorption suggests that the problem of separation and differentiation of parent and child remains a problem for the addict in his development out of addiction.]

S.F. *What did you do to merit punishment?*
J. Oh . . . anything, you know. We would go to people's orchard, you know, and we're not supposed to go in the field today to take watermelons today, but we go and we take them—anyway. She would tell us not to go to build swimming pools—swimming holes, but we would go and build them anyway . . . and uh . . . things like that. But, well, if you get it from him . . . you know . . . uh it—it was no good, you know? And uh I told him one time, you know, he was givin' me a whippin' and I said "Geez, this guy's tryin' to 1'll me." Really! You know. I could see—different, you know. "Why are you so mean?" You know? And uh he had three brothers and no sisters and all of them was just the opposite. All of them was just the opposite.
S.F. *Was he the oldest brother?*
J. He's the oldest brother. Right. And he has three others under him.
S.F. *What happened to his father?*
J. Well, his father died when he was a baby. Not a baby, but a little boy. And uh . . . his stepfather uh just died a few years ago. Uh . . . I don't know . . . my father—is somethin' seems to been wrong with his life. Because he has a brother—my father used to do things, you know, and his mother and dad had went out one day and left three boys home, and uh . . . one of his brothers, next to the youngest one, told him—had his shoes off, you know—and they had the chopping block on the place and told him to cut his toe off, and my

father took the ax and chopped his toe off. Now, today, he's got a toe missin'—really. And but they—they done it as kids, but I uh . . . was thinkin' after, you know . . . he said what kind of whippin' that uh . . . his stepfather did and . . . if I remember correctly, he somewhat resented the whippin' that . . . his stepfather gave him. . . . Because he think he whipped him too much . . . and he say uh . . . it would be there for a few days, you know. Seemed like every time he would think of it he would give him a spankin' for cuttin' the boy's toe off, and maybe—I never asked him did he feel it because it was his stepfather instead of his real father. So . . .

S.F. *Did you sometimes feel you had a stepfather too?*

J. Well . . . back then uh . . . I felt that it were . . . you know, and it took me a long time to accept the fact that uh he's still—he's my real father. And really, up to now, h—h—honestly speaking, I really haven't accepted fully now.

S.F. *Let me ask you another question, thinking back how you felt when you were a kid, when your father was around—not when he was absent. When he was around, did you feel anything about him, about yourself? Did you have any fears of any kind?*

J. Def—most certainly so!

S.F. *What were those fears?*

J. I could never be relaxed until he leaves. . . . We were doin' farmin' and I remember . . . and this is why today I always try to teach somebody just like a kid that's going to meet me at three o'clock, you know, when they get out of school. And uh my aunts tell me that uh I will always have good luck because I seem to have the gift to want to help somebody, you know? And teach somebody— have the patience to teach somebody. And this gets back to when I was a kid and he was goin' to teach me and my older brother how to thin out the cotton, you know, in the cotton grove. We had to chop the cotton down. We had never done this. Now this had to be demonstrated to us by an adult—somebody who know and uh—give us a chance at it and if we go wrong, show us again and explain it. So I— I—I—tells him that I could never forget that day that he carried me and my older brother out, goin' to teach us to chop cotton. And the first mistake we made uh . . . he kicked my brother and he snatched the—the—the hoe out of my hand and hit me with it, you know. And uh . . . that was the first mistake we made, you know? And uh from that particular point on, anything he would tell me to do, I would always do it. Now . . . not long after that he had the car, he had been drinking that Saturday and, you know, he was goin' to take grain and sell it and—and such things. So the car is parked in front of the house and the barn is somewhat—about a distance of a block —city block. And uh he wanted four bags of grain in the car, but I had so much fear for him, instead of my brother and I drivin' the car up to the barn, asking him if we could drive the car up to the barn, we, like fools, *lugged* it all the way up, you know? And uh I wound up with a bad back for a while, and uh we put these big bags of grain on our shoulders out of fear, you know. I carried one all by myself, and uh out of fear I used to carry fertilizer the same way, and uh . . . it—it's almost impossible for a kid to be able to lift two hundred pounds and move it, and that's how much those bags of fertilizer weighed, you know. And I would find myself uh—he'd tell me to do something and he'd yell, and I would have to run to do it because I'd be frightened, you know? And I would be—have with so much joy . . . when he leave, you know, that everything I wanted was released, everything was all right.

S.F. *Can you remember how old you were when you lost this fright?*

J. . . . Yes . . . the night that he slapped me and told me to get out of the house.

S.F. *That's when you lost it?*

J. That's when I lost it. I told him, at that particular point, I told him, "You wouldn't be safe ever puttin' your hand on me again, because I'm not goin' to set for no more." I—I was fifteen then.

S.F. *You weren't using drugs then?*

J. Uh . . . no—actually.

S.F. *No?*

J. I uh . . . had snorted a little, but it wasn't playin' no part—

S.F. *You hadn't had a shot or a snort that day?*

J. No, I don't believe I had. You see, what happened . . . it's a strange thing. I used drugs for a long time before I knew I was hooked.

S.F. *Right.*

J. You see what happened. I used to go two—three days sometimes without it. So, one day I had a terrible headache . . . and I don't know why I felt so bad and I didn't know what to do. So I'd say, well I got a headache and, you know, what the hell, I won't even go get no stuff. So, I was goin' and I see a little girl . . . that I knew and I used to go to her house, and uh she told me to come up. And I was tellin' her I felt bad, you know. I was goin' home. So she said, "Well, come and see mother for a moment." And, okay, I went up, and uh . . . the old lady looked at me . . . and she say uh . . . "Com' 'ere." Put the daughter in the other room and told me, she say, "You —you got a habit. You're hooked—you know that?" "What are you talkin' about?" You know? She say, "I know you're usin' junk, you know? I can see it—you're hooked. That's all you need is a fix. What do you shoot or snort?" And I looked at her, I said, "What the devil is this?" So, I told her, you know, I was snortin' and [Slight laugh] her mother was a drug addict, and she said, "Here, try this." And I snorted some, and I found out that I had a habit, what it was wrong with me because the minute I started snortin', the headache pains went away, the nervousness went away, and everything, and I—I'm strong again. And that was a time that I probably needed some to fix me up and didn't know about it.

S.F.   *Did you have headaches before then—before using drugs?*

J.   Yes. Yes.

S.F.   *Severe headaches?*

J.   Severe headaches—yes.

S.F.   *How often did they come?*

J.   Well . . . uh . . . every now and then. Sometimes a month would pass before I would have a headache. Uh . . . my sister was tellin' me uh when she came over to Riker's Island to visit me last year, she told me she said, "You know, I'm proud of you. You're in good shape." She's a little younger than I. I said, "What do you mean?" She say, "You—you have a very strong mind. You know, you fell on your head when you was a kid, you know." And I always asked her, "Did I really fall on my head?" You know? Because at one time, as a kid, I remember I could never figure out why I had what the doctors say was spasms . . . and I had it twice.

S.F.   *What do you mean you had spasms?*

J.   Uh . . . one time—I'm goin' to give you—tell you exactly what

I seen the first time it happened. We was at some people's house and uh it was a nice . . . summer day, and they had on the porch, they had a swing . . . you know. And uh . . . they didn't want, you know, me to run around the yard, you know? They wanted me to swing, you know, swing on the swing. Okay. The man and my father was sittin' over talkin' and I was in the swing, and the swing was rockin' and uh . . . all of a sudden . . . uh, just like you're sure as I'm seein' you sittin' there, I could visualize a big wheel like the kind that's on a farmin' tractor? And I would see the wheel rollin' toward me and I couldn't move and uh . . . I started screamin'. And the lady . . . she had some . . . what do you call tablets or some-thin'—ammonia, smellin' salts or somethin'. They gave it to me. So they put me in this car . . . and carried me to the doctor. Now the doctor say that I had heart trouble . . . and the next morning I wake up with chicken pox. Now . . . another time I was in bed and I waked up screamin'. I had a headache. And uh . . . my mother and father ran into the bed and uh I remember I was tellin' her I have a headache. "My head hurts. My head hurts." That's all I was sayin'. So they rushed me to the doctor this time . . . and uh . . . the same particular thing happened, you know. Like I came up the next morning, and I got this terrible, you know . . . breakin' out—this uh . . . popped again. So this was twice this particular thing happened, and both times the doctor said that I had heart trouble, and he told my mother this time, he say uh "His heart can't stand anything as strong as coffee, because if he drinks anything as strong as coffee, you know it might stop." And I was nine years old, I believe, nine.

S.F. *Was this down South?*

J. Right. And uh . . . I was tellin' my mother not long ago that same doctor died about fifteen years ago and uh . . . it wasn't so much the heart that was weak. It was the mind that was weak. I think he meant somethin' that I went through is a—is a father and son re-lationship, you know? Because my body over the past seventeen years, my body's consumed things that uh . . . it withstood so many things that people swear to God that I'm dead. I should have died. And that why I—I—I don't believe it was the heart at all. It was the mental sufferings that I was goin' through, and probably I might've been dreamin' that uh he was gettin' ready to whip me or somethin' and I was making an excuse. And I always told mother that—that uh I had dreamed sometime that daddy was givin' me a whippin', and I say uh I always would try to have a lie for him because I was somehow always afraid to tell him the truth. And uh I told her that I believed when I was screamin' I had a headache that uh he was goin' to whip me and I was screamin' I had a headache, and when I woke up I had a terrible headache, you know? But the doctor said it was heart trouble and I couldn't figure out why I had the chicken pox—one time it was the chicken pox, the other time it was a flu or whatever you call it, would be the result the next morning. But I would come with— the first time it was the chicken pox, the next morning I came up with the chicken pox. After havin' a spasm. It only happened twice . . . uh . . . and about the headaches I used to get, they used to carry me to the doctor . . . and the doctor couldn't find anything, and he say "Well, he'll grow out of it over the years." And actually I did. I grew out of it, but—

S.F. *When was the last time you recalled having headaches?*

J. Oh . . . in '63 when I got hurt in a subway station. I had fell off the platform in the Queens Plaza subway station in '63.

S.F. *How did that happen?*

J. I was . . . sick and dizzy—

S.F. *Were you high? Were you on stuff then?*

J. Yeah, I was on stuff . . . but—

S.F. *Goofballs or stuff?*

J. Yeah, I had had goofballs too, and I believe I had drunk some chloral hydrate before I left home from uh . . . Greenpoint in Brooklyn where I was livin'. But it was a snowy day and uh . . . a lot of people had tracked down, you know, from off the street and it was wet there. And uh I remember comin' down the stairs. I was real high . . . but I remember slippin'. And . . . I slipped on the stairs, but I wound up on the track, you know? When I slipped, I went . . . dizzy—completely, but I do remember slippin'. And uh . . . when I came to, they had called the hospital in uh—Elmhurst Hospital, and uh the doctors, everybody was there. And uh . . . I started to come to myself, you know, so he told me don't move, that I had fell and I might be hurt bad, you know. They was goin' to take me to the hospital. So they had me sittin' on the steps now and I was able to turn around, and I remember that I had slipped on the steps, and I asked the guy there, the one who—the man who took me off the tracks, "Did I fall all the way down these steps?" So he said, "Worse than that. You fell right off the platform." And somehow I got a headache when he told me that—that I had fell off the platform on the tracks, and I did find out from the time it had first happened until that particular time they were talkin' to me then, two trains had went through there. And uh . . . what happened when I fell, there was a train comin' into the station which was near the end of the platform. When the train makes it turn right in the station, you know? And uh . . . the men—there was three of them—what happened was, when they seen the train comin' in, you know, they all jumped down on the track and they said I was stretched across the track, and they thought I was electrocuted. They thought I was holdin' the third rail because that's where my hand was—underneath it. And they waited to, you know, the last moment 'cause they was afraid to touch me, you know. They was afraid, you know, they would get the shock too, and at the last moment they tell me that uh . . . the men talked between themselves. One of them got back on the platform and uh . . . one, you know, gave me a kick, you know. They found out I wasn't holdin' the third rail, and the two of them was able to throw me over and get back get on the side while the train was comin' in. The guy wasn't able to stop the train, and they told me that uh . . . it was just a split second that, you know, saved me. You know. And, oh, man! I started gettin' these terrible headaches and . . . they gave me some medication in the hospital. They kept me there seven hours and then discharged me, and gave me these pills and told me whenever the pain was very bad in the head that uh . . . get in bed and take one of these pills. But the pain would be so bad I would take two instead of one and . . . one day I had took the pills—it was on a Monday night and I had said I was goin' to see my mother on Tuesday morning. So I took the pills, you know, and I wake up and I *still* had a headache and uh . . . I took one more. And . . . I go out in the street and . . . somethin' seems to be wrong outside. I see people doin' shoppin' and the fish market is doin' big business, you know, and it looked strange to me people buyin' fishes on that day, and I found out it was Friday. And it was supposed to have been Tuesday morning, you know? And no matter what depended on it I could never remember what happened in between that time. And I found that when I started gettin' these headaches I used to try to take a lot of st—junk, you know, or somethin' to try to get rid of the headache. But . . . when I went away I was actually gettin' headaches then. I got busted in '64. But I—I went through a thing of not taking no medication and I found out that uh it was, you know, it was my heart that was doing it—had no headaches.

S.F. *Did you have headaches in jail?*

J. . . . Every now and then I'd have a slight headache because I wouldn't wear my glasses. I would see a movie or would watch TV and I would be able to know why I had a headache or what had happened or what I had done. I was watching TV and I'd go out in the ball park and, you know, be lookin' a long distance and uh I would wind up havin' a headache. And it happened a few times, I believe—

[Headaches seem an understandable physical effect of Justis' life style. The amount of rage that he experiences as well as the continual frustration, the exaggerated goals that he unconsciously sets for himself, and his idealization of himself and his mother, all these seem to me to set the stage for the headaches that he reports. In turn, these headaches undoubtedly gave him an added pretext for the use of drugs, a medical license, as it were. In this connection we notice that, as the discussion of headaches proceeds, Justis' associations take him back at once to his father and exploitation by his father.]

S.F. *I want you to talk a little more about this business of headaches and this dream you apparently dreamed about your father when you were a kid.*

J. Right.

S.F. *Tell me a little more about it. I know it's hard to remember but do you think there's a connection? That is, do you think that you sometimes have these headaches after a bad night?*

J. Well . . . not only after the bad night but also after, you know, the experience with my father. I remember once, somethin' . . . that hurted me very deeply. I used to work sometimes, you know, and I had worked once for four weeks with this guy who was buildin' this pasture up there on his farm, and Saturday he paid me. He paid me fifteen dollars on Saturday. Down South at that time that was a big salary, especially for a kid, and . . . when I got home I had to give it to my father. And I didn't get anything back, you know, nothing and my mother, you know, she tried to talk with him 'cause—because I had become very upset about it. "What the hell is this? You mean to say I worked all week and you're goin' to take my fifteen dollars, and didn't give me a dime back?" And it hurt me very much and I could find myself wanderin' out there in the field or out in the barn, figurin'—tryin' to think of somethin' wrong to do. Somethin' I could do to hurt my father that I wouldn't have to be around him to do. Hopin' that he would get hurt or somethin' would happen to him. As far as, say, hopin' someone would beat him up or somethin'. And he had a fight with a guy once, and came home, and the whole side of his face looked like it was opened up, but actually it was just one little scratch and it was the way it bled, you know? And him wipin' it with his hand, it was all over his face. And he came home and . . . I was very much frightened because he got a shotgun and he was goin' back and kill the guy with the gun. And my mother talked to him, you know. "You sit down and first I'm goin' to clean your face." You know? So, while she's cleanin' his face, I'm gettin' to feel different because she's wipin' blood away that's dry now, and I can't see no cuts and things, you know? Somebody's got to pay him for all this he's been doin' to me, I'm feelin'. And when she get finished, she told him that, "You know, you just got a pimple head the size of a match of a scratch here, and you're raising all this Cain and bull. You're goin' to go and kill a man." And I was angry myself, you know, because I wanted him to have had a big scar, you know, a wound, and didn't like the idea of my mother bein' able to talk him out of it—of him not goin' back, you know. I just wanted to see no sight of him. You know, because I was always afraid when he was around, and I would find myself, you know, bein' very much alone standin' out in the field and goin' out to the barn and I'd say, "You know? What is this, you know? I'm scared of my father. I can't ask him nothin'." I wouldn't dare ask him for any money or to go any place. I would ask my mother. And I used to tell her when she used to tell me, "You have to ask your father. Go ask your father." And I would say, "Mother, you ask him. You know I'm not goin' to ask him. You ask him. You know I can't ask him nothin'." And this I told my brother a few years ago, we was thinkin' back to the time we was down South and we, you know, not holdin' no grudge on this particular thing now, but we was talkin' about the time . . . we figured daddy used to play the shit on us, we used to say. He used to give us crops and say, "Five acres is there for you, and five acres is there for you." We were able to have any of these, you know. I remember when he made the excuse to us that the Agriculture Department, I believe, had to take away a lot of people's crops. They had too much on it. They was strict. And I've never been able to figure out why. And they came and they cut some away themself. They cut the amount of acres away that they said was too much, and that particular thing he said we could have it for our property. And he used that particular thing—that particular cop-out—that the circus had come to town. It came every year and this is the particular thing for us. When the circus came we weren't able to go, he say we had to move part of our crop, you know, and the other boys were able to go. And the last day of the circus was there, and my brother and I . . . people around the neighborhood were gatherin' their crops—their cotton to sell what you're supposed to sell. So on this particular day he had told us that the circus was next week and the man had called to say to pick the cotton. We call it crap cotton. That's what's left over, and say you ought to pick the crap cotton, and you can sell it and you can go to see the circus next week. Now it hurt me so, and I could never forget Ben Wolf. That was the name of a man on the circus. And this Saturday he had carried his kids to town with him to the circus, and my brother and I was pickin' this crap cotton. We were goin' to sell it and we would be able to go next week to the circus. And we was in the field, and when they came back from the circus that evenin', and a boy told me that, you know, "We wanted to stay longer, but they make you leave the circus at a certain time, you know." I wanted to scream. [Laughs] I say, "My daddy—you see what he done to me. We're here pickin' this crap cotton to sell it to go to the circus and he knew in the beginning the circus was closin' today."

S.F. *When you were a kid down South, what picture did you have of yourself? What were your ambitions?*

J. Well . . . a minister quite frankly. I always wanted to be a minister. I'll tell you what, the first time I can remember them mentionin' my mother's father. He was a minister and his name was Justis also. And . . . he—I never seen him, you know? And all the other family used to tell me I looked like him so much. That he was short and he always had a strong voice, and he was always demandin' because he was always tryin' to do right, you know? And he was a very good minister. And somehow, you know, never seein' him, I always wanted to be like him. I always felt I was goin' to be like my grandfather's boy, you know? And that's actually what I wanted to be, and I felt like—I found myself at times when I went to church . . . durin' the months of July and August, we used to have what you call Revival Meetings. It would last day and night for a whole week at one church. The next week it would be a whole week day and night at another church. Our church was in the middle of this and this would go on in July and August. And . . . I had went to church and I had told the particular minister there that I wanted to learn how to pray, you know? And I told him I thought it was a special thing to know how to pray and he asked me what kind of prayers do I want to pray, you know. The Lord's Prayer or what? What do you want to say? What do you want to thank the Lord for or what do you want to ask him for? And I say, I want to be able to know how to pray, and he told me, if you're sincere and want to pray, get down on your knees and pray. And that's how I learned to accept failure. I never can, you know? And if a person want to pray I like to see him kneel down.

S.F. *Do you pray nowadays too?*

J. Oh, yes, I'm crazy about the Lord's Prayer. And I set it up for singing. The lady used to play the piano for me, you know, and I was always proud to go to church, and I would—it was a funny thing, I would always want to be the center of attraction by sittin' on the back seat. And the night that I was—joined the Protestant church, you know, you have to stand up and talk, you know, and I was on the back seat, the back row of the church, and the church was a long church. And I remember when I was walkin' up to join the church, everyone was lookin' at me. And my mother had lost me, you know. She was there, but she had lost me—didn't know where I was. And she had no idea what was goin' to happen. She was three rows from the front, and she almost fainted when she seen me up there, you know. She told me how—how great it made her feel, you know, and they told me how proud I looked when I go up and shake the minister's hand, and you know . . . and really I thought I really was on the road of what I was goin' to be someday. I was goin' to be a minister.

S.F. *Did you inquire into it?*

J. Yes.

S.F. *At what point did you feel you could no longer be a minister?*

J. Well . . . when we came to New York.

S.F. *Really? Can you tell me why your folks decided to come up North? How old were you when you got here?*

J. I was . . . it was 1948. I think I was fifteen years old.

S.F. *In 1948. You came to New York—before you used any stuff. Right?*

J. Right. Now . . . I've asked my mother that, but I never really could find out, really, why they decided to leave, but I do remember that my father was sayin' once that all of a sudden he wanted to see one of his brothers who lived in the Bronx that . . . he hadn't seen his brother for quite a few years, you know, and he decided he was goin' to see his brother. And his brother told him "Well, why don't you move your family up, you know?" That's the best I've learned of why we decided to come, but I didn't want to come.

S.F. *You didn't want to come.*

J. Right. So what happened . . . he came November . . . '47, and my mother and two sisters and the baby boy came about the early summer—the next year '48—and my brother and I came in August of '48.

S.F. *Where did you stay?*

J. With my grandfather—my stepgrandfather and . . . I remember when my grandfather got the mail, and the tickets that came on a Thursday and we was to leave on Saturday comin' up. And they had difficulty 'cause I didn't want to go. I was goin' to run away. I didn't want to go. So when I got here, they had difficulty 'cause I didn't want to stay. That lasted two weeks. I couldn't hold any food down, I couldn't stand it, you know. I could see where I'd been taken out of a cultivated city, and put into a savage jungle. And I was comin' out of the country into the city, but it was just the difference. It was just the opposite. I was goin' into a wild jungle, you know, into the big city. And they wanted to keep me in the house for two weeks.

[Justis' lamentations in these lines indicate how strong were the negative effects upon him of the shock of different cultures; in particular, the transition from south to north. The image of the jungle of New York serves naturally as the backdrop for the development for justifying the kinds of things he did on drugs. However, ironically, as a con man, he tells us, later on he used his Southern accent to outwit the city slicks. Is it any accident that he retains the oral side of the South and builds it into a component of a manipulative pattern against the city?]

S.F. *What gave you the feeling of a jungle?*
J.   . . . Maybe—
S.F. *Are you sure this is how you felt then?*
J.   Yes. Definitely. Maybe the people around . . . well, I had my life cut out, you know? I was enjoyin' what I was doin' and . . . I was thinkin' ahead. Maybe I'd be a minister of the church I was baptized in . . . the particular church that I sang in the choir. Maybe I'd be minister of that church or whatever. My life was planned for this particular thing, and when they said leave here, you're goin' to New York City . . . New York City? Why we got to go to New York City? Why do I have to go to New York City? And, you know, they wouldn't let me stay, and when I got here . . . my resentment was there so strongly that I couldn't hold the food down or anything like that. And . . . everything frightened me, you know. This is not what I want. Where is our old church? Where is St. Paul's? And this is, you know, what I want—and it took about two weeks for me to accept that I couldn't go back, and I even thought of the possibility of, you know, *robbin'* in order to get some money to get back. Really! I wanted to leave, and I started to, you know, acceptin' it then because I started to findin' churches right away, and I also carried them.

But when I first came we only had two rooms, you know? And . . . that was also a problem. I can remember my house, you know? I can remember walkin' from my bedroom and by the time I'd get to the kitchen I'd walked a long distance.

S.F. *Down South, you mean?*

J. Right. And my stepgrandfather's house was so huge, we had room that . . . we used to invite people there just so somebody could use the rooms. The rooms never was used. Really. And this is the type of thing, I could walk from the porch to the front bedroom . . . back to the kitchen or the back porch or someplace . . . I'd be walkin' for a long time, you know? And here we have to live in this particular close quarters and things, you know? And I could never accept this, and they could never explain to me why they really consolidate me [?] from why they left, you know?

S.F. *How was school down South for you?*

J. School down South was different. Well, what happened . . . I built up somethin' in school that teachers was very strict, and they would give you a shellackin', but the thing that was most effective was, not only if I get a shellackin' from the teacher, I would get one from my father when I get home. You know? And, oh, man! That was somethin'. I remember the teacher slapped me across the face once— across the ear—somebody had said somethin' to me, and he was at the blackboard. And I had turned around to answer them, and the teacher caught me talkin' and hit me across the ear. And I told him . . . that I was goin' to, you know, kill him one day for hittin' me across my head, you know? And he didn't see the other person, but if he would have asked me, I would have told him, "Somebody asked me somethin' and I'm sorry, I didn't mean what I just answered. Really." And to add insult to injury . . . I got home and . . . my father whipped me again. And I said, "What are you whippin' me for?" So he say, "You know. It's 'cause you done somethin' wrong in school." So . . . he whipped me one time and he found out that he was wrong . . . you know? And . . . he told me, "Well, why didn't you tell me?" I said, "You didn't give me a chance to tell you. The first thing you done, you smacked me," and I fell in the corner, and the first thing I started doin' was pissin'. You know, water started comin' out. Really. And I say, "You didn't give me a chance to explain." So he say, "Well, you can hold a whippin' anyway because you probably did do somethin' wrong that I don't know about." You know? And I say, "What kind of understandin'—how is it that I'm going to accept it?" Really. And I used to stay frightened until they brought me to what I called a jungle—I mean a savage jungle, too. You know, takin' me to Siberia would have been better. Some place where I couldn't, you know, couldn't even see people.

S.F. *When you were a kid, did you wet the bed very often?*

J. Uh . . . no. But my kidneys were always pretty weak. It would happen I would, you know, somethin' would upset me. Such as him, you know. It would force me to do it. Right.

S.F. *To wet the bed?*

J. Right. If it didn't happen when he hit me, it would happen usually in bed. This particular thing got me so concentrated on bein' afraid of him that I would release my water in bed.

S.F. *What would happen then?*

J. I would have a terrific whippin' the next mornin'.

S.F. *From him?*

J. Right. You know, and actually every time he would do it, I would —this would be my concentration—to try to hold my water because that's what would happen each time. That I would be completely fightin' it up here, but here I would be completely unprotected.

S.F. *Can you remember the last time this took place that you wet the bed . . . how old you were then?*

J. Oh . . . maybe ten years old.

S.F. *Ten years old?*

J. Ten or twelve.

S.F. *Ten or twelve. This was down South?*

J. Down South, yeah. Uh . . . the night that he slapped me and he told me to get out of the house and I stood up to him—it happened then.

S.F. *You were fifteen then?*

J. Right. I was fifteen.

S.F. *That was in New York?*

J. Right. He hit me and I did feel myself pretty good.

S.F. *You did?*

J. Right. I did feel myself good.

S.F. *That was the last time?*

J. That was the last time, but at that particular point he could never hit me no more. Like I told him, "I'm not afraid of you any more 'cause I'd rather be dead than be fightin' mentally with you any longer."

S.F. *How long after you came to New York did that episode take place?*

J. Uh . . .

S.F. *Roughly.*

J. Roughly, the next summer.

S.F. *Actually, you were fourteen when you came to New York.*

J. I was . . . this might've been my sixteenth—right after my sixteenth birthday when this happened.

S.F. *Sixteenth birthday?*

J. Right. Let me count up my years. I was fifteen when I came. Right. This must have been my sixteenth birthday. Right.

S.F. *Can you remember roughly how long after you came to New York you took your first snort?*

J. Yeah. I took the same Christmas.

S.F. *You came in August and at Christmas of the same year you took—*

J. Right. But . . . I didn't see any more for a few months, you know? But actually that Christmas was the first snort—

S.F. *Were you lonely in New York?*

J. Was I lonely? Yeah, I was very much lonely. One thing that bothered me was the different religions. That bothered me.

S.F. *What do you mean?*

J. I remember a lady who went to a church and . . . they had the Shepherd—I—I was a . . . Soul Baptist, you know? And we had a particular religion that—it was that. I had never been to a Catholic religion. I never have been to a Catholic service. I didn't n'er have that teachin'. I've had the Protestant teachin'. I'm a Baptist. And all these strange religions and things . . . and things—in New York, people had these places. They want to pull you off the street and tell your fortune. You know? "What you want to tell my fortune?" You know? "Get rid of my father. You want to do somethin' for me—get rid of my father. Otherwise, you know, don't bother me. Why you goin' to do these strange rituals, you know?" And everything was so strange to me, you know, that I had to be experiencin' somethin' but it's a funny thing, I wouldn't drink at that time. I just wouldn't drink. For one thing I despised it, for another he drank . . .

[Notice the frequency with which the words "strange" and "understandin' " are repeated through the tapes often in what might appear to be inappropriate ways. Sometimes he is trying to express a narcissistic feeling but other times there is a genuine sense of the dread of living a life full of hostility that he knows might be turned against himself directly or indirectly.]

S.F. *How much money did you need—it wasn't very much I suppose in the beginning?*

[This third interview started with the request that Justis tell a little bit about the way in which he maintained himself on drugs.]

J. No uh . . . it wasn't very much money needed . . . uh . . . a job was all right—enough. Uh . . . it could get a lot of drugs—good drugs for little money then, you know. The amount you could get for three dollars when I started usin' would cost you thirty dollars now. And . . . it's no uh . . . the strength is so much different, you know. You could use it then—you could cut it a half a dozen times. It still was terrific stuff. You could triple your money uh . . . three or four times, you know, but uh . . . as the years went by . . . uh it has been cut now a hundred times before you get it and you definitely couldn't cut it any more. So, and it would cost you three or four times the amount that you were payin' for it then. But in 1951, when I went away to Lexington, I came out and I had a strange experience. I was uh partyin' with more than I was usin'. Uh . . . I was doin' a lot of stealin' and uh . . . I had a whole lot of money in 1951 when I came out of Lexington. And uh . . . I had spread so much money around buyin' junk and hookin' people up, you know, givin' 'em some—some uh dope to sell . . .

[Justis is obviously proud of the time that he was able like a Kwakiutl Indian to engage in conspicuous waste by "partying." The amount may or may not be exaggerated but the intent is clear. He himself next explicitly connects this period with increased involvement in the underworld. For many addicts a short period of illegal prosperity in their adolescence or early adulthood remains behind as a paradisaical memory that haunts them and gives them some residual strength and justification for feeling that they are not quite as bad as they look at present.]

J. . . . that uh I was windin' up partyin' a hundred dollars a day with it, you know, and that's givin' a whole lot of people, you know, wearin' and uh . . . I started gettin' on the wrong . . . uh . . . side of life by havin' this particular type of life with the—with the people I was associatin' with. They were uh musicians, they were actresses. They were a group that was in uh . . . I think you call it summer stock. They were playin' up in Boston, you know. At the time they were studying. They were still goin' through uh . . . school, you know, to be actresses and they were in Boston at a play, and they all came down and uh . . . I seem to uh enjoy this type of people, you know. Just the . . . just the psychological effect they took on me that they were musicians, actresses. I won't mention no names, but they were pretty big names and uh . . . I enjoyed this type of thing —associatin' with these type of people, you know. And I felt *so* important uh until the type of life I was goin' through before I definitely couldn't go back to there, you know. I uh that was the last thing I would do and still I wouldn't do it is go back to the same life that I was goin' through prior to uh that I was on junk. So . . . after associatin' with these type of people it became uh somewhat a demand that I had to stay on a certain level as far as hustling is concerned. I met a few people that were . . . uh professional con men. They were professional jostlers and uh . . . I had a little uh teachin' from these people. Uh . . . they would—

[The connection between the popular entertainment media and popular artists such as musicians and actresses, on the one hand, and the street addict, on the other, is a fascinating one. The addict not only gets the feeling of "mobility," but I think there is also the fact that the street addict who is a proletarian depending upon his wits and a stick, knife, or gun, feels a kind of kinship with people of talent who have no capital other than that talent, plus their equipment. It is no accident that musicians stand so high in the addict's regard. If one adds to this that musicians did smoke pot and use heroin in earlier years, then the connection is even made more intimate. The irregular lives of the entertainment people who are often night people also fits in with the irregular rhythms of the addict's life.]

S.F. *You actually asked them to help you or would they—*
J. Well, what had happened . . . uh . . . they all thought I had a lot of sense, I had a lot of courage . . . and uh . . . I somewhat lost my vocabulary over the years, but during that time, I had a pretty winnin' personality with the . . . people—especially those who had much more than I and uh . . . they believed that I had a natural gift—you know—that I could fool everybody. Well, one thing the con men told me is that with my Southern accent that uh you know, I could get far with this Southern accent because I definitely could fool a lot of people, you know, with the particular accent that I had. And uh, of course, me knowin' that the accent I had is uh . . . uh the real thing, you know. That's me. It's not somethin' that I'm tryin' to do if any time I speak and don't use an accent, it's because I'm tryin' *not* to. So, they wanted to uh introduce me to these particular games. The only handicap I had was my fingers was too short. But that was the only thing and that uh in time they could teach me to uh do that—overcome that small handicap and that uh . . . different con games they could teach me, you know. They called 'em the short con, the long con . . . and . . . the Murphy game where more people . . . was hit for that game than any game . . . out during that time was the . . . the uh Murphy, you know? Everybody was playin' the Murphy. But uh they figured that this Murphy was just for small stakes. They could hook me up on the . . . uh . . . big game. So . . . they started teachin' me and I started to . . . goin' around with these people and I found out that . . . the only thing that I had to do was to . . . play what you call stick man, you know.
S.F. *What do you mean?*

J.   Well . . . what happened uh . . . I wasn't actually the one who take off the sting, you know. I—I didn't have to be involved with the money. In other words, I would uh . . . do what you call put people on a crosstown bus, you know. I could uh . . . use uh my particular accent and have them believin' one thing . . . and the others was—would be takin' the sting off, you know? I could uh . . . transfer like—I could talk people into uh . . . goin' with a woman and uh . . . when the end came they never seen a woman and uh I never touched the money. They didn't give me no money and uh . . . someone else got the money and later we . . . we—we met up and I was makin' big uh money—

S.F.   *Murphy game?*

J.   This is uh one Murphy game. There was another one just a little different. And uh we also had a game they taught me as uh playin' shots, you know . . . jostlin'. And uh . . . they figured that I was better than anybody as it's been my stick—this particular thing. And uh . . . I want to explain again when I say the stick man is uh—draws all attentions to me . . . while they takin' off uh . . . we'll say the sting and uh take it off, you know, and they could cross and get the high sign and get stung, you know? And uh . . . I could uh talk my way out of the situation that I had talked my way into and uh . . . things like that built up a kind of confidence that uh . . . always uh . . . frightened me that I always had to use this on this particular people—this particular association. People that uh within the musical field or uh . . . some type of show business. Uh . . . when I would see them, you know, I would—my name was . . . known all over and uh . . . everybody somewhat uh would give me a standin' ovation when I would come in and uh . . . that put me on a pedestal that uh . . . uh . . . Now that I see how dangerous and frightenin' it was, but at the time I couldn't see any of it, you know. I was very important and these was the only people that seemed to . . . understood what I uh . . . was doin' or what I was tryin' to do. I could—I didn't have no sympathy for a man when I'd go out in the street and when—when I'd heist him—when I'd pick him off. I want to play the game on him . . . and uh, a few times uh . . . I had to go out . . . play the few games on a few men . . . and they were somehow somethin' hit them before the game was over and uh . . . I—I, you know, there was no sympathy, no kickback, you know. Like a few times you would find a lot of professional men who—by the way, you do find a lot of professional people who are professional thieves, you know.

S.F. *Really?*

J. Yes. And uh . . . in fact I know quite a few of them that uh—doctors and lawyers—that are very, ve-ery professional people and very professional con men.

[Regardless of the truth or falsity of this generalization about professionals being con men, what matters is that Justis is at once able to feel identification with a higher class and at the same time get a justification for feeling victimized by being arrested since these professionals presumably escaped.]

S.F. *Con men?*

J. Right. We say it's larceny, you know. Larceny uh . . . people think of larceny as bein' small model larceny, but uh larceny is larceny, you know. People do these things, and these people usually kick back when uh . . . they uh . . . you know, the people wake up to what's goin' on, but I was always—whenever someone would wake up I would like uh be anticipating this. And when someone wake up I would be ready to uh . . . you know . . .

S.F. *Be brutal?*

J. Right. Right. Use force. Right. And all this was because with a particular . . . hate that I had to—had built up for my father because of the relationship between he and I.

S.F. *Now, going back, were you ever arrested for this sort of con game you described?*

J. Well, yes. What happened . . . it was turned into a robbery because I wouldn't kick the money back . . . you know? The man waked up on one of these deals with—five bills, you know. And he asked for his money. He said, "Well, if you give me my money, I'll forget it." And I said that uh "I'm not goin' to give you anything back because I don't have anything of yours." This is the way I talked to him and uh I was on the subway. And uh where he made his mistake was he attempted to grab me and uh . . . when he did, you know, I socked him, you know. And uh by havin' so much hate at the time against men I could've socked him and left, but it was just like sockin' him and keep on sockin' him and uh . . . before I knew it . . . police was there in the subway . . . and uh he said I robbed him. So they charged me with robbery and, of course, the charge was uh reduced a little lower than uh armed robbery because I didn't have a weapon and uh I got a year out of it.

S.F. *What year was that?*

J. Uh . . . 1953. Right. Uh . . . if uh durin' that time uh when these things happened, if a person would never know that I took 'em, it always took some kind of effect on me. I think I wanted them to know or if they didn't find out uh that I had took them I would be quick to go right and take someone else, you know? Usually when a person take a sting off, they are satisfied, and they go and lay in the cut you'd say. But uh usually if anyone didn't dig that I was takin' them uh I would go and take off somethin' else, but usually if uh they would dig I would be somewhat satisfied . . . some kind of way. And uh I could always say uh, you know, if it was a man I took off it was all right because they *deserved* bein' taken off . . . you know. And uh when I started to gettin' a different . . . uh outlook uh . . . or shocked, you know—I have strange words that I use . . . wakin' up or shocked. You know? Uh . . . flip side and such, you know. The record when I say flip side, I mean the record is completely turned over and . . . it started to frighten me, you know? And uh it was a strange thing. I uh couldn't uh find things to . . . to try to compensate for what I had done in the past or the feelings I've had and I had to do all this without makin' the people aware . . . of what I had been doin' in the past. And . . . it . . . was even uh . . . yesterday that I had seen a man that I had tooken off. And uh . . . I seen him on the street, and I called him. He was across the street. "Hello there!" he called me and he came over and he started to talk. And after we talked, he told me he was glad to see me, and after we talked for about five minutes, he told me that uh "I'm amazed at you. You know. I'm proud to see you. You looks wonderful and you sound good, you know. Comparing your attitude from the last time I seen you," and we kept on talkin' and he told me that uh . . . he understood at the time when I had done somethin' to him. Now he

didn't understand, but his wife did . . . and she could relate somehow that I had a particular hate for men for some particular reason,
the reason I done this to him. And I could face her, you know, knowing this is the wife and this is the husband and after it happened—she
owned a hat shop—and I would go into her hat shop sometime and
stop and talk to her and she would see me walkin' the street past
there, and she would stop me and "Come in," you know, to speak
with her as if nothin' had happened and I knew she knew what had
happened to her husband, you know. That I had uh . . . took him
off and uh he lost a couple teeth by it and uh I started to talkin' to him
yesterday, and I laughed and say, "What are you wearin'—a partial
in your mouth?" And he laughed and he say uh "You wearin' one
too. Right?" So I said, "Yeah." So he asked me how did it happen. I
told him a man hit me with a ball bat. So he said, "Well, maybe uh
the man hated men who hit you with the ball bat at the time. Do you
forgive him?" I say, "I forgot him years ago—long time ago when it
happened, you know. Right after, I forgot it." So I started thinkin'
uh maybe the same thing happened to me happened to them, you
know? Maybe this was someone else who had the same type of relationship . . . who had no feeling toward men as far as not uh hurting them and uh just hit me with the ball bat, you know? And uh I
was lucky it didn't break my jaw, but it uh loosened uh some of the
teeth. But I could never bring myself to uh look for this particular
person to hurt him when I could very well see any man and uh con
him uh . . . if he resisted, you know, I—I would always be uh prepared uh be ready to try to knock him out or somethin' like that.

[Observe how the transition from verbal conning to physical assault
takes place under the spur of the drug need. The effect upon Justis
is that the world continually appears to be a jungle more so than it
does really for addicts of a different life style.]

J.   This fantastic feeling, you know, that uh . . . keeps you in a—
in a jungle where you . . . you have to fear everybody and you
workin' on another basis tryin' to get the others to fear you. Because
of uh you—you—you have to get back some way. I uh always said
I had to get back at what my father was doin' to me . . . and even

though my father, who's well, he's an old man now—he's old man,
I'd say he's fifty—four years old . . . and uh all of these things, I see
now that he wasn't responsible for. I can, you know, just see them
now. He—he's not responsible for those—because over the years he
turned out to be an alcoholic, you know? And uh . . . he—he's definitely not responsible for these . . . I wasn't responsible for mine,
I see now and I know that he wasn't responsible for his. It—it's a
matter of bein' able to understand somethin' uh, you know, someone
wakin' you up—uh . . . not bein' ignorant, you know?
S.F.   *Well, I was wondering, you talked about the con games; if you
were so full of hate, how is it you didn't go in for mugging? Or did
you?*
J.   I . . . I never said I didn't.
S.F.   *I see. Tell me about that.*
J.   Listen . . . I had a muggin' habit once.
S.F.   *Really?*
J.   Right. Well, it's a funny thing . . . uh I'm happy that it happened this way. Didn't nobody resist me too much. . . . You know
what I mean? And uh I was on 106th Street and Columbus once. This
was years ago, years ago—long time ago and uh it was rainin' one
evenin' and just where the bus turns on 106th Street and Columbus
to come to Manhattan Avenue I believe to make another turn . . .
uh I snatched this guy—a man. And uh I drug him over to the doorway. And I believe that was a bar . . . a side entrance or somethin'
they didn't use and uh, a strange thing happened, because when I was
draggin' him over I wasn't chokin' him too bad and he was tellin' me
"If you'll let me go, I will *give* you the money. You don't have to
fight for the money." And uh I was thinkin', if I let this guy go, he
might be a police even. He might come out with a gun, but I'm prepared to snuff him if he does. And I let the guy go . . . and the guy
went in his pocket and took his money out and handed it to me. And
he had forty-three dollars, I believe, that he gave me. And uh . . .
somethin' went wrong with me. I—I—I—was satisfied with the
money but I wasn't satisfied with him. Somehow he didn't resist no
kind of way and every particular time I had mugged somebody, none
of them resisted—none of them resisted. Uh . . . not too far from
the uh . . . I had went on and not gettin' no resistance from the first

guy, I snatched the guy and I drug him off the street into a hallway—not a hallway—the vestibule, you know? This someone's private house . . . and uh I turned around when I got him inside the vestibule and uh . . . was goin' in his pockets and he was like uh, you know, yellin' and carryin' on. So . . . the yellin' didn't bother me but he didn't try to hit me or stop me or anythin', but he was goin' in his pockets also. I was goin' in his coat pocket. He was goin' in his pants pocket and a funny thing happened. He was just pullin' money out . . . green, and droppin' it, and he wasn't givin' me no kind of fight and . . . only once did uh . . . well, what happened if somethin' else was happenin' and uh after . . . this particular thing happened I decided to take the guy's money. But uh . . . we had started a little misunderstanding with knives, you know, and uh I was able to stick him before he stuck me, and that—that—that made me take his money then, after it happened, but that was the only time, that uh durin' a muggin' or anything that uh anybody was hurt, you know? Because they never resisted, and this particular time that I had stopped the guy I was muggin' him in the beginning, but that was the last thing that I had done. After I had stuck him I say, "Well, I'll take your money now, you know, and you're lucky you're still alive." But he wasn't able to do anything then because I had s—s—s—you know, stuck with the knife, and he went into a different phase of a . . . uh shock, you know?

S.F. *When you went out mugging, when you had that habit, as you call it, did you always go out by yourself?*

J. Yes—*always!* Always by myself. You see what happened . . . uh, it's a funny thing, you know uh . . . I always figured . . . if uh . . . you tried to help me listen and uh . . . I tell you everything correctly, you can't help me unless I tell you somethin' that sounds fantastic, and then you'll be able to find somethin' missin' in there. Because if everything is still on the level uh you could never find nothin' wrong, no matter whether if it's somethin' runnin' fifty miles an hour and n—no—no faster than that, but if it's runnin' fifty miles per hour now and a half hour later it runs forty-nine, you'll be able to find something not functioning right. And uh . . . I've always went by myself because what had happened, and always happened to me by myself. Now, I could never find this happen to no one else that would affect me like it did. It had me completely on a different uh separate bag. I was by myself and uh . . . it was like a thrill. Whenever I take somethin' off I didn't want to share it with nobody. . . . As far as havin' a partner in what I was doin'. And uh . . . I would say uh to myself, well . . . John or Frank or George uh . . . now, uh . . . didn't hurt him or didn't hurt him, you know? Now . . . uh this is not *for* him. This is *me*—this is somethin' that I feel. I don't see . . . no one else bein' involved in it, you know? And everything I done I had so much hate, so much resentment that any particular thing that I went in to do I felt capable of doin' it with this —all this resentment and hate backin' me up. You know? And uh . . . I must emphasize strongly and many times that I've never been resented, and uh . . . I had . . . stuck a place up with a gun once and uh the people didn't resent uh didn't uh . . . do anything at all and uh when I got dough I went out, I got very angry because no one tried to do anything. And then I started callin' them names, you know, and tellin' 'em that the men—"Every man here is—is—is a punk," you know? Uh, you see, to the women "You see, the men don't even try to protect you." And *one* man stepped up and I shot at him— right away. And uh, you know, when I shot everyone fell on the floor and started screamin', but I went out. But uh . . . I seemed to uh . . . always wanted someone to . . . back down, to try to stop me because uh it—it's different now in the way I feel toward men. You —you—you believe that and—and people in general. Uh . . . I— I'm doin' a flip side now. I mean, anything is realistic. It's nothing fantastic. You know, there's nothin' strange. Some things become a problem, but it's not hard to analyze it and work it out. And uh I've always wanted some man any place to uh . . . try to stop me. Uh couple of times I hit a guy upside of his head with the pistol . . . uh . . . that's because he—he give me just a little bit of trouble. He wasn't fast enough for me.

S.F. *Weren't there women who did this to you also, who—*

J. Well . . . I—I—I never had any difficulty with women . . . because women, I don't know, Mr. Fiddle, uh, somethin' is strange and I'll probably be a lifetime tryin' to figure it out. I've always got a way with women and—and a way women seem to uh enjoy me in some fashion. Now, I've had a few women to say bad things about me, but they wouldn't do anything. I could feel somethin' different, you know. I could *act* different with women because what happened uh . . . what was so strong is the love I have for women—the female. Because I always figured every woman should be like—is like my mother because uh . . . my mother . . . I've always said my mother never sinned, if sin is what I believe sin is, my mother has never sinned. And uh she won't smoke, she won't drink, and she won't use uh . . . no kind of uh—uh—uh—profanity and uh she think everybody in the whole world is the same, you know. A total stranger —she would have the same feelin' with a total stranger as she would have with a newborn baby . . . you know? And uh I told that uh . . . many times that "You—you are too good, honey. You're too real—too pure. You should sin. You should have uh animosity toward something." But she never did, and I always felt that women uh were somethin' different. And uh it's a funny thing, I still feel that way today. Like uh . . . and a woman could win my heart any time. Really. I can't stand to see uh a woman bein' misused.

[In general the first person the con man cons is himself. In this instance Justis' exaggerated description of his mother's perfection fits into not only his pride but also into his need to appear to be sincere beyond words and to be the recipient of some special aura by virtue of his being the son of such a perfect woman.

His essentially Freudian interpretation of the Oedipal influences on him has a special point here. He is not thinking purely in causal terms when he says that his relationships to women are molded in the light of his relationship to his mother. He actually is thinking in moral terms and saying that the reason why he is such a good guy is that his mother is such a wonderful person. The overwhelming evidence which he gives is that in effect he selected women toward whom he could act in a fairly passive way although he might beat upon them once they were within his emotional field, as it were. The glibness with which he offers the Oedipal interpretation is for him probably a source of pride in that it shows understanding. But the fact of the matter is that his passive relationships to women were exploitative. He shows a desire to put psychological distance between himself and those women. His not having married may well have Oedipal roots. It is characteristic, however, that he stresses what he deems to be the positive values of the mother-son relationship in this context. By convincing himself that he is acting in the light of an idealized image—his mother—he gives himself the feeling of being unique and different from most other addicts who, it is obvious to him too, also exploit women for their money. When he does that, however, he submerges the exploitation into a larger frame—that he is a misunderstood knight.]

J.   And uh no matter what type of education or understandin' or teachin' that I get for the rest of my life I'll *always* feel this. That uh a woman, see—I—I came up from a child with this particular affection for—for women because of the early relationship with mother. It was two different cultures with mother . . . and dad. And durin' some of those years I asked my mother, "How could you put up with this guy this long? You got to be *more* than perfect to put up with the guy, you know, and uh . . . because of the . . . *shit* he does, you know." Like uh . . . I told her, you know that's not right what he do and you know—he would even revolt against her goin' to church sometime. He would uh make false accusation: "Well, uh you probably goin' to see your man," and this and that. And I would get *so* angry till I had told him once, "How the hell can you say she is goin' to see some man? And look at the children she bore for you— seven kids. And you say she's goin' to see some other man and she put up with your shit all these years, and you're accusin' her of goin' to see some other man." And uh . . . this is one of the things that happened four or five times, you know, during my early childhood that I had to leave home, you know, by him tellin' her to, you know, these particular things, to get out. And the last time it happened, I told him I wasn't leavin'. Now I told him "I'm puttin' my foot down and I'm not leavin' uh—uh—uh my mother with somethin' as wild as you are because I definitely hate you" and—and—and I have to— the same thing that I felt that he did for me—hated me. "You hate me and I hate you. You're a devil and I'm a devil, so you're not goin' to hurt her. I'm goin' to stay here and protect her because that's the sweetest thing in the world. And she *never* sinned and never done anything wrong, and uh . . . somehow she's tryin' to look after you. She's tryin' to hold this thing together. I don't know how she got mixed up with you in the first place." And she would tell him not to . . . say anything to me—not to argue with me because she know how upset and violent he would make me. She would always tell him uh, "Don't say anything to him and 'cause you know it will upset him." And he—there was a point where he couldn't say anything to me until I said somethin' to him, and uh I would sometimes try to communicate with him and I would say somethin', but I could see the . . . the unsteadiness in it, you know. He was overanxious and uncertain, you know, about it, that uh he would try not to show too much, and while doin' such he would, you know, show too much, and it usually would come out the same thing: "Listen uh I want you to uh . . . behave yourself when you go out," and right away, I would st-start my, you know . . . my shit. "There you go . . . givin' me that bullshit advice," you know, I would tell him. "You know I don't go for that. How are you goin' to try to tell me to do somethin' that's right," and it might be a time when he was drinkin' and that would really, you know, blast off, you know. "How the hell can you tell me somethin' when you're half drunk? You goin' to tell me not to use junk or you're goin' to tell me not to go with this crowd . . . and uh you're half drunk yourself. You're goin' to tell me to be in at ten o'clock or don't go out tonight, and you didn't even come home for the last two days? Now, how are you goin' to tell me this? You're tryin' to hold your family together and what are you goin' to tell me? Can you give me advice?" And this would uh . . . would uh . . . make me uh . . . you know, tryin' to cut myself off from him, you know? And uh . . . I—I would always be with a problem like I need a father. And uh . . . everytime I would go out I would see a kid with his father, and especially when I'd find out they was father and son, you know? That would really—really shock me, you know? Why couldn't I have the same thing with my father, and then right away I would start to . . . "That son-of-gun," you know. Really. And, like I say before, I always tried to say that he wasn't my father durin' that time because I say I do not believe that a father . . . uh would be the same way with his son. Uh . . . I told a lot of people

302 PORTRAITS FROM A SHOOTING GALLERY

the reason I haven't uh . . . got married . . . and raise a family . . .

S.F. *I wanted to ask you and forgot to ask you, have you ever been in the position of being a pimp?*

J. . . . Have I? Oooh, listen! . . . I had . . . was fortunate enough to have two brand-new automobiles by women who . . . uh . . . was my women. You know, I had three women at one time. And uh . . . I would never want anything like that again. I want one woman now. Really. Understanding woman . . . and that's all. And I don't want no woman to—to go hustlin' for me. I'm not goin' to refuse no woman who has a job . . . I love honest people now—and if a woman has a job and a woman would accept me uh . . . it's on the highest level, I would like to . . . raise a family but, as I said before, I've never went into that because a person has to be in my—my—my mind, top level. And this woman that I had, that bought me the first car, the other woman envied her. Now . . . one bought me a brand new Oldsmobile and the other one envied her so she went and bought me a Chrysler.

S.F. *You were hustling broads?*

J. Yes, yes, I was hustlin' broads.

S.F. *When they were on stuff?*

J. *Yes.* They was on stuff, but one—one of them uh . . . was a—a Lesbian . . . and she used to tell me *"For you—I'll—I'll pull you any women you want . . . for you."* Now . . . a man can't have a woman unless the woman want him. Really. If—if some guy would get sharp and go out and say he can pull any woman he want—he's a liar! If a woman don't want you, you can't have her, and this is what happened. She wanted me and she told me—well, it gave me such a boost that a few guys had been tryin' for years . . . to uh pull her, and these particular guys was uh pretty, you know, had a lot of money. They was in the underworld, but . . . uh these guys should have been the one who pulled the woman, if the woman was that particular type that would fall for a man who's got a lot. I didn't have a dime. I told her when I met her, "Why do you want me? I don't have a dime. Why do you want me? I would like to have you—yes. But why do you want me?" And uh . . . she couldn't explain it and uh, well, you know, like we matched. You know, we were *for* each other.

Okay. And she told me she would pull any woman in that I want.
And uh . . . I couldn't mention no names, but she pulled one particular girl and the girl was very, very attractive, and everybody went
for her. And uh . . . I was with her one night and she told me uh
she was going to show me . . . how . . . easy it was for her to do
for me and how easy it was for her to buy me the car—that it would
take no time at all to get the money. . . . So she called a guy . . .
and she spoke two different foreign language other than, you know
. . . what you and I are speakin' now. And she called the guy . . .
and talked with him for a few minutes and . . . while she was
talkin' he say "Well—okay." And go in his pocket . . . and he gave
her five ten-dollar bills. And she told him, "Okay. Well, I'll see you
later then." He said, "All right." So, she came back to me, and so I
said, "Now, what went on?" She say, "Well, I promised him . . . that
I would see him later . . . and uh . . . the guy don't know whether
I'll see him later or not." But she was *so* attractive, you know, and uh
every man would see her would uh, you know, start thinkin' of ways
to . . . you know, come up with a lie to his wife that he's got to go
uh meet his buddy about the golf bag . . . or the fishin' rod . . .
guy wanted to build a . . . put a—got to put a new hull on his boat.
Guys would start, you know, gettin' these ideas when they would see
her. Especially if she would uh . . . you know, smile or somethin'.
And she told me that uh that's how easy it was for her to get money
from people. And she say uh "As far as myself . . . I'll get this.
That's enough. I don't need any more." So, she say, "You my man.
That's all I need is a man, and you're the man that I want . . . because there's somethin' about the way you . . . use yourself . . .
your heart, your attitude—especially toward women that uh . . .
won, you know." And this girl put somethin' in me uh . . . somethin' that was *terrible* to even think of. I thought I was the greatest
person in the world with three women . . . two new automobiles.

[Here Justis is looking at himself from a distance and saying that
his apparent pride in his self was caused by the extreme attentions
given to him by these three women. This is a curious example of
the way in which symbiosis affects both the woman and the man.

One suspects that if one were to interview the women they would stress their generosity and show pride in the way in which they were able to dominate him.]

S.F. *Were they Negro . . . white?*

J. Uh . . . two of them was white. One of 'em, when I say she was white, people figured she was white. She was Spanish really. She was from uh . . . Spain and . . . she was the one who speak the different languages. And uh . . . didn't no one know she was Spanish, you know. She definitely didn't look Spanish. She looked more . . . I would say white than she did Puerto Rican—uh Spanish or whatever. But the other one was a colored broad that was a Lesbian, jaspers, you know? And uh when I first met her she told me right away, you know, "I take you, you know?" But it's a funny thing, she say, "I'd like to be your woman, but uh . . . uh I want it where you understand, that I have a woman myself." So I say, "Well, I—you know, I can read you, baby. Like you should have one, you know. I'll accept that. Why not? Uh . . . she'll be *your* woman, and both of you will be *my* women. Will *she* accept that?" "Sure, she'll accept that. She's my woman. She goin' to do what I say all the way." And uh when this thing is goin' on, I start to thinkin'. "Say, Justis, you— you're pretty swift, baby! [Laughs] You know? You pretty swift." It—it—it—hooked me up and uh . . . a funny thing, I stopped usin' junk on account of that.

S.F. *Really?*

J. Yes, I did. Uh . . . when I got pinched in '64 I wasn't usin' no junk. . . . That's the reason I started usin' junk. Now . . . uh . . . but I wasn't usin' no junk and that's all. I wasn't usin' no junk but I didn't know what to do. That—that's the time when I would drink and I would do a lot of smokin', you know, pot. And . . . what happened . . . two days before I gets pinched . . . uh Peggy . . . had an abscess on the leg where she had shot some junk in the leg. Bombitas, it don't mix with . . . and it caused a knot to come in the leg and get sore and I had to carry her to the hospital.

[The following are excerpts from the fourth tape.]

S.F. *Are there any characteristics about yourself that you don't like?*

J. Well, just a small amount of uh—maybe suspicious of others—just wonderin' how—what sort of level do I uh—deal on with them when I uh . . . put the present against the past, you know? And uh course since I'm buildin' up so much in myself that little fear seems to be wearin' down but it still exists to a certain extent.

S.F. *Can you explain to me about this fear?*

J. Well . . . uh . . . everyone that know about the past these are the people that I'm associatin' myself with now that the amount of fear that I had whether or not they would . . . uh . . . really accept me as uh—what I hope they would not uh . . . somethin' that's uh . . . can't do anything with. I've had some pretty bad showings in the past. It . . . uh . . . stuck with me a long time that I would be years tryin' to clean it up with these people and somehow I seem to have that little bit of uh . . . of easiness about it whether or not—how is the level between us—you know. Not the way I stand . . . how I can see . . .

S.F. *Which level are you talkin' about now?*

J. Everybody that I associate with. You, the whole staff over here. I uh . . . it was a big thing I was thinkin' of before of uh . . . when I decided to uh . . . go into this I was just wonderin', you know, uh . . . how would I be reaccepted. Now this played a major role in what happened when the urine specimen came back and right away I told all the guys in therapy that uh—I had a strange feelin' that the staff wouldn't look at me on the same level since this thing came up and uh—I've tried every day to observe everybody and just see but I couldn't see no change that I would put on a lower level. This played a major role in that really it's uh . . . it's uh . . . there's still a little bit of uncertainty there and I feel like it's only natural and it's gonna wear off completely in due time with the uh . . . sense of understandin' and control and such that uh . . . I'm—I'm buildin' up now and as I said before in time all that slackness be completely drown out.

S.F. *Uh . . . are there any other things that you don't like about yourself?*

J. Well . . . no, I can't say that I am because I'm—I'm tryin' to be preoccupied all the time with positiveness and—and, you know. It's very seldom that I see any negativeness. In fact I'm—I'm—I'm not doin' anything that I can say, well . . . somethin' I was sorry for doin'. Even if it's just a thought run through your mind . . . that's only natural but I have a positive defense for that.

S.F. *Do you ever feel any of the anger that you used to feel?*

J. I can see it. I can recognize it. I can remember the times when such things made me angry and I can uh—laugh now and say it's impossible for these things to happen again. The change that I start makin' in Riker's Island . . . guys that knew me from the street there . . . it was a long time before they would accept what I was doin'. They wondered why things don't excite me—don't upset me and why have I got to always go along with the yellin' the police do making us wash the windows and washin' the walls and I would never complain and uh . . . a incident happened—I had broke my glasses and I had two officers and two civilians and I was discussin' it with them and another officer came over—he thought that I was in trouble or somethin' and he say uh . . . no, whatever you say, I'm with him, this is the officer sayin' to the other officers and a civilian. He say uh . . . "This is the best inmate in the bakery. He don't argue, he don't bitch about nothin', all he do is just work-work-work. I don't think he can get angry." So everybody despised the officer and they couldn't understand for a long time why I didn't despise him because it's another defense that I've set up and all of these things that seem to given me headaches in the past has made me angry and all that it's impossible now. I know more about myself and it's impossible for things like that to . . . to upset me . . . make me angry. I . . . uh . . . funny thing what I get now what I call an angry it's just uh . . . maybe . . . uh . . . works in a condition where I would be nervous or I would sit and think and I would debate it. . . . I couldn't be impulsive . . . I couldn't be angry over it. I would have to debate it . . . anything that uh . . . would seem to come up and uh . . . I would find myself sometime, speakin' somewhat harsh but it's not through anger and the people that I'll be discussin' it with will see that it's not through anger that it . . . sometime in order to get a point over . . . I have to talk fast sometime or they would strongly demand it sometime but the others who you are associatin' with could see that it's not anger but it's a little amount of frustration only but it's not anger.

[Justis here makes explicit the mechanism by which he tries to separate frustration from anger: through communication. He uses the
con man's skill, talking, to break up the connection between being
frustrated and being angry. As soon as he experiences frustration
he talks it over, he talks and talks and talks.]

S.F.   *Are there differences in your feelings about sex off drugs now
compared to when you are on drugs?*
J.   Well . . . well, yes. I believe there is. It—it—just—it's hard to
explain, you know—it's two sides completely. When you're on drugs
and when you're off drugs. When you're off drugs you enjoy life no
matter what it is . . . I enjoyed gettin' wet Friday in the rain—I
enjoyed it, that's all. And uh—a lotta people I could see was angry
for gettin' caught in the rain . . . I got caught in the market and I
was really drenched when I got home but it didn't bother me. Really
. . . I was happy with life . . . enjoyin' life and—and—sex will be
the same way. So when you're competent at what you're doin' and
uh—whatever you might feel.
S.F.   *So now you are enjoying it more, you're saying. Which means
that when you're on drugs you really didn't enjoy it.*
J.   No. No enjoyment whatsoever.
S.F.   *No enjoyment at all. Have you ever been really in love with a
girl?*
J.   Well, no, I cain't say that I have. I couldn't say that I was really
in love 'cause I was never in my right mind. I was always under the
influence of drugs. And uh . . . I find now that love is something
that you can't put in one spot—you have to spread it around.
S.F.   *Ha-ha. What do you mean by that?*
J.   You have to . . . well maybe that's a stigma are visible and all
of it need attention so I can't disregard one and put all my love on
the other so I just have to . . . have to . . . split it up. You know,
give everything consideration and a certain amount of love . . . you
know . . . that I wouldn't get lovesick over one thing and neglect
and lose somethin' else.
S.F.   *At this point do you feel lovesick about anyone?*
J.   Well, no . . . I don't feel lovesick. I'm able to uh . . . uh . . .
how would I say this . . . to uh . . . leave in myself a lotta de-

mands . . . how would I use that phrase? Deny myself . . . there's a lotta luxuries that I realize that I have to deny myself of some kind of social entertainments or coeducational entertainments that I feel that I have to deny myself at times and I'm able to accept this—I'm able to jot this down in my book. I'm workin' on somethin' and insteada leavin' a loose link weak . . . just tighten it up, that's all. And then I use the braces of . . . uh . . . my past, so I say to myself a few times, "Well, do you just hafta go out tonight? Do you remember all of those nights in Elmira you didn't go out? All of those nights in Riker's Island you didn't go out? You—you didn't hafta go out and so you don't hafta go out now"—and sometime I go in and all I do is carve all evening when I leave here and stay in and five o'clock in the morning I'm fresh and new again, you know.

S.F. *You know what I wish you'd do, Justis, I wish you'd tell me if you can recall what happened after you left the hospital last time. How long did you stay in the hospital?*

J. I stayed a full cure at Manhattan General—three weeks, I believe.

S.F. *Right. And then what happened?*

J. And I came right back out and started usin' drugs again.

S.F. *What? The same day?*

J. The same day. Yes.

S.F. *What was behind that?*

J. I don't know why. It was one of the—weakest moments that I have had in my life I believe because it was a panic on.

[If drug addicts were purely rational hedonistic personages as the punitive police policy assumes, then during a panic period, when there is a shortage, Justis, coming out without a habit, would not go around looking for drugs. He would realize the odds were against finding any and, furthermore, would feel no strong urge to get them. But in point of fact, as the discussion unfolds we see that the drug meant something very special to him in this situation. He was extremely alienated and humiliated by his Welfare situation and the drug met the need for some kind of ego support.]

S.F. *There was a panic on in the street?*

J. Right.

S.F. *So that the stuff was hard to get.*

J. Right. So we ran around for maybe three days before we got any. I can't understand that but somethin' happened after usin' two weeks. I stopped usin' and then I was arrested uh . . . a month or so later. I wouldn't use but I had stopped usin' but that's all—I had stopped usin' drugs.

S.F. *Let's go back to the day you left. When you left did you want to take a shot?*

J. Did I wanna take a shot? I don't know whether I did or not because I . . . I would say when I left the hospital I had no intentions on usin' it but I never gave it any thought. I hadn't even took time to try to figure out the . . .

S.F. *And then what happened when you left the hospital? Did you go home?*

J. I went to Welfare. And uh . . . after I left the Welfare I went and got a room where something happened before I got to the Welfare— I went and got me a bottle of wine, you know, and sat there at the Welfare all day. Then after I left I went and got the room and uh— I throw my things on the bed and without even sittin' down and restin' just left and started lookin' for the dope right away.

S.F. *Can you remember what it was that made you do that?*

J. I can't say. I didn't have anything upstairs strong enough to hold the fort really and uh—it was just—but after a couple of weeks go by I got disgusted somehow . . . I say . . . uh . . . I don't need no more and . . .

S.F. *It was a panic period. That meant that that day you couldn't cop. But what did you do—go around talkin' to the guys?*

J. We was lookin' . . . ridin' cars and goin' to different neighborhoods. It took us two and a half to three days.

S.F. *Were you at all sick?*

J. Yes. I was sick really. Not only mental sick but I could feel physical sick.

S.F. *Even after the full cure you still felt something?*

J. Right. Right. Then I would get these strings of butterflies in the stomach—and uh—sniff in my nose . . . really I felt physically sick as well as mentally sick. Somehow I felt that I had to have it that I . . . I, you know . . . that's my shot.

[Justis again spoke about his Southern church experiences. We pick up his conversation as he generalizes.]

J.   Everytime I would go to church I would be able to get uh . . . uh . . . what I call now that I have a new lease on life on what I was believin' in what was singin' to . . . to blot in there . . . the stigma that was causin' . . . I was able to . . . to . . . to wear that stigma down, to tear down that wall when I make an appearance in church and so I would say uh . . . well, he could be as mean to me as he want to be and still not stop me from goin' to church. He don't have to be here with the car when it's rainin' or snowin' I'm still going . . . that's uh . . . I'm gonna be there that's the only good thing there is and uh—maybe I took that blood after my mother and her father was a minister also and maybe I . . . I just got that blood after her side. She's very religious herself. My mother always has been.

[It is remarkable how similar Justis' discussion of the effects of religion upon him is to the discussion in the very first tape of what heroin meant to him. Is this not some unwitting corroboration of the orthodox Marxian theory of religion as the opiate of the masses? In each case he is talking about a traditionalistic mode of behavior, the old-fashioned Southern church and the ritual-bound conventionalized life of the addict.]

S.F.   *When you came up North, that was in the summer in '48, there was a period before you went to school, right? What were you doing then around in the city?*
J.   Dyin' in it and tryin' to find a way to get back, really. I couldn't say really what I was doin'. Everything were a different, different world altogether. Buildings, the street, people and no one were friendly . . . everybody was strangers and I wondered why did they take me from civilization and put me into a jungle. This is how I felt and there wasn't much that I could say that I done constructive . . . even thinking nothin' . . . that I could say that I done.
S.F.   *Were you able to find any new friends?*
J.   Well, a few . . . only when I started goin' to school but they were seem to be a different type of people than the people down

South. Everybody had a different way, you know? How they look in the streets and on Sunday and no one is goin' to churches . . . bottles is coming outta the bars and backyard . . . I seen people drunk all over the street. This bothered me, y'know? And I say uh . . . and I had to be brought to a jungle like this? And it . . . it just was a different world altogether and nothing . . . I couldn't do anything to standin' there I was confident I could make it through what I wanted to do or anything else constructive.

S.F. *Mm. Uh-hmm. These friends that you formed—did they come to your house?*

J. They did then, yes.

S.F. *Were you at all invited to be part of a gang?*

J. Well, yes, but uh . . . that I never approved of being a gang of the type that they had in New York and I couldn't find no good clubs you know to uh . . . join. And I just refuse any type of gangs.

S.F. *Why?*

J. Because they were violent gangs. They were just for fightin' and robbin' and I had none of these evil thoughts then. So I refused to become a member.

S.F. *When you were a kid down South what was the reputation you had among neighbors and friends?*

J. I was . . . well, one thing I was one of the greatest singers in the church and the hardest worker . . . I used to pick more cotton than everybody and I would keep feuds goin' in the neighborhood where men are tellin' my father that they bet their boy could pick more cotton than I . . . it was uh . . . somethin' I loved to do . . . you know. Just this particular type of work that I was doin' . . . pickin' the most amount in a day and uh . . . could nobody pick more than I.

S.F. *You had feuds with people . . .*

J. Well, no, not to the point where anyone would be angry or anything but uh . . . if it were in a feud between me and the guys that I were always racin' with it was just like the association between a young boy and a young girl. Puppy love . . . just like that, uh-huh. It didn't mean anything much. But it gave me great joy.

[At this point Justis offered some recitations, essentially poems by Longfellow, such as he gave down South.]

S.F. *Tell me, how do you feel about being on parole? Is it of any value to you?*

J. Yes. Well—it doesn't bother me really. It doesn't bother me. Well, for one reason I never believed the parole people could be interested so much in and uh . . . a parolee, you know? From what I see now when I go down, my parole officer is proud—is proud of me and another member of the Exodus House program. He has two parolees in Exodus House. Now, one of the greatest things in the world that he want is to see us make it, really. They very interested over there and they is very, very decent and understanding . . . that uh . . . he's not like a parole officer, he's like somebody tryin' to help, really and uh . . . he's very proud in his office to see us and if we meet up down there goin' to see him when uh . . . I'm sittin' down he'll ask me where's my friend and I'll say he's outside and he say go out and send him right in and usually he tells me I won't keep him so you can wait for him and you know we go together and that . . . that . . . helps a whole lot . . . you have to see some of these things, be part of some of these things to really know it, really understand it and I have been on parole quite a bit but this is the uh first time that I been able to understand the Parole Commission 'cause I—I—'cause there's a few parole officers down there that I've seen them givin' their guys a lotta trouble. Ralph [another member of Exodus House] —he has a parole officer, he's havin' a lotta difficulty with him really, everybody has difficulty with that particular parole officer but the Parole Commission itself and some of the others are very understandin' and makes parole very helpful to me. It's like I'm not only am I learnin' about myself and seein' things here I'm learnin' to understand and be understood on the same level with the parole people, you know?

[For many minutes Justis rambled on about his troubles with the Welfare Department, his attitude toward church and jail, parole, etc. Then we went back to discussing his behavior on drugs.]

S.F. *You mean that even taking a shot didn't calm you down?*

J. Well, it calm me down—yes. But I had built up such a terrible hatred for life in general, you know, that uh—it would be easy to get me to a breaking point where I would do something that, you know, something heavy, you know? But . . . there has been quite a few times that uh—insteada doin' somethin' I say what the hell I gotta go and take off first and I go and take off and I say what the hell, what the . . .

S.F. *But it did cut down a little bit on the—the violence.*

J. Right. Right.

S.F. *But at the same time the life that you were leading was causing you to get violent.*

J. Right. It calls for being violent. Only the ruthless survive, you know? And you had to be . . . be that way in order to survive.

S.F. *It's rather peculiar that the way of life in your case promoted violent tendencies but the use of the drug appeased the violence. Fantastic, isn't it?*

J. Mostly indeed. I think drugs saved my life.

[In saying that heroin saved his life Justis is not only indulging in characteristic hyperbole but he is also showing how it is a magical woman who comes to save addicts despite themselves.]

S.F. *Really! How did that happen?*

J. By the time I started to use it I had uh—well, I was cut off from my *real* life that I had expected to have, I got to a point where I guess I just started to get evil and when I first started to use drugs a couple of years I was—began to get real mean until people like school kids, people in the neighborhood said that they bet that I wouldn't live to get twenty-one years old so right after that time you know I really got hooked, you know.

S.F. *What is it that you were doing that they accused you of being mean?*

J. I was mean, you know just like—uh I get to the breakin' point, you know, be ready to fight, you know . . . so uh . . . a lotta people said I wouldn't live to get twenty-one years old and I made 'em all liars, you know, 'cause dope was cuttin' down on the violence, you know. That's why I say it saved my life really. 'Cause a person in the street usin' drugs he's got to be violent to a certain extent. I seen three junkies get hooked up in the street the other day two of them held the one and they try to cut his eye out.

S.F. *Really!*

J. Yes . . . tore his shirt off him. I was across the street. I just sat on my stoop . . . I didn't get near . . . and the police, funny thing, the police passed twice and seen it and stopped but they pulled away. Every time they pull up one of the guys would take the knife and go and hide underneath the truck, you know? So when the police would pull off they would go get the knife and stick in the guy again. So the last time the police came up they threw the knife down and they had to let the guy go and the guy started runnin' so people was walkin' aroun' the block to see if they would find the guy 'cause they figgered the guy would run around the block and fall dead, you know? Many times they had scufflings but he didn't show up, you know? And this is the kind of thing . . . an . . . an . . . 90 percent of the people that's has to do those things out there usin' drugs can be trained really. They really are not that bad. It's just that they *has* to be in order to su-survive. Probably, probably . . . probably that sold him some dope no good or probably beat them for their stash or something, you know? But they had to—they *had* to do that there because they were in that life and that's how they survive. You got to . . . got to make up a lotta things, you know, you gotta practice goin' through the mirror and practice and think I got to do this if it means goin' away for ten years with it. Like uh . . . a guy beat me for my dope and I got to break his leg, I got to break his arm or somethin' even if I have to go away for ten years I got to do this.

S.F. *Why? What's involved in it?*

J. Survivin' in it. That's the thing a drug addict has to build up, you know? In order to survive. So you can be violent in two ways. You can be natural violent, I mean through . . . through ignorance, but the others has to be through uh . . . going through on the streets you have to . . . there are all kinds of situations and every situation has to adjust and that's how they has to adjust to situation of drugs to be very very violent and that violence that they be and only pertaining to the life . . . life in the street and using drugs. So . . . so . . . if a person is weak out there usin' drugs and has no evilness toward that a person bein' shrewd, always connin' him, con him all the time slick, you know, gotta be smart, be able to think fast, gotta get this quick dollar, ya gotta beat the other man to it, right? And ya got to be mean violently in order to hold it or somebody'll try to take it from you, so you gotta protect what you have there and ooh! believe me you wind up killing somebody and that's somethin' that these guys were tryin' to do to that guy over there right in the street. And they . . . they had to project this thing so bad until one guy's holdin' him and the other guy's got the knife and the guy you know keeps him in front of him so the guy won't cut him, you know? And uh . . . the other guy is tryin' to run around so he could cut him so the guy that's holdin' him told him, "No, don't cut him, give me the knife," and he took the knife from his partner and you know and stick the guy on the other side and people was yellin'. They were right in front of a filling station. People were yelling, you know, and when the police car passed, somebody yelled and called and they looked back but they didn't stop. They may go turn around and come back and they just parked across the street and they sat so the guy still holdin' the guy in the collar and when the police pulled off he had his brother get his knife in front of the truck, you know, and give it back to him to work on the guy some more. That's how they had to survive . . . they had to survive.

[Justis is explicitly describing and outlining what might be called the survival theory of ethics. Taking a view that life in the underworld is comparable to Thomas Hobbes's "War of All Against All," he comes to the conclusion that violence and the ability to take violence are functional. His own style of life therefore makes sense within the confines of the "jungle." On the other hand, life outside of this society has tended to prove meaningless to him until his recent entry into Exodus House.]

S.F.   *Was it this way all along or did things get worse or better as the years went on?*
J.   Ooh . . . it gets worse as the years go on because uh . . . what happen is . . . a person can either get weaker or somethin' or stronger or somethin' . . . what I'm sayin' is if I uh . . . if I have to beat somebody up today for misusin' me or somethin' I'm prepared to beat him up the next day if necessary and whoever he bring along with him, two, three, four, five, whoever it is. So this doubles as the

days go on, as the time go on and uh . . . in other words, if I get enough of every time somebody do me wrong and right away I break his head, so I do this a half a dozen times, see, so I . . . I . . . it's nothin' to me now like uh . . . I'd just as soon as break his head as look at him 'cause if he cross me I'm gonna do it right away . . . no waitin' and uh . . . 'cause I got five or six notches in my gun already so at this point, since that doesn't bother me. The next step I'm on now I'm on the next level . . . I'm on the level now of shootin' . . . I'm on the level now of even killin' him maybe, and so when you get past that stage, well, when you get to the level where you . . . you know, all this built up . . . it's trouble, you got more and more every day, I feel.

S.F. *But in your case, even though things have gotten worse and worse, something happened to you that made you want to get out of that.*

J. I was afraid.

S.F. *Afraid? What do you mean? That's interesting.*

J. Afraid. Now . . . because I was too . . . I feared nothing . . . I wanted to fear something . . . I—I—I got to the point where I would say uh . . . that uh . . . I wasn't afraid for that but I refuse to let anybody take my life; now go on on this, you know . . . I'm not caring about that goof over there or that guy over there . . . him lookin' for me with no gun, you know? I'm not afraid to die but I tell you what I'm gonna do when he meet me and he got one I'll have one also so I say I got to fear somethin' . . . I'm scared to death . . . I gotta get outta this really so uh . . . I was afraid of my own self, really, because I was beginning to feel which was a fact that uh . . . I had no control over myself. I had no control over myself. It's like I would say of some cases uh . . . I would be hopin' that nothin' would happen to me because I don't know what I would do, you know? And uh . . . I was actually afraid of myself.

S.F. *You mean you were afraid to go to jail for life?*

J. For life or somethin'. I figgered that I wouldn't, you know . . . didn't have control enough to say whether . . . so what the guy beat me for $100 . . . I'll have to . . . you know, I'll let him get away with it or I get on away from him or somethin'. I knew I didn't have enough control to do anything like that and uh . . . what would happen where I really would have no control *if* a guy, say . . . a guy runs away with my money and I ketch him and maybe I got the knife or a stick or somethin' and uh . . . the guy started pleadin' with me and uh . . . he don't have any money to give me but he pleads with me . . . wins me by pleadin' with me and if I let him get away he promise me that he'll come up with the money. Now, he can get away but the very moment that he shows just a little bit of resentin' . . . uh . . . gonna stop . . . I have no control over myself then at that point because the moment he stop and say, "Oh, man, you're like uh . . ." that—at that particular moment he'll be in trouble . . . he'll be in trouble. Like I would be afraid because if . . . even to get into those situations because I know I have no control over myself.

S.F. *But you say that during those times, even though you are using heroin, you still have this fear of losing control?*

J. Oh, yes.

S.F. *Heroin wasn't enough to control you?*

J. Well, yes . . . it done a big job of controlling. It did bring the control down to a lower level and it would keep me from uh . . . you know, the point where I would uh . . . kill somebody and think nothin' of it . . . you know. . . . I couldn't do anything like that but uh . . . it did tone me down quite a bit.

S.F. *So it didn't remove the rage but cut it down.*

J. Right. Now, it cut down the—the—thing that I came up with . . . the type that was in me before—that I had to live with—built up inside me before I started usin' drugs. Now another one took over after I got out there in the streets, you know, chasin' the bag and uh . . . runnin' into all these strange people and uh . . . I developed another one out there and that's the one you has to live with out in the streets. It's the way to survive—you gotta survive out there. But the one that it toned down was the one that was pushed inside me over the years.

S.F. *Let's suppose that you needed money, right? You are on drugs. This is years back and suppose someone said to you, look I'll give you two choices, whichever one you want will be all right: (1) assaulting or threatening to assault or mug somebody for money or (2) conning him out of the money. Now, either way you get the same amount of money—the question I have for you is this—which one of these two ways would you prefer if you had a choice?*

J.   I have to con. I have to talk him out of it. Definitely. Now, there would be time though, I must tell you this, that I would prefer muggin' it . . . there would be a time. Because sometime a con game is gonna take you maybe hours . . . maybe all day or all night . . . maybe two days, right, for gettin' this money so now I might want to win it now . . . usually very few dope fiends can be con men . . . you . . . you lose the con game after a while when you start in usin' dope . . . case you get impatient . . . you see they invent games they call long con and short con, you know. Some of the games last uh . . . goin' outta the city . . . it took me six months one time to get some people's money and they will swear today that I didn't get it . . . everybody else coulda got it but me . . . they wouldn't believe that I got it really . . . and it took me six months to get 'em. Now, I was able to prolong this work this long time but there are times when I got to have money that I would say, oh, the hell with you now, talkin' this lane outta this money, I'll take this money off now, you know? And I would go and take it but I prefer talkin' him out of it because I . . . I've walked away from people and they beg me, please, here—and they give me the money and I felt good. I thought I was great but I was losin' this by usin' dope and I used to tell myself—baby, why don't you travel across country with a couple of people and you just talk people outta money—that's all you have to do—ha-ha. Talk 'em outta money 'cause uh . . . I've seen people . . . I've left them and disappeared from them—they found me and come and give me the money and I say, Justis, you are somethin', baby, you not like uh . . . you can talk J.C. out of his money! You know? Why don't you stop usin' dope? Because there were times I would go out an' throw a brick where I could've been patient and uh . . . but dope made me uh . . . dope came up before— Do you have this on? [Here Justis is checking to see if the tape recorder is on]—and uh . . . I would go . . . I shouldna tipped that old dude off like that, I coulda, you know, talked 'im outta half of the money but instead I go and I say well, 'cause if the man is givin' ya one the man is not gonna give ya all of it—if a man give ya money and saves somethin' but he's certainly not gonna give you all of his money but if you take anybody's money you're takin' it all.

Here is a man whose very language bubbles and froths under the force of his emotional states. Sometimes the very tapes he made—and he made six in all—border on the incoherent and at other times they spray color and tempo upon the listener's ears.

As a boy Justis was divided between rage and love. The rage was generated by what he felt was his father's mistreatment of both himself and his mother. The love derived from his symbiotic tie to his mother. He was torn from the traditional Southern surroundings, which gave him a sense of integrity and a measure of satisfaction, and brought to New York. It took many interviews fully to get Justis to describe the months after he came to the big city, but the picture is one of great depression during this period of confusion and resentment. The fact that he took his first snort of heroin during the Christmas season is, I think, no accident. He was yearning for reintegration to a traditional environment and was receptive to his brother's and his neighbor's son's offer of heroin. That he got immediate satisfaction was due not merely to the drug's pharmacological traits but as much to the life situation in which he found himself. Under heroin the paranoid style, with emphasis on rage and violence, took over. Heroin permitted him to act as though he were fighting his father. More exactly, the addict culture with its pretexts and spurs to get money gave him the channel in which to express this hostility.

But this same addict life gave Justis a way to use one of the talents that lay within him, his gift of gab: his capacity to use language to manipulate people. This gift he had had down South, and now, using a Southern drawl, he was able to set up con games by which to get money. Two life styles were fused in Justis and apparently without inconsistency. However, there is no doubt that he preferred the con game as time passed and he became more and more full of fear because of the repercussions of his reputation. A rumor spread about his death because the rumormongers really hoped and expected that he would die a violent death.

He was apparently frightened more and more by his own conduct, experiencing more and more estrangement from himself as well as from the world around him—both addicted and nonaddicted. Even the use of language to con others involved him more and more in the pseudo life pattern, in the feeling of not being for real. This feeling was intensified by his encounter with the Exodus House staff in prison and out and I believe that he found our program at a time when he sorely felt the need for more valid contact with social reality. Our stress on existential encounter, for example, and the necessity to be true to himself seem to have had special meaning for him at this point of his life.

On the other hand, Justis has a long way to go because the very processes and life style that I believe attracted him to Exodus House, in turn, limit his growth. As long as his verbal defenses can operate he has his rage under control. But this very dependence upon language limits the degree to which he will open himself to frightening self-encounter that he has not fully made even in the group therapy. What the future holds depends upon the rhythm of his growth and his growing self-acceptance with all his past and uncertain future. Would he be able to handle the sexual conflicts that he sought to cover up by his too facile recollections about being pursued by women? Should the defensive conning structure be broken too abruptly, it is always possible that he may revert to the use of drugs in order to control the rage if the rage itself has not been sufficiently diminished. However, at the time of this writing his prospects look quite good.

PART III

THE CHALLENGE OF ADDICTION

CHAPTER 1

The Unity and Diversity of Addiction

The sockets of their eyes were caves agape; their faces death-pale, and their skin so wasted that nothing but the gnarled bones gave it shape.

—DANTE*

Throughout this book we have seen, as interwoven threads, the unity and the diversity of addiction. It will be useful if in this concluding section I will make more explicit the different threads and the manner in which they are interrelated.

The unity of addiction derives first of all from the fact that it is an exaggeration of a state of modern man alienated, free, and even hollowed out, somewhat as shown in Dante's image of the glutton. The existentialist features of addiction that I have outlined form an idealized image that gives an impression to outsiders of great uniformity. A second source of unity is the fact that addicts share in one way or another a jumbled yet structured culture with its own language, mythology, codes, and hierarchy. A third factor, of course, is the pharmacological one, the fact that addicts subject themselves to a common drug. Finally, there is the psychological unity which some people have expressed in the misleading conception of an addictive personality which may well turn out to be the kinds of predictable responses that can be found because the drug induces in the addict a set of pseudo needs such as the need to get the fix

* From the *Purgatorio*, Canto XXIII, "The Gluttons," translated by John Ciardi.

to remove the symptoms. Here, too, would be the famous impatience, impulsiveness, and low tolerance of frustration so often found in the addict.

Now, these social, psychological, and pharmacological sources of unity are matched by equivalent forces of the same levels making for diversity.

Though the remote outsider, be he a layman or a professional, tends to accentuate the tendencies toward a monolithic structure, the addicts themselves stress how different each addict is. The ideology of individualism is itself a force for diversity. I have pointed out that there are different life styles; and in fact the same role, for example, pushing, is performed differently by different men. Many men are forced to push, but when a man who is essentially a retreatist pushes and goes through numerous contortions in order to avoid the police, he has to quell his anxiety. Others, such as the flamboyant paranoid, will test the acuity and acumen of the police by pushing right under their noses and laughing about it. Their life styles modify the sameness of the roles within the market context.

Again let us note that existential anguish, while common to all addicts, has different places in the personal economy of different addicts. For example, take the three men whose portraits I have detailed: for Billie and his depressed life style anguish is the very hub of existence, giving tone and grayness to it all; for Justis and his paranoid style anguish is but an underlying pretext giving a rational basis to his hostility and grievances; for Manny's obsessional form of existence anguish is a proper emotion to be experienced by one who falls mightily short of his goals, ideals, and norms. For another addict the retreatist anguish may be a source of detachment.

Again, the tendency of wanting everything one wants right away, which underscores the addict's relationship to his drugs, is modified by his constitution—"his system"—as well as by his life style. Moreover, the more successful the addict the more heroin he is likely to get and the more he is likely to develop a big habit which makes him all the more impulsive. These individual features of a man's life will, therefore, diversify this apparently monolithic trait.

A new factor which affects both the unity and the diversity of addiction is, of course, state intervention.

I might also note that merely because a man is fitted by his "style of life" to commit a certain type of crime, it does not necessarily follow that he will choose to commit it. For example, two men may pursue what I have called the pseudo life, but only one may choose to become a con man. The other may become a burglar, rationalizing that his habit is too large and too strong for him to engage in the long, time-consuming maneuvers required of the "big con." However, and I am thinking of an actual case, it turns out that such a burglar will not break down doors or crack windows, but instead engages in artful strategies for securing copies of keys to enter noiselessly only luxurious apartments.

This diversity and unity of addiction mirrors a kind of "deviant cultural pluralism" that has been permeating the general American society in recent years by which such groups as homosexuals, nudists, conscientious objectors, and others are allowed to feel that they have, more and more, a legitimate place in the general framework of the American idea. This trend runs counter to monolithic and monopolistic trends in the United States. Correspondingly, totalitarian trends in addict society squeeze down on the forces toward diversified life styles. Which of these internal forces will dominate in addict society is uncertain, but clearly the kind of programs that are subsidized for treating addicts will play a part in this internal battle. If punitive programs win out, then totalitarian trends will tend to be favored, but if the treatment programs themselves are more diversified, then the richness of these men and women will come more and more to the surface, and I would speculate there would be an enhancement of their chances for re-entry into the general American scene.

CHAPTER 2

Treatment

Obstacles to Effective Public Management of Addiction

There are a number of reasons why addiction to drugs is liable to remain in the public eye for the next decade or so.

Whether there be fifty thousand or a hundred thousand or many hundreds of thousands of addicts in the United States, the fact is that, thanks to a combination of punitive laws, the appeal of drugs such as heroin, and the development of an underworld distributing organization, an addict culture has been evolving over the past fifty years. Located predominantly, but not exclusively, in ghetto areas, it is continually replenished by new recruits and new quantities of drugs. Stretched over the United States, but particularly over the large metropolitan centers, it tends to be self-perpetuating, offering its own rewards. In fact, having its own codes, hierarchy, language, mythology, life styles, and modes of interaction, it offers to its inhabitants an alternative to the dominant American society. It cannot be crushed by the imprisonment of addicts because, as the experience of certain prisons shows, as the percentage of addicts rises the chances for the enlistment of the prison system into the addict society itself increase. Nor do hospitals contribute more. This addict culture is a continual obstacle to traditional ways of publicly managing the addiction problem.

In both the ghetto and the nonghetto areas of the big cities an observer is likely to find among the youth varying kinds of antipolice feelings. It is fashionable, indeed, in certain suburban areas to flout the police to an extent that one may ask if involvement in the criminal law is not becoming more and more a part of the ritual of passage from childhood into adolescence and adulthood. At any rate, this strong antipolice sentiment seeks for its symbols and finds in drug use a conspicuous, daring, and satisfying method of expression. It seems that the more the police are successful in apparently reducing the quality of the drug the more likely is drug use to be tinged with a degree of nonchalant prestige.

Leaving aside the question of personality or life patterns, I would say that the problem of excessive or illegal use of existential drugs and especially of heroin has to be linked to the prevalent and increasing urbanization of modern America in the relation it bears to the variety of groups of different ethnic, class, and religious backgrounds having different degrees of adaptation to the problems urbanization brings. I think that social scientists as well as laymen have been too eager to find one central problem, for example, socioeconomic deprivation, to account for drug use when, in fact, the widespread stresses generated by metropolitan life are differently experienced by these groups. Secularization and the scientific revolution, the spread of a consumption-centered life, intensified status competition among individuals in the big city, interracial conflict and the civil rights revolution, and the rapidly changing fashions in urban societies generate substitutes for life itself. These trends are likely to have different effects in different parts of the city. Until we have the basic research needed to describe these effects, we can only speculate on the differences in the stresses and strains in life, and hence in the receptivity in the use of drugs in the big city. Cutting across all these trends would be the rising resort to illegality or the apparently rising resort to illegality even among those who are ostensibly on the side of law and order. I refer in particular to the manner in which nonaddicts of varying stations benefit from the drug traffic in and out of the ghetto areas. These people are conscious and unconscious obstacles to effective management of the problem and are stimuli to drug involvement.

What might be called the revolution in drug technology illustrates the special importance of secularization. A significant fraction of our scientific establishment devotes its time to the production of drugs which turn out to be habit forming or addictive or at least to be existential in the sense that their use radically modifies the course of their users' lives. This proliferating technology produces an ever-widening range of options for those who are otherwise predisposed to use drugs. In the field of addiction and drug use, supply tends to create demand as well as vice versa so that in a special way secularization increases the momentum of drug use.

Men of good will may well differ on the best route to ex-addiction. Specifically, because of the complex nature of addiction and of addicts themselves it is likely that every method offered, from the administration of drugs to halfway houses, is likely to appeal and be useful to some groups of addicts. Of course, there are some addicts who might benefit from any one of a number of treatment modalities so that for them particularly it is a question of philosophy of life as to whether they choose to try to live life with or without drugs. Until we have more research and more frank discussion of what actually are the results over a long period of time of different programs, it is likely that these philosophies will continue to differ.

There is a notable contrast between the large amount of space in periodicals and newspapers devoted to addiction and the large amount of time devoted to it on television and radio, and in the great apathy of a large percentage of the electorate toward large-scale, significant action about it. More exactly, public interest seems to be moody, going up and down in a rather unpredictable fashion. One is reminded of the widespread interest in the United States in love and the really surprisingly low number of real behavioral demonstrations of an interest in it. Americans talk about addiction but do little about it themselves. This is but one of the reasons why it becomes a political football and one hears all manners and varieties of politicians sounding as though they were experts and making extravagant claims and promises, depending upon their particular conversion to one or another solution. The lack of firm high interest in this problem is a serious obstacle to its management.

These social philosophies, in turn, have been embodied in agencies and institutions and have come to serve as the moral backbone for different personalities in the field of addiction treatment. Hence there are not only ideological conflicts, but conflicts of a political nature having to do with the funding of organizations. Historically, the bane of addiction treatment has been the short-lived nature of organizations and projects in this field. It would be unfortunate if, as a result of differential access to propaganda, the public were to fund one or two types of programs exclusively and ignore other kinds of programs that proceed without the benefit of publicity and public relations men.

Perhaps the most pervasive and most neglected obstacle to the management of addiction is the inadequate funding of basic research in this field. A corollary or collateral aspect of this problem is the tendency to assume that the best kind of research is that conducted by medical men. If the point of view within this text has been correct, that there are social, psychological, biological, and pharmacological aspects to this problem, then what is needed is an integrated team effort of combining the social and physical sciences looking toward the development of a coherent interconnected set of concepts which will do justice to all four levels of the problem. Lacking such teamwork, what results are scattered, often isolated, and too often banal bits of very specialized research that do little to penetrate to the essence of addiction in our society. Moreover, a good deal of research is spent on the symptoms of drug use and its effects and not enough on the cultural matrices which surround drug use and perpetuate it.

I cannot avoid speaking also of the social context of addiction research which impedes progress. Obviously, the fact that drug use is illegal has tended to make many of the addicted highly suspicious of the nonaddicted investigator who necessarily would have to be told in some way of the criminal aspects of the life of the addict. Much of what is now known about addiction has understandably come from ex-addicts. This kind of material, however, is subject not only to the error of memory but to the even more delicate error that many ex-addicts tend to assume that what was true in the past is true in the present, so that they give the unwary investigator the impression of a static addict life. Nothing is further from the truth.

Another problem might be called the sociological Heisenberg principle of indeterminacy. By this I mean that in order to study, for example, a treatment program effectively, a full team would be required. However, it is very likely that the very size of the team may itself affect the treatment process itself. Even in a considerably organized, fairly large establishment such as the Synanon House, a team of investigators would not only be a possible drain upon funds which the organization would like to use for therapy, but it would also make significant changes in the interaction of some of the groups into which the team penetrated. To what extent this would be true, one can only conjecture, but it must be reckoned as one of the factors which may limit or serve as an obstacle to addiction research, and hence ultimately to the management of the problem.

Finally, we should not overlook an important value change everywhere evident in modern urban civilization, a change toward a "synthetic bias." Whether it be in the matter of fluoridation or the use of vitamins and additives, one notices that more and more city people have tended to accept the use of synthetics as the substitute for a "more natural" way of life. This long-term trend would, of course, include the resort to existential drugs. However, it is my opinion that the 1960's will also be known as the decade in which a countersynthetic movement got under way in the cities themselves. The precise outcome of these two trends is hard to predict at this point. We are all too much in it.

The Dynamics of Treatment

There have been a number of phases in the history and treatment of the urban drug addict since the first epidemic period of 1945–1950 during which youthful addiction was first brought sharply to the attention of the police and health authorities. In the beginning much stress was placed upon detoxification and rehabilitation in hospitals and upon rather primitive community facilities that were oriented toward alleviating the addict's sufferings. This phase was succeeded by the still current interest in a variety of treatments oriented around halfway houses and comparable group-oriented structures. However, the apparent failure of the earlier methods taught us much about the addict and the ex-addict that points up the need to explore some of the reasons why a man goes back on drugs. With such knowledge we may be able to forestall or delay his relapse to drugs by providing countermeasures in our programs.

Let us suppose that we are dealing with men who have been either detoxified in a hospital or "dried out" in jail so that they have no problem of physical addiction. Now the problem has been that even under these conditions men have recurrently relapsed. What are some of the reasons?

ALIENATION FROM BOTH ADDICT AND NONADDICT SOCIETY

If we talk to men living out in the open community who have just been released from an institution and are trying to stay off drugs we are recurrently struck by their loneliness. They complain that they don't dare associate too much with drug addicts because this will be a sure way to go back on drugs; on the other hand, they still are called "junkies" by the people who knew them in the past. They get few invitations to join the square society and, contrariwise, are continually being offered a free fix by some enterprising friend. How many men have ironically commented on the fact that when they used to need a fix they could never get one, and now that they want to stay off the offers appear? We must remember that the veteran addict is likely to have alienated his family and his close friends because he probably has sponged upon them or even stolen from them. He may have done this more than once, so they, having been gulled once or more, are reluctant to reinvest themselves and their property and their time in his uncertain future. They lack confidence in him, and he becomes not only lacking in confidence but exceedingly lonely. It is an easy temptation to resolve this question by going back on drugs.

THE FORCE OF SEDUCTIVE SIGNIFICANT FIGURES

On the other hand, this problem of loneliness may be solved for a man who has a mother who has been loyal to him and has visited him in jail, for example, every month or a wife who has done the same. Then the problem becomes not one of loneliness but of being overcontrolled by a person who is really using him for some deep emotional need or resolving some basic anxiety that itself needs treatment. In short, he is being used as a psychological couch by a patient who is willing to pay him for his "love." He discovers that he cannot control his own life even if he wants to. The seductive figure will even find ways and means of involving him in drugs as a price of keeping him close. Anyone who has worked with addicts knows many stories of how a seductive figure has actually put enough money into an ex-addict's hands to suggest to him that it would not be wrong for him to take a shot.

AMBIGUITY IN FAMILY ROLES

For the man who has been married and on drugs, coming back and trying to reassume his family responsibilities as an ex-addict may well precipitate a problem of power dynamics. On drugs there was no question: his wife was master and mistress of the household even if she was seducing him. She probably worked or at least was the homemaker, according to the Department of Welfare's budget description, and he was a sojourner. Now, full of high hopes and emptied of heroin, he tries to assume his role as master of the household. He may find that his wife has grown in social size and now enjoys her authority as head of the household. She is not so likely to cater to his whims. Some men find this change of situation to their liking because they claim they need the discipline which a strong woman gives them. Others cannot adjust to this break with traditional conceptions of husband-wife inequality. These ex-addicts experience in their lives a sense of unease and a temptation to resort to drugs to resolve their emotional disturbances.

FAILURE IN JOB ADAPTATION

As part of a program they have thought through before, perhaps even as made necessary by parole, the ex-addict may have a job. It is upon this economic base that he hopes to reconstruct his life with or without his previous family. He discovers that he has great difficulty in adapting to the disciplines of the job. He may, for example, come late, tend to take long breaks, work unevenly, and want to quit work early. Or his inability to take abrupt orders from a tactless boss or the joshing of his work associates leads him to avoid close contact with them. He discovers that he is tempted to drink too much during lunch hour, before work, and after work. His absentee rate starts to rise. All these factors in turn, of course, make it likely that he will be in trouble with his employer. If he is docked for poor work, lateness, and absenteeism, as is liable to happen, it would mean financial trouble. He may borrow money from the bookkeeper or timekeeper in advance, and this will throw out of whack what little planning he does. Most important of all, he will resent the fact that the job is beneath him.

EXCESSIVE EXPECTATIONS AND OVERCONFIDENCE

One of the recurrent complaints made by ex-addicts is that the jobs they get are boring, beneath them, and low-paying. Often ill equipped for competition in the job market, they are forced to accept residual positions. Only a few ex-addicts are lucky enough to have some family or friendly connections in a union or through a friendly employer who will endure their whimsical work patterns and not fire them. Every day of work means that much more of a discrepancy between a man's self-image and the image that is involved in his work as a menial. How long can he keep on lying to himself or lying to others about what he is doing? How much irritation can he take from a boss or a foreman for whom he has little respect and whose every error in judgment he records and fumes about?

An ex-addict is likely to become overconfident in the early weeks or months of his abstinence from drugs. A vicious circle can occur that has the appearance of being a virtuous one. As he gets to stay off drugs he makes friends and also repersuades his family that he is a new man. They, in turn, after a while are so delighted that they reward him for his success in staying off drugs. This, in turn, feeds back and bolsters him in his confidence about himself. Many men under the impact of genuine gratification and congratulations overestimate their strength and ability to control the drug. It is in this situation that they are likely to agree to a walk with a scheming addict or a visit to his home just to be sociable. Chance encounters such as the one that G. described play havoc with a man who overestimates just how much of an ex-addict he really is.

INCIDENTAL REBUFFS, INCIDENTAL INSULTS, AND CHANCE COMMENTS

There is no holding of people's tongues and no way in which an ex-addict can insulate himself from the barbs and comments that people will make off and on drugs. An ex-addict may be in a bar and overhear a comment by someone who knows him, addressed to a third party: "Once you are an addict, you are always an addict." He cannot be sure the comment is made about him or made even for him to hear, but it leaves its mark. The pattern of "signifying" permits a person to play conversational billiards in such a way as to appear not to be hurting another, and yet do so. The ex-addicts may have to learn how to ignore these comments. Some have a harder time than others and experience verbal insults as body blows. Enough of these can, as they say, "shake up" a man.

THE TEMPTATIONS OF THE ADDICT CULTURE

Finally, there is the powerful influence of the addict culture itself in the form of associations, the conditioning of ten, fifteen, or more years of drug addiction, and involvement with drug addicts. As I remarked earlier, every addict carries his own body memory with him, and even if he consciously forgets or claims to forget what it meant to be a drug addict or denies that he has urges to use drugs, there still is close to him this body which has experienced the rush or buzz of the drug and the resolution of earthly griefs by drug use.

There are also temptations for a man without money to engage in the sale of drugs. But this apparently economic temptation may itself mask the hidden desire to resume use of drugs. The ex-addict knows that only a few men can sell drugs and not use after they have been addicted more than once. Then, too, as I have indicated, his old friends are here; here, too, hours of work are not governed by a boss nor must the addict kowtow to a boss every day for eight hours; here he can resolve his family problems by justifying nonparticipation on the grounds that he is an addict, and here he can ignore the barbs and insults around him by narcotizing them out of existence. The temptations in the addict culture are great. The question is, are they insuperable?

NEEDED: "THERAPEUTIC FIELDS"

If we review those factors which bring about readdiction we have to come to at least one conclusion: that a basic reason why addicts relapse is that they treat themselves as "normal" individuals able to function in society if given the chance. The fact of the matter is that many of them are quite unstable and emotionally disturbed. The six kinds of lives I have outlined earlier do not by any means exhaust the spectrum of disturbances which one encounters in working with addicts, but they are enough to indicate how romantic and, indeed, quixotic is the idea that many an addict retains while in jail of his chances for unaided readjustment to society. If an addict is going to stay off drugs for any length of time, he, his fellows, his family, and his friends must accept, if only implicitly, the reality of another idea: re-entry to civil nonaddict society must be through "therapeutic fields." By this term I refer to a set of dynamic relationships and processes oriented toward mental health of which an ex-addict can form a part and to which he can contribute. The term "therapeutic community" has recently come into vogue and refers to a particular and ideal form of therapeutic field such as a small hospital or a ward run professionally along the lines of good fellowship and orientation to health. But therapeutic fields are more general and include looser formations than those of the therapeutic community.

Any good comprehensive program for the rehabilitation of addicts actually generates a therapeutic field. It attracts potential ex-addicts by reaching out for them as well as encouraging them to reach out in turn; it selects specific groups for treatment, sends them through a period of induction, generates an atmosphere that embraces even families and friends of the addicts, and step by step restores the addicts to self-confidence and a place in society. It is a field in that it seems to radiate out via social relationships beyond its immediate clientele and personnel to serve as sort of a beacon for strangers who want to help and be helped. New York City apparently has a significant fraction of the total addict population in the United States and is now, and will be, increasingly dotted by a series of therapeutic fields to the point where it is possible that under the leadership of Dr. Efren Ramirez, the Narcotics Coordinator, it may come to be one interrelated therapeutic field. Until that happens, however, it is more useful to consider the individual treatment fields as part of a total spectrum or market and to consider how the different autonomous programs appear in the eyes of addicts.

MAINTENANCE PROGRAMS

Currently there are a number of hospitals in New York such as Beth Israel and Metropolitan which offer selected candidates the opportunity to be detoxified and then retoxified on increasing dosages of the drug methadone. Thanks to research at Rockefeller Institute under Drs. Dole and Nyswander, it has been rediscovered that methadone exercises a blocking effect on heroin so that the correctly stabilized former heroin addict no longer will experience his preferred drug no matter how much he injects into his system. From this discovery Drs. Dole and Nyswander have concluded that it would make sense to give heroin addicts a daily dosage of the drug and then let them function as normal citizens. Methadone is a slower-acting drug than heroin so that only one injection is required daily and there is not the usual manipulation practiced if one were to try to maintain the same man on, say, heroin or morphine. This program has been given considerable support at federal and local levels, and by middle 1966 well over one hundred fifty men and women were said to be on this program, which reportedly has a very high rate of success in keeping its men coming back for their dosages. Figures on what the men do are somewhat unclear, if not misleading, but there seems to be little doubt that the crime rate among these men was reduced on the average. From various reports there was evidence that some of the former heroin addicts were sometimes using other drugs such as barbiturates and amphetamines, whether orally or by needle, but clearly there was no need for them to enter the heroin market and get reinvolved in the frantic search for money.

This program has attracted various kinds of addicts and seems to rest basically on the addicts' theory that if only one could maintain an addict so as to give him chemical security the addict would be able to function well. As a result, the methadone program, at least in Beth Israel, has a minimum of psychotherapeutic intervention. From the point of view I have been expressing, a program such as this, which is essentially chemotherapeutic, holds a pessimistic image of addicted man, for it seems to imply—and many men so interpret it—that an addict will tend to remain an addict, for methadone is an addictive drug.

It is further assumed seriously that the methadone addict is indistinguishable from a normal person. Psychomotor and psychometric tests are said to have been unable to differentiate the addicts from non-addicts. However, detailed interviewing by me of a number of addicts on methadone programs reveals the presence of psychosexual difficulties, psychological feelings of narcotization, and so on which need to be explored. Finally, there is the ethical question of whether it is proper to maintain a man on drugs and not give him a genuine opportunity to be treated in a comprehensive program so that he might find out why he is using drugs and how he can get rid of the habit and live a natural life.

If the methadone program is at the minimum level of the therapeutic field, what is called the cyclazazine program can incorporate more elements of a therapeutic community in addition to using a blocking drug. It is much more recent in origin on a more limited scale. Since late 1965 Metropolitan Hospital has been giving oral dosages of this powerful blocking agent, not only building up men in their chemical tolerance but also introducing an intense group atmosphere. Passes are given two days a week for work and a variety of recreation and group therapeutic treatment is available throughout the week. This program stands between the methadone treatment and the halfway-house program.

HALFWAY-HOUSE PROGRAMS

The term "halfway house" may refer to an actual house or simply to a kind of program, as has been true of Exodus House. There may be transitional and permanent halfway-house systems. Let me contrast the two typical programs, Synanon with its minor variant Daytop Lodge, on the one hand, and Exodus House, on the other. It will be seen that there is much that these two groups have in common but also much that is different. Only long-range research will determine the ways in which these therapeutic fields may be superior to each other and/or to maintenance programs generally.

Synanon is now familiar to many interested citizens, for it is the most publicized of all addiction treatment programs in the United States. Let me, therefore, simply sketch out some of its dominant structural traits. First of all, recruitment is voluntary, but the addict has to prove by his behavior and sometimes by actual money contributions that he is ready to enter treatment in a serious way. If he is allowed to enter—and this is deemed a privilege—then he can expect no medication on the house premises. Some men have kicked cold turkey at Synanon House and others have come there from hospitals and prisons so that kicking was not the problem.

Synanon is run by a group of ex-addicts under an ex-alcoholic, and special pains are taken to demonstrate that this elite group does not need professional collaboration, though it welcomes professional learners. The system as a therapeutic field has commanded the highest respect from a diversity of observers. The group process is used in a variety of ways through "synanons" (discussion groups) or through "haircuts" (brutal sessions involving total verbal attack on a deviant, in which ex-addicts have at it with each other). Physical violence is tabooed and only talk and proper conduct are permitted for therapeutic and control value. Synanon does not believe that an addict from New York can stay in New York and stay off drugs, so New York addicts are transferred to California and apparently, hopefully, eventually California addicts will be settled on the East Coast. The Synanon organization has various estimates of how long it expects a man to stay in a house, but the general tenor of the comments suggests that an indefinite stay is demanded of most if not all of the men and women who go there. Whole families have been formed and have moved into Synanon, but at the same time it is felt to be more therapeutic for a man to cut off his ties and, like a monk, become a new man in the family of Synanon House.

The organization has grown and it is oriented in the direction of becoming self-sufficient economically and socially. It has its own ideology, language, history, and mythology; in short, it has its own culture, and its ideal is to produce a Synanon City. The elite group who run this organization are bold men, and they have considerable courage and character. It is to be lamented that at times they have been extravagant in their claims or have been disingenuous. A detached observer gets conflicting reports even from those who claim to be in favor of the Synanon principle as to the percentage of "cures." In general it is wise for laymen not to look for any reasonably scientific and valid evaluations of any program until it has a sufficient number of men off drugs and in the community for five years, the period used by cancer specialists to determine that a cancer cure has been effected. (By this criterion it is impossible, as yet, to evaluate validly any of the programs working with addicts.)

While words are important in Synanon, performance is the canon by which a man is judged. Particular scorn is shown for processes involving pure insight. Instead, it is hoped that by the group process a man will become less alienated from himself, less stupid, less absurd, less concerned with his own problems and more concerned with becoming a functioning member of society.

Recently Synanon has entered prisons such as Nevada Penitentiary and set up groups there. Apparently provision is being made for transferring some parolees directly to Synanon out in the open community. The Exodus House program has systematized the connection between the halfway house and the prison as a part of an interesting experiment to see if a halfway house can work in the open community in a drug market area. Originally known as the East Harlem Protestant Parish Narcotic Committee, Exodus House has been involved with drug addicts since the 1950's, first under the direction of the Rev. Norman C. Eddy, and since the early 1960's under the direction of the Rev. Lynn Hageman. Like Synanon, it is a voluntary organization and, like Synanon, it emphasizes the importance of staying off drugs as a basic prerequisite for living a good life.

Exodus House program has two parts. The mass program is a referral program involving the sending of men to hospitals and for other services deemed desirable. As part of this mass program, staff members have gone to prisons, especially to Riker's Island and the House of Detention. Since late 1964, however, the main emphasis of the House has been intensive treatment of a few men who eventually would be living in a halfway-house setting.

A unique system of induction has been developed, modeled in part on a program evolved by Dr. Efren Ramirez and his associates at the psychiatric hospital in Rio Piedras in Puerto Rico. Essentially, the program consists in having tried and tested in attendance ex-addicts who go to New York prisons, in particular Riker's Island and Greenhaven, and set up intraprison programs. Each prison program has three stages called "C," "B," and "A" groups. The "A" group is elite, and each level represents a higher degree of functioning as judged by the ex-addicts. As they progress from "orientation," the "C" group, then to the intermediate "B," and then to the "A" pretherapy groups, the men are oriented to the Exodus House program and to the idea that it is possible to stay off drugs in the open community. A reality orientation is stressed rather than psychiatric probing in depth. The Rev. Stephen Chinlund directs and participates with the ex-addicts in the prison program.

The same ex-addicts are employed in the House, where there is a comparable three-stage induction period. In "orientation" are men who are off drugs, who come from across the street or from different prisons, or, again, from hospitals where they may have been detoxified. Once more they go through a candidacy period. Once they have established themselves, they move into dynamic encounters with ex-addicts. Discussion is led by another ex-addict in pretherapy sessions. Then, when the staff deems them ready for *candidacy* in the workshop program, they are also simultaneously seen in groups run by a psychiatrist. After several weeks, if it is deemed wise, they are seen in several intensive interviews by the sociologist, and then, if all goes well, they are permitted to enter the intensive workshop scene. Here they work six days a week, seven hours a day, receiving what is nominal rehabilitation pay. This 42-hour workweek is broken up by continuing group therapy and bull sessions led by the minister or the workshop foreman. Recreation is provided along with tutorial sessions, discussion periods, and Bible study sessions. In short, the objective is to fill the seven days of the week with meaningful interaction with people, things, and ideas.

As with Synanon, this program is young and cannot be fully evaluated although there are already some encouraging signs. Like Synanon, this program seems to depend upon the formation of a kind of elite group, able to withstand the rigors and temptations of the street. In contrast to Synanon, of course, Exodus House believes that proximity to the drug market may be turned to an advantage by a program with high morale. Whereas Synanon would insulate and make a man dependent upon itself ("hook them on Synanon"), Exodus House believes in the gradual maturation and moving out of the individual into the open community as an independent functioning individual. While great stress is placed upon staying off drugs, relapse is not treated as a fatal blow or a source of excommunication. It is punished, for example, by demotion to a lower level, but the major stress is placed upon understanding the nature of the relapse and discovery of a better way of handling both the situation and the temptation to use drugs. Unlike Synanon, too, there is room for the professional both as leader of the group and for individual discussions.

The relationships between the professional and the ex-addicts generally are cordial, with each learning from the other. The ex-addict groups deal with the problems of adaptation to welfare or to the House, whereas the psychiatrist and his group try to deal with the deeper trends in the addicts' conduct.

Individual encounters with the professional staff supplement the group processes. They are used during the screening process for emergencies while a man is a candidate, for feeding ideas, stimulation through the individual into the different groups, for emergencies such as slips that take place where the man is unable to talk about the slips, and, finally, for certain individual problems that a man may feel he is unable to speak about in the group context. In general, the goal of the individual encounter is to find the best way to help the man relay the problem to the group whether it be pretherapy or therapy group. As with Synanon, the goal is the achievement of a therapeutic community and, as with Synanon, it is too early to say whether this form of therapeutic field does resocialize the potential ex-addict so that he can function under the strains of a complex civilization as a free-moving individual.

Commitment and Responsibility Within Therapeutic Fields

Earlier in this book I underscored some of the parallels between the life of the addict and the *descriptions* and theories of the existentialist thinkers. In closing, let me now seek to tie in some of their prescriptive concepts to the treatment of the addict. Granted that we have to fight the alienation of the addict, that we have to teach him to take frustrations and disequilibria on the job, at home, in the street, and so on, and that, finally, we have to induce him to grow toward maturity, we must ask what imperatives should be placed upon him and what expectations are reasonable in a therapeutic field. It is interesting to notice that those programs, such as Synanon and Exodus House, which demand that the man "make it on the natch," all insist on a strong commitment to positive health and growth. It is as though the therapeutic field were in conflict with the self-medicating claims of the drug or addict field, and that part of weaning a man away from the addict culture must be his demonstration to the staff of a treatment program that he is willing to sacrifice, to commit himself and a fraction of his life to undoing the damage done to him in the years of addiction or even before that, and to build, however painfully, a new and stronger self. How to get this commitment and how to distinguish it from a pseudo commitment is solved differently by various groups. Both Synanon and Exodus House make use of a time criterion. In both cases a man cannot be sure when he will be really accepted as a full-fledged member and given responsibilities. In both he is carefully observed not only for his words but for his conduct, and in both he is subject to group criticism to find out "where he is at." To be part of such a program, a man must join voluntarily. To make "rehabilitation" compulsory is to doom the effort from the start. (But even a prison may be a treatment setting.)

Significantly also, in each the objective is to get an all-around, all-week program so that a man can truly be said to live *for* the organization as well as in it. Put otherwise, the objective in a genuinely therapeutic field is to make a vocation of the field. The man in the program gives his all and in return receives as much as he needs from the program. His strength blends with the program strength in a kind of mutual radiation.

It follows, too, that the commitment of the man who wants to be in the program has to be matched by those who are staff. In Synanon, these are ex-addicts themselves and in Exodus House they are the veteran ex-addicts plus professionals. In each case a kind of elite model sets the norms of the group's conduct. In all such total programs the commitment of the staff is itself a fact to be observed as much as commitment of the potential ex-addicts.

It is part of the nature of the therapeutic field that it furnishes a consistent and comprehensive picture of a way of life to the ex-addict, a set of associations both mental and social that can completely absorb his energies. If we bear in mind this comprehensiveness as well as the transitional nature of the halfway house,* we can see how such programs can act as a buffer between prisons and hospitals, and how, if there is a graduated weaning-away process, a man can spend several years of his life trying to enter, entering, staying within, and gradually leaving and cutting his ties to these groups. The future will let us know whether, in fact, addicts can form and preserve an existential commitment of this type out in the open community and on a voluntary basis. Meanwhile we can look to diversified forms of halfway houses in and around communities with high drug use. Only future research will be able to evaluate fairly and accurately the comparative merits of different systems of variables such as we have used to describe Synanon and Exodus House.

Playing out their changing roles within the addict culture, and shaping them in part according to their circumstances and in part according to their life styles, the addicted represent a distinctive and modern form of social deviation. In their lives one sees pharmacollogical, biological, psychological, and social forces that knit together as if they were culminating a long historical evolution that applies, however differently, to both the West and the East. It appears that

* Whether Synanon is "transitional" is a matter of semantics and reality. The issue is too complicated for comment in this space.

no nation in modern times may consider itself safe from drug abuse and addiction. Hopefully, these pages have stimulated the reader as a citizen and family member to promote the basic research needed on all four levels of the problem. Only through detailed and systematic knowledge, if then, can a larger measure of security be obtained from this social problem.

GLOSSARY

Bag, to be in a. To be of a particular infatuation, persuasion, or mood.

Beat. Cheat.

Bing, in the. In solitary confinement.

Bombitas. An amphetamine compound, Desoxyn.

Boosting. Shoplifting.

Boss. Excellent; very, excellently.

Burn out. Overexploit.

Bust. Arrest.

Buzz, bust. Arrest; sensation from heroin.

Carried. Transported, accompanied.

Chippie. Using freely on occasions when available.

Ciba. Doriden, a hypnotic. The other drugs are barbiturates.

Clitch. Clincher.

Coke. Cocaine.

Commissary. Things brought into hospital ward by private purchase.

Con games, "short" and "long." Petty vs. grandly designed confidence game. "Big con" is a synonym for "long con."

Cop. Buy drugs.

Dope fiend. Drug addict. The term may be used humorously by the drug addicts themselves or with a sense of self-denigration.

Five bills. $500.

Flip side, to do the. Reverse one's field.

Four-twenty-two. Older statute regulating possession of drugs. Now 3305.

Going down. To be going well; to be happening.

Goof something, to. To make a mess.

Half load. Fifteen bags of heroin.

Horse. Heroin.

Jasper. Lesbian.

Kick. 1. Withdraw. 2. Thrilling habit.

K.Y. United States Public Health Hospital at Lexington, Kentucky.

Lame. Square.

Lay in the cut. Watch a situation unobserved prior to any action.

Mainline. Inject needle into vein.

Market. Drug market.

Murphy game. Con game involving a promise of a nonexistent female; pseudo pimping.

O.D. Overdose.

Panic. Stringent shortage of heroin on the street.

Partying. Enjoying heroin sociably; sharing it with others. Also used in referring to Bacchanalian service festivities.

Put someone in a crosstown bus. Put someone in a dilemma.

Rap. Talk.

Roguey. Poorly dressed; unkempt.

Salt shot. Injection of salt believed by many addicts to be effective in resuscitating an addict after an overdose. (Milk shots also are used.)

Score. Illegal money-making transaction.

Set of works. The needle, dropper, etc., used for injecting heroin.

Seventeen-fifty-one. Felonious possession of drugs.

Seventeen-forty-seven B. Possession of barbiturates.

Shooting gallery. A place in which an addict who pays for the right is allowed to inject his heroin; e.g., an apartment or a basement.

Skin-popping. Subdermal or intramuscular injection.

Speedball. Mixture of cocaine and an opiate; e.g., heroin or morphine.

Stick. Preferred way of doing something.

Sting. Illegal venture; a crime against property.

Taken off, to be. To be robbed of one's drugs or money.

Take off.   Inject oneself.

Take-off artist, also called "off artist."   One who takes another's money or heroin by force or threat of force.

Thirty-three-o-five.   Possession of narcotics; misdemeanor.

Throw a brick.   Commit an illegal act.

Throwing rocks.   Committing crimes.

Toast.   A ballad about "the life," the underworld and gray world through which the addicted pass for a period of time; generally handed down in prisons and hospitals.

Upside of a head.   On the side or on top of his head.

Violated.   Arrested for parole violation.

Works.   See Set of works.

INDEX

Index

Abstractions
  experience preferred to, 49–50
  significance of, to obsessional addict, 176
Absurdity, 77
  addict's awareness of his own, 63
  existential, 46–47
Addict life styles, 324–25, 343
  types of, 21–31
  See also specific life styles
Addiction, addicts' first realization of, *see* Dependency—on drugs, realization of
Adolescents, 38, 159
  as addicts, 290, 330
    angry-depressed addict, 245–46
    antipolice sentiment of, 327
    depressed addict, 92–111, 146–49
    paranoid con man, 256–58, 270, 313
  gangs of, 146, 156, 311
  LSD meets needs of, 34
  strive for significance, 65
Aggression (violence), 224, 338
  of barbiturate addicts, 63
  in case histories, 146, 156
    aggression against friends, 124–29
    aggressive drive, 251
    of angry loser, 159–60
    depression-aggression complex, 246–47

Aggression (violence)—*Continued*
  of Lesbian, 169
  of paranoid con man, 255, 259, 262, 266, 268–69, 272–75, 281, 286–88, 293–95, 297–99, 301, 311, 312–18
  parental aggression, 103, 104–5, 107, 175, 245, 250, 255, 268, 272–74, 281, 286–88
  of obsessional addict, 200, 207, 217–18, 222
  interracial, 327
  of juvenile gangs, 311
  passive-aggressive behavior, 60
  stereotyping of, 11–12
  See also Anger; Crime
Alcohol, 9, 162–63, 299, 311
  addicts' use of, 36, 208, 251, 257, 263, 289, 304, 309
  as chemical depressant, 3
  ex-addicts' use of, 333
  in family backgrounds, 103–4, 106–7, 250
  See also Alcoholism
Alcoholism, 19, 40, 42, 44, 70, 338
  in addicts' families, 106, 162, 245, 258–61, 267–68, 270–72, 275, 289, 296, 301
  d.t.'s from, 51
  social drinking shields, 81–82
Alienation, 39, 44–45, 53, 83–84
  absurdity resulting from, 46

Alienation—*Continued*
  from distribution hierarchy, 71
  exaggerated state of, 323
  homelessness as, 51
  of hustlers, 62
  in paranoid life style, 320
  during rehabilitation, 331
  therapy for, 339, 342
Allport, Gordon W., and P. E. Vernon, *Study of Values*, 47
Allstate Insurance Company, 142–43
Ambiguity, 43–44, 46
  in family roles, 332
  magic in, 68–69
Amnesia, temporary, 129–30, 133–34, 279–80
Amphetamines, 3–5, 28, 62–63
  ex-addicts' use of, 336
  experience of time in addicts to, 34
  hyperactive addicts to, 63
  as stimulants, 62
Anger (rage, resentment), 104, 156
  over addiction, 45
  in addicts' life styles, 25–27, 29
  of angry-depressed addict, 245–47
  of angry loser, 158–61
  heroin alleviates, 148, 312–13
  homosexuality expresses, 169
  of isolated prostitute, 163–64
  of obsessional addict, 171, 206–7
  of paranoid con man, 257, 258, 268, 270, 280–81, 285, 289, 298, 306–7, 317, 319–20, 324
  at present time, 53
Anguish (suffering), 35–42, 49, 249, 324
  of addicts' hunting, 38
  of contingency, 37–38
  of depressed addict, 129, 154, 324
  education in, 15
  intrinsic, 41–42
  in market conduct, 38–39
  of nodding, 36–37
  of paranoid con man, 277
  systems of impotence and, 40–41
  therapeutic relief of, 330
  vicarious enjoyment of another's, 222
Anxiety (fear), 60, 66, 332

Anxiety (fear)—*Continued*
  addict life styles respond to, 25, 27, 29–30, 324
  in case histories, 159, 168, 251, 253
    of depressed addict, 103, 107, 130, 144, 156
    of manipulator, 248–49
    of obsessional addict, 175, 179, 193, 196, 213, 241
    of paranoid con man, 255, 274–75, 281, 287–88, 292, 294, 305, 316, 319–20
Arendt, Hannah, 52
Art, 39, 54, 83
  iconoclastic existential, 53
  prison training in, 192
  produced by addicts, 16, 18, 50, 253, 261–62
  retreatist addict's talent for, 166
  social contact with world of, 222, 290–91
Atavism, 38
Auburn State Prison (N.Y.), 192
Authenticity, yearning for, 53–54

Barbiturates (goofballs), 3–4, 278, 304
  addicts to
    depressed, 121–23, 129–30, 133–40, 142–44, 156
    irrational magic of, 69–70
    life styles of, 63
    obsessional, 211–13
    retreatist, 166
  brain damage from, 9
  effect of, 106–7, 123
  ex-addicts use, 336
  experienced as stimulant, 28–29
  heroin diluted with, 59–60
Barrett, William, *Irrational Man*, 49
Baudelaire, Charles, 50
Bed-wetting, 287
Beggars, 60
  case history of, 138
  social position of, 48, 57–58
Bellevue Hospital Center (New York City), 121–22
Beth Israel Medical Center (New York City), 336–37

Biondo, Victor, 265
Blindness, 160–61
Bombitas, 62, 211–12, 304
  addiction to, 123
  defined, 345

California addicts, 338
Chicago *Defender,* 158
Chinlund, Rev. Stephen, 340
Choice
  of addictive life, 223
  existential, 47–49
  passivity toward, 161
Christian Science Monitor, 264
Cibas, 121, 135, 137
Cigarette smoking, 9, 51–52, 208
Cocaine (coke), 3, 11, 28, 123, 182,
  184, 241
  bombitas compared to, 212
  cost of, 62
  effects of, 179–81
Color, *see* Race
Commitment
  premature, 47
  in therapeutic fields, 342–44
Communications media, *see* Mass
  communications
Compulsion, *see* Obsessional life style
Conditioning, 8, 50*n*
Conflicts
  physical, *see* Aggression
  psychological, 31, 62
    magic cures for, 66
    paranoid con man's, 259–60, 271,
    320
    between personalities, 216–17
  of rehabilitative organizations, 329,
  342
Connection, The (Gelber), 26–27
Connections, 57, 139, 169, 182, 225–
  26, 235
  for barbiturates, 122
  of good hustlers, 60, 79
  hierarchy of, 71–72, 75
Consciousness-expansion, 3–4, 18
Contingency, 37–38, 46, 49
Cooking-up process, illness from, 50
"Cool" state, 82
Cough medicine, 166, 170

Creeps, 48, 56–58
Crime
  case histories of, 166, 169, 251
    angry loser, 158, 159–60
    depressed addict, 98–100, 109,
    119–20, 137–39, 146, 151–56
    isolated prostitute, 163–64
    obsessional addict, 184–87, 190–
    92, 205, 208, 216–19, 233, 241
    paranoid con man, 244, 253, 273,
    285, 289–94, 296–99, 304, 309,
    317–18
  increase of juvenile, 327
  possession or use of drugs as, 4, 58,
    61
    alienation and, 44–45
    possession of marijuana, 6–7
    ritual quota of arrests, 51
  reduced by methadone experiments,
    336
  related to addiction, xiii, 12, 19,
    71–79, 227, 325
    addict's view of crime, 17
    assessment of victim's worth, 78
    drugs produce criminal courage,
    64
    magical aspects, 69–70
    passive life style and, 27
    pressure on addicts and, 56–62
    pride in criminal cunning, 84–85
    racketeering, 71–76, 232
  See also Imprisonment; Police
Curse of the necessary extra dimension, *see* Necessary extra dimension
Cyclazazine programs, 337
Cynicism, 37, 41, 46

Dante Alighieri, *The Divine Comedy,*
  323
Death, 77, 233, 277
  existential attitude toward, 52, 54
  false rumors of, 238–39, 253, 319
  of grandparents, 144, 267, 273
  from overdosage, xiii, 239
  of parents, 158–59, 162, 165, 174,
  198, 246, 250
  violent, 163, 245, 316–17, 319
  See also Suicidal tendencies

Daytop Village (Lodge), 7, 338
Dechemicalization, *see* Detoxification
Dependency, 65, 67
  on addict culture, 240–41
  in addict life styles, 27, 31
  on drugs, realization of
    depressed addict, 149–51
    obsessional addict, 182–83, 223
    paranoid con man, 275–76
    stone addict, 166–67
  interdependency, *see* Symbiosis
  of parents, 176
  of pushers, 222
  on Synanon, 341
Depressants, 54, 62, 241
  alcohol as, 3
  heroin as, 28
Depressed life style, 22–23, 28–29,
  202
  angry-depressed pattern, 245–47
  of angry loser, 158–61
  of isolated prostitute, 162–64
  of paranoid con man, 319
  taped interview illuminates, 89–157,
    324
    mother's financing of son's habit,
      98–99, 109–10, 116–17, 125,
      142, 148, 157
    relapses into drug use, 94, 119–
      21
    split personality structure, 91–92
Desoxyn, *see* Bombitas
Despair, 27, 49
Destruction, 255
  in addict life styles, 25–26, 28, 29
  self-destruction, 29, 47; *see also*
    Suicidal tendencies
Detoxification (withdrawal), 63, 166,
  190, 264, 330–31, 340
  addict's description of, 186
  defined, 33
  dread of, 66
  experimental programs of, 90, 336
  sex drive during, 112
  stereotyped picture of, 12–13
  See also Hospitalization
Deviation
  sexual, *see* Homosexuality

Deviation—*Continued*
  social
    addiction, 343–44
    cultural pluralism, 325
Dewey, John, 187
Diplomat, Hotel (New York City),
  203
Disgust, *see* Nausea
Dispensability (contingency), 37–38,
  46, 49
Dole, Dr., 336
Don Quixote, myth of, 40, 80–86
Doriden, 5, 34, 63, 135, 137
Double binds, 260
Dreams
  of depressed addict, 108–9, 112
  nightmares, 249, 277–78, 280–81
Drives, 33
  sexual, *see* Sexual relations
  for success, 251
Drug technology, proliferation of,
  327–28
Dummy shots, 68

East Harlem Protestant Parish Narcotics Committee, xiv, 89; *see*
  also Exodus House
Eddy, Rev. Norman C., xiv, 253, 339
Education, 65, 82, 204, 221–22, 254–
  56, 259, 261, 340
  case histories of formal, 158, 243,
    246
  of depressed addict, 90, 92, 101
  of obsessional addict, 174–77,
    186–87, 189, 192, 198, 208,
    223, 241
  of paranoid con man, 255–56,
    258, 286
  of retreatist addict, 165–66
  criminal, 290–92
  prison, 192
  self-education in psychiatry, 186–
    87, 241
Einstein, Albert, 32
Elitism, addict, 81–86
Elmhurst Hospital (N.Y.), 278
Elmira State Reformatory (N.Y.),
  308

Employment, 181–82, 342
  addicts' records of, 166, 248, 250–51
  angry loser, 158–60
  depressed addict, 110, 148
  isolated prostitute, 163–64
  obsessional addict, 177–78, 183, 185, 187–89, 192–95, 196–99, 205, 213–14, 219
  paranoid con man, 243–44, 280–82, 311
  drug magic and, 64–65
  failure to adapt to, 332–33
  in halfway houses, 339–40
Escape, 76, 256; see also Retreatist life patterns
"Everything is Everything" (slang), 38–39
Ex-addicts, 15, 19, 68
  as inadequate research subjects, 329
  spot ambiguities, 68
  view addicts, 15, 19
  See also Rehabilitation
Excitement, 65, 80, 92
  in case histories
    of depressed addict, 150, 156
    of Lesbian, 168–69
    of obsessional addict, 213, 216, 218, 241
  thrill of mugging as, 298
Existential drugs, 3–7, 18, 80–81, 342–43
  addiction to, 36–37, 42–54, 156–57
    of obsessional addict, 197, 241
    obstacles to therapy for, 327–28, 330
    sense of uniformity, 323–24
    uniqueness of experience, 49–50, 65
  depressed life style and, 29, 156–57
  lack of pharmacological data on, 9
  necessary extra dimension of, 31–42
  produce change in outlook, 94
  responsibility projected onto, 249
Exodus House, xi–xii, xiv, 15, 42, 89, 251, 263–65, 315
  angry-depressed patient of, 247
  discourages pot-smoking, 7

Exodus House—Continued
  exploitation of, 249
  as halfway house, 337, 339–43
  Lesbian patient of, 169
  obsessional patient of, 171, 195, 241–42
  parolees as patients of, 312, 339
  penitentiary sessions of, 253, 263–64, 320, 340
  screening of applicants to, xv, xvii, 253–54, 340–41
Expectations, excessive, 333–34
Exploitation, 37, 243
  of angry-depressed addict, 246–47
  of angry loser, 159–60
  by being "into something," 56–57, 78–79, 231
  by conning, 293–95, 299–300, 314, 317–19
  in depressed addict's case history, 127–29, 134, 139, 157
  exploitative lawsuit, 142–43
  feeling of emotional exploitation, 112–15, 116
  by manipulation, 248, 259
  in obsessional addict's case history, 219, 231–34
  exploitation of others, 236–38
  self-exploitation, 232–34
  by parents, 280–82
  in pseudo life style, 168–70, 248–49
  by pushers, 48
  of self, 42, 232–34
  in totalitarian structure, 75–76, 78–79
  See also Crime

Families, 64, 236
  of addicts in therapy, 331–33, 334–35
  alienation from, 59, 331
  case histories of, 243–44, 250
    angry-depressed addict, 245–47
    angry loser, 158–59, 160
    depressed addict, 95–111, 113, 116–17, 120–21, 125–26, 132–33, 134–36, 138–39, 141–44, 147–48, 151, 154, 156–57

Families—*Continued*
    exploitative Lesbian, 168, 170
    isolated prostitute, 162–64
    obsessional addict, 172–77, 183,
        197–98, 200–3, 205–6, 208–10,
        218–21, 223, 228–29, 239–42
    paranoid con man, 254–55, 258–
        61, 262–63, 266–77, 279–89,
        293, 295–96, 299–301, 310–11,
        319
    retreatist addict, 165–66
    synthetic life style and, 248–49
  overlays practiced on, 68
  in Synanon, 338
Fashion, 151, 193, 227
  absence of, *see* Greasy junkies
  anxiety over inadequate, 255
  importance placed on, 85
Fear, *see* Anxiety
Feeling, absence of, 46
Fences, 59, 69, 166
54th Street Employment Agency, 192
Flunkies (fools), 57, 150
Freud, Sigmund, 187

Gelber, Jack, *The Connection,* 26–27
Goofballs, *see* Barbiturates
Greasy junkies, 27, 57, 84
  depressed addict as near, 136, 140,
    157
  magical appearance of, 70
Guilt, 24, 42, 98, 166, 239, 249
  over addiction, 45, 137, 223

Hageman, Rev. Lynn L., xiv, 339
  "Foreword," xi-xii
Halfway-house programs, 328, 330,
    337–42; *see also* Exodus House;
    Synanon
Hallucinogenic drugs, 3–7, 28, 54,
    249; *see also specific halluci-
    nogens*
Harlem Hospital (New York City),
    141–42
Hashish, 6, 249
Heidegger, Martin, 43, 52–53
"High," *see* Nodding
Hobbes, Thomas, "War of All Against
    All," 315

Homosexuality, xvii, 56, 83, 325
  female, 169–70, 302, 304
  latent, 241, 243
Hospitalization, 13, 77, 326, 330, 338,
    343
  case histories of, 166
    depressed addict, 89, 121–22,
      126, 141–42, 156
    obsessional addict, 173, 189–90,
      195
    paranoid con man, 258, 261–64,
      279, 308–9
  elitism demonstrated in, 85
  reduces size of habit, 63
  as therapeutic field, 335, 339–40
Hunting economy, 38, 47, 49
Hustlers, 78–79, 157, 223–24
  confidence men as, 290–94
  pressures on, 55–62
Hyperactivity, 62–63
Hypnotic drugs, 28–29, 166

Identity, 221, 262, 293
  deprivation of, 245–47
  magic acquisition of, 66–68
Identity crisis, 22
I.I.P.'s (Invisible Illegal Personages),
    71–76
Illness (disease), 46, 69, 143, 178
  addiction stereotyped as, 12
  allergies, 256
  as endemic to addiction, 36–37, 50
  of family members, 116–17, 261,
    269
  hepatitis, xiii, 148–49
  from injections, 147, 180–81, 304
  from lack of drugs, 58–60, 66
    of depressed addict, 109, 124–26,
      128, 149–50
    of obsessional addict, 183, 189
    of paranoid con man, 276, 309
  psychosomatic, 171–72, 193–94,
    276–80, 285, 306
  from sniffing of drugs, 267
  withdrawal, 186
Impotence, system of, 40–41
Imprisonment, 13, 37, 46, 48–49, 89,
    232, 325–26, 331, 338, 343

Imprisonment—*Continued*
addicts' information network on, 77, 78–79
case histories of, 158–60, 163–64, 246–47
depressed addict, 99–100, 119–20, 151
obsessional addict, 184–87, 190–92, 199, 205, 224, 235, 241
paranoid con man, 253, 256–57, 261, 263, 280, 294, 306, 312, 316
elitism stifled during, 85
history of parental, 245
of pushers, 73
rehabilitation from addiction during, 253, 263–64, 339–40, 342
Individualism, 39, 48–49, 73–74, 324
Informers ("rats"), 48, 61, 167, 238
Integration, psychological, 65–66
Intelligence, 18, 50, 167, 169, 221–22
of obsessional addict, 171
special claims of, 82
Intramuscular injections, *see* Skin-popping
Intravenous injections, *see* Mainlining

Language, 38–39, 50, 254, 323
of barbiturate addicts, 212
of con man, 285, 291–92, 318–20
disdain for hip, 167
knowledge of foreign, 171, 177, 187–88, 243, 303–4
magical, 67–69
of Synanon, 339
Life (magazine), 3–4
Loneliness, 44, 62, 288
of angry loser, 160–61
of ex-addicts, 331
of isolation, 162–67, 190–91
of obsessional addict, 191
Louria, Donald B., "Preface," xiii–xiv
LSD-25, 3–4, 18, 34, 39, 249

Magic markets, 63–70, 79, 81, 313
Mainlining, initiation into, 93, 146, 181
Marijuana (pot), 11, 28, 163, 180, 182, 304

Marijuana—*Continued*
changes sense of time, 34
excitement from smoking, 216
as existential drug, 3–4, 6
introduction to use of, 178–79, 246, 250
lack of pharmacological data on, 9
musicians' use of, 291
Market, drug, 145, 159–60, 308, 326–28
conduct in, 38–39, 226–27, 290–94
diversity of, 324
reaction to panics, 160, 308–9
growth of, 326
halfway houses' policy toward, 338, 341
imperative of, 74
law of supply and demand in, 328
located in Puerto Rican ghetto, 178*n*, 241
purity (impurity) of drugs on, 59–60, 75, 118, 259, 289
role of take-off artists in, 61
upper echelons of, 71–76, 115, 169, 231–35
See also Connections; Hunting economy; Pushers
Markets, magic, 63–70, 79, 81, 313
Marriage, 247, 249, 332
addicts' views on, 112–14, 259, 301–2
obsessional addict, 196–97, 202–5, 214–15, 230–31
Oedipal feelings prevent, 299–302
Mass communications, 18, 41, 42, 232
fail to arouse public, 328–29
publicize Synanon, 338
Maturation (age, growth), 56, 145, 320
through therapy, 341–42
Men's House of Detention (the Tombs) (New York City), 190, 340
Methadone retoxification experiments, 14, 90, 112, 336–37
Metropolitan Hospital (New York City), 89, 126–27, 253, 336–37
Mind-expansion, 3–4, 18

Money-and-heroin relationship, 77–80, 115–16
Morphine, 3, 32, 336
Murphy game, 291–92, 346

Narcissism, 257, 259, 289
Narcotics, Federal Bureau of, 72
Nembutal, 121, 135, 137
Nausea (disgust), 36–37, 102
  existential, 45–46, 49, 54
Necessary extra dimension, curse of the, 31–42, 79–80, 90–91
  anguish of, 35–42
New York City, 4–7, 82, 159, 245–46
  addict population of, 336
  cost of addiction in, xiii
  crime network of, 75
  Negro addicts of, 162, 166
    as urban migrants, 158–59, 245–46, 254, 256, 284–88, 310–11, 319
  Puerto Rican ghetto of, described, 96–98, 177
  rehabilitative programs in, xiv, 336–37; see also Exodus House
New York State, xiv, 11, 41, 338
Nietzsche, Friedrich, 43, 49
Nodding (narcotic "high"), 32, 35–36, 62, 70, 77, 83
  addicts describe, 90, 118, 121, 136–37, 181
Nothingness, existential, 36, 53–54

Obsessional life style, 23, 29–31, 65
  taped interview illuminates, 171–242, 324
    autodidactic psychiatry, 186–87, 241
    indifference to exploitation, 231–35
    overconformity, 192–94, 238
    role of control, 206
    role of respect, 174, 179, 182, 196, 199–200, 204, 219
O.D., see Overdosage
Oedipal feelings, 29, 268–69, 299–302
Opiates, 5, 20, 249, 310; see also Morphine
Overconfidence of ex-addicts, 333–34

Overdosage (O.D.), 118, 122, 138, 146, 211, 239
  percentage of deaths from, xiii
Overlays (role-playing), 68, 70, 227–28

Paranoid life style, 23, 25–26, 51, 69, 167, 324
  alienation in, 44
  of con man, 253–320, 324
    addict sibling of, 266–67, 319
    expression of love of children, 257, 261
    fear of losing control, 316–17
    nonresistant prey of, 296–98
  paranoid-depressed, 246–47
Passivity, 135, 161, 243–44, 299
  as addict life style, 23, 26–28, 60
Personality cycling, 31
Pharmacology, 9, 21, 28–29, 64, 319, 323, 329
  cultural pressure vs., 62–63
  technological advances of, 327–28
Police, 6–7, 48–49, 57, 64, 77, 169, 184, 294
  addicts' views of, 16–17, 38, 74
  alleged misintervention by, 151–56
  antipolice sentiment, 326–27
  choice of career with, 197–98
  crimes in presence of, 69–70, 123, 138, 324
  denial of exploitation by, 235
  ignore display of violence, 314–15
  I.I.P.'s betray addicts to, 76
  plan arrests of pushers, 73
  pride in outwitting of, 84–85, 324
  "prison," 306
  pushers' attitudes toward, 61, 324
  ritual arrests by, 51
  stereotype addicts, 12–13
Pressure, 55–63, 77, 80, 166, 251, 254
  causes prostitution-drug complex, 164
  denial of exploitative, 233–34
  magic market relieves, 64, 68, 70
  negative response to, 168, 223–24
  release from, 227, 238
Pseudo life style, 23–25, 248–49, 320, 325

Pseudo life style—*Continued*
of Lesbianism, 168–70
magical language in, 67–68
Psychiatric Hospital (Rio Piedras, Puerto Rico), 15, 82, 340
Psychiatry, 22, 50–51, 64, 99, 341
absent from methadone experiments, 337
aggressive attitude toward, 251–52
for barbiturate addict, 122
for obsessional addict, 172, 173, 187, 190
for paranoid con man, 269–70, 320
self-education in, 186–87, 241
stereotyped addicts, 14
Psychochemical drugs, *see* Existential drugs
Public Health Hospital, U.S. (Lexington, Ky.), 89, 173, 189–90, 289, 346
Puerto Rico, 82
addicts' childhoods in, 94–96, 101–2, 108, 172–76, 197–98, 207–8, 220
Punishment, 25, 36–37, 47, 239
drug use as, 27
halfway-house methods of, 341
legal, *see* Imprisonment
parental, 101, 208, 272–74, 286–87
Pushers, 5, 17, 56–57, 78, 115
arrests of, 37, 73
case histories of, 160, 243, 249–51
depressed addict, 115, 122–23, 125
obsessional addict, 191–92, 220–22
of defective heroin, 59–60
diversity of types of, 324
ex-addicts as, 334
misconceptions about, 11, 13
pressure on, 61
in racketeering hierarchy, 72–73
sense of responsibility of, 48–49
social status of, 58
waiting for, 52–53

Quinine, 68–69

Race (color), 158, 162, 244–45, 250, 253, 304

Race—*Continued*
depression over, 113
feeling of persecution about, 166
identity crisis due to, 22
as obstacle to therapy, 327
Rage, *see* Anger
Ramirez, Dr. Efren, 265n, 336, 340
Reality, 40–41, 62, 64, 70–80, 320
absence of, *see* Alienation; Magic markets
addict life styles and, 25, 27
existential concern with, 49, 51, 53–54
Regressive tendencies, 31
Rehabilitation, xiv, 7, 47, 257, 325–44
assessment of skills in, 82
change of language in, 67n
desire for instant, 193
existential elements of, 51
financing of, 40–41, 329–30, 338
Lesbianism hampers, 169–70
motivation for, 54, 74, 223, 247
necessary extra dimension and, 33–34, 79–80
obstacles to public-managed, 326–30
oppressive sense of time during, 53
psychosomatic illness during, 171–72, 193–94
relapse to addiction foils, 331–35, 341
screening of candidates for, 85–86, 251, 338, 340–41
for welfare recipients, 158, 162
See also Exodus House; Hospitalization; Imprisonment; Synanon
Religion, 31, 44, 138, 327, 340–41
existentialist position on, 53
of obsessional addict, 229–30
of paranoid con man, 255–56, 257, 258–60, 283–85, 288, 310–11
Renegade criminals, 71–72, 75
Research, 327–30, 336, 338
Resentment, *see* Anger
Responsibility, 189, 213–16, 235, 246, 249, 296, 342
absence of, 14, 135, 137, 172, 215–16
existential, 47–49, 52
marriage as, 196–97, 204–5, 332

Responsibility—*Continued*
toward parents, 103–4, 110–11, 116, 206
Retoxification experiments, 14, 90, 112, 336–37
Retreatist life patterns, 23, 30, 165–67, 324
Riker's Island (New York City correctional institution), 120, 185–86, 188, 190, 247, 276, 306, 308
Exodus House sessions at, 253, 263–64, 340
Role-playing (overlays), 68, 70, 227–28

Sartre, Jean-Paul, 35–37, 43, 49, 51–52
concept of nausea of, 45
Seconal, 121, 137
Self-contempt, 160–61
Self-sabotage, 47
Sensitivity, special claims to, 82–83
Sexual relations, 8, 62, 64, 249
case histories of, 159, 163, 165, 168–70, 243–44, 247
depressed addict, 111–14
obsessional addict, 180, 209–10, 241
paranoid con man, 298–99, 302–4, 307–8, 320
diminished interest in, 33, 111–12, 180, 247
extramarital, of parents, 102–3, 262
heroin distorts, 84
illegal, xiii, 56, 163–64, 302
of methadone addicts, 337
See also Homosexuality
Skin-popping, initiation to, 92–93, 146
Sniffing of drugs, 267, 275–76
introduction to, 288, 319
Social causes of addiction, 21, 327–30
addicts' theories of, 16–17, 26, 99
to existential drugs, 4–5
relapses to addiction, 8
Social deviation, *see* Deviation—social
Social workers, 51, 64, 78

Sociological Heisenberg principle, 329–30
Sociological jargon, 50
Speedballs, 180–81, 184, 346
Spiritualism, 230–31, 288–89
Stereotyping of addicts, 10–19, 62
Stimulants, 9, 28, 54, 62, 249
cocaine as, 179–80, 241
Stone addicts, defined, 166
Subdermal injections, *see* Skin-popping
Substitute culture, 71–80
Suffering, *see* Anguish
Suicidal tendencies, 28, 106, 118–19, 122, 235
Survival theory of ethics, 314–17
Symbiosis, 116, 273, 303–4, 319
Symbolism, 172, 175, 240
drug, 65, 327
of slang term "horse," 84
Synanon, 7, 15, 330
as halfway house, 338–39, 341–43
Synthetic bias, 330
Synthetic instinct, 32–34

Take-off artists, 61, 200, 243, 293–95
Therapeutic fields, 335–42
Therapy, *see* Psychiatry; Rehabilitation
Time, 34–35, 51–53, 80, 157, 224–25
Tolerance levels, 35–36, 42, 59n
Totalitarianism, ersatz, 71–80, 325
Tuinol, 121, 133, 135, 137, 211

Uncertainty, 43–44, 54, 68–69, 305
Unmasking process, 50–51, 53
Urbanization, 326–27
by migration, 158–59, 245–46, 254, 256, 284–88, 310–11, 319

Vernon, P. E., *see* Allport
Victims, addict, 169, 243–44, 251
con man as, *see* Paranoid life style
—of con man
Violence, *see* Aggression
Vomiting, 36–37

Welfare, Department of, 158, 162, 164, 308–9, 312, 332
Withdrawal, *see* Detoxification

ABOUT THE AUTHOR

Seymour Fiddle is a sociologist, educator, and attorney. For more than a decade he has worked in ghetto areas in various capacities. From 1954 to 1957 he worked with the New York Department of Welfare, and from 1957 to 1960 he served with the Domestic Relations Court. He joined Exodus House, formerly known as the East Harlem Protestant Parish Narcotic Committee, in 1960 and is currently a research sociologist there.

The author has earned degrees in sociology at the City College of New York and at Columbia University. He has taught at Douglass College in New Brunswick, and later at the Columbia School of General Studies. A graduate of the New York Law School, Mr. Fiddle is a member of the Bronx County Bar Association. He has published in several journals and lectures widely.

Born in New York City, the author currently lives there with his wife and two daughters.